HEMATOLOGY
A Pathophysiological Approach
Third Edition

HEMATOLOGY
A Pathophysiological Approach

Third Edition

Bernard M. Babior, M.D., Ph.D.

Member and Head, Division of Biochemistry
Member, Division of Hematology/Oncology
Department of Molecular and Experimental Medicine
Research Institute of Scripps Clinic
Scripps Clinic and Research Foundation
La Jolla, California

Thomas P. Stossel, M.D.

American Cancer Society Professor of Medicine
Harvard Medical School
Director, Experimental Medicine Division
Senior Physician, Hematology-Oncology Division
Brigham & Women's Hospital
Boston, Massachusetts

CHURCHILL LIVINGSTONE
New York, Edinburgh, London, Madrid, Melbourne, Tokyo

Library of Congress Cataloging-in-Publication Data

Babior, Bernard M., date
   Hematology : a pathophysiological approach / Bernard M. Babior,
Thomas P. Stossel. — 3rd ed.
      p.   cm.
   Includes bibliographical references and index.
   ISBN 0-443-08939-6
   1. Hematology. 2. Blood—Pathophysiology. I. Stossel, Thomas P.
II. Title.
   [DNLM: 1. Hematologic Diseases—physiopathology. WH 100 B114h
1994]
   RB145.B23 1994
   616.1'5—dc20
   DNLM/DLC
   for Library of Congress   93-44656
                                                                  CIP

© **Churchill Livingstone Inc. 1994, 1990, 1984**

Distributed in the United Kingdom by Churchill Livingstone, Robert Stevenson House, 1–3 Baxter's Place, Leith Walk, Edinburgh EH1 3AF, and by associated companies, branches, and representatives throughout the world.

The Publishers have made every effort to trace the copyright holders for borrowed material. If they have inadvertently overlooked any, they will be pleased to make the necessary arrangements at the first opportunity.

Acquisitions Editor: *Kerry Willis*
Copy Editor: *Elizabeth Bowman-Schulman*
Production Supervisor: *Patricia McFadden*
Desktop Coordinator: *Robert Quattro*

Printed in the United States of America

First published in 1994   7 6 5 4 3 2 1

Preface

Hematology, the study of the blood, is in our not unbiased view the most beautifully rational and therefore the most intellectually satisfying of all the disciplines of medicine. Hematology achieved this status because blood can be studied in the laboratory more easily than any other human tissue. Through a simple venipuncture, the physician-scientist can obtain the material needed to understand how normal blood works and what goes wrong when the blood is diseased. Because of the availability of this human tissue, more has been learned about disease mechanisms in hematology than in perhaps any other area of medicine. Through this knowledge of mechanisms, logic and order has been brought to the bewilderingly complex field of hematology, and the modern approach to the patient with a disease of the blood has been developed.

Our plan in writing the first edition of this introduction to hematology was to make this inherent connection between mechanisms and diseases as clear as possible. To achieve this goal, we found it necessary to organize the book in a way that differed from the way many hematology books were put together. Many of the innovations were well received and have been retained. The major approaches in our book are the following:

1. We discuss as far as possible normal function side by side with diseases pertinent to that function. High-affinity hemoglobins, for example, are treated in one of the first chapters in the red cell section—the chapter on the binding of oxygen to hemoglobin—not in a later chapter on mutant hemoglobins. By a similar token, discussion of the mechanisms of destruction of senescent red cells is not presented in a preliminary chapter on red cell turnover, but is deferred to the chapter on extravascular hemolysis, which is one of the later chapters in the red cell section. This close association between the normal and abnormal serves as an ongoing "clinical correlation" that emphasizes the way in which the principles of normal function are applied to hematological diseases. In this integrated approach, we have done our best to see that these principles are introduced in a logical order, so that by the time the discussion has reached diseases with complicated pathophysiology (e.g., sickle cell anemia or disseminated intravascular coagulation), most of the relevant principles will have been explained.

   As hematology has advanced, however, many areas of physiology and pathophysiology have merged, so that it has become necessary to introduce some general principles in advance of their application to specific diseases. Stem cells and hematopoietic hormones, for example are generally relevant to nearly every aspect of hematology, and therefore are introduced in Chapter 1. Growth factors, oncogenes, the cell cycle, and ways to affect them in the treatment of neoplastic disease are pertinent to all the hematologic malignancies, and a chapter (Ch. 21) combining this information was reconstructed from separate bits in the previous edition and placed before the first chapter on hematological malignancies.

2. We employ a classification of hematological diseases that emphasizes pathophysiological mechanisms. This modified classification places a number of diseases into categories somewhat different from those traditionally used. The most extensive modifications are the introduction of a category called *stem cell diseases*, in which are included several disorders affecting all three blood cell lines that were heretofore squeezed uncomfortably into categories designed for conditions involving only one cell line (e.g., chronic myelogenous leukemia, paroxysmal nocturnal hemoglobinuria, and essential thrombocythemia), and the addition of a category called immune-mediated blood cell destruction, into which are placed all diseases caused by the immunological destruction of blood cells, regardless of the cell line affected. Other modifications include the distribution of the mutant hemoglobins into functional categories more explicitly than usual and division of the acute thrombocytopenias between immune cytopenias and disseminated intravascular coagulation/thrombotic thrombocytopenic purpura. Those familiar with the traditional classifications of hematological disorders will probably recognize other modifications as well, mostly minor.

3. We have discussed fully certain rare diseases that shed light on pathophysiological principles in a particularly straightforward way. One example of this is our treatment of the α-thalassemias, a group of conditions that provide a striking example of the clinical ramifications of molecular genetics, although they are of relatively minor clinical importance in the United States.

By the time most students get around to the initial study of the blood they will (it is hoped!) already have received instruction in biochemistry, cell biology, immunology, and physiology. This background was not taken for granted in our explanations of principles. Rather, we have attempted to provide further information concerning aspects of hematology about which the readers may already have been instructed in another context (for example, the morphology of blood cells and the structure of hemoglobin and of immunoglobulins). The molecular biology of cell proliferation and differentiation and the principles of immunology are inextricably bound to hematology. Therefore, we provide considerable information on these topics. This material is presented both to jog the memories of informed readers and to show them how their previously acquired knowledge can be applied to the medical discipline of hematology. Repetition is the mother of learning.

True to its history, the science of hematology has moved rapidly, and we have tried to incorporate important new advances into this edition. Of particular note are discoveries in molecular genetics that have radically improved our understanding of hematologic growth factors and blood coagulation proteins, not to mention better comprehension of their structure and function. The order of chapters and deployment of content has been changed somewhat to accommodate current mental processes of practicing and teaching hematologists: the chapters on principles of neoplasia and its therapy followed by stem cells and stem cell disorders were reorganized. In addition, we responded to criticisms of earlier editions by providing more information about therapies. We hope that the changes in the text will allow the book not only to continue to serve as a useful introduction to clinical hematology for medical students but also as a source of review for physicians in training and in the practice of hematology and related disciplines.

We are grateful to colleagues who have provided suggestions and criticisms of the book. In particular, we thank Drs. Scott Berkowitz, Frank Bunn, Gregory Del Zoppo, Lawrence Schulman, and Marc Shuman. We again acknowledge our families, Shirley, Greg, and Jill Babior, and Anne, Scott, and Sage Stossel, for their support, which we needed to see yet another revision of the book through to its realization.

Bernard M. Babior, M.D., Ph.D.
Thomas P. Stossel, M.D.

Contents

Section III
White Blood Cells and Their Diseases / 263

An Overview of the Blood

The discipline of hematology encompasses the circulating blood and the function of blood cells throughout the body. Robert Burton, in 1628, characterized the blood as a "hot, temperate, red humor whose office is to nourish the whole body to give it strength and color being dispersed by the veins through every part of it." That elegantly simple and apt description of the blood can now be embellished by our deep understanding of the biology of this most excellent humor.

The mass of the circulating blood is 5 to 7 percent of our body weight. The blood is a suspension of cells, called the *formed elements*, in *plasma*, a solution of protein and salts. The blood and the circulatory system, the conduit of sluices, gates, and alleyways through which the blood courses, were required for the evolution of complex higher organisms. In these organisms the blood provides for nutrition, oxygenation, the cleansing of wastes, and the defense of body tissues against a relentless assault by microbes.

THE COMPONENTS OF THE BLOOD

Our bodies are 70 percent water, our cells all function in a watery environment, and the blood is responsible for bringing adequate hydration to all our tissues. Plasma, the blood fluid, also contains dissolved ions that are cru-

cial for cell functions. These ions are principally sodium, potassium, chloride, hydrogen, magnesium, and calcium. As discussed in Chapter 4, the plasma also transports iron, which is vital for crucial tissue enzymes but is particularly important for the structure and function of red blood cells.

The proteins of the blood plasma can be broadly divided into three classes: *carrier proteins*, *immunoproteins*, and *coagulation proteins*. The carrier function of plasma proteins is threefold. First, the plasma proteins can bind molecules in the plasma, thereby diminishing the nonspecific diffusion of these molecules into the tissues or their nonspecific interaction with blood and tissue cells. Second, complexes of carrier proteins and molecules bound to them may be recognized by particular cells with a high degree of specificity. In this way molecules such as iron can be directly targeted to cells that require them, as discussed in Chapter 4. Finally, plasma proteins can diminish the toxic effects of certain molecules in the plasma by binding to them and by carrying these neutralized toxins to specific sites, where they can be eliminated. Examples of these three carrier functions are evident for the plasma proteins described in the following paragraph.

The chief plasma protein is *albumin*. Comprising two-thirds of the mass of plasma protein (the normal concentration value is about 4 g/dl), albumin is the major source of the osmotic pressure of the plasma. In this sense albumin can be said to be a carrier of water, and when the serum albumin level declines, the tissues of the body become edematous. Albumin is also a carrier of many compounds, examples of which are bilirubin and other bile pigments (described in Ch. 5), and of free fatty acids. Albumin does not bind all such molecules with very high avidity, but because of the high albumin concentration, the proportion of these molecules that remains uncomplexed in the plasma is small. Other carrier proteins are the *lipoproteins*, which transport cholesterol, triglyceride, and phospholipid between tissues. Two plasma proteins are particularly important for the transport of nutrients needed by the blood. One of these proteins is *transferrin*, an iron-binding protein described in Chapter 4, which carries iron to developing red blood cells. The second carrier is a class of proteins called *transcobalamins*, proteins that transport cobalamins, vital cofactors for DNA synthesis in blood cells and other tissues. The cobalamins are described in Chapter 6.

Another set of carrier proteins complex to substances that may not ordinarily be present in the plasma but appear following injury or tissue destruction. *Haptoglobin is* a protein that binds hemoglobin if this principal red blood cell constituent appears in the plasma because of red blood cell destruction (Ch. 9). A protein with a similar function is *hemopexin*, which binds to free heme released from denatured hemoglobin (Ch. 9). Two proteins, *alpha-1-antiprotease* and *alpha-2-macroglobulin*, bind and neutralize proteolytic enzymes released from destroyed tissues and phagocytic leukocytes (Ch. 18). The protease–antiprotease complexes are avidly cleared from the circulation by mononuclear phagocytes (Ch. 18). These antiproteases also function in the tissues. Injury and inflammation frequently increase the permeability of blood vessels, allowing plasma constituents to leak into the injured area. The antiproteases participate in the neutralization of proteolytic enzymes activated by the injury and inflammatory processes (Ch. 18). Another "anti-inflammatory" plasma protein is a copper-binding protein called *ceruloplasmin.*

Ceruloplasmin participates in the detoxification of oxygen-derived free radicals that are released during inflammation by phagocytic cells (Ch. 18). In addition, ceruloplasmin is required to prevent the accumulation of copper in tissues, where it can have toxic effects. A congenital disorder in which ceruloplasmin is absent, *Wilson's disease, is* associated with extensive tissue damage, including red blood cell destruction.

Aside from nutrition, defense is the major function of the blood. Both cells and humors participate in this defense. The blood humors active in defense against invading microorganisms are the immunoproteins, the *immunoglobulins*, and the *complement proteins*. These proteins are described in Chapter 17.

One of the tasks of the blood is to maintain the integrity of its conduit, the vascular system. As in defense against infection, cells and humors cooperate in this endeavor. The humoral arm of this defense is the *coagulation system*, a series of plasma proteins that interact to produce gelatinous plugs for sealing breaks and leaks in the vasculature. As described in Chapter 13, a variety of conditions activate the coagulation proteins. The solidification of plasma as a result of this activation is due to the formation of a network of strands composed of the protein *fibrin*. Between the strands of fibrin are water, salts, and the majority of plasma proteins. By centrifugation of the clot, these compounds can be squeezed out; collectively they are called the *serum*. One of the stimuli for blood coagulation is contact of the plasma with foreign surfaces such as glass or plastic. Therefore, any attempt to remove blood from the vascular system results in activation of the clotting system unless coagulation is inhibited in some way. For a number of diagnostic procedures involving blood and for blood transfusion (Ch. 31), it is inconvenient to have clotting occur. Therefore blood is often *anticoagulated*. The coagulation system is very dependent on the presence of ionized calcium (Ch. 13), so that if calcium is lowered by means of a suitable chelating agent coagulation is inhibited. Blood can be drawn into a container containing a sufficient quantity of sodium citrate or else ethylenediaminetetraacetic acid (EDTA) to complex all the free calcium, and it will not clot. A system of proteins complementary to the coagulation proteins inhibits the coagulation system. It prevents the whole circulation from clotting up at once, if exposed locally to one of the many coagulation activators, and it also breaks down formed clots when they are no longer needed. This system is called *the fibrinolytic system*. The components and interactions of the coagulation and fibrinolytic systems are described in Chapters 13 and 16.

THE FORMED ELEMENTS

Tbe bulk of the formed elements, about one-half the blood volume, is composed of *red blood cells (erythrocytes)*. The function of these anucleate biconcave discs is to carry oxygen to the tissues and to return to the lungs carrying carbon dioxide. The red blood cells function totally within the vasculature. Chapters 2 through 12 describe the structure, function, and disorders of these *erythroid cells*. The normal function of *white blood cells (leukocytes)* is to defend the organism against infection. In contrast to the red blood cells, the vasculature is merely a highway for white blood cells, which function mainly in the tissues. The white blood cells are divided into two main categories: the *phagocytes*, cells capable of engulfing particulate matter, and the *lymphocytes*. Both phagocytes and lymphocytes are nucleated ameboid cells capable of locomotion within the tissues. Chapters 18 through 26 describe the structure, function, and disorders of white blood cells.

The *platelets* are disc-shaped anucleate fragments released from a giant cell called the *megakaryocyte*. Platelets, the structure, function, and disorders of which are described in Chapter 14, work with the coagulation proteins to defend the vasculature in case of tears or leaks.

The formed elements of the blood are easily visualized by means of the *blood smear* (Fig. 1-1). A drop of blood is obtained by pricking the finger or else taken from a tube of anticoag-

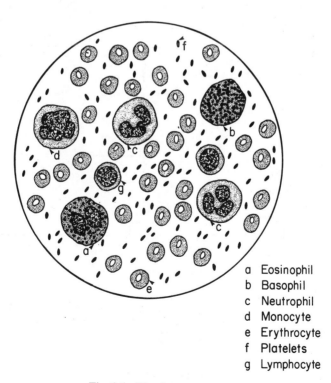

a	Eosinophil
b	Basophil
c	Neutrophil
d	Monocyte
e	Erythrocyte
f	Platelets
g	Lymphocyte

Fig. 1-1. Blood smear.

ulated blood, smeared out on a glass slide or coverslip, and allowed to dry. The dried smear is then stained with *Wright's stain*. This stain is a mixture of dyes dissolved in methanol. During initial exposure of the smear to the dye, the cells are fixed by the methanol and the cell nuclei and certain cell components stain blue. After a few moments, water buffered to an alkaline pH is added, which causes the red blood cells and parts of other cells to stain red. The coloration of cell components described in this text all refer to Wright's-stained cells. Although the Wright's-stained blood smear is the benchmark for description of formed elements of the blood, increasingly these cells are enumerated in clinical laboratory by automated electronic cell counters that discriminate different cells on the basis of their size and shape, DNA content, and reactivity with fluorescently labeled reagents that bind to specific receptors on the cell surface.

THE LIFE HISTORY OF THE FORMED ELEMENTS

Of the many body cells, blood cells are among those with the highest rate of self-renewal or *turnover*. Each blood cell type has a somewhat different reason for requiring this high rate of turnover. In the course of their meanderings through the circulation, the erythrocytes are subjected to mechanical and oxidant stresses that lead to their destruction. Furthermore, evolution has had to allow for the replacement of red blood cells in case of bleeding following injuries. Phagocytes function continuously in tissues invaded by microorganisms. This invasion is an unending process, particularly in the gastrointestinal tract, oral cavity, and skin, which are zoological gardens teeming with microbial species. In dealing with these microbes, phagocytes are destroyed and must continually be replaced. Lymphocytes

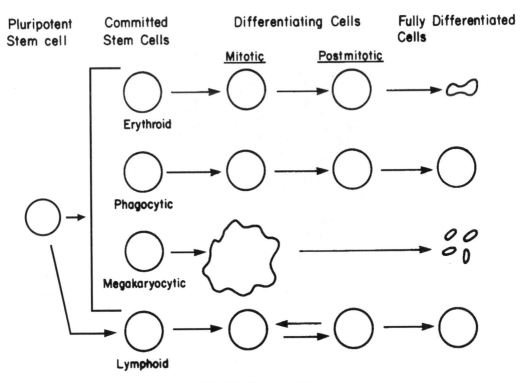

| Pluripotent Stem cell | Committed Stem Cells | Differentiating Cells | | Fully Differentiated Cells |
| | | Mitotic | Postmitotic | |

Erythroid

Phagocytic

Megakaryocytic

Lymphoid

Fig 1-2. Hematopoiesis.

perform complex immunological functions requiring that discrete lymphocyte populations amplify themselves on demand (Chs. 19 and 20). Finally, platelets are consumed during the process of coagulation and must be replenished. Even in the absence of overt injury, the coagulation system functions at a low level to maintain the integrity of the vascular system.

Except for an early portion of fetal life, the *bone marrow is* the site of production of most blood cells. The ultimate source of blood cells is the *pluripotent hematopoietic stem cell.* This cell (which is discussed further below) is present in very small numbers, replicates itself, and differentiates into *committed* stem cells destined to differentiate into erythroid, phagocytic, megakaryocytic, and lymphoid cells (Fig. 1-2). Hematopoieitic precursors are also progenitors of *osteoblasts* and *osteoclasts* involved in bone turnover. Fibroblasts, endothelial cells, and fat cells, which constitute the *stroma* of the marrow, are derived from other lineages. Only cells differentiated beyond the stem cell stage can be recognized by their morphological appearance. Early in their differentiation these cells are capable of cell division and are therefore defined as the *mitotic compartment* of blood cells. The more mature forms of differentiation and the fully differentiated erythroid and phagocytic cells, which are incapable of mitosis, are called the *postmitotic compartment*. Although, as described in Chapter 22, there is evidence that stem cells may circulate in the blood, it is primarily the completely mature blood cells that leave the bone marrow and can be observed in the peripheral blood.

Figures 1-2 and 1-3 illustrate that the lymphoid cells are in many respects exceptions to statements that have been made above. First, lymphoid cells, unlike erythroid phagocytic and megakaryocytic forms, do not necessarily follow a unidirectional development from mitotic stem cells to end cells. Rather, lymphoid cells can oscillate between mitotic forms and dormant "memory" cells capable of

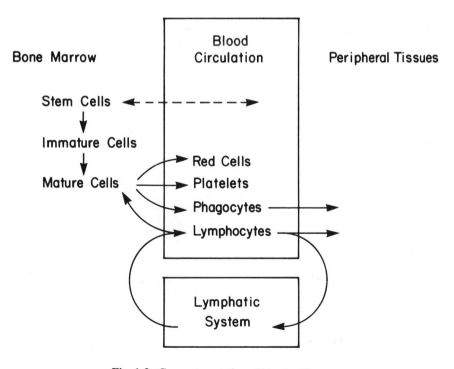

Fig. 1-3. Compartmentation of blood cells.

recruitment into a mitotic pool on demand. Second, lymphoid cells percolate back and forth between various compartments, the bone marrow, the blood and lymphatic circulations, and the tissues. In contrast, erythrocytes and platelets released from the marrow live out their life spans in the blood. Phagocytes enter the tissues and do not return to the blood.

In the bone marrow, blood cells develop in *sinuses* lined with endothelial cells, fibroblasts, and abundant fat cells. The bone marrow is a rich mixture of blood cells of all types in all stages of maturation. A sample of bone marrow stained with standard histological dyes reveals a beautiful variety of cell shapes, colors, and sizes. Easiest to identify are occasional megakaryocytes, distinctive for their large size and multilobed nuclei (in contrast with osteoblasts or osteoclasts, which have multiple separate nuclei). Most of the other cells visible are developing phagocytes, principally polymorphonuclear leukocytes, and developing erythrocytes. The phagocytes outnumber the erythrocytes by a ratio of about 3:1. Mature cells leave the marrow by creating gaps in the endothelial lining of the sinuses and enter capillaries in continuity with the circulation. The bone marrow, with its remarkable diversity of cellular forms, resembles a tropical coral reef.

In a child the entire bone marrow contains growing blood cells (*hematopoietic tissue*). However, of the total mass of bone marrow in an adult, only a fraction contains substantial amounts of hematopoietic tissue, although the absolute amount of this tissue is the same in adults and children. The locations of this *red marrow*, as it is called from its appearance, are illustrated in Figure 1-4. The rest of the marrow contains principally fat and is therefore called *yellow marrow*.

Examination of a bone marrow sample is an important procedure in hematology because it affords a view, albeit relatively qualitative, of blood cell production. It is quite simple and not too painful to put a suitable needle into the bone marrow (Fig. 1-5) and obtain a small quantity of marrow tissue. Figure 1-4 shows

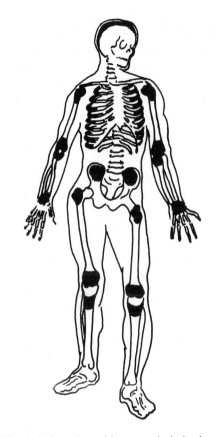

Fig. 1-4. Location of hematopoiesis in the adult bone marrow.

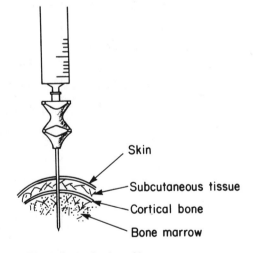

Fig. 1-5. Aspiration of bone marrow.

that there is considerable red marrow in the pelvis. For this reason the posterior superior iliac spine is a site frequently selected for bone marrow sampling. Another location often used is the sternum. The two techniques employed for sampling are the *aspirate* and the *biopsy*. Aspiration through the needle into a syringe disrupts the bone marrow structure but obtains cells in a relatively dispersed form suitable for staining and examination with Wright's or Wright–Giemsa stains. The details of cellular structure are well visualized by this approach, and a general impression of the relative numbers of different cell types in the sample can be obtained. The aspirated marrow sample can also be innoculated into appropriate media for determining whether certain infectious organisms, such as typhoid bacilli, mycobacteria, or fungi, are present. The overall architecture of the bone marrow, however, is not readily appreciated by this approach. Furthermore, "sticky" elements, such as tumor cells or fibrotic lesions, cannot be aspirated, and if the bone marrow contains no hematopoietic tissue, as in aplastic anemia (Ch. 22), the attempt to aspirate will yield a "dry tap." The biopsy, in which a core of marrow is acquired, overcomes some of the limitations of the aspirate and complements it. The biopsied tissue must be decalcified, fixed, and stained with histological dyes, such as hematoxylin and eosin, before visualization. These treatments render the morphology of individual cells considerably less distinct than the stained cells of aspirates. However, it is possible to discern the principal types of bone marrow cells in the fixed specimen. Most importantly, the biopsy sample reveals the architecture of the bone marrow. The presence of clumps of tumor cells, fibrosis, or aplasia is readily appreciated. The decalcification process takes many hours, thereby delaying the opportunity to observe the sample. By placing the biopsy sample on a glass slide before placing the sample in fixative solution, it is sometimes possible to obtain a "replica" of the marrow on the slide that can be observed immediately after staining. This procedure is called a *touch preparation*.

THE REGULATION OF BLOOD CELL RENEWAL

As mentioned above, the high turnover of blood cells is in part geared to the capacity to respond to stress, for example, blood loss (erythrocytes and platelets) and infection (white blood cells). The events leading to the increased demands for blood cells usually occur at sites distant from the bone marrow, the organ of blood cell production. Accordingly, feedback mechanisms involving circulating humors exist to signal the distant bone marrow to increase its output on demand. In addition to factors acting over great distances, others mediate communication between cells locally; collectively these endocrine and autocrine hormones are designated *cytokines*.

The primary signal regulating red blood cell production (*erythropoiesis*) is the tissue oxygen tension (Fig. 1-6). A fall in tissue oxygenation, resulting from anemia or pulmonary insufficiency, is followed by an increase in red blood cell production (Ch. 3). The link between tissue oxygen tension and bone marrow red blood cell production is the glycoprotein hormone *erythropoietin*, which is produced by the kidney. Erythropoietin circulates in the blood and is also excreted into the urine. When tissue oxygenation decreases, the activity of erythropoietin in the plasma and urine rises. The action of erythropoietin is to accelerate the commitment of pluripotent stem cells into erythroid development and to enhance the rate of division and maturation of red cell progenitors. Since the kidney is the major source of erythropoietin, loss of renal tissue results in anemia because of erythropoietin deficiency, and intravenous infusions of erythropoietin correct this anemic state.

Growth factors also have an important role in regulating phagocyte and lymphocyte production (Table 1-1). These factors were initially recognized as glycoproteins in the blood and urine that promoted the growth and differentiation of blood cells in tissue cultures. These hematopoietic hormones caused committed

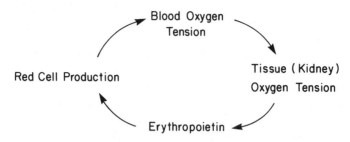

Fig. 1-6. Regulation of erythropoiesis.

stem cells in samples of bone marrow or blood to develop into colonies of mature phagocytic cells and were therefore named *colony-stimulating factors* (CSFs). CSFs act on stem cells to enter the cell renewal cycle from a dormant state and to differentiate into their mature phenotypes, and they also may enhance some of the mature cell functions. Other agents have been discovered as components in tissue culture media that induced lymphocytes to divide and grow. The CSFs and lymphocyte growth factors can be highly specific for particular cell types: granulocyte (G)CSF, for example, promotes the development of granulocytes whereas macrophage (M)CSF yields monocyte and macrophage colonies. Other cytokines have overlapping activities, such as GM-CSF, which promotes the development of granulocyte *and*

Table 1-1 Hematopoietic Cytokines

Factor	Target Cell(s)	Actions
Erythropoietin	Erythroid precursors	Erythroid cell growth
G-CSF	Phagocyte stem cells and neutrophils	Development of neutrophils
M-CSF	Phagocyte stem cells	Development of mononuclear phagocytes (MNP)
GM-CSF	Phagocyte stem cells	Development of all phagocytes
Stem cell factor (SCF)	Multipotent stem cells and mast cells	Growth of stem cells and mast cells
Interleukin 1α and β (IL-1)	Multiple	Induces G-CSF, M-CSF, IL-6; promotes growth of all blood cell lineages; induces fever, acute phase proteins (Ch. 17)
Tumor necrosis factor (TNF)	Multiple	Similar to IL-1; toxic for some tumor cells
Interleukin-2 (IL-2)	T lymphocytes	T-cell growth factor; activates NK cells
Interleukin-3 (IL-3)	Many stem cells, basophils	Growth of all blood cells
Interleukin-4 (IL-4)	B lymphocytes, mast cells	Growth factor for B cells, mast cells and eosinophils; induces IgE
Interleukin-5 (IL-5)	Phagocyte stem cells	Growth of eosinophils
Interleukin-6 (IL-6)	Multiple, especially B cells and osteoclasts	B cell growth; differentiation of stem cells into all lineages
Interleukin-7 (IL-7)	B lymphocytes, thymocytes	B cell growth, thymocyte differentiation
Interleukin-8 (IL-8)	Neutrophils	Released by MNP; a chemotaxin (Ch. 18)
Interleukin-9 (IL-9)	T lymphocytes, others	Potentiates other growth factors
Interleukin-10 (IL-10)	T lymphocytes	Suppresses cytokine synthesis, immunosuppressive
Interleukin-11 (IL-11)	Stem cells	Growth of leukocytes and megakaryocytes
Interleukin-12 (IL-12)	Cytotoxic lymphocytes, others	Activation of lymphoid cell cytotoxicity; antiviral activity
Interferon-γ	Phagocytes, lymphocytes, other	Increased class major histocompatibility complex (MHC) class II expression; MNP activation; antiviral activity
Interferon-α	Multiple	Regression of malignant myeloid stem cells; antiviral activity
Tumor growth factor	Multiple	Inhibits hematopoiesis and inflammation

monocyte colonies. Table 1-1 summarizes the spectrum of activities of cytokines active in blood cells. The emergence of molecular cloning techniques has facilitated the identification and characterization of these growth factors, which are also known as *interleukins*. White blood cell growth factors are produced by a number of tissues, including fibroblasts, mast cells, and macrophages. Stimulation of the latter two cell types in inflammatory states may induce the secretion of CSFs and interleukins. Cytokines act on target cells directly or, in some cases, when they are displayed on the extracellular matrix laid down by bone marrow stromal cells.

It is important to respect the complexity of growth factor interactions and not to take too literally the value of various flow diagrams depicting blood cell proliferation and differentiation: the cytokines work in combination, they work on multiple cell types and at different states of cell differentiation, they induce one another, and more factors must exist than have hitherto been recognized.

As discussed in Chapter 18, the interaction between microorganisms and tissue results in the elaboration of a number of mediators of inflammation, some of which include the immunoproteins discussed above and in Chapter 17. These mediators can also increase the production of phagocytic leukocytes and call forth these cells into the blood and into the tissues where they are needed (Fig. 1-7). Chapter 20 discusses how lymphoid cells are recruited by exposure to foreign substances to differentiate and acquire the capacity to produce immunoglobulins and then undertake other immunological functions. It also discusses how this recruitment is amplified following repeated exposures to the offending agents. Finally, anemia and bleeding bring about an increase in the number of circulating platelets. Whether this action is in part mediated by erythropoietin, or is totally the responsibility of some as yet unidentified humor, called thrombopoietin, is not known (Fig. 1-8). It is unclear whether the putative platelet growth regulator acts positively like CSFs and erythropoietin to stimulate platelet production or is rather released by platelets and inhibits megakaryocytes in a suppressive feedback loop.

The cytokines, which stimulate the growth and development of blood cells and also influence their function, work by binding to specific externally disposed *receptors* on the plasma membrane of their target cells. Some of the cytokine receptors have unique structures, but many of them share features with each other. GM-CSF, interleukin-3, and interleukin-5 receptors consist of two polypeptide chains that penetrate the plasma membrane, one of which is shared (designated the β-chain) and one of which is unique (the α-chain); the latter determines the specificity of the ligand for the receptor. Engagement of cytokine receptors by growth factors leads to metabolic changes inside the cell that initiate a cascade of events leading to cell growth, cell differentiation, or

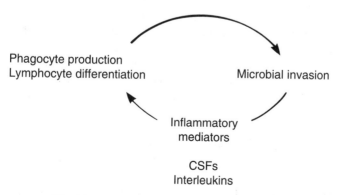

Phagocyte production
Lymphocyte differentiation

Microbial invasion

Inflammatory
mediators

CSFs
Interleukins

Fig. 1-7. Regulation of white blood cell production.

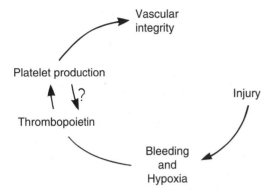

Fig. 1-8. Regulation of platelet production.

both. This process, known as *signal transduction*, is of general relevance to many receptor-mediated cell responses. Signal transduction is discussed in the context of platelet physiology (Ch. 14) phagocytic cell function (Ch. 18), and the complex programming of events by which lymphocytes acquire specific recognition of antigens and respond to this recognition (Chs. 19 and 20). Signal transduction mechanisms are important in controlling whether immature hematopoietic cells proliferate or differentiate, and aberrant signalling processes are often responsible for the malignant behavior of neoplastic cells, discussed in Chapter 21.

STEM CELL PHYSIOLOGY

Before the sixth week of gestation of the human embryo, blood cells appear in the yolk sac. Thereafter, the liver becomes the site of blood cell production until week 20, when hematopoiesis takes place in bone marrow, the origin of synthesis of blood for the remainder of the human life span. Under certain pathological conditions, the bone marrow ceases to be a hospitable site for blood cell production; hematopoiesis may then return to the liver and to other organs, a condition called myeloid metaplasia. These changes in the location of hematopoiesis reflect the place where the soil is fertile for growth, replication, and differentiation of the hematopoietic pluripotent stem cell. These cells have the capacity both to dif-

ferentiate into all types of blood cells—the erythrocytes, granulocytes, lymphocytes, and platelets—and to renew themselves. The rate of renewal and differentiation of stem cells must keep pace with the death rate of peripheral blood cells under various states of demand to maintain the peripheral blood cell concentration at a level compatible with the proper functioning of the organism.

The pluripotent hematopoietic stem cell is present in normal bone marrow in very small concentrations. The ratio of such stem cells to nucleated bone marow cells is about 1:2,000. Both the physiologist and the clinician usually evaluate the stem cell by its offspring, the differentiated blood cells. In experimental systems, described below, researchers define stem cell activity by the progeny they produce in experimental animals and in tissue cultures. Clinicians infer from cell lineages that fail to develop or that show abnormal maturation including malignant (cancerous) behavior which stem cells have been subjected to pathological alterations. Several types of stem cells can be defined by these approaches (Fig. 22-1, Ch. 22).

In mice subjected to about 9 Gray of ionizing radiation (1 Gray is the radiation dose yielding 10^{10} ionizations/gr of tissue), which is sufficient to destroy all hematopoiesis, and then given intravenous infusions of bone marrow from untreated mice, colonies of blood cells appear in the spleen. These discrete colonies contain erythrocytes, phagocytes, lymphocytes, and megakaryocytes, indicating that the donor infusion must have contained hematopoietic progenitor cells capable of differentiating into all blood cell types. Such pluripotent stem cells can replicate themselves as required to respond to peripheral demands for differentiation into cells committed to the production of erythroid, phagocytic, and platelet lines. Physiologists refer to these cells as *colony-forming units, stem cell*, or simply CFU-S.

Recent research has permitted study of very early stem cells, and a pluripotent stem cell has been cultivated from mice. Although this feat has not been accomplished in humans, evidence strongly implies that a marker for human stem cells is a surface protein called *CD34**, which permits use of antibodies to this structure as a way of obtaining enriched stem cell populations by the technique of fluorescence-activated cell sorting.* A growth factor required for the proliferation of stem cells was identified by studying two unrelated mouse strains that had hypoplastic anemia, mast cell deficiency, sterility, and melanocyte depletion. Both mouse strains had complementary mutations in a growth factor system known as stem cell factor, which is normally produced by bone marrow stroma. One strain, Sl/Sl^d, did not produce stem cell factor, whereas the other, W/W^v, had a mutant unresponsive stem cell factor receptor. As expected, normal fibroblasts cured the defects in Sl/Sl^d but not in W/W^v mice. In addition to stem cell factor and other cytokines that promote stem cell proliferation, inhibitors of stem cell growth, which are members of the transforming growth factor β (TGFβ) family of cytokines, have also been identified.

Another important development is the ability to grow mouse embryonic stem cells (ES cells) in tissue culture in the presence of a cytokine called *leukemia inhibitory factor (LIF)*. ES can be induced to differentiate into hematopoietic cells in vitro by removal of LIF and cultivation in various combinations of other cytokines or else used to create mice with altered hematopoietic cell genes. This system has enabled researchers to identify a gene, designated GATA-1, which encodes a DNA-binding protein that programs erythroid differentiation of hematopoietic stem cells.

The cultivation of bone marrow or peripheral blood in an appropriate medium can lead to the formation of colonies of cells differentiating into either phagocytic, erythroid, or megakaryocytic cells. These culture techniques are therefore believed to select for the expression of committed stem cells, designated CFU-C. The cultivation of bone marrow or peripheral blood in semisolid medium leads to the growth of discrete colonies containing cells having the morphology of phagocytes, polymorphonuclear leukocytes, and macrophages. This procedure recruits colony-forming units for granulocytes and macrophages (CFU-GM). Growth of peripheral blood or bone marrow in plasma clots to which is added a source of erythropoietin leads to the outgrowth of different types of colonies containing erythroid cells. Large clusters of immature erythroid cells are defined as primitive burst-forming units, erythroid (BFU-E), named for the resemblance of these colonies to sunbursts. Smaller colonies are designated mature burst-forming units, erythroid; small cell colonies containing erythroid cells are believed to be the expression of relatively more mature erythroid stem cells, called CFU, erythroid (CFU-E). Appropriate cultivation techniques can also lead to the selection of stem cells committed to growth into megakaryocytes, CFUs, megakaryocytic (CFU-M) into lymphocytes or, depending on the culture conditions, either macrophages or B cells. Such culture systems also point to the existence of a progenitor cell common to erythroid, myeloid (phagocytic) and megakaryocyte lineages (indicated by the bracket in Fig. 1-2).

The relevance of these culture systems to hematopoiesis in humans and in experimental animals was initially evident from the fact that the presence, absence, or number of CFUs obtainable from the bone marrow or peripheral blood often changes in parallel with alterations in the production of blood cells in the intact organism. Subsequently, humoral factors were shown to stimulate growth of particular blood cells, both in animals and the culture systems. Recently, the activity of hematopoietic hormones has been directly and stunningly demonstrated in humans by the infusion of

---

*Throughout this text and elsewhere the reader will frequently encounter the designation *CD* followed by a number, which identifies a cell surface antigen. The convention *CD* (for "*cluster of differentiation*") has evolved from international workshops in which antibodies provided by investigators are tested against cell targets and those that react with the same cell surface structure. These antibodies may react with different portions of the surface molecule, but they are "clustered" in that they all react with a particular surface antigen.

recombinant erythropoietin and of CSFs, with subsequent enhancement of erythro- and myelopoiesis, respectively, and cytokine therapy is now widely used in the treatment of anemia and hematologic malignancies. Current clinical trials of these agents are testing combinations of such cytokines as well as novel genetically engineered constructs expressing the receptor-binding domains of more than one hematopoietic hormone.

Stem cells can be harvested from peripheral blood as well as from bone marrow. This fact suggests that the stem cells may sense the environmental demands for differentiation and replication by coursing through the blood and peripheral organs, as well as waiting in the bone marrow for humoral signals to provide this information. This circulation of stem cells might also explain how leukemic cells and other malignant stem cells are almost invariably found throughout the bone marrow at the outset of clinical disease. Furthermore, it explains how infusions of bone marrow stem cells into the peripheral blood can lead to engraftment of the bone marrow during the procedure of bone marrow transplantation (Ch. 32).

THE SCOPE OF HEMATOLOGY

The foregoing discussion has provided an overview of and set the stage for the detailed description of the structure and functions of the blood in the remainder of this text. We close this introductory chapter by considering for whom this information can be useful.

In one guise, hematology is a subspecialty of internal medicine. Practitioners of this form of hematology are specialists in dealing with diseases of the blood. They diagnose and treat anemias, coagulation disorders, and malignant neoplasms of blood cells. The treatment of malignancies of the blood, discussed in Chapters 21 to 29 and 32, is similar to the

treatment of a variety of solid tumors. Conversely, the therapy of solid tumors often has profound effects on the blood. For these reasons, the disciplines of hematology and oncology have always been closely related and in recent years have become even more closely linked. Another close relationship exists between hematology and immunology. Abnormalities of the numbers and functions of white blood cells often cause a patient to become abnormally susceptible to infection, a state defined as *immunodeficiency*. On the other hand, perversion of the immune system so that it destroys normal blood cells, a state defined as *autoimmunity,* is frequently encountered in medical practice.

Another aspect of hematology is *blood transfusion therapy*. Replacement of whole blood and blood components is a major medical enterprise, occurring during surgery and following injury. Not only are blood components infused into patients, but, increasingly, abnormal proteins are removed from patients with various diseases. All the procedures described in Chapter 31 are performed in transfusion services that are present in all but the smallest hospitals. Furthermore, in the United States there is a regional network of blood transfusion centers organized by the American National Red Cross. This very active dimension of hematology has enormous medical and economic ramifications.

Finally, nearly every physician is, in a sense, a "hematologist." Because of its access to all tissues of the body, the blood is often one of the first sources of information that indicate changes in the state of health and the development of specific diseases. Changes in the number or appearance of formed elements and in the levels of plasma components are extremely useful to all clinicians. It is not surprising, then, that diagnostic hematology laboratories are consulted by nearly all clinicians and that the total impact of the work of these laboratories on the cost of health care is considerable.

In closing this chapter, we want to emphasize to all physicians the utility of analyzing the blood. Examination of a Wright's-stained specimen of blood under the microscope may be the first clue to a dangerous depression in the number of circulating platelets and alerts the clinician to the possibility of bleeding. A large number of "bluish" red blood cells on the smear indicates the presence of *reticulocytes*, young red blood cells, which increase in number when bleeding is occurring. The smear can indicate the presence of elevated numbers of circulating phagocytes and changes in the appearance of these cells, which suggest existence of bacterial infection. In some instances, together with other information, the presence of a specific infection may be suggested. For example, parasitic microorganisms, such as the plasmodia of malaria, may be directly observed. The aggregation of red blood cells on the smear might suggest alterations in the levels of plasma proteins (Ch. 17). Peculiarities in the shapes of the red blood cells can mean the presence of vascular injury, liver disease, or overwhelming infection. We emphasize that the examples given here are not diseases limited to the province of the "hematologist" but are conditions that any physician is likely to encounter. The blood is truly a window into our state of health, and the peripheral blood smear affords a practical and simple glance into that window.

SUGGESTED READINGS

Baum C, Weissman IL, Buckle AM, Tsukamoto A (1992) Identification and isolation of a candidate human hematopoietic stem cell. Proc Natl Acad Sci USA 89:2804

Cumano A, Paige CJ, Iscove NN, Brady G (1992) Bipotential precursors of B cells and macrophages in murine fetal liver. Nature 356:612

Dinarello CA, Wolff SM (1993) The role of interleukin-1 in disease. N Engl J Med 328:106

Erslev AJ (1991) Erythropoietin. N Engl J Med 324:1339

Galli SJ (1993) New concepts about the mast cell. N Engl J Med 328:257

Goldberg MA, Dunning SP, Bunn HF (1988) Regulation of the erythropoietin gene: evidence that the oxygen sensor is a heme protein. Science 242:1412

Handin RI, Lux SE, Stossel TP (1994) Hematology. Function and Disorders of the Blood. JB Lippincott, Philadelphia

Lieschke GJ, Burgess AW (1992) Granulocyte colony-stimulating factor and granulocyte-macrophage colony-stimulating factor. N Engl J Med 327:28

Ogawa M (1993) Differentiation and proliferation of hematopoietic stem cells. Blood 81:2844

Sanderson CJ (1992) Interleukin-5, eosinophils, and disease. Blood 79:3101

Shadduck RK (1992) Clinical applications of granulocyte-macrophage colony-stimulating factor. Semin Hematol 29 (suppl. 3):1

Simon MC, Pevny L, Wiles MC et al (1992) Rescue of erythroid development in gene targeted GATA-1 mouse embryonic stem cells. Nature Genetics 1:92

Spangrude GJ, Smith L, Uchida N (1991) Mouse hematopoietic stem cells. Blood 78:1395

Taga T, Kishimoto T (1992) Cytokine receptors and signal transduction. FASEB J 7:3387

Westerman MP (1981) The bone marrow: structure, function and pathology. Semin Hematol 18:177

Wiles MV, Keller G (1991) Multiple hematopoietic lineages develop from embryonic stem (ES) cells in culture. Development 111:259

Zipori D (1992) The renewal and differentiation of hemopoietic stem cells. FASEB J 6:2691

Zucker-Franklin D, Greaves MF, Grossi CE, Marmont AM (1988) Atlas of Blood Cells. 2nd Ed. Lea & Febiger, Philadelphia

Section I

Red Blood Cells and Their Diseases

To survive, the tissues of the body must receive a steady supply of oxygen from the atmosphere. One of the functions of the blood is to provide this supply of oxygen. This function is performed by the red cells, which take up oxygen as the blood flows through the lungs and release it when the blood reaches the tissues.

For maximum delivery of oxygen, the blood must contain the right proportion of red cells to total volume. Too low a proportion decreases the amount of oxygen that can be carried by the blood; too high a proportion thickens the blood, impeding its flow through the tissues. It is not surprising, then, that the proportion of red cells in the blood is closely regulated and stays within rather narrow limits under normal circumstances.

Red blood cell disorders typically present as abnormalities in the proportion of red cells to total blood volume. Most common by far are those in which this proportion is low. These are the *anemias*. The anemias include many different red cell disorders, some of which are quite prevalent. Most of the hematological conditions seen in daily practice are anemias of one kind or another. Other disorders show an abnormally high proportion of red cells, but these are seen much less frequently than the anemias.

2

Red Blood Cell Diseases: Red Cell Production, Red Cell Indices, and the Reticulocyte Count

Red cells are the oxygen-carrying elements of the blood. They are highly flexible biconcave discs filled with hemoglobin (Fig. 2-1). Flexibility is necessary to permit them to pass through the very narrow vessels they must negotiate as they pick up oxygen from the lungs and deliver it to tissues. Hemoglobin is the protein that actually carries the oxygen.

RED CELL PRODUCTION

Like all the cells of the blood, red cells arise from a population of incompletely characterized marrow stem cells that start out with the capacity to become any cell in the blood or lymphatic system but then commit themselves to a single line—in this case, the red cell line. The daughters of these now-committed stem cells differentiate into red cells by passing through a series of stages identifiable under the microscope as successively more mature red cell precursors. Eventually they mature fully and are released into the blood stream as young erythrocytes. After circulating for a period of time, the erythrocytes are removed from the bloodstream and destroyed.

The earliest red cell precursors, though not recognizable under a microscope, can be detected by marrow culture, a technique in which bone marrow cells are grown in soft agar containing suitable nutrients and hormones. Two types of red cell precursors have been identified by this technique: the CFU-E (colony-forming unit, erythrocyte), a single cell that gives rise to a tight cluster of hemoglobinized cells as it proliferates and differentiates; and the BFU-E (burst-forming unit, erythrocyte), an earlier cell whose descendents, after wandering a short distance, mature into closely spaced CFU-Es that eventually appear as a group of hemoglobinized cell clusters—a so-called burst (Fig. 2-2). The CFU-E is thought to be the immediate precursor of the pronormoblast, the earliest erythrocyte precursor that can be identified under the microscope.

As they differentiate further into erythrocytes, the red cell precursors undergo three major changes: (1) they accumulate hemoglobin; (2) they lose their protein-synthesizing apparatus (including all their RNA) and their mitochondria; and (3) their nuclear chromatin condenses into a functionless mass, with contraction and finally extrusion of the nucleus.

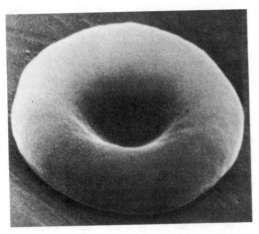

Fig. 2-1 A normal red cell, seen under a scanning electron microscope. (From Wintrobe MM et al [1974] Clinical Hematology. 7th Ed. Lea & Febiger, Philadelphia, with permission.)

These changes are responsible for the changes in the appearance of the red cell precursors as they pass through the various stages of differentiation (Fig. 2-3). The earliest detectable stage is the pronormoblast, a large cell consisting mostly of a large, purplish nucleus with finely divided chromatin and a couple of dark-staining nucleoli, wrapped in a rim of cytoplasm that is colored a deep rich blue because it contains a very large amount of blue-staining RNA but hardly any pink-staining hemoglobin. Next the red cell precursor becomes a basophilic normoblast, then a polychromatophilic normoblast, and finally an orthochromatic normoblast. As it shrinks in size, its nucleus condenses and contracts, and its cytoplasm turns from blue to pink as RNA is replaced by hemoglobin. Last comes the

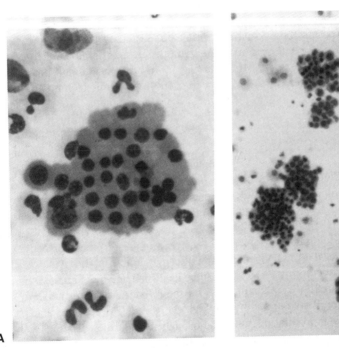

A

B

Fig. 2-2. Detection of early red cell precursors in bone marrow cultures. (**A**) A cluster of hemoglobinized cells generated by a CFU-E (colony-forming unit, erythrocyte). (**B**) A closely spaced group of such clusters produced by a BFU-E (burst-forming unit, erythrocyte). (From Zucker-Franklin D, Greaves MF, Grossi CE, Marmont AM [1988] Atlas of Blood Cells. 2nd Ed. Edi Ermes, s.r.l., Milan, with permission.)

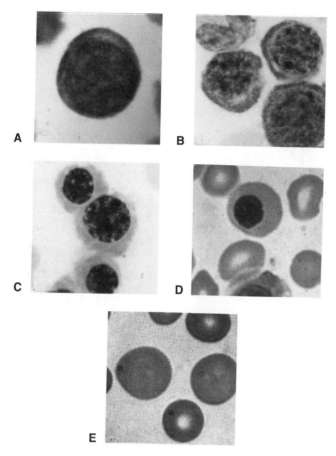

Fig. 2-3. Stages of maturation of a red cell progenitor. (**A**) Pronormoblast. (**B**) Basophilic normoblast. (**C**) Polychromatophilic normoblast. (**D**) Orthochromatic normoblast. (**E**) Erythrocyte. As the cell matures its size diminishes, its nucleus shrinks, its chromatin condenses, and it acquires hemoglobin. (B,C: From Wintrobe MM et al [1974] Clinical Hematology. 7th Ed. Lea & Febiger, Philadelphia, with permission; A, D, E: From Lessin LS, Bessis M [1972] Morphology of the erythron. In Williams WJ et al [eds] Hematology. McGraw-Hill, New York, with permission.)

extrusion of the nucleus—by now nothing more than a small, dark, round, structureless mass—and the release of the red cell into the bloodstream. The newly released red cells still contain a few mitochondria and a little RNA, but these disappear within a day or two to produce the fully mature red cell.

Of the four precursor stages—pronormoblast, basophilic normoblast, polychromatophilic normoblast, and orthochromatic normoblast—the first three consist of cells that are able to divide. These cells are said to be in the mitotic compartment (Fig. 2-4). Division and maturation occur at the same time, so a single normoblast will generate several basophilic normoblasts, each of which will produce several polychromatophilic normoblasts, and so forth. The result is that the percentage of red cell precursors in the marrow is much greater for the later stages than for the earlier stages.

It takes about 3 to 5 days for a pronormoblast to become a red cell. Once in the bloodstream, this cell will live for about 4 months. It will then die of old age, and its remains will be degraded for reuse.

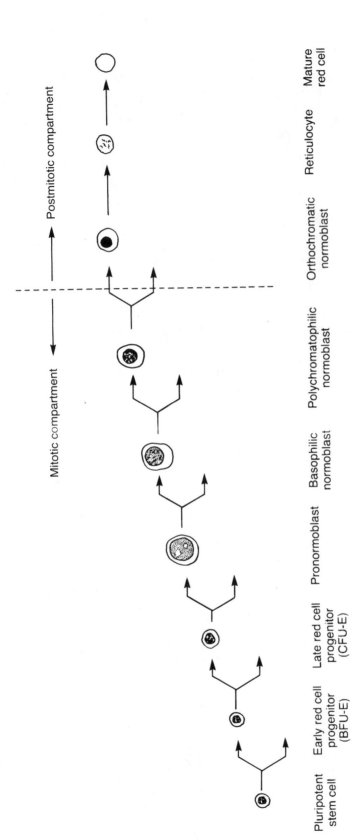

Fig. 2-4. Red cell differentiation.

The production of red cells is normally controlled fairly tightly, with the fraction of the blood volume occupied by the red cells (this fraction is known as the *hematocrit*) being maintained in the vicinity of 40 to 45 percent. It is probably not a coincidence that 40 to 45 percent also happens to be the hematocrit range that affords the best delivery of oxygen to the tissues. This optimum range is dictated by two properties of the blood that affect oxygen delivery: its hemoglobin content, which determines how much oxygen the blood can carry, and its viscosity, which influences how rapidly the oxygen-laden blood can flow through the tissues. The hemoglobin content, which is equivalent to the oxygen-carrying capacity of the blood, increases linearly with the rising hematocrit. The viscosity also increases with a rising hematocrit, but in a more complex way, the change being rather small as the hematocrit increases to about 50 percent, but very large as it exceeds this value (Fig. 2-5). Over the flat

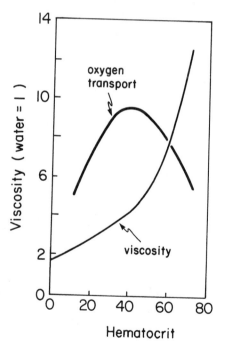

Fig. 2-5. Effect of the hematocrit on blood viscosity and oxygen transport. (Adapted from Erslev AJ, Gabuzda TG [1975] Pathophysiology of Blood. WB Saunders, Philadelphia, with permission.)

portion of the viscosity curve, oxygen delivery to the tissues goes up smoothly as the hematocrit rises, because the oxygen-carrying capacity of the blood increases while the blood viscosity stays nearly the same. In the region of the steep portion, however, oxygen delivery actually falls as the hematocrit rises, because the increase in the oxygen-carrying capacity of the blood is more than offset by the impedance to tissue blood flow caused by the rapidly increasing blood viscosity. The relationship between these factors is such that oxygen delivery to the tissues is maximum at a hematocrit of 40 to 45 percent.

Red cell production is controlled by several growth factors. The earliest stem cells, those that have not yet committed themselves to a particular line, are regulated by *interleukin 3* and *granulocyte-macrophage colony-stimulating factor (GM-CSF)*, two growth factors that are made in the marrow and act locally (see Ch. 1). Once committed, however, the red cell precursors fall under the control of a glycoprotein hormone called *erythropoietin*. This hormone is manufactured mainly by the kidney (Fig. 2-6), although a small amount is also made by the liver. Its production by the kidney is inversely related to the renal oxygen tension; it is increased when the renal oxygen tension is low and depressed when the renal oxygen tension is high. The hormone is carried by the circulation to the bone marrow, where it augments red cell production by increasing the number of stem cells committed to the red cell line and by shortening the time required for these committed stem cells to mature into reticulocytes (Fig. 2-7).

Erythropoietin is the main factor responsible for the compensatory increase in red cell production that occurs when the oxygen content of the blood drops, as occurs, for example, in anemia, at high altitudes, and in pulmonary diseases that impede the passage of oxygen from the lungs to the red cells. The drop in blood oxygen content leads to a decrease in the renal oxygen tension, which in turn causes erythropoietin production to rise. As a result, the bone marrow is stimulated, thereby increasing red

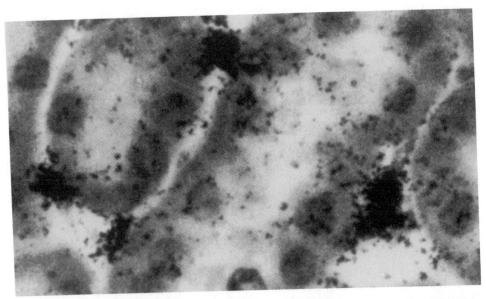

Fig. 2-6. Erythropoietin is produced in the kidney by a minor population of juxtaglomerular cells. In this cross section of kidney, the cells that contain erythropoietin messenger RNA (i.e., the cells that secrete erythropoietin) are marked by silver grains. (From Semenza GL, Koury ST, Nejfelt MK, Gearhart JD, Antonarakis SE [1991] Cell-type-specific and hypoxia-inducible expression of the human erythropoietin gene in transgenic mice. Proc Natl Acad Sci USA 88:8725, with permission.)

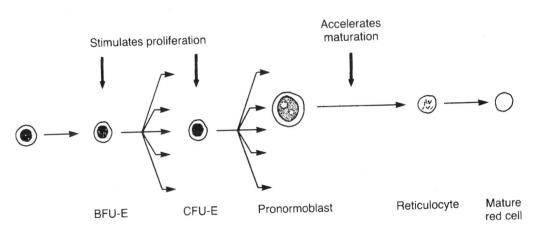

Fig. 2-7. The action of erythropoietin.

cell production. The marrow has the capacity to increase red cell production by a factor of 7 to 8 when maximally stimulated.

RED BLOOD CELL DISEASES: THE RETICULOCYTE COUNT AND THE RED CELL INDICES

Diseases of red cells are by far the most common of the hematological disorders. Almost without exception, these diseases cause a quantitative alteration in the blood hemoglobin level—usually a reduction (anemia), less often an increase (erythrocytosis). An abnormal blood hemoglobin value is the sign that points to the existence of a red blood cell disorder.

Once the presence of a red blood cell disorder has been established, its nature must be determined. This is accomplished by analyzing the clinical and laboratory features accompanying the abnormality in blood hemoglobin in the affected patient. Most of these features are discussed in the chapters that deal with the specific disorders. Two, however, are of general utility in the evaluation of red blood cell diseases, so it is appropriate to present them here, before discussing the specific disorders. These features are the *reticulocyte count* and the *red cell indices* (Wintrobe indices).

The Reticulocyte Count

The RNA of the protein-synthesizing apparatus is degraded as the red cell precursor reaches maturity. Degradation is well under way at the time the cell leaves the marrow, but it does not reach completion until the cell has been in the circulation for a day or two. Newly released red cells therefore contain RNA that is not found in older cells. Because of this RNA, these new cells can be identified morphologically. On a routine smear, which is ordinarily prepared with a hematoxylin-containing stain called Wright's stain, the tinting of the residual

RNA by the hematoxylin gives the new cells a distinct bluish cast. Cells with this bluish cast are known as *polychromatophilic cells*. If instead of Wright's stain the smear is prepared with new methylene blue or brilliant cresyl blue, the RNA precipitates as a deep blue-staining reticulum of strands and clumps. Cells containing these precipitates are known as reticulocytes (Fig. 2-8). Polychromatophilic cells and reticulocytes are two morphological aspects of the same cell population—that is, red cells that have been released from the marrow 1 to 2 days earlier. These normally constitute about 1 percent of all red cells in the blood.

Reticulocytes are important in the clinical evaluation of the anemias because they provide crucial information on the rate of red cell production. Anemias can be divided into two broad classes: those caused by increased red cell loss from the blood, and those associated with decreased red cell production by the marrow. When an anemia results from increased red cell loss, the marrow compensates by increasing red cell production. New cells are released from the marrow in greater than normal numbers, so the reticulocyte count increases. Conversely, when an anemia is caused by a decrease in red cell production, the release of

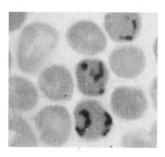

Fig. 2-8. Reticulocytes. Their dark-staining precipitates distinguish them easily from the homogeneously stained older cells. (From Lessin LS, Bessis M [1972] Morphology of the erythron. In Williams WJ et al [eds] Hematology. McGraw-Hill, New York, with permission.)

new cells falls below normal, and the reticulocyte count decreases.

Red Cell Indices

Among the features that distinguish one type of anemia from another are the average size and hemoglobin content of the affected red cells. These properties of the red cell are generally expressed in terms of the three red cell (or Wintrobe) indices:

Mean cell volume (MCV), expressed in femtoliters (fl)

Mean cell hemoglobin (MCH), expressed in picograms (pg) per red cell

Mean cell hemoglobin concentration (MCHC), the approximate percentage of the red cell mass that is made up of hemoglobin

Only two of these indices are independent, however; the third can be calculated from the formula

MCHC = 100 x (MCH/MCV)

The way in which these indices are determined depends on the method used for quantitating red cells in the blood. As a rule, red cells are quantified using automated counters. The measurements obtained by these counters are the blood hemoglobin (measured in g/100 ml blood); the red cell count (cells/ μl blood); and the MCV. Automated counters can also determine the *hematocrit* (sometimes called the *packed cell volume*), which is defined as the percentage of the total blood volume occupied by the red cells. They usually do this by calculation, multiplying the MCV by the red count (with an appropriate correction for the units in which these figures are expressed). Alternatively, they may measure the hematocrit by centrifugating the blood to separate the red cells from the plasma and then measuring the appropriate volumes. Indices are calculated directly by the instrument.

When automated counters are not available, red cells can be quantitated by hand, using simple equipment. The measurements obtained are the hematocrit, the blood hemoglobin, and the red cell count.

Using results obtained from automated counters, red cell indices other than the MCV may be calculated according to the formulas:

$$MCH = \frac{10^7 \text{ x hemoglobin}}{\text{red count}}$$

$$MCHC = \frac{10^7 \text{ x hemoglobin}}{\text{red count x MCV}}$$

Normal values are as follows:

MCV 80–96 fl
MCH 27–33 pg
MCHC 33–35%

Table 2-1. Classification of the Anemias by Mean Cell Volume (MCV)[a]

Microcytic (MCV low)		Macrocytic (MCV high)		
Disorder	Chapter	Disorder	Chapter	Normocytic (MCV normal)
Iron deficiency anemia	4	Megaloblastic anemia	6	Most other anemias
Thalassemia	10	Hemolytic anemia	8,9	
Sickle cell anemia and related disorders	11	Anemia of liver disease	8	
Sideroblastic anemia	5	Anemia of hypothyroidism	7	

[a]Although this classification scheme is highly useful as a general guide to the diagnosis of anemia, it must be borne in mind that exceptions to these rules do occur.

The red cell indices are important because they form the basis for an extremely valuable classification of the anemias by pathophysiological category. In the most useful version of this classification, the various anemias are grouped by red cell size into three categories: microcytic (small cell), normocytic (normal size), and macrocytic (large cell). Accordingly, although all three Wintrobe indices are routinely obtained in anemic patients, the only index usually needed to classify an anemia is the MCV. The classification of anemias by MCV is given in Table 2-1.

Often, anemias are described in terms of the amount of hemoglobin in the red cells as assessed under the microscope. Cells that look deficient in hemoglobin are termed "hypochromic"; those with normal amounts of hemoglobin are designated "normochromic"; and those with excess hemoglobin are termed "hyperchromic." In practical terms, though, the apparent quantity of hemoglobin in a red cell viewed through a microscope is determined by the size of the cell. Accordingly, microcytic anemias are hypochromic, normocytic anemias are normochromic, and macrocytic anemias are hyperchromic. It is a common practice to use adjectives describing both cell size and hemoglobin content when classifying an anemia—for example, iron-deficiency anemia is generally referred to as a hypochromic microcytic anemia—but little seems to be gained by this dual terminology.

Between the reticulocyte count and the red cell indices, it is usually possible to place an anemia into one of a small number of fairly narrowly defined pathophysiological categories. These pathophysiological categories are the point of departure for the discussions of anemias and other red blood cell disorders presented in the succeeding chapters.

SUGGESTED READINGS

Adamson JW (1991) Erythropoietin: its role in the regulation of erythropoiesis and as a therapeutic in humans. Biotechnology 19:351

Bernstein A, Forrester L, Reith AD et al (1991) The murine W/c-kit and Steel loci and the control of hematopoiesis. Semin Hematol 28:138

Erickson N, Quesenberry PJ (1992) Regulation of erythropoiesis. The role of growth factors. Med Clin North Am 76:745

Graber SE, Krantz SB (1978) Erythropoietin and the control of red cell production. Annu Rev Med 29:51–66

Groopman JE, Molina JM, Scadden DT (1989) Hematopoietic growth factors. Biology and clinical applications. N Engl J Med 321:1449

Houwen B (1992) Reticulocyte maturation. Blood Cells 18:167

Krantz SB (1991) Erythropoietin. Blood 77:419

Nathan DG (1990) Regulation of hematopoiesis. Pediatr Res 27:423

Orkin SH (1990) Cell-specific transcription and cell differentiation in the erythroid lineage. Curr Opin Cell Biol 2:1003

Quesenberry P, Levitt L (1979) Hematopoietic stem cells. N Engl J Med 301:755

Surgenor DM (1974–1975) Red Cell. 2nd Ed. Vols. 1 and 2. Academic Press, Orlando, FL

Sytkowski AJ (1991) Control of erythropoietin production. Blood Rev 5:15

3

Hemoglobin and Oxygen Transport: Disorders of Oxygen Binding

Hemoglobin is the oxygen-transporting protein of the red cell. By weight it composes about 30 percent of the erythrocyte, a concentration high enough that 1 ml of oxygen-saturated packed red cells holds the equivalent of about 0.5 ml of oxygen gas. The hemoglobin picks up oxygen as the red cell passes through the lungs, unloading it when the red cell reaches the capillaries of the tissues. The oxygen-binding properties of hemoglobin are such that it can unload its oxygen even at the relatively high oxygen tensions that prevail in most tissues.

Hemoglobin is actually a family of molecules whose members differ slightly in primary structure. In the context of oxygen binding, however, the most important hemoglobin by far is hemoglobin A, which constitutes more than 95 percent of all the hemoglobin in the normal adult red cell. The following discussion deals with the properties of hemoglobin A. The oxygen-binding properties of other normal hemoglobins differ only in detail from those of hemoglobin A. Clinically important features of oxygen binding by the minor hemoglobins are discussed in connection with diseases of hemoglobin biosynthesis in Chapter 10.

STRUCTURE OF HEMOGLOBIN

The hemoglobin molecule is a tetrameric protein of molecular weight (MW) 65,000. It consists of two types of peptide chains: the α- and β-globin chains. These assemble to form a tetrahedral molecule containing two chains of each kind ($\alpha_2\beta_2$) (Fig. 3-1). The molecule is held together mainly by interactions between dissimilar chains. Because the chains interact less firmly with one of their dissimilar neighbors than they do with the other, the hemoglobin molecule contains a natural plane of cleavage, which will be seen to be important in the regulation of oxygen affinity, and along which the molecule can split into $\alpha\beta$ dimers when it is sufficiently dilute. The portion of the molecule

$$\alpha + \beta \rightarrow \alpha\beta \text{ (tight)} \rightarrow \alpha\beta\cdots\alpha\beta$$

lining this plane of cleavage is known as the $a_1\beta_2$ region.

A globin chain itself, containing approximately 150 amino acids, is arranged in a precisely defined configuration resembling a long, thin sausage tied in an elaborate knot (Fig. 3-2). Within the knotted chain, regions of particular functional importance can be identified.

27

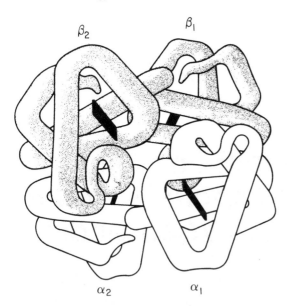

β_2 β_1

α_2 α_1

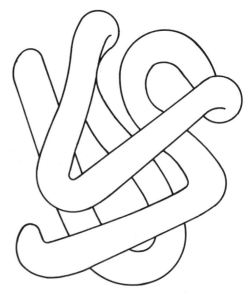

Fig. 3-1. The hemoglobin tetramer. The molecule consists of two $\alpha\beta$ dimers that combine to form the complete hemoglobin molecule. The region where the two dimers come into contact is known as the $\alpha_1\beta_2$ region. (Modified from Dean J, Schechter AN [1978] Sickle-cell anemia: molecular and cellular bases of therapeutic approaches. N Engl J Med 299:752–763, with permission.)

Fig. 3-2. A globin chain: the knotted sausage. (Adapted from Wintrobe MM et al [1974] Clinical Hematology. 7th Ed. Lea & Febiger, Philadelphia, with permission.)

are critical in giving hemoglobin its very remarkable oxygen-binding properties (Fig. 3-4).

The Heme Crevice

Heme is the large, flat, iron-containing disc that actually carries the oxygen molecule. It binds to a specific region of the globin chain, the heme crevice, by strong but noncovalent forces. Of note are two special histidines in the crevice. Each is directly opposite the iron, one in front and one in back of the ring (Fig. 3-3). The one in back is attached directly to the iron through one of its imidazole nitrogens, while the one in front is separated from the iron by a space large enough to accommodate an oxygen molecule. It will be seen that these histidines permit hemoglobin to bind oxygen reversibly.

The $\alpha_1\beta_2$ Region

The $\alpha_1\beta_2$ region is important because interchain interactions that occur within this region

The Region of the β-Chain N-Termini

The β-chain N-termini region contains a pocket lined with positively charged groups consisting of the two terminal amino groups of the β-chains together with positively charged side chains of nearby lysine and arginine residues. This pocket represents a binding site for 2,3-diphosphoglyceric acid (2,3-DPG), a major physiological regulator of the oxygen affinity of hemoglobin. Occupation of this binding site by 2,3-DPG tends to draw together the two $\alpha_1\beta_2$ regions of the hemoglobin tetramer.

FUNCTION OF HEMOGLOBIN

The function of hemoglobin is to bind oxygen reversibly, delivering it from the lungs, a

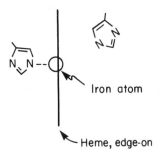

Iron atom

Heme, edge-on

Fig. 3-3. The environment of the iron atom in hemoglobin. Oxygen binds to hemoglobin by combining with the iron atoms.

region of high oxygen tension, to the tissues, a region of much lower oxygen tension. As mentioned earlier, the oxygen-binding site is the iron of the heme group. This iron is in the ferrous (Fe^{2+}) form, and in the normal course of events it takes up and releases oxygen atoms without undergoing a change in valence. This is a remarkable feature of hemoglobin, because the iron of free heme is very readily oxidized to

the ferric (Fe^{3+}) state, and hemoglobin containing Fe^{3+} heme, commonly called methemoglobin, is unable to transport oxygen. Stabilization of the iron in the Fe^{2+} state is somehow connected with the special histidine residues at the heme-binding site; disruption of this histidine-iron relationship can result in the rapid oxidation of the hemoglobin iron (see the discussion of hemoglobin M, below).

Oxygen Affinity

The molecule that transports oxygen from the lungs to the tissues is faced with a dilemma. On the one hand, it must take up as much oxygen as possible when passing through the lungs. On the other hand, it must unload much of its oxygen at tissue oxygen tensions high enough to support life. Hemoglobin solves this dilemma through its remarkable oxygen-binding properties. The relationship between the PO_2 and hemoglobin oxygen saturation is S shaped (Fig. 3-5), so hemoglobin is able to

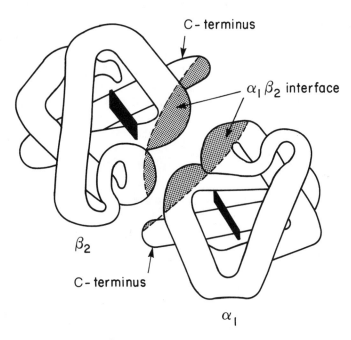

C- terminus

$\alpha_1\beta_2$ interface

β_2

C- terminus

α_1

Fig. 3-4. An $\alpha_1\beta_2$ interface. Hemoglobin has two of these.

load up nearly completely in the lungs and yet can release a substantial fraction of its oxygen at the relatively high oxygen levels in the tissues. Specifically, tissues generally take up about 25 percent of the oxygen brought to them by the blood, so that hemoglobin leaving the tissues is about 75 percent saturated. The oxygen saturation curve shows that this corresponds to a tissue PO_2 value of about 40 mm, well within the life-supporting range. Were the relationship between PO_2 and oxygen saturation hyperbolic in shape (i.e., more typical for the binding of a small molecule to a protein), then hemoglobin would be unable to unload the amount of oxygen required by the tissues until the PO_2 fell to around 2 mm—clearly a metabolic catastrophe that is prevented by the sigmoidality of the hemoglobin oxygen-binding curve.

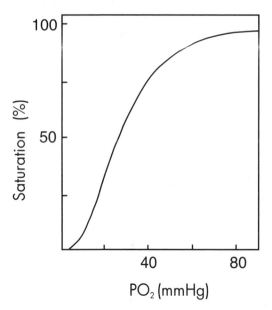

Fig. 3-5. How the oxygen saturation of whole blood varies with oxygen tension. The sigmoidal shape of the curve is critical for hemoglobin function, permitting hemoglobin to become almost fully oxygen saturated in the lung and yet unload oxygen as required at the relatively high oxygen tensions prevailing in the tissues. (Adapted from Bunn HF, Forget BG, Ranney HM [1977] Human Hemoglobins. WB Saunders, Philadelphia, with permission.)

The characteristics of the saturation curve for this and other hemoglobins are frequently summarized by two numerical parameters. The first is the oxygen tension at 50 percent saturation, known as P_{50}. This is a measure of the inherent oxygen affinity of the hemoglobin; the tighter the oxygen is held, the lower the P_{50}. It is clear from the foregoing discussion that tissue oxygen tensions will correlate roughly with P_{50}, other things being equal.

The second parameter is the Hill coefficient, a number derived from the oxygen-binding curve. This coefficient measures the "S-ness" of the saturation curve. The hemoglobin saturation curve is S-shaped because oxygen binds to hemoglobin in a cooperative fashion. The hemoglobin molecule that is already partly saturated has a higher affinity for oxygen than does a hemoglobin molecule that is completely free of oxygen. Thus the uptake of one oxygen molecule by hemoglobin will facilitate the uptake of the next. It can be shown mathematically that if cooperativity were perfect—that is, if one molecule of hemoglobin were to take up four molecules of oxygen before the next were to take up its first oxygen molecule—then the oxygen saturation curve would obey the relationship: saturation $\approx (PO_2)^4$ (at low and intermediate levels of saturation, where the arithmetic is not affected by the depletion of free oxygen-binding sites) (Fig. 3-6). If there were no cooperativity, the oxygen saturation curve would obey the relationship: saturation $\approx (PO_2)$. For intermediate degrees of cooperativity, the power to which PO_2 is raised would take on an intermediate value (i.e., a value between 1 and 4). This exponent thus gives a measure of the degree of cooperativity, which in turn is an index of how effectively hemoglobin can unload oxygen to tissues. The Hill coefficient is an estimate of this exponent. It is determined from the Hill plot, a way of plotting saturation against PO_2 that expresses cooperativity in an unusually clear and straightforward manner (Fig. 3-7). The Hill coefficient is simply the slope of the Hill plot at the point where the curve crosses P_{50}. The steeper the slope, the greater the Hill coefficient, and the higher the

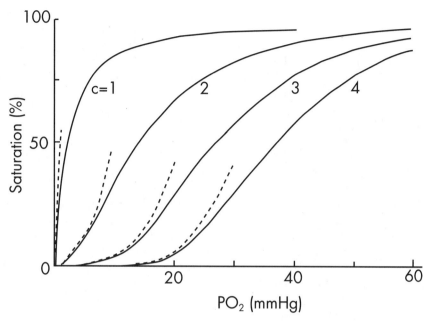

Fig. 3-6. The theoretical oxygen-binding curve of hemoglobin, assuming perfect cooperativity (*right*), intermediate levels of cooperativity, or no cooperativity (*left*). At low levels of saturation, each curve comes very close to the relationship: saturation ≈ $(PO_2)^c$ (*dotted line*). The greater the degree of cooperativity, the greater the value of the exponent c, making this exponent an index of cooperativity. At high levels of saturation, the curves fall away from these relationships because of the progressive depletion of unoccupied binding sites as the hemoglobin takes on its load of oxygen.

degree of cooperativity in the binding of oxygen of hemoglobin.

The Hill coefficient for hemoglobin A is about 3. Some of the abnormal hemoglobins to be discussed later in this chapter have abnormally low Hill coefficients. This defect in cooperativity adds to the difficulties with oxygen transport in patients burdened with these abnormal hemoglobins.

The molecular basis for cooperativity lies in the fact that hemoglobin exists in two conformations, known as the T and R states, whose oxygen affinities differ from one another (Fig. 3-8). The T (taut) state is characterized by a relatively low oxygen affinity and a close fit between the two $\alpha_1\beta_2$ regions, while the R (relaxed) state has a relatively high oxygen affinity and a wider $\alpha_1\beta_2$ separation than the T state.

In the absence of oxygen, the equilibrium between the two conformers favors the T state.

The binding of oxygen to a molecule in the T state induces structural changes that tend to cause the molecule to flip to the R state, whose affinity for oxygen is now higher than it was originally (Fig. 3-9); thus the binding of one oxygen increases the likelihood that a subsequent oxygen atom will bind to the molecule. The greater the number of oxygens bound to a hemoglobin molecule, the more likely it is to be in the R as opposed to the T state. Conversely, a hemoglobin molecule that for one reason or another finds itself in the R state—for example, a molecule in which the $\alpha_1\beta_2$ faces have been permitted to move apart because of, say, the loss of some protons (see below, the Bohr effect)—will bind oxygen more tightly than one fixed in the T state. It is important to recognize that the relationship between conformation and oxygen binding is reciprocal. Uptake or release of oxygen by hemoglobin will alter the proportion of T to R,

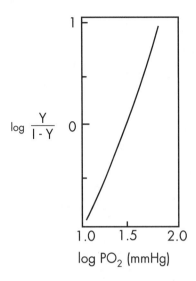

$\log \dfrac{Y}{1-Y}$

log PO$_2$ (mmHg)

Fig. 3-7. The Hill plot for whole blood. Y is the fractional oxygen saturation. By definition, the curve crosses P_{50} at $Y = 0.5$ (i.e., half-saturation). It can be calculated that when $Y = 0.5$, $\log [Y/(1 - Y)] = 0$. The slope of the curve at this point is the Hill coefficient. (Adapted from Bunn HF, Forget BG, Ranney HM [1977] Human Hemoglobins. WB Saunders, Philadelphia, with permission.)

and an alteration in the proportion of T to R will change the oxygen affinity of hemoglobin.

Regulation of Oxygen Affinity

The fitness of hemoglobin as an oxygen-transporting protein is further expressed in the fact that its oxygen affinity is adjustable, varying with its environment. Its alterations in oxygen affinity generally serve to improve the efficiency of oxygen delivery to the tissues. Two mechanisms are responsible for most of the variation in oxygen affinity: the Bohr effect and the effect of 2,3-DPG.

THE BOHR EFFECT

A fall in pH leads to a decrease in the oxygen affinity of hemoglobin (Fig. 3-10). This effect of pH on oxygen affinity is known as the Bohr effect. The Bohr effect facilitates the unloading of oxygen in the tissues. The rela-

tively low pH of actively metabolizing tissues causes a fall in the internal pH of red cells passing through such tissues. The fall in oxygen affinity that results from this drop in pH increases the ease with which oxygen moves from the red cells to the tissues. In the lung, the pH rises, favoring the uptake of oxygen by the red cell.

The Bohr effect occurs because the interaction between the $\alpha_1\beta_2$ faces of the hemoglobin tetramer is strengthened when the molecule takes up protons in response to a fall in pH. The strengthening of this interaction stabilizes the low-affinity (T) conformation of hemoglobin. The fall in oxygen affinity is caused by the stabilization of the T state over the R state as the pH drops.

2,3-DPG

The red cell is unique in containing a glycolytic shunt that permits the accumulation within the cell of large quantities of 2,3-DPG. 2,3-DPG is produced from 1,3-diphosphoglyceric acid, a glycolytic intermediate that normally goes directly to 3-phosphoglyceric acid during the conversion of glucose to lactic acid. The enzyme responsible for the formation of 2,3-DPG is diphosphoglycerate synthetase. The same enzyme can convert 2,3-DPG to 3-phosphoglyceric acid, another glycolytic intermediate. The overall pathway is known as the *Rapoport-Luebering shunt* (Fig. 3-11).

2,3-DPG binds to hemoglobin in the pocket formed by the N-termini of the β-chains (Fig. 3-12). This reduces the affinity of hemoglobin for oxygen by forming a bridge between the two $\alpha_1\beta_2$ faces, stabilizing the T state. The effect of 2,3-DPG on the oxygen affinity of hemoglobin is shown in Figure 3-13. It is probably the most important regulator of the day-to-day oxygen affinity of hemoglobin, providing a baseline setting around which short-term fluctuations in oxygen affinity such as those due to the Bohr effect can take place. Depending on circumstances, the 2,3-DPG concentration will vary so as to promote the normal delivery of oxygen to tissues when the system is stressed.

Deoxy

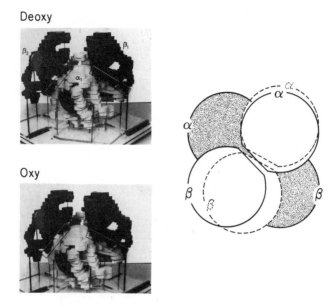

Oxy

Fig. 3-8. The two conformations of hemoglobin. In the molecular model, the $\alpha_1\beta_2$ contact areas are enclosed in boxes. The diagram is a highly simplified scheme of the conformational differences between deoxyhemoglobin (*solid lines*) and oxyhemoglobin (*dotted lines*), as seen in the molecular models. The diagram shows how one of the two $\alpha\beta$ dimers rotates with respect to the other on oxygenation of hemoglobin. Besides rotating, the two dimers move closer together by about 1 Å when hemoglobin takes up oxygen. (*Left:* From Muirhead H et al [1967] J Mol Biol 28:117, with permission. *Right:* Modified from Perutz MF [1979] Regulation of oxygen affinity of hemoglobin. Annu Rev Biochem 48:327, with permission.)

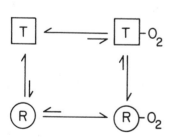

Fig. 3-9. Relationship between hemoglobin conformation and oxygen binding. The preferred conformation of oxyhemoglobin (*right*) is the R conformation, whereas the preferred conformation of deoxyhemoglobin (*left*) is the T conformation. As a result, factors that stabilize the R conformation over the T conformation will favor the binding of oxygen to hemoglobin, whereas factors that preferentially stabilize the T conformation will drive oxygen off the hemoglobin molecule.

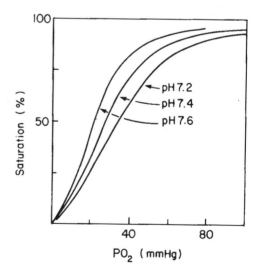

Fig. 3-10. The Bohr effect. How the oxygen affinity of hemoglobin changes with pH. (Adapted from Wintrobe MM et al [1974] Clinical Hematology. 7th Ed. Lea & Febiger, Philadelphia, with permission.)

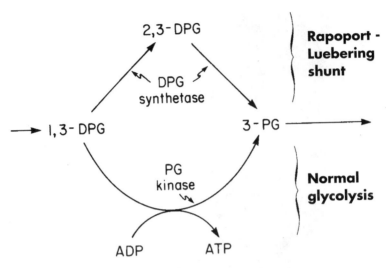

Fig. 3-11. The Rapoport-Luebering shunt.

For example, 2,3-DPG levels rise under conditions of hypoxia, promoting more complete unloading of oxygen in tissues to offset the decrease in the amount of oxygen carried by the blood. Similarly, 2,3-DPG levels increase in anemia. Unlike changes in intracellular pH, however, the changes in 2,3-DPG concentration take place over hours to days, a rate consistent with the role of the compound as a sort of thermostat for oxygen affinity.

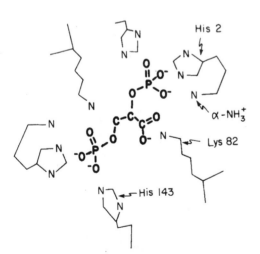

Fig. 3-12. The 2,3-disphosphoglycerate pocket is formed by the N-termini of the two β-chains plus some nearby histidines and lysines. (Adapted from Arnone A [1974] Structure of inositol hexaphosphate-human deoxyhaemoglobin complex. Nature 249:34, with permission.)

DISORDERS OF OXYGEN AFFINITY

Certain diseases are characterized by an alteration in the affinity of hemoglobin for oxygen. These diseases fall into two broad classes: those caused by an inherited abnormality of hemoglobin structure, and those caused by abnormalities involving 2,3-DPG.

Hemoglobinopathies

Many hematological disorders result from inherited abnormalities of hemoglobin. Some are caused by defects in the rate of synthesis of structurally normal hemoglobin molecules (i.e., the thalassemias). Most, however, are caused by the production of hemoglobins in which amino acid substitutions in one of the globin chains results in a molecule with aberrant prop-

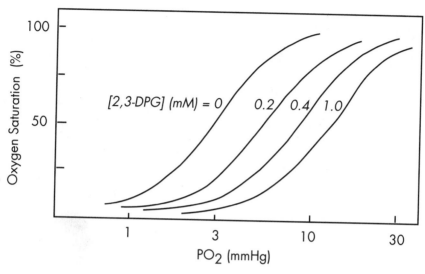

Fig. 3-13. The effect of 2,3-DPG on the oxygen affinity of hemoglobin. (Adapted from Benesch R, Benesch RE [1969] Intracellular organic phosphates as regulators of oxygen release by haemoglobin. Nature 221:618, with permission.)

erties. The precise functional abnormality depends on the nature and location of the amino acid substitution. Some substitutions, for example, lead to a hemoglobin that crystallizes in the red cell; others result in a molecule that is easily denatured under physiological conditions. The substitutions discussed here result in a hemoglobin whose oxygen-binding properties deviate from normal.

HIGH-AFFINITY HEMOGLOBINS

Most hemoglobins with abnormal oxygen affinity bind oxygen too tightly. Tissue oxygen tensions are therefore lower than normal, leading to the release of erythropoietin, the hormone that stimulates red cell production. Clinical manifestations are largely due to the increase in erythropoiesis that results from the action of this hormone of the bone marrow.

The disease is expressed as one type of familial polycythemia. Its inheritance pattern is autosomal dominant, for reasons that will be discussed below, so that on the average half the family members will be affected by the condition. Hematocrits may range as high as 70, but

levels around 60 are more common. Other signs and symptoms are discussed in the chapter on polycythemia (Ch. 12).

In addition to the increased hematocrit and red cell mass, laboratory manifestations include an arterial oxygen saturation exceeding 90 percent and a normal serum uric acid. (Uric acid, a breakdown product of purine metabolism, is often elevated in conditions of accelerated myelopoiesis, some of which also show polycythemia.) The bone marrow examination shows an excessive number of normal red cell precursors. Hemoglobin electrophoresis is sometimes helpful, because in about one-half of affected patients the mobility of the abnormal hemoglobin in an electric field is different from hemoglobin A. The best clues to the disease are listed on page 36.

The diagnosis is made by demonstrating an abnormality in hemoglobin oxygen affinity. This is usually done with intact red cells, although measurements made with hemolysates have the theoretical advantage that effects of oxygen affinity regulators are minimized. The oxygen dissociation curve of red cells from a patient with hemoglobin Bethesda

$(\alpha_2\beta_2^{145\ his\ \to\ tyr})$,* a typical high-affinity hemoglobin, is compared with that of normal red cells in Figure 3-14A. The shift of the curve to the left is very apparent. What is less apparent in this figure, but becomes very evident in the Hill plot (Fig. 3-14B), is the biphasic nature of the oxygen dissociation curve. This is because the red cells from these patients actually contain both the normal and the high-affinity hemoglobins, so the oxygen dissociation curve reflects the combined properties of both hemoglobins. Inspection of the left-hand segments of the Hill plot indicates a P_{50} for hemoglobin Bethesda of about 2.8 mmHg and a Hill coefficient of about 1.

The fact that clinically significant high-affinity hemoglobin disease occurs when only part of the hemoglobin A is replaced by the abnormal hemoglobin explains why this condition is inherited as an autosomal dominant trait. For part of the hemoglobin A to be replaced by an abnormal hemoglobin, it is only necessary for an individual to inherit a single mutant hemoglobin gene from one parent. The disease is therefore transmitted by a single affected parent: the autosomal dominant mode of transmission.

The diagnosis of high-affinity hemoglobin disease is generally confirmed by family stud-

---

*Amino acid substitutions in mutant hemoglobins are indicated by abbreviations of this sort. This particular abbreviation means that the β-chain of hemoglobin Bethesda contains a tyrosine instead of the normal histidine at position 145. In hemoglobin Chesapeake, another high-affinity hemoglobin, leucine replaces arginine at the 92 position of the α-chain. This substitute is abbreviated $\alpha_2^{92arg\to leu}\beta_2$.

ies, and the workup is terminated there. It is possible to identify the amino acid substitution by purifying the abnormal hemoglobin and examining its structure, but this is almost never done except for research purposes.

To date, more than 40 different high-affinity hemoglobins have been reported. The locations of the altered amino acids in several of these high-affinity variants are shown in Figure 3-15. The alterations cluster in the $\alpha_1\beta_2$ region and the nearby C-terminal ends of the globin chains, just the right locations to disrupt the R $\leftrightarrows$ T transitions that play so important a role in the binding of oxygen to hemoglobin. It is not surprising that alterations affecting these regions give rise to hemoglobins with altered oxygen-binding properties.

Treatment is not necessary in most patients. If problems arise due to high blood viscosity, phlebotomy may be useful to reduce the hematocrit and relieve symptoms.

LOW-AFFINITY HEMOGLOBINS

Patients have been described whose hemoglobins show sharply reduced oxygen affinity. Oxygen binding is ordinarily sufficiently poor that the abnormal hemoglobin is largely in the deoxyhemoglobin form even at normal arterial oxygen partial pressures. Deoxyhemoglobin is an off-colored hemoglobin that imparts a dusky bluish hue known as cyanosis to the skin and nail beds when it is present in the blood in sufficiently high concentrations (>5 g/dl). Such concentrations are routinely found in patients with low-affinity hemoglobins. These patients therefore present with chronic cyanosis. Cyanosis is also seen in family members, since, like high-affinity hemoglobin disease, and for the same reason, low-affinity hemoglobin disease is transmitted as an autosomal dominant trait. The hematocrit and red cell mass are usually normal, an uncommon feature in diseases associated with chronic cyanosis, in which hematocrits tend to be high.

As with high-affinity hemoglobins, the diagnosis of a low-affinity hemoglobin is made by measuring the oxygen dissociation curve. The changes are opposite those seen with high-affinity hemoglobins; the dissociation curve is

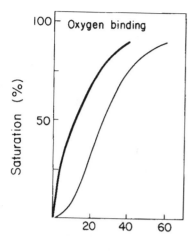
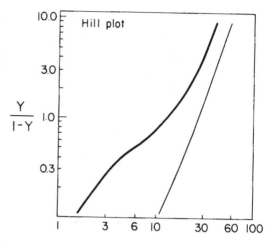

PO$_2$ (mmHg)

Fig. 3-14. (*Left*) The oxygen dissociation curve of a patient with hemoglobin Bethesda, a high-affinity hemoglobin. (*Thick line*) Patient cells. (*Thin line*) Normal cells. The patient's oxygen dissociation curve is not only shifted to the left, but has a peculiar graceless shape. This is because the curve is actually the sum of the oxygen dissociation curves of two hemoglobins, the high-affinity hemoglobin and hemoglobin A, both of which are present in equal amounts in the red cells. (*Right*) The biphasic Hill plot for red cells from the patient with hemoglobin Bethesda. The two hemoglobins in the red cells take up oxygen independently, so that the high-affinity hemoglobin has become largely saturated at a point where the normal hemoglobin has taken up very little oxygen. Each of the two segments can therefore be regarded as a full Hill plot for one of the two hemoglobins. Seen in that way, it becomes clear that one of the two hemoglobins is half-saturated when one-quarter of the total hemoglobin is in the oxy form (*Y*/(1 - *Y*) = 0.25), and the other is half-saturated at the three-quarter point (*Y*/(1 - *Y*) = 0.75). The P$_{50}$ values can be read off the Hill plots at these points. For the plot shown, these are 2.8 mm (Hb Bethesda) and 26.5 mm (Hb A). (Adapted from Bunn HF, Forget BG, Ranney HM (1977) Human Hemoglobins. WB Saunders, Philadelphia, with permission.)

shifted to the right, not the left, and the P$_{50}$ values from the biphasic Hill plot are high and normal, not low and normal.

Low-affinity hemoglobins are rarer than high-affinity hemoglobins. As with the high-affinity hemoglobins, the amino acid alterations that give rise to low-affinity hemoglobins occur largely in the $\alpha_1\beta_2$ region of the molecule.

This condition does not require treatment.

Alterations in 2,3-DPG Concentration

A number of conditions are characterized by changes in red cell 2,3-DPG levels that lead to alterations in the binding of oxygen to hemoglobin (Table 3-1).

By far the most important factor affecting the level of 2,3-DPG in the red cell is the acid–base status of the patient. 2,3-DPG rises with alkalosis and falls with acidosis, a consequence of the effect of pH on the enzyme responsible for its production and consumption. If the acidosis or alkalosis lasts long enough, the 2,3-DPG eventually reaches a level at which it compensates almost exactly for the Bohr effect caused by the acid–base disturbance, restoring the hemoglobin oxygen affini-

Table 3-1. Conditions Causing Abnormalities in Red Cell 2,3-DPG Levels

Increase	Decrease
Alkalosis	Acidosis
Hypoxia	Shock
Anemia	Hypophosphatemia
Hepatic cirrhosis	Bank blood
Uremia	

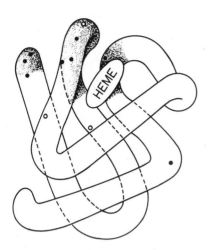

Fig. 3-15. Locations of the amino acid substitutions in some hemoglobins with abnormal oxygen affinity. The region of the $\alpha_1\beta_2$ interface is stippled. (•) High affinity. (○) Low affinity. (Modified from Wintrobe MM et al [1974] Clinical Hematology. 7th Ed. Lea & Febiger, Philadelphia, with permission.)

ty to normal. The increases in 2,3-DPG observed in hypoxia and in cirrhosis of the liver appear to be caused by the accompanying respiratory alkalosis; the increase seen in anemia may also be caused by that factor, at least in part. Acidosis is responsible for the fall in 2,3-DPG in patients in shock. The fall in 2,3-DPG levels in bank blood, which is stored in an acid anticoagulant, may also be an example of the effect of acid on red cell 2,3-DPG levels.

Other factors affect red cell 2,3-DPG as well. 2,3-DPG rises and falls with the serum phosphate, accounting for its increase in uremia and its decrease in hypophosphatemia. Inherited deficiencies in glycolytic enzymes are rare causes of abnormal 2,3-DPG levels (e.g., pyruvate kinase deficiency). An inherited deficiency of DPG synthetase causes an isolated drop in 2,3-DPG, with erythrocytosis secondary to the resulting increase in the in vivo oxygen affinity of normal hemoglobin.

METHEMOGLOBINEMIA

When oxyhemoglobin dissociates, the oxygen almost always leaves the same way it arrived—namely, as an oxygen molecule. Every once in a while, though, the oxygen takes an extra electron with it when it goes. The products of this aberrant dissociation reaction are superoxide (O_2^-), which is rapidly destroyed in the red cell, and a form of hemoglobin in which the heme iron has been oxidized by one electron from Fe^{2+} to Fe^{3+}. This form of hemoglobin, known as methemoglobin, is unable to take up oxygen. It must therefore be converted back to deoxyhemoglobin if the red cell is to retain its capacity to carry oxygen to the tissues.

The reduction of methemoglobin back to hemoglobin is accomplished in the red cell by a short electron-transport chain that transfers an electron from NADH to the heme iron atom (Fig. 3-16). Reading backward from methemoglobin, the components of the chain are cytochrome b_5, a heme enzyme that passes the electron to methemoglobin, and methemoglobin reductase (more accurately NADPH-cytochrome b_5 reductase), a flavoenzyme that takes the electron from NADH and gives it to the cytochrome. In the normal red cell, the rates of methemoglobin formation and reduction are such that methemoglobin amounts to less than 1 percent of the total hemoglobin in the cell. In certain diseases, this balance is altered, and methemoglobin accumulates in the red cell. This condition is known as *methemoglobinemia*. There are three categories of diseases in which methemoglobinemia occurs: hemoglobin M, methemoglobin reductase deficiency, and ingestion of oxidizing agents.

HEMOGLOBIN M

Hemoglobin M refers to a group of mutant hemoglobins whose iron atoms are fixed in a partly oxidized state. In these hemoglobins, there is a mutant chain (α or β) that has lost its ability to stabilize the heme iron in the reduced state because of an amino acid substitution in the vicinity of the metal. This chain remains perpetually in the methemoglobin form, so hemoglobins containing this chain will always be partly oxidized.

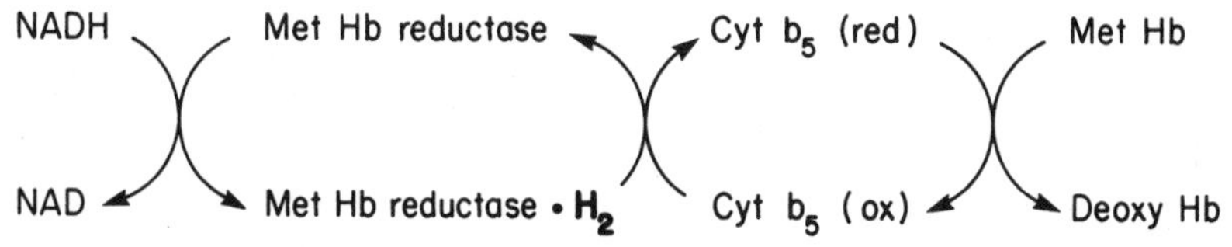

Fig. 3-16. The reduction of methemoglobin. This is the normal route of methemoglobin reduction. The electron donor for this pathway is NADH.

There are five known types of hemoglobin M (listed in Table 3-2). It is of interest that in four of these five types, one of the two iron-coordinated histidines is placed by a tyrosine.

How much mutant chain is actually present in hemoglobin M red cells? In the heterozygote, about 25 percent. This can be understood by considering a patient who is heterozygous for, say hemoglobin $M_{Saskatoon}$, a β-chain mutant. Red cells from this patient will contain equal quantities of α- and β-chains. All the α-chains will be normal, as will one-half the β-chains. The other half of the β-chains will be mutants, because the heterozygote makes the normal and mutant β-chains in roughly equal amounts. Accordingly, this patient's red cells will contain globin chains in the proportion: $2α$ to $1β^A$ to $1β^M$.

Methemoglobin levels in patients with hemoglobin M are equivalent to the level of the mutant chain. Red cells in affected heterozygotes therefore contain about 25 percent methemoglobin. This level is high enough to be clinically significant (for clinical manifestations, see below). Consequently, hemoglobin M is a disease seen in the heterozygote—that is, a disease transmitted as an autosomal dominant.

METHEMOGLOBIN REDUCTASE DEFICIENCY

Methemoglobin reducase deficiency results from a deficiency of the NADPH-cytochrome b_5 reductase. Methemoglobinemia occurs because the rate of spontaneous methemoglobin production, slow though it is, is fast enough to outstrip its rate of reduction in these defective cells.

Table 3-2. Hemoglobins M[a]

Hemoglobin	Substitution
M_{Boston}	$α58^{his→tyr}$
$M_{Hyde\ Park}$	$β92^{his→tyr}$
M_{Iwate}	$α87^{his→tyr}$
$M_{Saskatoon}$	$β63^{his→tyr}$
$M_{Milwaukee}$	$β67^{val→glu}$

[a] The substitution in $M_{Milwaukee}$ is the only one not involving the special histidines near the heme iron. It is nonetheless a heme crevice substitution, as can be seen by comparing its position with that of $M_{Saskatoon}$.

Methemoglobin reductase deficiency is inherited as an autosomal recessive trait. It is not seen in heterozygotes because their reductase levels, though decreased, are high enough to handle the normal methemoglobin load without difficulty. Methemoglobin levels in homozygotes with this disease generally range between 10 and 40 percent. The fact that methemoglobin is reduced at all seems to be due to the presence in the red cell of a group of NADPH-dependent reducing systems whose normal functions have nothing to do with hemoglobin but which can reduce metheoglobin slowly in a pinch.

INGESTION OF OXIDIZING AGENTS

Certain oxidizing agents produce methemoglobinemia by entering the red cell and oxidizing the hemoglobin directly. Such agents include inorganic nitrite (NO_2^-), the classical source of which is contaminated well water; organic nitrites, which are used to produce methemoglobinemia in the treatment of cyanide poisoning; and chlorate (ClO_3^-), a constituent of safety match heads.

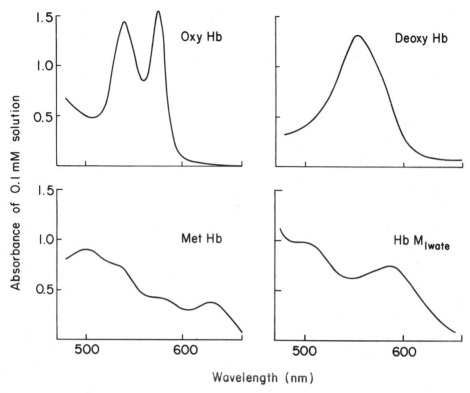

Fig. 3-17. Hemoglobin spectra. Oxyhemoglobin is bright red; the others are dark. The methemoglobins all have the same brownish hue in the test tube, but the spectrum of "normal" methemoglobin is different from that of the M methemoglobins because of the differences in the environment of the heme iron. (Adapted from Bunn HF, Forget BG, Ranney HM [1977] Human Hemoglobins. WB Saunders, Philadelphia, with permission.)

Clinical Manifestations

The hallmark of methemoglobinemia is *cyanosis*. The bluish cast to the skin, most often caused by deoxyhemoglobin, is also seen when the blood contains sufficient amounts of circulating methemoglobin, the other off-colored hemoglobin. It is generally easy to distinguish between deoxyhemoglobinemia and methemoglobinemia: Deoxyhemoglobinemia is almost invariably associated with diminished arterial oxygen tension, while the partial pressure of oxygen in methemoglobinic blood is normal (though the oxygen *saturation* of the arterial hemoglobin is reduced, because methemoglobin does not bind oxygen), and the cardiorespiratory diseases that cause arterial hypoxemia are absent. Furthermore, most patients with methemoglobinemia tend to be clinically well, since their modest methemoglobin levels have little practical effect on the oxygen-carrying capacity of their blood; serious problems do not appear until methemoglobin levels reach 40 percent or so.

It is in patients with acquired methemoglobinemia that trouble occurs. When methemoglobin reaches very high levels, oxygen transport by the blood is grossly deranged: the methemoglobin chains are no longer able to carry oxygen, and the normal chains in extensively oxidized hemoglobin molecules (i.e., molecules in which two or three of the four chains are in the methemoglobin form) are fixed in their high-affinity configuration and

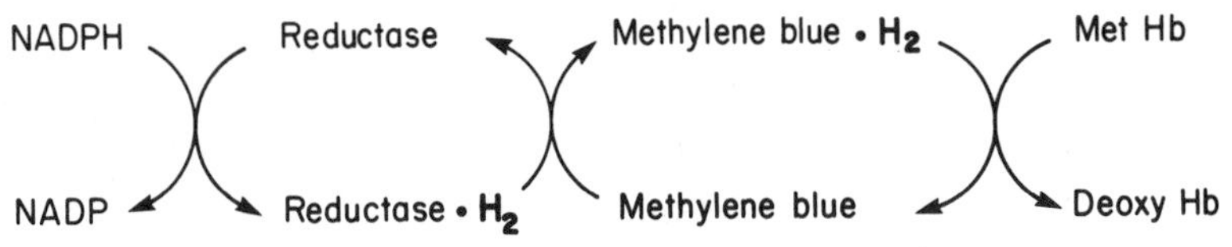

Fig. 3-18. Methylene blue-mediated reduction of methemoglobin. The electron donor for this pathway is NADPH.

cannot release their oxygen to the tissues. Any patient whose methemoglobin level exceeds 60 percent is in mortal danger from anoxia. Methemoglobinemia of this degree constitutes a medical emergency that must be dealt with instantly.

The diagnosis of methemoglobinemia should be considered in any patient exhibiting cyanosis. For any patient who is both cyanotic and sick, acquired methemoglobinemia must be considered, because it is a life-threatening illness that can be cured by immediate treatment. Congenital methemoglobinemia should be suspected in a cyanotic patient who is otherwise healthy, especially if the cyanosis was present at birth or appeared in early childhood, as expected for congenital diseases. A normal arterial oxygen pressure (not hemoglobin saturation) provides an important clue to methemoglobinemia. An even more important clue is the color of drawn blood, which is dark red to brown and does not change on shaking in air. In chronic methemoglobinemia the hematocrit will be elevated, a response to the diminished oxygen-carrying capacity of the blood, but red cell survival does not seem to be compromised by uncomplicated methemoglobinemia (contrast this with the red cell destruction of oxidant hemolysis). The diagnosis is made by demonstrating the presence of methemoglobin in the blood by spectrophotometry (Fig. 3-17) or by electrophoresis. The cause is then established by measuring methemoglobin reductase or by looking for one of the five types of hemoglobin M, or, if acquired, from the history.

Therapy depends on the cause. Acquired methemoglobinemia can be treated by methylene blue, a harmless reducing agent that enters

Clinical Features Associated with Congenital Methemoglobinemia

Cyanosis since infancy
Good health otherwise
Normal arterial oxygen saturation
Off color of drawn blood

the red cells and passes electrons from an NADPH-dependent reductase to methemoglobin (Fig. 3-18). If methemoglobin levels are high enough to cause life-threatening hypoxia, a procedure known as exchange transfusion, in which the patient's blood is replaced with normal blood, may be required. Methemoglobin reductase deficiency is also treated with ascorbate or methylene blue. Treatment is not necessary, however, in mild cases of the disease. No treatment is available for *hemoglobin M* disease, but none is needed.

SULFHEMOGLOBIN

Sulfhemoglobin is an altered form of hemoglobin that is produced when blood is exposed to powerful oxidizing agents, especially in the presence of sulfides. It is thought to arise when methemoglobin generated by the oxidizing agent undergoes a futher reaction with a nearby -SH group (either a cysteine residue or an exogenous sulfhydryl compound). Unlike methemoglobin, sulfhemoglobin cannot be turned back into normal hemoglobin, so the oxygen-carrying capacity of any hemoglobin that has been converted to sulfhemoglobin is irretrievably lost.

Clinically, sulfhemoglobinemia usually results from exposure to an oxidant drug (e.g., dapsone or an aniline derivative such as phenacetin). Cyanosis is generally the only finding. The diagnosis is made by spectrophotometry, a method that distinguishes sulfhemoglobinemia from other causes of cyanosis. Treatment is usually unnecessary except for withdrawal of the offending agent, but patients with a life-threatening level of sulfhemoglobin may require exchange transfusion.

SUGGESTED READINGS

Adamson JW (1975) Familial polycythemia. Semin Hematol 12:383

Adamson JW, Finch CA (1975) Hemoglobin function, oxygen affinity and erythropoietin. Annu Rev Physiol 37:351

Bellingham AJ, Grimes AJ (1973) Red cell 2,3-diphosphoglycerate. Br J Haematol 25:555

Bunn HF, Forget BG (1984) Human Hemoglobins. 2nd Ed. WB Saunders. Philadelphia

Cook JD, Lynch SR (1986) The liabilities of iron deficiency. Blood 68:803

Finch CA, Lenfant C (1972) Oxygen transport in man. N Engl J Med 286:407

Golde DW, Hocking WG, Koeffler HP, Adamson JW (1981) Polycythemia: mechanisms and management. Ann Intern Med 95:71

Hanash SM, Ricknagel DL (1980) Clinical implications of recent advances in hemoglobin disorders. Med Clin North Am 64:775

Harrison BD, Stokes TC (1982) Secondary polycythaemia: its causes, effects and treatment. Br J Dis Chest 76:313

International Hemoglobin Information Center variants list (1990) Hemoglobin 14:249

Jaffé ER (1981) Methaemoglobinaemia. Clin Haematol 10:99

Jaffé ER (1986) Enzymopenic hereditary methemoglobinemia: a clincal/biochemical classification. Blood Cells 12:81

Lenfant C, Sullivan K (1971) Adaptation to high altitude. N Engl J Med 284:1298

Mansell M, Grimes AJ (1979) Red and white cell abnormalities in chronic renal failure. Br J Haematol 42:169

Mansouri A, Lurie AA (1993) Concise review: methemoglobinemia. Am J Hematol 42:7

Nagel RL, Bookchin RM (1974) Human hemoglobin mutants with abnormal oxygen binding. Semin Hematol 11:423

Perutz MF (1979) Regulation of oxygen affinity of hemoglobin. Annu Rev Biochem 48:327

Perutz MF (1987) Molecular anatomy, physiology, and pathology of hemoglobin. p.127. In Stamatoyannopoulos G, Nienhuis AW, Leder P, Majerus PW (eds.): Molecular Basis of Blood Diseases. WB Saunders, Philadelphia

Perutz MF (1990) Mechanisms regulating the reactions of human hemoglobin with oxygen and carbon monoxide. Annu Rev Physiol 52:1

Stephens AD (1977) Polycythaemia and high affinity hemoglobins. Br J Haematol 36:15

4

Heme Formation: The Supply of Iron. Iron Deficiency and Iron Excess

Heme is a complex molecule consisting of four pyrrole groups joined by one-carbon bridges into a large ring that contains an iron at its center (Fig. 4-1). It has many roles in biological systems, serving as the oxygen-carrying component of hemoglobin and as an electron carrier for a variety of enzymes that catalyze oxidation-reduction reactions. Because of its central importance in the function of the red cell, abnormalities in heme production are associated with well-defined hematological diseases.

Heme production involves two basic processes: the acquisition of iron and the synthesis of the heme itself. Problems with the former give rise to conditions of iron deficiency or iron overload. These are discussed in this chapter. Problems with the latter present as porphyrias and sideroblastic anemias, which are discussed in Chapter 5.

IRON METABOLISM

Every day the normal adult destroys about 15 ml of senescent red cells and produces an equal quantity of new red cells to replace them. For the daily production of new erythrocytes, about 15 mg of iron is required. Almost all this iron is drawn from stores laid down when old red cells are destroyed. The movement of iron back and forth between the red cells and the iron storage pool involves a sequence of steps called the *iron cycle*. A small but critical fraction of red cell iron is obtained from the diet.

Iron Cycle

The iron cycle is illustrated in Figure 4-2. It can be considered arbitrarily to begin with the uptake of iron by transferrin. This is a plasma protein to which almost all the circulating iron is bound. It carries two atoms of ferric (Fe^{3+}) iron, binding them so avidly ($K_d = 10^{-30}$) that the plasma contains virtually no free iron.

The red cell precursors obtain their iron from circulating transferrin. On the surface of these cells are binding sites for transferrin, the so-called transferrin receptors. Precursors as late as reticulocytes possess transferrin receptors, their number declining as the cell matures; fully mature erythrocytes, however, have no transferrin receptors. Iron-loaded transferrin binds to these receptors, which are then carried into the cell along with their cargo by an invagination of the surface membrane that seals and breaks free to form an intracellular

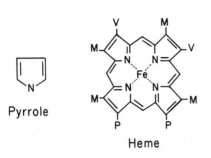

Pyrrole

Heme

Fig. 4-1. Pyrrole and heme. The heme is composed of four pyrroles fused into a large ring. The letters at the periphery of the ring refer to substituents attached to the carbons indicated. The substituents are M, methyl; V, vinyl ($-CH=CH_2$); P, propionyl ($-CH_2CH_2COOH$). (The structure and biosynthesis of heme are discussed in Ch. 5.)

vacuole (Fig. 4-3). Fusion of the vacuole with a lysosome followed by acidification releases the iron from the internalized iron–transferrin complexes. The liberated iron then makes its way into the cytoplasm, while the vacuole migrates to the cell surface, rejoining the outer membrane and returning the now unloaded transferrin molecules to the plasma. During this passage, the iron is reduced from ferric to ferrous.

In the red cell precursor, the newly acquired iron atom may follow one of two paths. It may become incorporated directly into a molecule of heme, or it may be reoxidized and taken up into a molecule of ferritin. Ferritin, a storage form of iron, consists of a core of ferric hydroxide encased in a protein shell composed of 24 identical subunits. The empty shell,

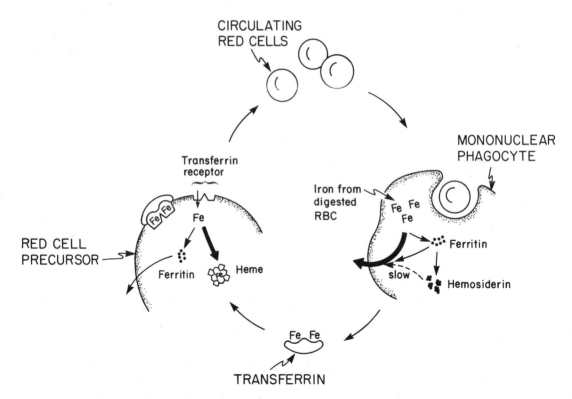

Fig. 4-2. The iron cycle. In the blood, iron circulates in association with transferrin, its carrier protein. It is delivered by transferrin to the red cell precursors, where most of it is incorporated into hemoglobin. These mature and are released as circulating red cells. After 4 months, these cells are removed from the bloodstream by mononuclear phagocytes, which digest them and return their iron to transferrin, either directly or after storing it for a while as ferritin/hemosiderin.

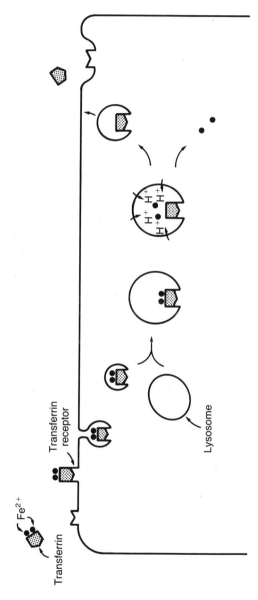

Fig. 4-3. Iron transport into cells. A circulating transferrin molecule loaded with iron binds to a transferrin receptor on the cell surface. The membrane in the region of the loaded receptor invaginates and detaches to form a small vacuole that carries the receptor and its bound cargo into the cytoplasm of the cell. The vacuole fuses with a lysosome to form a combined vacuole whose interior then acidifies, releasing the iron from the transferrin. The iron passes into the cytoplasm, while the vacuole fuses with the plasma membrane, returning the transferrin receptor to the cell surface and liberating the now unloaded transferrin molecule back into the surrounding fluid.

known as *apoferritin*, is filled atom by atom with iron, so that ferritin molecules with widely varying core sizes are present in red cell precursors and other storage iron-containing cells.

In normal red cell precursors, the storage iron may be seen as a few tiny grains of Prussian blue-staining material representing microscopically visible aggregates of ferritin. Cells containing these aggregates are known as *sideroblasts*. They may represent up to 50 percent of all red cell precursors in the normal marrow. Almost all this surplus iron is extruded from the precursors before they leave the marrow, explaining why very few circulating red cells contain ferritin granules. It is important to distinguish these normal marrow sideroblasts from ringed sideroblasts, a type of iron-containing red cell precursor seen only in the sideroblastic anemias.

Mature erythrocytes circulate for about 4 months. They are then taken up by mononuclear phagocytes, primarily in the spleen, and are disposed of by these cells. During the course of destruction of the outdated red cells, the heme is freed from the globin, the ring is opened, and the iron is released into the phagocyte. Most of this iron is delivered immediately to plasma transferrin. However, a portion stays behind in the phagocyte, where it becomes incorporated into ferritin. In a normal person on a normal diet, substantial quantities of ferritin accumulate in the cells of the mononuclear phagocyte system. During the course of time, some of this ferritin undergoes partial degradation, forming heterogeneous aggregates known as *hemosiderin* (Fig. 4-2). The combination of ferritin and hemosiderin in the mononuclear phagocyte system represents the major iron storage pool of the body. It is readily visible on Prussian blue-stained smears of bone marrow, where it is described as "stainable iron." From this storage pool, iron is released to plasma transferrin as necessary. The transfer of iron from the phagocyte to the circulating transferrin completes the iron cycle.

A recurring theme in the iron cycle and in the mechanism of gastrointestinal iron absorption is the series of changes in oxidation-reduction state that iron undergoes during the course of its movements. These changes make sense if the following rule is kept in mind: Iron is trivalent (ferric) when it is bound, or about to become bound, to a carrier (transferrin or ferritin); otherwise it is divalent (ferrous).

Absorption of Iron

Although the vast majority of the iron is retained in the body as it moves from one compartment to another, a small amount—1 to 2 mg—is lost every day; the iron cycle is not a fully closed loop. Iron is lost from the gastrointestinal tract in the form of blood and sloughed epithelium. Secretions and exfoliated skin also account for a small fraction of the loss. Menstruating women lose iron each month in the menstrual flow, and a pregnancy costs nearly 1 g, as iron is transferred to the newborn and the placenta and is lost with blood at delivery.

These losses are replenished by absorption of iron from the diet. Dietary iron is supplied largely as heme, but also as inorganic iron derived from nonheme iron-containing enzymes and storage iron. Both forms of iron can be absorbed throughout the length of the small intestine, but because the first encounter between iron and the gut epithelium takes place in the upper small intestine (duodenum and upper jejunum), most iron absorption takes place there. Heme is absorbed as such, while the inorganic iron is reduced to the divalent form (Fe^{2+}) before being absorbed, in a reaction facilitated by the low pH of the stomach.

In the intestinal mucosal cell, a complex series of events takes place (Fig. 4-4). The heme is split open just as it is in the mononuclear phagocyte, and its iron is released as Fe^{2+} to join the Fe^{2+} taken up as such by the mucosal cell. This Fe^{2+} then follows one of the two paths. Some is transported out of the mucosal cell to be oxidized in the plasma, then to bind to transferrin and enter the iron cycle. The rest is oxidized to Fe^{3+} to be incorporated into ferritin, which remains sequestered in the mucosal cell until the cell is shed from the tip of the intestinal villus.

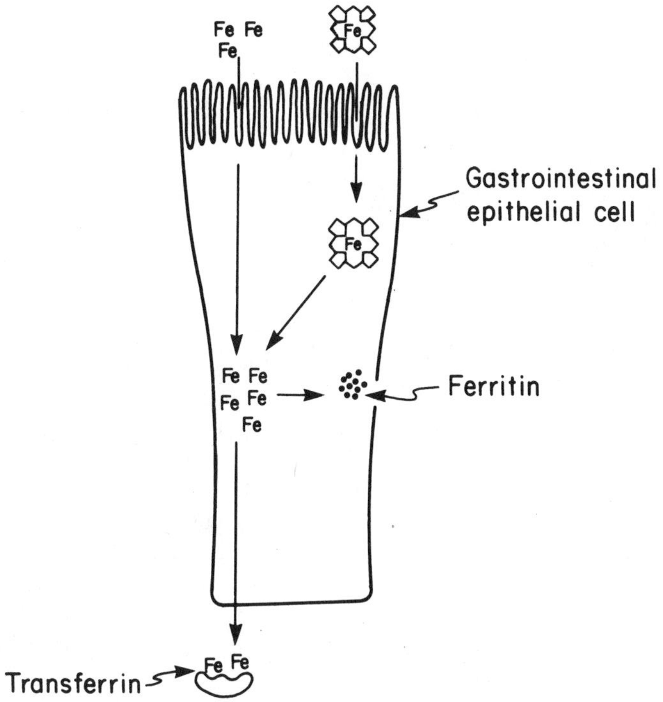

Fig. 4-4. Absorption of iron by the intestinal epithelial cell. Some of the iron taken up by the cell is passed into the bloodstream. The rest is sequestered as ferritin, which is lost when the cell is sloughed into the intestinal lumen.

The total body iron load is regulated at the level of intestinal absorption. Under normal circumstances, the amount of iron transported into the blood is a small fraction of the amount ingested, the fraction falling as the ingested load rises (Fig. 4-5). This fraction is such that on the usual diet, iron absorption is equal over time to iron losses, so the total amount of iron in the body remains roughly constant. Under conditions of stress, however, the mucosal cell alters its capacity to absorb iron. Two kinds of stresses elicit this response from the mucosal cell:

1. *Alterations in body iron stores.* Iron absorption changes to correct for deviations in iron stores in either direction. When stores are low, iron absorption increases. When stores are overloaded, iron absorption falls, sometimes to very low levels.

2. *Alterations in red cell turnover.* Mucosal cells somehow sense the rate of red cell produc-

tion and adjust their iron absorption accordingly, regardless of the state of the iron stores. Iron absorption increases sharply in anemias characterized by the destruction of red cells (e.g., immune hemolytic anemias) or their precursors (e.g., thalassemia), disorders in which red cell formation can be increased as much as six- to sevenfold. Conversely, iron absorption falls when red cell formation is depressed. The paradoxical augmentation in iron absorption in the face of greatly increased iron stores can add substantially to the problems faced by iron-overloaded patients with hypoproliferative anemias (discussed below under hemochromatosis).

Despite many years of research on the cellular basis for these alterations in iron absorption, their mechanism remains largely obscure. The amount of iron a mucosal cell is capable of transporting into the blood stream seems to be

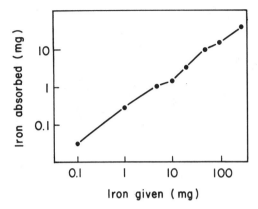

Fig. 4-5. Relationship between iron ingestion and iron absorption. (Adapted from Fairbanks VE, Beutler E [1972] Iron metabolism. In Williams WJ et al [eds] Hematology. McGraw-Hill, New York, with permission.)

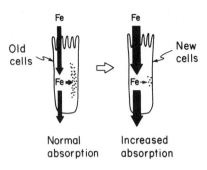

Fig. 4-6. Regulation of intestinal iron absorption. Intestinal epithelial cells live for 2 days, and then are sloughed off and replaced. Because of this rapid turnover, it is possible to change the absorptive properties of the entire intestinal epithelium within 48 hours by replacing the current cells with cells possessing new characteristics. This appears to be how iron absorption is regulated. Iron absorption is increased by replacing the epithelial cells with a new crop that takes up more iron from the gut and delivers a greater proportion of the iron to the bloodstream, as opposed to the inert ferritin pool. Absorption is decreased by replacement with cells having the opposite properties.

programmed into the cell at birth, by a mechanism that is not understood (Fig. 4-6). Part of the variability in iron transport appears to depend on the amount of intracellular Fe^{2+} transported into the blood, as opposed to the amount sequestered as ferritin; how the decision is made as to the partitioning of Fe^{2+} between transport and ferritin is not known.

Ferrokinetics

Useful clinical information can be obtained by measuring the movement of iron through its various pools. This is done by administering ^{59}Fe intravenously and measuring the distribution of isotope among these pools as a function of time. These measurements permit determination of how rapidly iron is transferred from plasma to tissues, what fraction of this iron is incorporated into the red cells, and how much of the iron is held by the marrow, liver, and spleen, the major storage organs.

The plasma iron transfer (PIT) rate measures the amount of iron moving from plasma to tissue in a day. This value is calculated by multiplying the fractional iron turnover in plasma by the total amount of plasma iron. The fractional iron turnover is equal to the fraction of total plasma iron that moves into the tissues in a given interval of time. The plasma iron concentration does not change in that interval of time because the iron lost into tissues is replaced by an equal quantity of iron from stores and from the diet. The fractional iron turnover, however, can be measured by measuring the rate at which ^{59}Fe is lost from the plasma, since there are no tissue stores of radioactive iron to replenish the supply, permitting the one-directional flux to be measured directly. The procedure is to give ^{59}Fe intravenously, and then follow its disappearance from plasma over time. From this disappearance curve, which is exponential for the first few hours and falls on a straight line in a semilog plot, the half-time for disappearance is measured. This half-time is usually expressed in minutes. Dividing this figure into 0.693 (the reciprocal of e, the base of the natural logarithms) and multiplying the result by 1,440 (the number of minutes in a day) gives the fractional turnover expressed in its most useful form: the fraction of plasma iron turned over per day. When this figure is multiplied by the total plasma iron (plasma iron concentration x plasma volume), the result is the PIT rate, the complete formula of which is

$$PIT \ (mg/day) = \frac{1,440 \ x \ 0.693 \ x \ \text{total plasma iron}}{t_{1/2}}$$

A low plasma iron turnover implies sluggish red cell production, as in certain hypoproliferative anemias; a high plasma iron turnover means more rapid than normal erythropoiesis and is seen especially in conditions associated with the destruction of red cells or their precursors.

The red cell iron utilization rate (RCU) measures the fraction of the iron transferred from plasma to tissues that is actually incorporated into circulating red cells. To make this measurement, a quantity of ^{59}Fe is given intravenously, and the amount of label in the total of the circulating red cells is measured after 14 days. This interval is long enough so that no labelled red cell precursors would be left in the marrow. The amount of label in all the red cells is determined by measuring the radioactivity in 1 ml of packed red cells and multiplying by the red cell mass. Normally the RCU is 80 percent; the remaining 20 percent is accounted for by incorporation of iron into other tissue proteins and by the destruction of iron-labeled red cell precursors in the marrow before release (ineffective erythropoiesis).

The amount of iron in the marrow, liver, and spleen can be measured by scanning after injection of ^{59}Fe. (Marrow iron is measured by scanning the sacrum.) Normal values, expressed as the fraction of the value measured shortly after injecting the isotope, are given in Figure 4-7. The early reciprocal changes in blood and marrow iron represent the incorpora-

tion of iron into red cell precursors followed by its release into the circulation in the form of new erythrocytes. Liver and spleen iron represent part of the 20 percent that does not get into the red cells. Characteristic changes in these patterns in disease states are discussed in connection with the diseases themselves.

IRON DEFICIENCY

The amount of iron in the diet is only slightly greater than the amount necessary to replace the small quantities lost through normal processes. Even a modest increase in these daily iron losses will lead to iron depletion unless measures are taken to increase the amount of iron taken in with the diet. Iron deficiency is therefore an exceedingly common condition, probably the commonest of all causes of anemia.

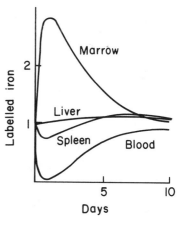

Fig. 4-7. Movement of labeled iron through various tissues during the first 10 days after administration. Characteristic changes in these patterns are seen in patients with shortened red cell survival (hemolytic anemia), destruction of red cell precursors in the marrow (ineffective erythropoiesis), or diminished red cell production (aplastic anemia). (From Finch CA et al [1970] Ferrokinetics in man. Medicine 49:17, with permission.)

Causes

Increases in iron requirements occur under a variety of circumstances. Any of these may lead eventually to iron deficiency, even on a normal diet.

PHYSIOLOGICAL INCREASE IN IRON REQUIREMENTS

The normal adult male requires 1 to 2 mg of iron a day to make up for iron lost from the gastrointestinal tract and through other processes. In other populations, however, iron requirements are substantially greater (Fig. 4-8). Children require unusually large amounts of iron during the first 5 years and during early adolescence, periods of exceptionally rapid growth. During their reproductive years, women require an additional 1 mg of iron a day to make up for menstrual losses (about 50 ml blood/month), and each pregnancy uses up about 0.7 g of iron, which must be replaced through the diet. Iron deficiency in these populations is frequent.

GASTROINTESTINAL BLEEDING

Gastrointestinal bleeding is by far the commonest pathological cause of increased iron losses. Any bleeding lesion may lead to iron deficiency, including peptic ulcer, drug- or alcohol-induced gastritis, hookworm, inflammatory bowel disease, or cancer. Cancer of the right side of the colon is notorious for presenting as an isolated iron deficiency anemia in the absence of other signs or symptoms.

> **Causes of Iron Deficiency Anemia**
>
> Increased requirements
>   Early childhood and adolescence
>   Women during the reproductive years
> Losses from the GI tract
> Losses from urine or sputum (rare)

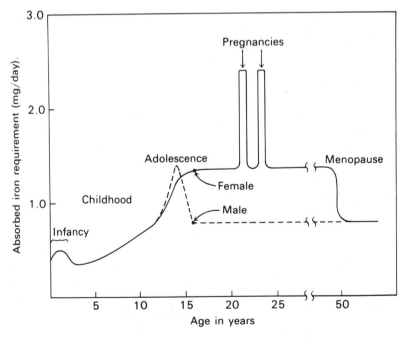

Fig. 4-8. Iron requirements throughout life. (From Wintrobe MM et al [1974] Clinical Hematology. 7th Ed. Lea & Febiger, Philadelphia, with permission.)

MENOMETRORRHAGIA

A large number of gynecological conditions can cause abnormally heavy menstrual periods (menorrhagia), nonmenstrual bleeding from the uterus (metrorrhagia), or both. Iron deficiency attributable to excessive vaginal blood loss is the rule in these conditions.

OTHER CAUSES

Chronic loss of iron in the urine or sputum is an occasional cause of iron deficiency. Iron deficiency anemia has been produced in hospitalized patients by enthusiastic withdrawal of samples for blood tests.

MANIFESTATIONS

Iron Deficiency Anemia

The major manifestation of iron deficiency is a characteristic anemia. The red cells are small, pale, and irregularly shaped (Fig. 4-9); indices show a hypochromic microcytic anemia. Marrow red cell precursors may also be pale and moth-eaten. Under ultraviolet light the cells fluoresce because of the accumulation of abnormal amounts of iron-free porphyrins (iron-containing porphyrins do not fluoresce). The white count is normal, but platelets are often increased, and the spleen and lymph nodes may be slightly enlarged in an occasional patient.

· The basis for this clinical picture is the lack of iron to incorporate into heme. With the deficiency of heme, the cells grow poorly, an abnormality perhaps related to the finding that heme deficiency can retard protein synthesis by causing the reversible inactivation of the enzyme responsible for elongating the peptide chain. Nevertheless porphyrin synthesis continues, with the result that porphyrins containing zinc instead of iron at the center accumulate in the iron-deficient red cells. In iron deficiency anemia, the red cell precursors also seem to undergo an extra division before extruding their nuclei, another factor causing a reduction

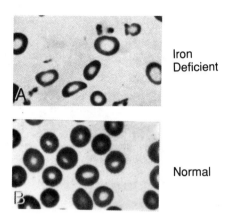

Iron Deficient

Normal

Fig. 4-9. Blood smear in iron deficiency anemia. (**A**) Iron deficiency. (**B**) Normal. In iron deficiency, red cells are small and misshapen, and the area of central pallor is disproportionately large because the cells are deficient in hemoglobin. (From Wintrobe MM et al [1981] Clinical Hematology. 8th Ed. Lea & Febiger, Philadelphia, with permission.)

in the size of the red cell; the reason for this extra division is unknown.

Alterations in the Iron Cycle

Alterations in the iron cycle designed to compensate for the iron-depleted state also take place in iron deficiency and can be detected by appropriate tests. These alterations are the earliest manifestations of iron deficiency, preceding the development of the anemia.

In iron deficiency, storage iron falls for two reasons: (1) iron is transferred from the storage pool to the red cell precursors, and (2) ferritin production drops. The drop in ferritin production is caused by a fall in tissue iron that leads in turn to the loss of iron from a specific repressor protein, changing the protein into a form that binds to apoferritin mRNA and blocks translation (Fig. 4-10). Iron deficiency as the cause of an anemia is indicated by the absence from the marrow of storage iron (detectable as stainable marrow iron; Fig. 4-11) or by a reduction in the level of serum ferritin (the most reliable noninvasive index of storage iron).

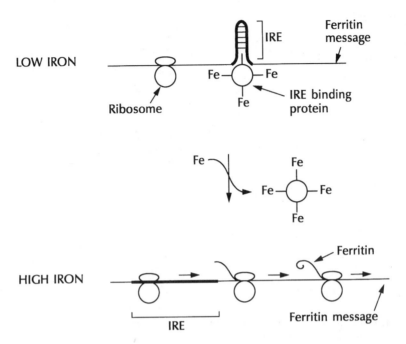

Fig. 4-10. How ferritin production is regulated by iron. Regulation depends on an interaction between a short stretch of bases in the apoferritin messenger RNA known as the *iron responsive element* (the IRE) and an iron-binding protein known by the accurate but long-winded name of *iron responsive element binding protein* (or IRE-binding protein). At low iron levels the IRE-binding protein contains three iron atoms. In its three-iron form it inhibits ferritin biosynthesis by binding to the iron-responsive element of the apoferritin messenger RNA and blocking translation. As iron levels rise, the IRE-binding protein takes up a fourth atom of iron and is released from the apoferritin messenger, making the messenger available for translation.

Iron absorption from the small intestine increases, as does the serum transferrin, although the amount of iron carried by the transferrin is reduced. The transferrin-bound iron is measured as the serum iron, and the total transferrin as the total iron binding capacity (TIBC); the serum iron:TIBC ratio in iron deficiency anemia is less than 1:6. The marrow is avid for iron, so ferrokinetic measurements show an increased PIT and an increase in the amount of iron that appears in the marrow at early times.

Other Signs and Symptoms

Patients with iron deficiency anemia sometimes show fatigue and lethargy out of propor-tion to their degree of anemia. This might be attributable to depletion of iron from iron-requiring enzymes, as has been shown in iron-deficient animals by a correlation between physical endurance and tissue levels of the nonheme iron enzyme glycerol phosphate dehydrogenase. The tongue becomes smooth and sore. Pica, a peculiar desire to eat substances such as ice, laundry starch, and clay, is also seen in iron deficiency anemia. No one knows why. Koilonychia, or spooning of the fingernails, is occasionally seen in severe iron deficiency. Finally, some patients with severe iron deficiency, particularly women, may acquire a web high in the esophagus, with dysphagia; this lesion, which is thought to be pre-malignant, resolves when the iron deficiency is corrected (Fig. 4-12).

Management

The first principle of management is to find out the reason for the patient's iron deficiency. The diagnosis of iron deficiency anemia is easily made by measuring the serum iron, TIBC, and ferritin; it may be confirmed by measuring iron stores, since a low serum iron, the hallmark of iron deficiency anemia, is also seen in the anemia of chronic disease, but in this condition iron stores are full. The source of iron loss must be established in every patient, paying special attention to occult blood in the stool as a clue to chronic gastrointestinal blood loss. This must be done even in a woman with a history of seven pregnancies and 25 years of heavy menses; she, too, may have a bleeding ulcer.

Iron deficiency is treated by replacement therapy and by correcting the iron-losing condition, if correction is indicated. Iron is usually replaced orally, with therapy continuing well beyond the point at which anemia is corrected, in order to replenish depleted stores. The amount of iron that the body can assimilate by this route is small, even in severe iron deficiency, so the response is relatively slow. Generally, a reticulocyte response does not reach a peak until 10 days after treatment is begun, and the anemia is not fully corrected for weeks. Occasionally, parenteral iron therapy is useful; this is ordinarily given by injection into the gluteus, a painful procedure, but may be administered intravenously slowly and with great care to avoid the sometimes fatal hypotension that may result from anaphylaxis or from too rapid infusion of the iron with resulting acute iron poisoning. Iron stores are rapidly repleted by the parenteral route, but its hazard is sufficient that it should be used as little as possible.

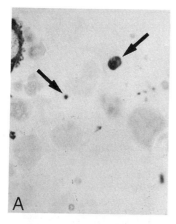

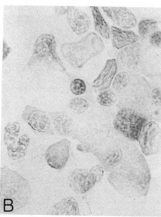

Fig. 4-11. Absence of stainable marrow iron in iron deficiency anemia. The "stainable iron" is the hemosiderin in the mononuclear phagocytes, a storage pool drawn on when iron requirements exceed iron intake. Prussian blue stains these hemosiderin granules a deep, intense blue (**A**, *arrows*). Disappearance of this hemosiderin is the first sign of iron deficiency (**B**).

The Diagnosis of Iron Deficiency

Hypochromic microcytic anemia
Low serum iron
High total iron-binding capacity (TIBC)[a]
Low serum ferritin[b]
Absent marrow iron stores[b]

---

[a]In iron deficiency, TIBC may be high, normal or low. High values are very suggestive of iron-deficiency anemia; normal or low values are of no help in making the diagnosis.
[b]The best indicators of iron deficiency.

HEMOCHROMATOSIS

It is not uncommon to see patients with modest increases in iron stores resulting from the anemia of chronic disease or from diseases associated with increased erythropoiesis. The occasional patient accumulates a tremendous load of storage iron, depositing the excess iron not only in the mononuclear phagocytes, but also outside the phagocytes in locations such as hepatocytes and cardiac muscle cells, where the metal causes potentiallly fatal tissue damage. Generally speaking, patients with modestly increased stores of iron deposited primarily in the mononuclear phagocytes are said to have hemosiderosis, while patients with greatly increased iron stores and substantial deposits outside the phagocytes are said to have hemochromatosis. The distinction between these two disorders is somewhat arbitrary but is useful because the term hemochromatosis implies a dangerous predisposition to iron accumulation that will require therapeutic removal of iron either immediately or at some time in the future.

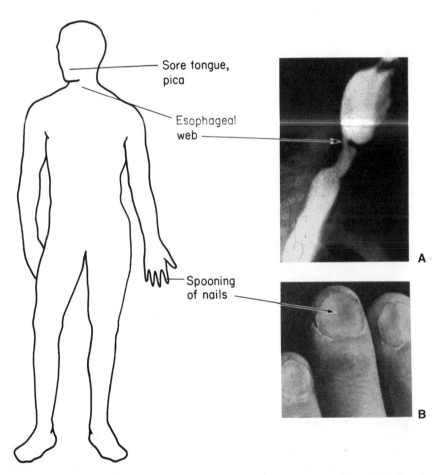

Fig. 4-12. Auxiliary manifestations of iron deficiency. (**A:** From Hutton GF [1956] Plummer Vinson syndrome. Br J Radiol 29:81, with permission. **B:** From Rosenbaum E, Leonard JW [1964] Nutritional iron deficiency anemia in an adult male. Ann Intern Med 60:683, with permission.)

Causes of Hemochromatosis

CHRONIC TRANSFUSION THERAPY

Patients with forms of anemia for which there is no effective specific therapy sometimes require transfusion on a chronic basis to maintain their hematocrits at a level sufficient to prevent secondary complications, such as congestive heart failure or ischemic disease. Each unit of blood contains 250 mg of hemoglobin iron. It is easy to see how such a patient, who may require an average of 1 unit of blood a week and who can only eliminate iron by the usual physiological mechanisms, can quickly accumulate iron to the point of hemochromatosis.

INCREASED IRON ABSORPTION

If enough iron accumulates through gastrointestinal absorption, hemochromatosis may develop. In some instances, this condition is thought to result from a combination of hepatic cirrhosis, which leads to augmented iron absorption, together with an abnormally large quantity of iron in the diet. This combination is most frequently seen in alcoholics, especially those who drink red wine, a beverage rich in iron. In other instances, hemochromatosis results from an inherited defect in which the gastrointestinal mucosa is unable for some reason to regulate iron absorption in a normal manner.

Manifestations

CLINICAL

Cardiac

The accumulation of iron in the heart leads to serious cardiac disease (Fig. 4-13). Both the operation of the myocardial conduction system and the strength of contraction of the muscle itself are compromised. Abnormal cardiac rhythms are therefore frequent, and heart failure with its symptoms of fluid retention and shortness of breath is a common occurrence. Studies in severely affected patients show a heart that is diffusely enlarged, beating rapidly but with little force. The clinical picture is that of a generalized cardiomyopathy that develops over the course of months to a few years and is

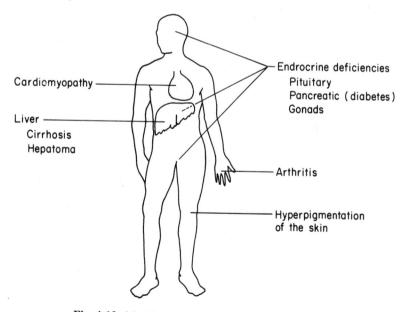

Fig. 4-13. Manifestations of hemochromatosis.

The Diagnosis of Hemochromatosis

High serum iron
Excessive iron stores
    High serum ferritin
    Increased marrow iron stores
    Increased iron in the liver biopsy[a]
Increased iron mobilization by chelators

---

[a]Quantitation of iron in the liver biopsy is the best way to diagnose hemochromatosis.

refractory to standard therapy for arrhythmias or heart failure. More than one-half the patients with untreated hemochromatosis die a cardiac death.

Hepatic

The accumulation of iron in the liver leads to cirrhosis and liver failure. Cirrhosis is expressed clinically as an enlargement of the liver and spleen and the development of increased pressure in the portal venous circulation, with dilated veins at the lower end of the esophagus (esophageal varices) that can rupture and bleed, sometimes massively. Liver failure leads to a rise in serum bilirubin with jaundice because of the inability of the affected organ to handle the breakdown products of hemoglobin; a defect in coagulation because of an impairment in the production of certain clotting factors made by the liver; a fall in albumin production, leading to the retention of fluid that, because of increased portal venous pressure, accumulates mainly in the peritoneal cavity as ascites; and in severe cases stupor or coma because of the failure of the liver to destroy toxins generated by bacteria in the gastrointestinal tract and absorbed into the bloodstream. Hepatoma is a frequent consequence of hemochromatosis of the liver. Most patients with untreated hemochromatosis who do not die from their heart disease will die of liver disease.

Endocrine

The other major clinical manifestations of hemochromatosis involve the endocrine system. Like the cardiac and hepatic disease, the endocrine abnormalities seen in hemochromatosis are thought to result from the destruction of cells by iron deposits. The glands affected are the pancreatic islets, the pituitary, and the adrenals. Islet cell disease leads to diabetes mellitus, a common complication of hemochromatosis. Pituitary disease causes hypogonadism, a problem to which the hepatic disease also makes a contribution. Adrenal insufficiency occurs, but is rare.

Other

Involvement of the skin by hemochromatosis causes increased pigmentation resulting from an increase in dermal melanin, not hemosiderin. The combination of diabetes and increased skin pigmentation has been termed "bronze diabetes." An arthritis typically affects the joints of the hands.

LABORATORY

The increased iron stores in hemochromatosis are reflected in the laboratory. Serum iron is high, while the serum transferrin (measured as the TIBC) is normal, so the ratio of serum iron to TIBC is increased. Serum ferritin, the best noninvasive indicator of iron stores, is higher than normal, as is the stainable marrow iron. Liver biopsy specimens are loaded with iron; this is apparent both under the microscope and by direct measurement, which shows that liver iron may be increased above normal by a factor of 20 or more. Finally, the amount of iron appearing in the urine after administration of the chelating agent desferrioxamine is greatly increased by hemochromatosis.

Chelation

Chelation is a means by which excess iron (or other metals) can be removed from the body. The term "chelation" refers to the ability of compounds that possess several metal-binding groups to attach to a metal ion by more than one of these groups. Such chelation complexes can be so tight that the metal ion is trapped and removed from the environment, for all practical purposes.

Desferrioxamine is a chelating agent that reacts with iron to form a very tight complex (Fig. 4-14). In both its free and iron-bound forms, the agent is relatively nontoxic and is rapidly excreted in the urine, making it useful in the diagnosis and management of iron overload states. Only a very small fraction of the body iron is available for complexation by desferrioxamine at a given time, so that after a single injection of desferrioxamine only a small amount of iron (about 0.01 percent of total body stores) appears in the urine (Fig. 4-15). This chelatable iron, however, exchanges with the nonchelatable iron in the storage pool (i.e., ferritin and hemosiderin). As a result, when desferrioxamine is given by continuous infu-

sion, substantial amounts of iron can be unloaded over the course of a day, because of the continuous movement of iron from the storage pool through the chelatable pool and into the urine as the desferrioxamine complex. Single injections of desferrioxamine followed by measurements of urine iron are therefore useful in making the diagnosis of hemochromatosis, because the urine iron level after a dose of desferrioxamine is a good measure of iron stores. Treatment with desferrioxamine requires long-term infusions, however, because only in this way can clinically significant reductions in iron stores be achieved.

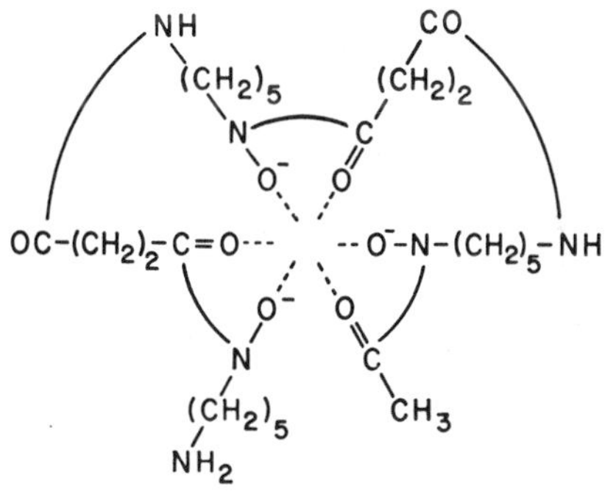

Management

The management of hemochromatosis involves the removal of the excess iron from the patient. The method used depends on whether or not iron accumulation resulted from chronic transfusion therapy.

CHRONIC TRANSFUSION THERAPY

Hemochromatosis attributable to chronic transfusion therapy is treated by long-term subcutaneous infusion of desferrioxamine using an infusion pump to deliver the chelating agent. Daily overnight infusions delivered by a portable pump that can be used at home are given initially. When iron stores reach normal levels, treatment may be given less frequently.

Fig. 4-14. Desferrioxamine. The iron-binding element of desferrioxamine is the hydroxamic acid residue

$$\begin{array}{cc} O & OH \\ \| & | \\ -C- & N- \end{array}$$

a group having an unusually high affinity for iron. The desferrioxamine molecule contains three of these groups. They are close enough to each other so that a single iron atom bound to desferrioxamine is held by all three at once. (Modified from Emery T [1971] Hydroxamic acids of natural origin. In Meister A. Adv Enzymol 35:125, with permission.)

IDIOPATHIC HEMOCHROMATOSIS

Patients with hemochromatosis not caused by transfusion therapy are managed by phlebotomy. The program is similar to the infusion pump program in that the frequency of therapy is high early in the course of the disease and is reduced substantially after normalization of iron stores. It is important to investigate family members of patients with idiopathic hemochromatosis as well, because relatives with asymptomatic increases in iron stores may benefit

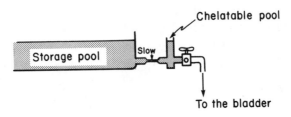

Fig. 4-15. Removal of iron by chelation. Giving a single injection of desferrioxamine is like drain-ing the chelatable pool once. This pool empties quickly and completely, and then refills slowly from the storage pool. Because the chelatable pool contains only a tiny fraction of the iron, draining it once has little effect on total iron stores. Infusing desferrioxamine continuously is equivalent to draining the chelatable pool on a continuous basis. As iron moves from the storage pool into the constantly emptying chelatable pool, it is steadily drained away. Under these conditions, iron stores will slowly but inevitably decline.

from treatment to forestall clinical disease. Tissue typing, normally used in marrow trans-plantation (Ch. 32), can help identify family members at risk, because there is a very close genetic linkage between the gene for idiopathic hemochromatosis and the tissue type HLA-A3.

PROGNOSIS

In following patients with hemochromato-sis, the best measure of iron stores is the fer-ritin level (Fig. 4-16). Serum iron generally does not fall until late in the course of therapy.

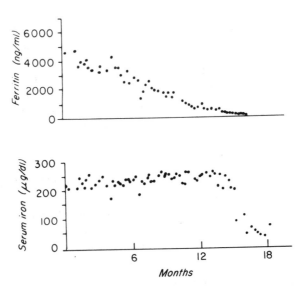

Fig. 4-16. Changes in iron during the treatment of hemochromatosis. Ferritin levels fall steadily. Serum iron remains elevated until iron stores are near normal. (From Milder MS et al [1980] Idiopathic hemochromatosis, an interim report. Medicine 59:34, with permission.)

Treatment will correct the cardiac disease and hepatic cirrhosis, with a substantial prolongation of life, but diabetes appears to be permanent, and the incidence of hepatoma in patients treated successfully for hemochromatosis remains high.

ANEMIA OF CHRONIC DISEASE

In disorders associated with chronic inflammation, including chronic infections, malignancies, and connective tissue diseases such as rheumatoid arthritis, a characteristic anemia often develops. This anemia has two features: a decrease in red cell production and an impairment in the transfer of storage iron from mononuclear phagocytes back to the hematopoietic tissues. Both of these features are thought to result from the effects of certain cytokines that are released in these disorders.

The cytokines are a family of peptides containing dozens of members, including among others the interleukins, the interferons, and certain hematopoietic growth factors. The cytokines act as mediators in a fantastically tangled network of interactions that serve to regulate cells engaged in host defense (e.g., endothelial cells, lymphocytes, hematopoietic cells, hepatocytes) and in growth and repair (proliferating cells of any type). These cells secrete the cytokines in response to infections and other forms of tissue injury, and at the same time are regulated by these cytokines, both their own and those produced by other cells.

In the anemia of chronic disease, the cytokines responsible for suppressing red cell production are the *interferons*, which act directly on the red cell progenitors to inhibit their proliferation. The abnormalities in iron metabolism, however, are caused by two other cytokines: *interleukin-1* and *tumor necrosis factor*. These two cytokines act on many types of cells including mononuclear phagocytes after being secreted by mononuclear phago-

cytes that have been activated by an encounter with T lymphocytes that themselves have been activated by the binding of antigen to receptors on their surfaces—a clear if oversimplified illustration of the labyrinthine ways of the cytokines, their sources, and their targets. One of the effects of interleukin-1 and tumor necrosis factor is to stimulate apoferritin synthesis by mononuclear phagocytes. This excess apoferritin directs newly mobilized iron into the storage pool, thereby blocking its release from the mononuclear phagocyte and hindering the red cell precursors in their quest for the iron they need to make hemoglobin (Fig. 4-17).

The anemia in this condition develops fairly rapidly (2 to 4 weeks), but remains mild; hematocrits below 30 are distinctly unusual. The red cells usually look normal on the smear, but in some cases they may be rather small and pale, perhaps because of their iron-deficient state. Since the anemia is caused by a decrease in red cell production by the marrow, reticulocyte counts are normal to low. The serum iron is low, but the serum iron binding capacity (i.e., transferrin) does not show a compensatory increase in iron deficiency. Instead, it drops too, and the paradoxical combination of a low serum iron and a low iron binding capacity is the hallmark of the anemia of chronic disease.

There is plenty of iron around, however—in fact, more than normal. It is all locked away in the mononuclear phagocytes as storage iron. The superabundance of storage iron is manifested clinically as an elevation in serum ferritin and a marrow that on staining is loaded with iron, completely the opposite of the iron-free marrow seen in iron deficiency anemia.

As to management, there is little that can be done, and little that needs to be done. Transfusions are not warranted by the degree of anemia seen in the uncomplicated condition and should not be given. Iron therapy is obviously useless. Erythropoietin will work if given in high enough doses, but is not worth the expense. The best therapy is to treat the underlying condition; alleviate this, and the anemia will cure itself.

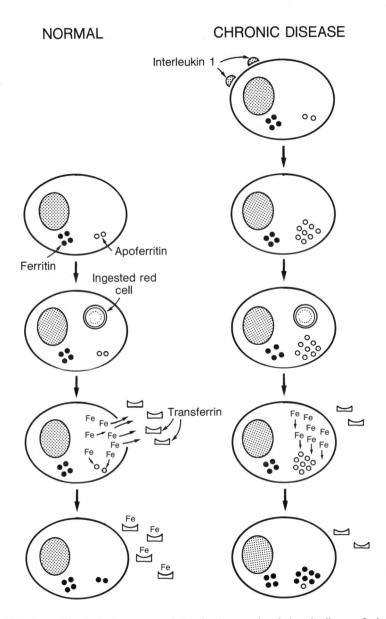

NORMAL   CHRONIC DISEASE

Interleukin 1

Apoferritin

Ferritin

Ingested red cell

Transferrin

Fe

Fig. 4-17. Proposed basis for iron accumulation in the anemia of chronic disease. In inflammatory states, a cytokine is released that stimulates the synthesis of apoferritin by mononuclear phagocytes. As a result, some of the iron released into the phagocyte during the breakdown of ingested red cells is not secreted into the plasma, its usual fate, but instead is taken up by the extra apoferritin to form ferritin, the storage form of iron. Iron stores are thereby increased at the expense of the iron supply available for red cell production.

SUGGESTED READINGS

Aisen P, Brown EB (1977) The iron-binding function of transferrin in iron metabolism. Semin Hematol 14:31

Bentley DP (1985) Iron metabolism and anaemia in pregnancy. Clin Haematol 14:613

Cartwright GE (1975) Sideroblasts, siderocytes, and sideroblastic anemia. N Engl J Med 292:185

Cartwright GE, Lee GR (1971) The anaemia of chronic disorders. Br J Haematol 21:147

Cook JD, Skikne BS (1987) Intestinal regulation of body iron. Blood Rev 1:267

Cox TM (1990) Haemochromatosis. Blood Rev 4:75

Crichton RR (1977) Ferritin: structure, synthesis and function. N Engl J Med 284:1413

Dallman PR (1986) Biochemical basis for the manifestation of iron deficiency. Annu Rev Nutr 6:13

Dallman PR, Beutler E, Finch CA (1978) Effects of iron deficiency exclusive of anaemia. Br J Haematol 40:149

Drysdale J, Dugast I, Papadopoulos P, Zappone E (1991) Intracellular iron metabolism. Curr Stud Hematol Blood Transfus 58:148

Finch CA (1982) Clinical aspects of iron deficiency and excess. Semin Hematol 19:1

Finch CA, Deubelbeiss K, Cook JD et al (1970) Ferrokinetics in man. Medicine 49:17

Green R (1991) Disorders of inadequate iron. Hosp Pract [Off] 26:25 (suppl. 3)

Harrison P (1977) Ferritin: an iron-storage molecule. Semin Hematol 14:55

Hershko C (1987) Non-transferrin plasma iron. Br J Haematol 66:149

Hershko C, Pinson A, Link G (1990) Iron chelation. Blood Rev 4:1

Jacobs A (1979) Iron chelation therapy for iron-loaded patients. Br J Haematol 43:1

Jacobs A, Worwood M (1975) Ferritin in serum. Clinical and biochemical implications. N Engl J Med 292:951

Klausner RD, Rouault TA, Harford JB (1993) Regulating the fate of mRNA: the control of cellular iron metabolism. Cell 72:19

Massey AC (1992) Microcytic anemia. Differential diagnosis and management of iron deficiency anemia. Med Clin North Am 76:549

Means RT Jr, Krantz SB (1992) Progress in understanding the pathogenesis of the anemia of chronic disease. Blood 80:1639

Milder MS, Cook JD, Stray S, Finch CA (1980) Idiopathic hemochromatosis. Medicine 59:34

Modell B (1979) Advances in the use of iron chelating agents for the treatment of iron overload. Progr Hematol 11:267

Van Campen D (1974) Regulation of iron absorption. Fed Proc 33:100

Woods S, DeMarco T, Friedland M (1990) Iron metabolism. Am J Gastroenterol 85:1

Worwood M (1990) Ferritin. Blood Rev 4:259

5

Heme Formation: Biosynthesis of the Tetrapyrrole. Porphyrias and Sideroblastic Anemias

Heme biosynthesis, although complicated at first glance, is actually a straightforward process involving a logical sequence of biochemical steps. The process can be divided into three stages: (1) the synthesis of the five-carbon building block from which heme is made, (2) the formation of a tetrapyrrole from this building block, and (3) the conversion of this tetrapyrrole into the heme molecule. Disorders of the latter two stages give rise to the porphyrias, a group of diseases in which the relationships between the biochemical and clinical manifestations are unusually well worked out. Disorders of the first stage appear to be responsible for many of the characteristic features of the sideroblastic anemias, but these diseases are not nearly as well understood as the porphyrias.

BIOSYNTHESIS OF HEME

The stages involved in the formation of a heme molecule are (1) the production of δ-aminolevulinic acid (ALA), the building block; (2) the formation of the first tetrapyrrole by

two successive condensation reactions, the first producing a monopyrrole from ALA, and the second producing the tetrapyrrole from four monopyrroles; and finally (3) the conversion of this tetrapyrrole into heme. This sequence is outlined in Figure 5-1.

The Building Block

ALA is produced by the enzyme ALA synthetase in a reaction in which glycine and succinyl CoA are joined end to end. The reaction requires pyridoxal phosphate, a point of clinical importance (Fig. 5-2).

The First Tetrapyrrole

This is synthesized in two steps. The first step is the condensation of two molecules of ALA to form the monopyrrole porphobilinogen (PBG); this reaction is catalyzed by PBG synthetase (Fig. 5-3). The first tetrapyrrole is then formed by the one-step condensation of four PBGs, catalyzed by an enzyme with the unin-

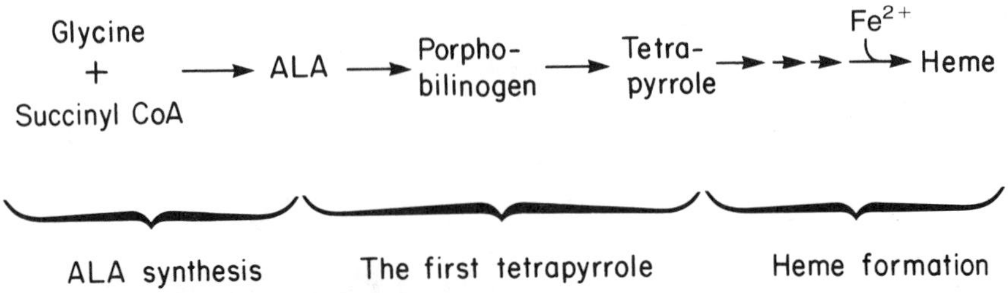

Fig. 5-1. Three stages of heme biosynthesis.

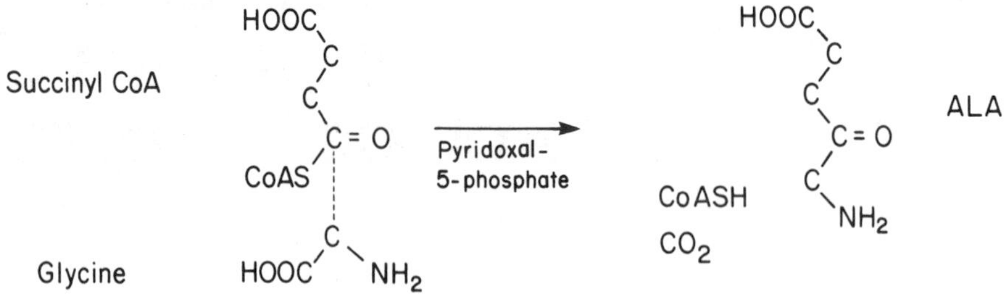

Fig. 5-2. The production of δ-aminolevulinic acid (ALA) by the condensation of glycine and succinyl coenzyme A (CoA).

formative name *PBG deaminase*, so called because it splits an ammonia out of each PBG molecule during the condensation (Fig. 5-4). The product of the two successive condensation reactions is called uroporphyrinogen (UROGEN). The suffix -ogen refers to the fact that the tetrapyrrole is partly reduced, with the one-carbon bridges each containing two hydrogen atoms.

Hanging from the pyrrole ring of each PBG molecule are two carboxylic acid side chains: an acetate (A) and a propionate (P). PBG deaminase acting by itself causes the PBG monomers to condense in a head-to-tail manner, so that the order of the side chains around the tetrapyrrole ring is as follows: A—P—A—P—A—P—A—P—. This compound, known as UROGEN I, is normally made in small amounts, but cannot be further metabolized: it is a dead-end product. The true precursor of heme is UROGEN III, a molecule in which the order of side chains is A—P—A—P—A—P—P—A— (Fig. 5-4). It is produced by the combined action of PBG deaminase and a second

enzyme, cosynthetase. Thus the order of the substituents around the periphery of the tetrapyrrole, seemingly a trivial matter, is actually of considerable physiological, and as will be seen, clinical significance.

To summarize, PBG is formed by the condensation of two ALA molecules in a reaction

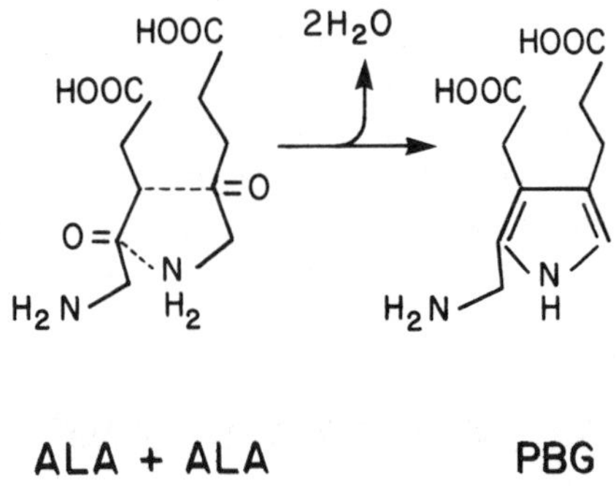

ALA + ALA   **PBG**

Fig. 5-3. The first tetrapyrrole. Porphobilinogen (PBG), the first tetrapyrrole, is formed by the condensation of two molecules of ALA. This reaction is catalyzed by PBG synthetase.

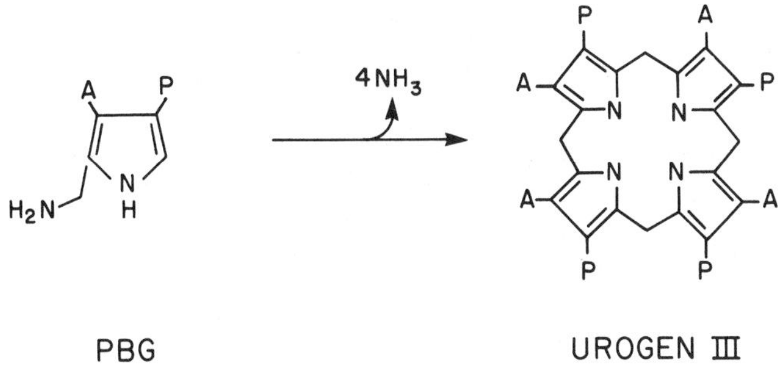

Fig. 5-4. Formation of UROGEN III by the condensation of four molecules of PBG. This reaction is catalyzed by two enzymes: PBG deaminase and cosynthetase.

catalyzed by PBG synthetase. Four PBG molecules then condense to yield UROGEN. When condensation is catalyzed by PBG deaminase plus cosynthetase, the product is UROGEN III, which can be metabolized further to heme. When condensation is catalyzed by PBG deaminase alone, the product is UROGEN I, a dead-end metabolite.

Heme

Heme is produced by three successive modifications in the tetrapyrrole followed by the insertion of an iron atom to yield the final product (Fig. 5-5). In the first modification, CO_2 molecules are removed from the acetate side chains to produce coproporphyrinogen III (COPROGEN III), containing four methyl groups (M) instead of the four acetates. The order of side chains in COPROGEN III is M—P—M—P—M—P—P—M—. The four CO_2 molecules are all removed by a single enzyme, coproporphyrinogen synthetase.

In the next modification, the two nonadjacent propionate side chains are oxidized. Oxidation of these chains is accompanied by the departure of two more CO_2 molecules. The product is protoporphyrinogen IX (PROTOGEN IX), containing vinyl groups (V) instead of propionyl groups in two of the peripheral locations. The order of side chains in PROTOGEN IX is M—V—M—V—M—P—P—M—. The enzyme catalyzing this reaction is coproporphyrinogen oxidase.

The final modification is the oxidation of the ring. Four additional double bonds are created to produce the fully oxidized porphyrin, protoporphyrin IX (PROTO IX). This reaction is catalyzed by protoprophyrinogen oxidase.

Finally, heme is produced by the enzyme-catalyzed insertion of an iron atom into the center of the porphyrin ring. This reaction is catalyzed by ferrochelatase.

The four steps involved in the conversion of UROGEN III to heme are summarized in Table 5-1.

PORPHYRIAS

The rate of porphyrin synthesis is tightly controlled by the intracellular concentration of free heme, which regulates its own production by acting as a feedback inhibitor of ALA synthetase. When the activity of one of the porphyrin-synthesizing enzymes is decreased, the resulting slowdown in heme synthesis causes the release of this feedback inhibition, with an increased flow of precursors into the porphyrin synthetic pathway. This increase in flow, combined with the restriction in the rate of one of the porphyrin synthetic steps, causes the accumulation of the intermediate whose further metabolism is restricted by the enzymatic defect (Fig. 5-6). All the intermediates in the porphyrin biosynthetic pathway are toxic compounds whose accumulation leads to disease. The diseases produced by these intermediates are the porphyrias.

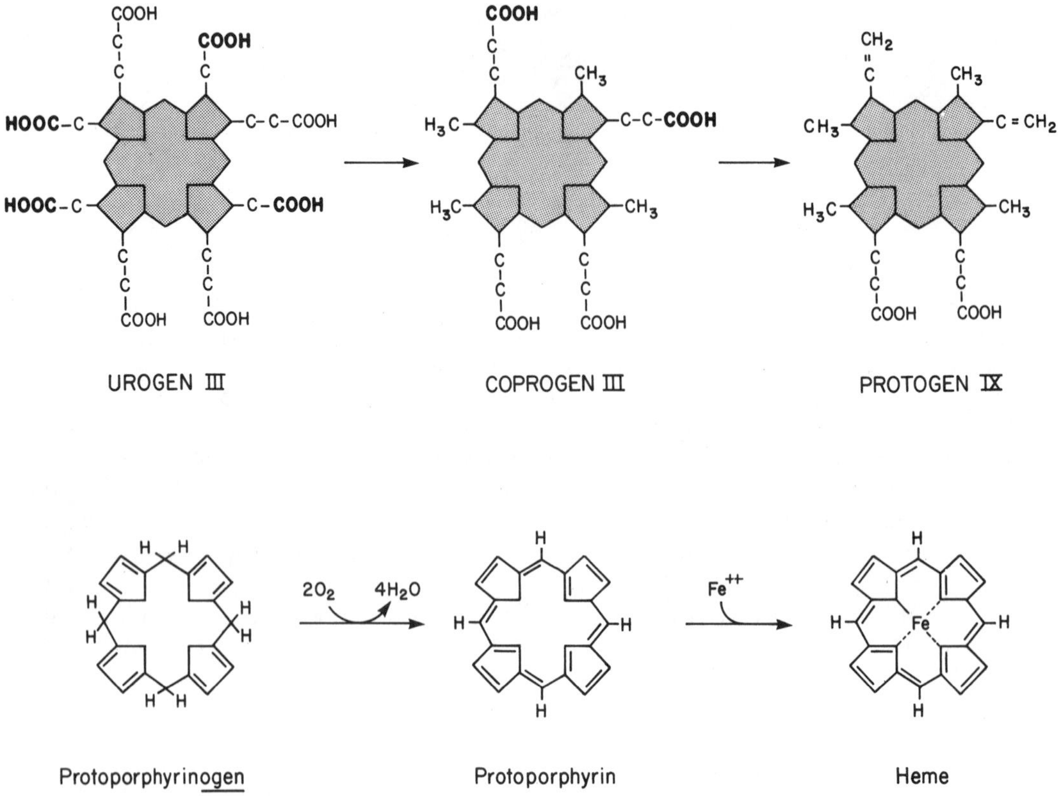

Fig. 5-5. Conversion of UROGEN III to heme. (**Top row**) Side-chain modifications, leading successively from UROGEN III through COPROGEN III to PROTOGEN IX. (**Bottom row**) Last two steps in heme synthesis: the oxidation of protoporphyrinogen to protoporphyrin and the insertion of the iron. For clarity, the nitrogens and most of the hydrogens have been omitted and the side chains have been left off the figures in the bottom row.

The porphyrias are a confusing group of conditions, because there is a different form of porphyria for each enzyme, and these different forms vary in their manifestations depending on the nature of the intermediate that accumulates. There is, however, a series of logical principles that can serve as a guide through this rather bewildering thicket of diseases:

1. A 50 percent reduction in the activity of one of the porphyrin-synthesizing enzymes is often enough to lead to symptomatic porphyria. Inheritance therefore tends to be *autosomal dominant.*

2. PBG causes neurological abnormalities, possibly because PBG or a metabolite can mimic a normal neurotransmitter. Tetrapyrroles, however, act mainly in the skin, where they are deposited and cause a photosensitivity dermatitis whose severity varies depending on which compound accumulates.

Table 5-1. The Conversion of UROGEN III to Heme

Step	Reaction	Enzyme
UROGEN → COPROGEN	4 Acetate→4 methyl	Uroporphyrinogen decarboxylase
COPROGEN → PROTOGEN	2 Propionate→2 vinyl	Coproporphyrinogen oxidase
PROTOGEN → protoporphyrin	Oxidation of the ring	Protoporphyrinogen oxidase
Protoporphyrin → heme	Insertion of iron	Ferrochelatase

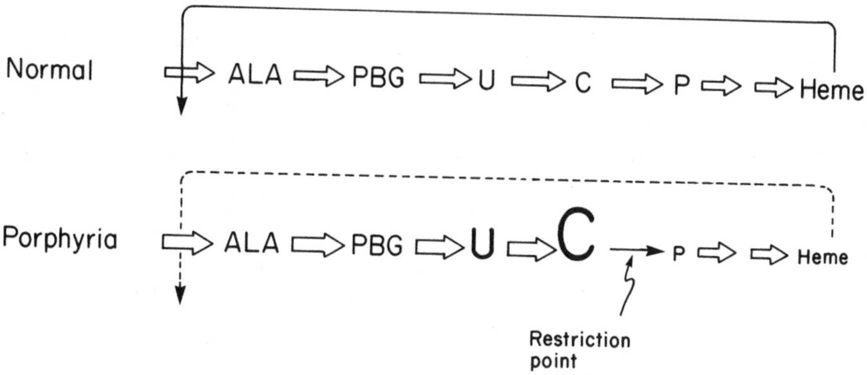

Fig. 5-6. The origin of porphyria. (**Top**) Normal situation. Heme feeds back on the enzyme that makes ALA, controlling ALA production. (**Bottom**) Porphyria attributable to a deficiency of COPROGEN oxidase. Heme production is decreased. This lifts the feedback inhibition of the ALA- forming enzyme, causing ALA production to increase. Intermediates down the line, however, accumulate behind the partial block. These increased quantities of intermediates push heme synthesis back toward normal, but their toxicity also causes the signs and symptoms of porphyria. U, UROGEN; C, COPROGEN; P, PROTOGEN.

3. Porphyria is generally diagnosed by measuring the excretion of heme precursors in the urine and stool. The distribution of a precursor between the urine and the stool depends on its water solubility, which is related to the number of negatively charged carboxyl groups at its periphery (Fig. 5-5). PBG and UROGEN, which contain two carboxyl groups/pyrrole, are excreted in the urine. COPROGEN, which contains one carboxyl group/pyrrole, is excreted partly in the urine and partly in the stool. Later precursors are excreted entirely in the stool.

Acute Intermittent Porphyria

Acute intermittent porphyria (AIP) is caused by a partial deficiency of PBG deaminase, the tetrapyrrole-forming enzyme. Under normal circumstances, patients with this disease are usually clinically well, and only small amounts of precursors accumulate. When a deficient patient is stressed, however, levels of PBG and ALA build up, provoking one of the recurrent attacks that characterize the disease (Fig. 5-7). The symptoms of the attack are widespread, but they can all be ascribed to abnormalities of the nervous system (Fig. 5-8). Psychosis and convulsions indicate disease of the cerebral cortex. Instability of temperature and blood pressure are caused by brain stem disease; this may lead to death. Abdominal and pelvic pain that can be so severe as to mimic an acute abdomen are thought to be caused by dysfunction of the autonomic nervous system. Acute peripheral neuropathy, most typically an acute paralysis involving one or more motor nerves, may also be seen, and respiratory paralysis leading to death can occur in this condition.

Several types of stresses can precipitate attacks of AIP (see box on p. 68). They may occur during the menstrual period, and in fact women are generally more susceptible to

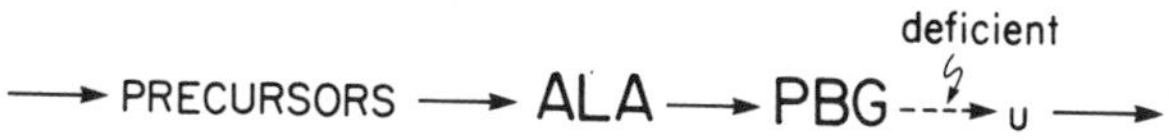

Fig. 5-7. Site of the blockade of porphyrin synthesis in acute intermittent porphyria.

attacks of AIP than are men. Infections and acidosis may initiate attacks of AIP. Attacks are characteristically precipitated by certain drugs, of which barbiturates are the most frequent offenders. These AIP-precipitating drugs have in common the capacity to induce the formation of hepatic drug-metabolizing enzymes, including cytochrome P-450, and it is thought that the attack results from the increase in heme formation that is required to provide the cytochrome with its prosthetic group.

The diagnosis of AIP is made by demonstrating the presence of ALA and PBG in the urine. These are invariably found in the urine during the course of an attack, and are usually present between attacks too, though in smaller amounts. On the other hand, tetrapyrroles are not found in either the urine or stool at any time during the course of this disease; their presence should raise doubts about the accuracy of the diagnosis. Carriers may be detected by demonstrating reduced levels of red cell PBG deaminase, and they should be warned about drugs that might precipitate attacks.

> **Factors Precipitating Attacks of Acute Intermittent Porphyria**
>
> Menstrual periods
> Infections
> Acidosis
> Drugs
>   Barbiturates
>   Birth control pills
>   Others

The management of AIP has been at least partly rationalized on the basis of an understanding of the precipitating factors and the control of the heme biosynthetic pathway. Between attacks the patient should be on a high carbohydrate diet to prevent minor degrees of acidosis that increase susceptibility to an attack; drugs that can precipitate attacks should be scrupulously avoided. An attack is treated with intravenous heme,

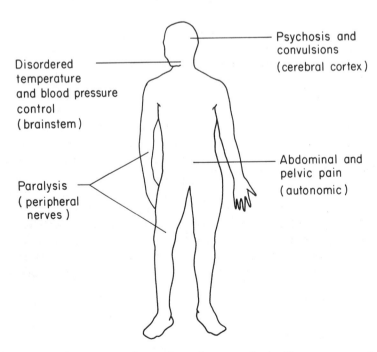

Fig. 5-8. Signs and symptoms of acute intermittent porphyria. These occur as attacks. They are thought to be caused by the neurotoxicity of PBG or its metabolites.

which terminates the attack by blocking ALA synthetase (Fig. 5-6).

Porphyria Cutanea Tarda

Porphyria cutanea tarda results from a reduction in the activity of UROGEN decarboxylase, the enzyme that converts UROGEN to COPROGEN (Fig. 5-9). The disease is sometimes caused by an inherited deficiency of UROGEN decarboxylase, but most often it occurs as a sporadic disorder in patients with cirrhosis of the liver. In these patients, the enzyme itself is present in normal amounts, but its activity is partly blocked by an inhibitory metabolite that is produced in response to the excess iron that accumulates in the parenchymal cells of cirrhotic livers. In a few cirrhotics, the resulting fall in the activity of the decarboxylase is enough to cause an accumulation of precursors and the onset of symptoms.

The precursors that accumulate are tetrapyrroles, as expected from the location of

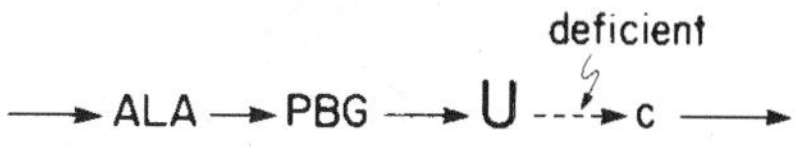

$$\longrightarrow \text{ALA} \longrightarrow \text{PBG} \longrightarrow \text{U} \overset{\text{deficient}}{\dashrightarrow} \text{c} \longrightarrow$$

Fig. 5-9. Site of the blockade of porphyrin synthesis in porphyria cutanea tarda.

the block in porphyrin synthesis. The tetrapyrroles are UROGEN III and some partially decarboxylated products that arise because of the incomplete decarboxylation of UROGEN by the decarboxylase, a single enzyme that removes all four CO_2 molecules in the course of converting UROGEN to COPROGEN. The accumulation of the tetrapyrroles leads to a dermatitis in sun-exposed portions of the skin that may be very severe, with painful bullae that heal with scarring, irregular increased pigmentation, and hair growth in affected areas (Fig. 5-10).

A clue to the presence of porphyria cutanea tarda is provided by clinical examination of the urine from suspected patients. The heme precursors excreted in the urine of patients with porphyria cutanea tarda are porphyrinogens,

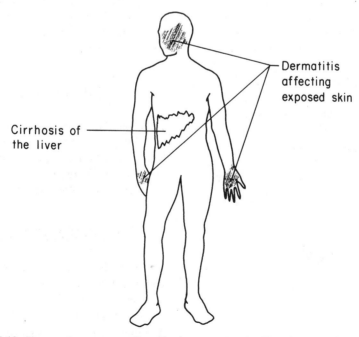

Cirrhosis of the liver

Dermatitis affecting exposed skin

Fig. 5-10. Signs and symptoms of porphyria cutanea tarda. Hepatic cirrhosis is a contributing cause of the disease. The dermatitis is caused by the deposition of porphyrins in the skin, sensitizing it to damage by the sun.

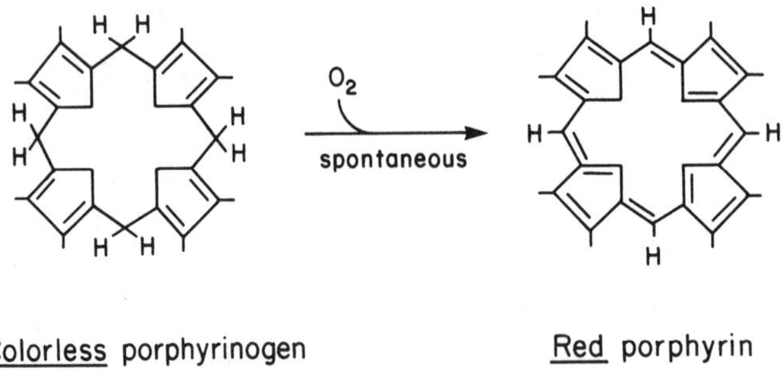

Colorless porphyrinogen   Red porphyrin

Fig. 5-11. Spontaneous oxidation of a porphyrinogen to a porphyrin in voided urine. The side chains and nitrogens are omitted for clarity.

which are tetrapyrroles containing a partially reduced ring (see above). Porphyrinogens are colorless, so that freshly voided urine containing these compounds is normal in color. On standing, however, the porphyrinogens in this urine undergo oxidation to the corresponding porphyrins, which are deep red (Fig. 5-11). Urine from patients with porphyria cutanea tarda therefore turns dark with time.

The diagnosis is made by the method used to diagnose all porphyrias: the demonstration of porphyrin precursors in the urine or stool. In porphyria cutanea tarda, precursors are found in both, the relative proportions varying with the number of carboxyl groups as discussed above. Owing to their susceptibility to oxidation, however, the -ogen precursors are not found as such, but will have been converted to the fully oxidized porphyrins by the time the measurement is made. Thus UROGEN III, a major component of the porphyrin precursors excreted in porphyria cutanea tarda, is found mostly in the urine, where it is detected as uro-

porphyrin III. Partially decarboxylated precursors, however, appear in both urine and stool as fully oxidized 5- to 7-carboxyporphyrins. This is summarized in Figure 5-12.

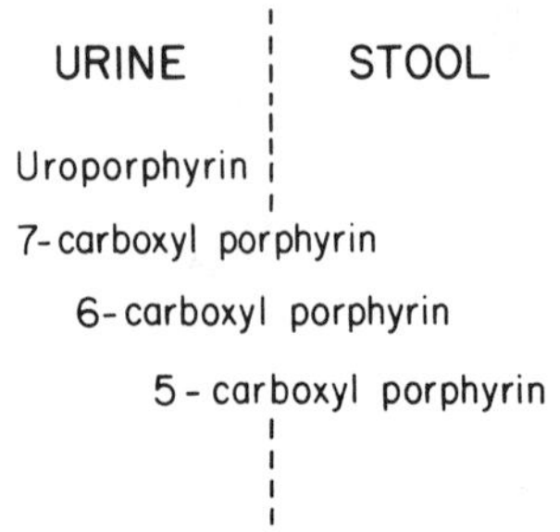

On the basis of pathogenetic mechanisms, a rational approach has been developed for the management of porphyria cutanea tarda associated with cirrhosis. The mainstay of treatment is phlebotomy, which by removing excess iron from the liver relieves the inhibition of the decarboxylase and permits precursors to flow normally into heme. Treating the underlying cirrhosis will also alleviate the porphyria, but this is usually much less successful because of the difficulty in eliminating the cause of the cirrhosis, usually alcohol.

Other Porphyrias

Porphyrias have now been associated with deficiencies of each of the enzymes of the heme synthetic pathway, except for ALA synthetase. The features of these porphyrias are summarized in Table 5-2.

URINE	STOOL
Uroporphyrin	
7-carboxyl porphyrin	
6-carboxyl porphyrin	
5-carboxyl porphyrin	

Fig. 5-12. Porphyrin excretion in porphyria cutanea tarda.

SIDEROBLASTIC ANEMIAS

The sideroblastic anemias are a group of conditions in which the incorporation of iron into heme is impaired. Uptake of iron by the red cell precursors is intact, however, and iron accumulates in these precursors in a characteristic pattern. The basis for the problem with iron metabolism is not well understood, but

Table 5-2. The Porphyrias

Deficiency	Disease	Products Excreted[a]	Manifestations[b]
PBG deaminase	Acute intermittent porphyria	ALA–PBG[c]	N
UROGEN decarboxylase	Porphyria cutanea tarda	U, decarboxy U	D
Cosynthetase	Erythropoietic porphyria	U I (not U III)	D (very severe)
COPROGEN oxidase	Hereditary coproporphyria	C, ALA–PBG	N, D
PROTOGEN oxidase (?)	Variegate porphyria	C, P, ALA–PBG	N, D
Ferrochelatase	Erythropoietic *proto*porphyria	P	D

[a]Principal compounds: U, uroporphyrin; C, coproporphyrin; P, protoporphyrin. U is found mainly in the urine, C and P mainly in the stool.

[b]Manifestations correlate with the products excreted. N, neurological: attacks like those in acute intermittent porphyria. D, dermatological: solar dermatitis.

[c]ALA and PBG are always excreted together in the hereditary porphyrias.

there is some evidence that it may be associated with a defect in the formation of ALA, the starting material for heme synthesis. The concept of a defect in ALA formation provides both a rationale for understanding the pathophysiology of sideroblastic anemias and a thread that ties together a number of otherwise unrelated facts about the diseases. They will therefore be discussed within the context of this idea.

Ineffective Erythropoiesis

The sideroblastic anemias, as well as the megaloblastic anemias, thalassemias, and certain hematological malignancies, are characterized by an aberration in red cell formation known as *ineffective erythropoiesis*. This term is used to describe the destruction of red cell precursors in the marrow before they can mature fully to appear in the blood as reticulocytes.

The occurrence of ineffective erythropoiesis has been established by observing the fate of newly synthesized heme over the course of time. Newly made heme can be tagged by administering isotopically labeled glycine to a subject. A portion of the labeled glycine is incorporated into heme, while the rest is rapidly metabolized by other routes. The labeled glycine is thus available only for a short period of time, and only those heme molecules that were synthesized during that short time interval will carry the label.

The tagged heme is then incorporated into proteins—mostly hemoglobin, but also heme-requiring enzymes, of which the most abundant by far is the cytochrome P-450 of the liver. When these proteins are degraded, the heme is converted into bilirubin, which is excreted in the bile. Tagged bilirubin will appear when proteins containing tagged heme molecules are degraded. It is possible, therefore, to determine the lifetime of heme-containing proteins by measuring the interval between the administration of labeled glycine and the appearance of labeled bilirubin in the bile. This method, of course, only indicates that some heme-containing proteins have been degraded; the identity of the degraded protein must be determined by other types of studies.

The fate of newly synthesized heme has been followed in humans, using ^{13}C-labeled glycine (Fig. 5-13). Three peaks of labeled bilirubin appear in the bile. The first two are the so-called early labeled peaks. They appear 1 to 4 days after the tagged glycine is given and contain about 15 percent of the total excreted label. The first peak has been shown to result from the breakdown of cytochrome P-450, while the second is from hemoglobin that has been degraded during the destruction of red cell precursors in the marrow—that is, from ineffective erythropoiesis. The third peak, by far the largest, appears about 4 months after the labeled glycine is given and is caused by the destruction of the cohort of red cells that had formed in the marrow at the time the tagged heme was available. From the ratio of the sec-

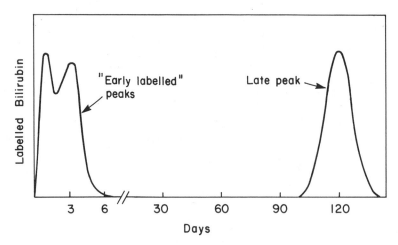

Fig. 5-13 Fate of newly synthesized heme in humans, as measured by the production of labeled bilirubin from heme tagged in vivo with labeled glycine. A small fraction of the new heme is in the liver, where it is incorporated mostly into cytochrome P-450; turnover of this protein accounts for the first of two "early labeled" peaks. Almost all the rest of the new heme is made in the red cell precursors. About 10 percent of these are destroyed before they leave the marrow, their heme producing the second of the two "early labeled" peaks. The rest develop into red cells, which enter the bloodstream and circulate for about 4 months. They are then destroyed, producing the late peak of labeled bilirubin. (Note the change in scale on the x-axis.)

ond and third peaks, it can be calculated that ineffective erythropoiesis accounts for about 10 percent of total red cell production under normal conditions.

In patients with sideroblastic anemias and the other anemias listed above, the percentage of red cell precursors destroyed in the marrow is much greater than normal. In especially severe cases, ineffective erythropoiesis may amount to 90 percent of total red cell production. This increase in ineffective erythropoiesis could in principle be diagnosed by the tagged heme method. This method, however, is not practical for the routine investigation of anemic patients. At the bedside, ineffective erythropoiesis is generally diagnosed from the results of the bone marrow examination combined with ferrokinetic data (see box below). As expected from the very high rate of erythropoiesis necessary to maintain an adequate hematocrit in this condition, the marrow is grossly hypercellular, with almost no fat, and the myeloid:erythroid ratio is shifted far in the direction of the red cell series. The increased marrow iron requirement necessary to meet the demands of erythropoiesis is reflected in ferrokinetic measurements, which show a greatly increased plasma iron turnover and an increase in the amount of iron taken up by the marrow.

Diagnosis of Ineffective Erythropoiesis

Hypercellular marrow with a disproportionate increase in the red cell series (increased erythroid/myeloid ratio)
Increased plasma iron turnover
Erythrocyte iron turnover < 70 percent of plasma iron turnover
Increased uptake and retention of iron by the marrow[a]

[a]See Figure 5-14 for further details.

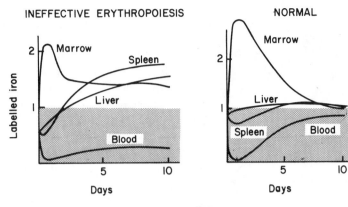

Fig. 5-14. Movement of labeled iron through various tissues during the first 10 days after administration in a patient with ineffective erythropoiesis. Note especially that after 8 to 10 days there is more iron in the marrow and less iron in the blood than is seen in normal circulation. (From Finch CA [1982] Clinical aspects of iron deficiency and excess. Semin Hematol 19:1, with permission.)

In this respect, the ferrokinetics of ineffective erythropoiesis are the same as those of iron deficiency. They differ, however, in that most of the iron in ineffective erythropoiesis does not end up in the red cells, but remains in the marrow, where the hemoglobin-containing precursors are destroyed. This is most apparent in the fact that the erythrocyte iron turnover, instead of being 80 to 90 percent of the plasma iron turnover, is considerably lower, indicating that a substantial amount of the iron taken up from the plasma did not reach the peripheral blood. Studies of iron distribution show that iron is preferentially retained by the marrow at the expense of the peripheral blood (Fig. 5-14). All the ferrokinetics can be understood in the context of a marrow that is taking up iron avidly to make cells of the erythropoietic series, most of which are destroyed in situ before thay can be released into the bloodstream.

Causes

In understanding the causes of sideroblastic anemia, it is useful to have a rationale to explain its characteristics—especially the iron accumulation, which is its most typical feature. Such a rationale is available, although it must be emphasized that for most forms of sideroblastic anemia the supporting evidence is at present rather skimpy and indirect. Nevertheless, this rationale is presented, because it provides a convenient way of thinking about these conditions and pulls together a lot of information about what otherwise appears to be a rather heterogeneous group of diseases.

The sideroblastic anemias can be considered in terms of a blockade in heme synthesis at the level of ALA production (Fig. 5-15). This blockade occurs so early in the heme biosynthetic pathway that monopyrroles and

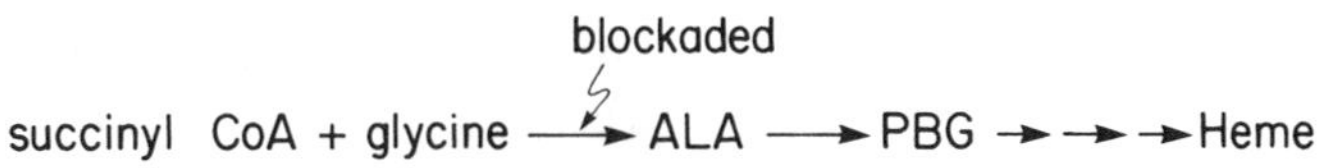

$$\text{succinyl CoA} + \text{glycine} \xrightarrow{\text{blockaded}} \text{ALA} \longrightarrow \text{PBG} \rightarrow \rightarrow \rightarrow \text{Heme}$$

Fig. 5-15. Sideroblastic anemias may be caused by a blockade in the synthesis of ALA.

Causes of Sideroblastic Anemias

Drugs
  Alcohol
  Antituberculosis drugs
  Lead
  Others
Inherited
Idiopathic (stem cell mutation)

tetrapyrroles are prevented from accumulating. Instead, iron accumulates, perhaps because it is taken up by the red cell precursors at a near-normal rate, but cannot be disposed of by the usual route of incorporation into heme.

As to causes, the sideroblastic anemias arise either spontaneously or as the side effect of a drug. Many of these causes can be understood in terms of the rationale presented above.

DRUGS

Most drug-related sideroblastic anemias are caused by one of two types of agents: alcohol, or certain agents used against tuberculosis. The latter include isoniazid (INH), cycloserine, and pyrazinamide. What these appear to have in common is an antagonism against pyridoxal phosphate, the cofactor necessary for the synthesis of ALA. The antipyridoxal effect of INH has been especially well shown and results from the addition of INH to pyridoxal phosphate to form a compound excreted in the urine. With alcohol, there may be interference with the conversion of the vitamin pyridoxine to the coenzyme pyridoxal phosphate.

OTHER CAUSES

Most of the non-drug-related sideroblastic anemias appear to arise through the replacement of the normal hematopoietic stem cells by a line of mutant stem cells that have acquired a defect in heme production, resulting in a sideroblastic state. Such a sideroblastic anemia—actually a form of myelodysplasic syndrome (see Ch. 22)—generally develops in late middle age. It can be a premalignant condition, with some patients going on to develop acute myelogenous leukemia. A small percentage of patients with this condition respond to very large doses of pyridoxine.

Sideroblastic anemia may also be inherited, presenting in childhood. The mode of transmission may be autosomal dominant, autosomal recessive, or X-linked. It has recently been shown that X-linked sideroblastic anemia is due to an inherited deficiency in ALA synthase.

Manifestations

Sideroblastic anemia looks at first like a disease caused by a deficiency of precursor cells in the bone marrow (i.e., a hypoproliferative or hypoplastic anemia). It is characterized by a low hematocrit combined with a reticulocyte count that is low for the degree of anemia, a combination suggesting that marrow red cell precursors are lacking. On the peripheral smear, the cells usually look smaller than normal (Fig. 5-16), an appearance borne out by microcytic red cell indices. A significant minority of patients, however, have cells that are larger than normal (macrocytosis), and a few show both microcytes and macrocytes, a so-called dimorphic smear. A characteristic feature of the red cell is basophilic stippling, a finding that results from incomplete degradation of RNA as the red cell matures. Normally, the RNA in the red cell precursor is broken down to its nucleotides when the cell reaches maturity. Residual RNA is found only in the youngest circulating cells (see reticulocytes, Ch. 2), and then only in small amounts. If RNA degradation is impaired, however, red cells containing large amounts of RNA will be present in the circulation. In these cells, the nucleic acid can precipitate as visible deep blue aggregates when the smear is stained with

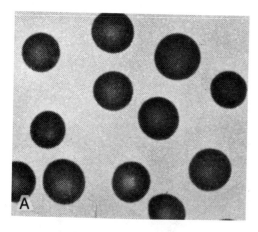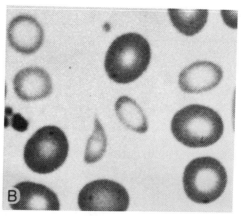

Fig. 5-16. Peripheral smear in sideroblastic anemia. **(A)** Normal smear. **(B)** Sideroblastic anemia. The red cells are irregular in shape (poikilocytosis). Some are small and pale; others appear to be slightly macrocytic. This dual population is characteristic of sideroblastic anemia. Basophilic stippling is seen in an occasional cell. (From Wintrobe MM et al [1974] Clinical Hematology. 7th Ed. Lea & Febiger, Philadelphia, with permission.)

Anemias in Which Basophilic Stippling May Be Seen

Sideroblastic anemia
Megaloblastic anemia
Thalassemia
Sickle cell anemia

Wright's stain.* Cells containing these aggregates are said to display basophilic stippling. This morphological abnormality is typical of sideroblastic anemia and is seen in several other forms of anemia as well.

The bone marrow examination establishes the diagnosis of sideroblastic anemia. Contrary to what might be expected from the hypoproliferative picture in the periphery, the marrow is packed with red cell precursors. Furthermore, the mononuclear phagocytes of the marrow are

---

* Wright's stain is the stain used for routine blood smears. It can precipitate high concentrations of RNA, but it cannot precipitate the small quantity of RNA in a reticulocyte; for this, new methylene blue or brilliant cresyl violet is needed.

loaded with iron in the form of hemosiderin, a consequence of the high rate of local destruction of red cell precursors (i.e., the abnormally high level of ineffective erythropoiesis). Most importantly, it is in the marrow that the diagnostic cell of sideroblastic anemia is found.

The diagnostic cell is a ringed sideroblast. This red cell precursor accumulates large quantities of iron in the mitochondria, a situation that does not occur in normal erythropoiesis. When an iron-stained marrow sample is examined under the light microscope, the ringed sideroblast appears as a nucleated red cell precursor with a necklace of coarse, iron-containing granules around the nucleus (Fig. 5-17). Electron microscopic examination shows these iron-containing granules to be the mitochondria, which cluster around the nucleus in this cell, giving it its characteristic "ringed" appearance.

The accumulation of iron in the mitochondria of these cells may have to do with the fact that the incorporation of iron into heme takes place in mitochondria. The iron is supplied by a mitochondrial iron-transporting system that normally seems to maintain a balance between the iron supply and the rate of porphyrin formation, since there is little free iron in the

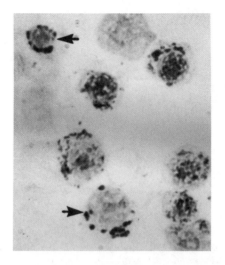

A

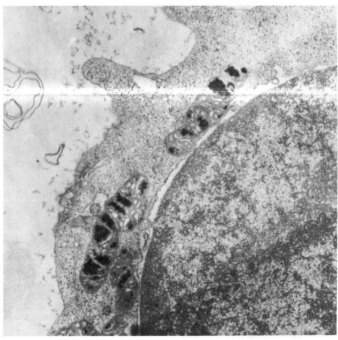

B

Fig. 5-17. Bone marrow in sideroblastic anemia. **(A)** Prussian blue stain. The marrow is packed with red cell precursors. Iron (dark granules) is abundant. The ringed sideroblast (*arrows*) is a red cell precursor with a necklace of prominent iron granules around the nucleus. These granules are iron-filled mitochondria **(B)**. (**A:** From Castoldi GL [1981] Erythrocytes. p. 33. In Zucker-Franklin D et al [eds]: Atlas of Blood Cells: Function and Pathology. Edi. Ermes s.r.l., Milan, with permission. **B:** From Wintrobe MM et al [1974] Clinical Hematology. 7th Ed. Lea & Febiger, Philadelphia, with permission.)

mitochondria of normal red cell precursors. It is conceivable that an impairment in porphyrin synthesis out of proportion to any change in mitochondrial iron transport occurs in sideroblastic anemia. In that event, iron would pile up in the mitochondria, because no porphyrin is available to which it can be transferred.

Other general features of sideroblastic anemia have to do with abnormalities in iron metabolism. Serum iron is high, and transferrin saturation is greater than normal, because iron stores are elevated and iron absorption from the small intestine is increased in association with the increase in marrow erythropoietic activity. Serum ferritin is high, another indication of increased iron stores. Ferrokinetics are altered in the characteristic way.

Features may also be seen that are specific for the cause of the sideroblastic anemia. For example, a history of alcoholism or antituberculosis therapy may be obtained. Family studies may provide evidence for an inherited condition. In the spontaneously appearing sideroblastic anemias, other hematopoietic lines may be shown to be involved, indicating a stem cell abnormality (Ch. 22).

Management

Once the diagnosis is made, the management of sideroblastic anemia is straightforward. If the anemia is iatrogenic, the drug can

---

Clinical Iron Measurements in Sideroblastic Anemia

High serum iron
Normal total iron–binding capacity (equivalent to a normal transferrin level)
High transferrin saturation
High serum ferritin

---

be discontinued, unless its use is essential to the patient's welfare. High-dose pyridoxine should always be tried in spontaneously acquired sideroblastic anemia, although the likehood of success with this form of treatment is not great. In sideroblastic anemias that do not respond to these measures, transfusion may be used, but it must be remembered that hemochromatosis is a serious consideration with chronic transfusion therapy, particularly in anemias with ineffective erythropoiesis in which iron stores are expanded by the nature of the disease itself.

LEAD

Lead inhibits several of the enzymes of the heme synthetic pathway, affecting PBG synthetase as well as enzymes catalyzing later steps. Perhaps because of its effect on these enzymes, chronic lead poisoning causes a disease exhibiting features of both sideroblastic anemia and porphyria. Porphyrialike features include a motor neuropathy and a characteristic pattern of recurrent abdominal pain with constipation (so-called lead colic); coproporphyrin and ALA (but no PBG, an important distinction from the inherited porphyrias) are excreted in the urine. The anemia of lead poisoning is a typical sideroblastic anemia, with microcytosis, basophilic stippling, an elevated serum iron, and ringed sideroblasts in the marrow. Red cell porphyrin is increased, probably reflecting the inhibition of ferrochelatase by the toxic metal.

Other manifestations of chronic lead intoxication include renal failure, hypertension, and gout. Psychosis may also result from chronic lead poisoning; the decline of the Roman empire has been attributed in part to psychosis among the Roman rulers arising from their practice of drinking wine from lead vessels. The "lead line" is a bluish-black deposit seen in the gingival margin; such a line is highly suggestive of intoxication by lead or other heavy metals, but it is seen only in patients with poor dental hygiene. Acute lead poisoning may lead to an acute encephalopathy with greatly increased intracranial pressure, papilledema, and coma. .

Lead poisoning typically affects persons exposed to the metal in the course of their work. It used to be particularly common among painters, because of the lead-based pigments at one time present in paints. The paint content has changed, so that lead poisoning in painters is not the problem it once was. Lead-containing paint, however, may still be found on the walls of old houses. This paint represents an insidious source of lead poisoning in children, who flake it from the walls and eat it because of its sweet flavor. In working up any child displaying signs of lead poisoning, this possibility must always be kept in mind.

The diagnosis of lead poisoning is made by the demonstration of elevated lead levels in the blood or urine. The condition is treated by chelation therapy with calcium EDTA and by removal of the patient from the source of poison.

SUGGESTED READINGS

Berris P, Graf BJ, Miescher PA (1983) Primary acquired sideroblastic and primary acquired refractory anemia. Semin Hematol 20:101

Besa EC (1992) Myelodysplastic syndromes (refractory anemia). A perspective of the biologic, clinical, and therapeutic issues. Med Clin North Am 76:599

Cartwright GE (1975) Sideroblasts, siderocytes, and sideroblastic anemia. N Engl J Med 292:185

Clin Haematol (1980) The porphyrias. 9, no. 2

Cullen MR, Robins JM, Eskenazi B (1983) Adult inorganic lead intoxication: presentation of 31 new cases and a review of recent advances in the literature. Medicine 62:221

Elder GH, Smith SG, Smyth SJ (1990) Laboratory investigation of the porphyrias. Ann Clin Biochem 27:395

Felsher BF, Kushner JF (1977) Hepatic siderosis and porphyria cutanea tarda: relation of iron excess to the metabolic defect. Semin Hematol 14:243

Kramer S, Becker DM, Viljoen JD (1977) Enzyme deficiencies in the porphyrias. Br J Haematol 37:439

Lindenbaum J, Roman MJ (1980) Nutritional anemia in alcoholism. Am J Clin Nutr 33:2727

Moore MR, McColl KE, Fitzsimons EJ, Goldberg SA (1990) The porphyrias. Blood Rev 4:88

Mufti GJ, Galton DA (1986) Myelodysplastic syndromes: natural history and features of prognostic importance. Clin Haematol 15:953

Mustajoki P (1978) Variegate porphyria. Ann Intern Med 89:238

Nusbaum NJ (1991) Concise review: genetic bases for sideroblastic anemia. Am J Hematol 37:41

Pasanen A, Tenhunen R (1986) Heme synthesis in sideroblastic anaemias. Scand J Haematol, suppl. 45:69

Sassa S (1990) Regulation of the genes for heme pathway enzymes in erythroid and in non-erythroid cells. Int J Cell Cloning 8:10

Straka JG, Rank JM, Bloomer JR (1990) Porphyria and porphyrin metabolism. Annu Rev Med 41:457

Yunis AA, Salem Z (1980) Drug-induced mitochondrial damage and sideroblastic change. Clin Haematol 9:607

6

DNA Replication and Hematopoiesis: Megaloblastic Anemias

In most tissues of the body, cell division is a rare event, taking place only as needed to replace losses due to damage or to provide an increase in organ mass to handle a functional overload (e.g., the hypertrophy of the remaining kidney that follows unilateral nephrectomy). In a few tissues, however, cell division is a continuous process. These tissues include the hematopoietic system, the gastrointestinal epithelium, the epidermis, and the germinal epithelium of the testis. In all these tissues, normal function involves a continuous loss of cells, so constant production of new cells is necessary to maintain the tissue in a normal state.

The key event of cell division is the synthesis of new DNA. This process occurs only in an occasional cell in slowly dividing tissues, but it is the rule in the hematopoietic system and the other continuously dividing tissues. All these tissues are therefore sensitive to damage by factors that disrupt DNA synthesis, in contrast to slowly dividing tissues, which tend to be resistant to such factors.

In the hematopoietic system, impaired DNA synthesis is expressed clinically as a characteristic disorder of hematopoiesis known as *megaloblastic anemia*. The term *megaloblastic* refers to the abnormally large (megalo-) red cell precursors (blasts) that populate the marrow in this disorder. Megaloblastic anemia is most often caused by a deficiency of folate or cobalamin, the two vitamins necessary for normal production of deoxyribonucleotides. Drugs that inhibit DNA synthesis may also cause megaloblastic anemia. Occasionally, megaloblastic anemia appears as a manifestation of an acquired stem cell disorder.

MEGALOBLASTIC ANEMIA

Unlike most of the conditions discussed so far, megaloblastic anemia involves all three hematopoietic cell lines—red cells, white cells, and platelets. This is because all three lines are produced continuously by the marrow, and as a result all three lines are affected when a megaloblastic state develops because of a disturbance in DNA synthesis. Accordingly, wide-ranging abnormalities are seen in the peripheral blood of patients with megaloblastic anemia. In addition, a diagnostic cell appears in the marrow—an abnormal red cell precursor known as the megaloblast.

In the peripheral blood, a macrocytic anemia is the rule. By mean cell volume (MCV), the red cells are large; in some cases they are huge, exceeding the normal MCV by 50 percent or more. The blood smear contains many macroovalocytes—the oversized, elliptical, hemoglobin-stuffed red cells characteristic of megaloblastic anemia—but also contains many cells that are smaller than normal. Gross macrocytosis is virtually diagnostic of megaloblastic anemia, but minor degrees (MCV increased by up to 10 percent) occur in some sideroblastic anemias, in the anemias of hypothyroidism and liver disease, and in anemias with large numbers of circulating reticulocytes, which are bigger than mature red cells and will cause an increase in the MCV.

As to the other formed elements, the white blood cell count may be low because of neutropenia, and the platelet count may be reduced as well. "Hypersegmented polys"—neutrophils with more than the normal three to five nuclear lobes—are seen on the smear in many cases (Fig. 6-1). This abnormality is caused by a defect in nuclear segmentation, and not, as was formerly postulated, by the release of hypermature neutrophils from the marrow.

The anemia in megaloblastic anemia is caused by ineffective erythropoiesis. Accordingly, the marrow is packed with red cell precursors, yet the reticulocyte count is low for the degree of anemia and in many cases is reduced in absolute terms as well. The serum bilirubin is elevated because of the increase in the "early label" peak caused by the degradation of hemoglobin released when red cell precursors are destroyed in the marrow. The serum iron is increased as well. The serum lactate dehydrogenase reaches remarkable heights because of the release of the enzyme from the red cell precursors as well as from leukocyte and megakaryocyte precursors, which are also thought to be destroyed in the marrow (ineffective myelopoiesis and thrombopoiesis).

The hallmark of megaloblastic anemia is the *megaloblast*. This cell, seen in the marrow, is a red cell precursor in which DNA synthesis is retarded (the common feature of megaloblastic anemia), while protein and RNA synthesis proceed at a normal rate. The result is a cell in which cytoplasmic differentiation has out-

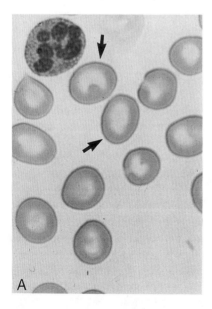 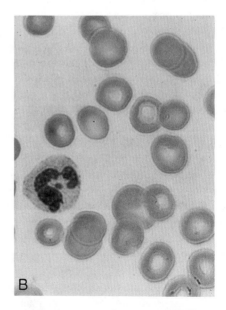

Fig. 6-1. Blood smear in megaloblastic anemia. **(A)** Megaloblastic smear. This field shows several macroovalocytes *(arrows)* as well as a neutrophil with more than five lobes in its nucleus (a "hypersegmented poly"). The typical variability in red cell size is also evident. **(B)** A normal smear for comparison.

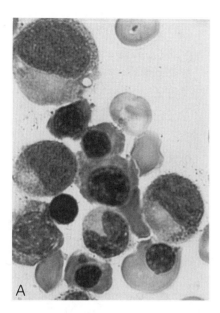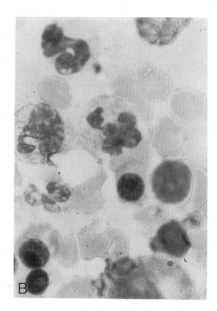

Fig. 6-2. Marrow in megaloblastic anemia. (**A**) Megaloblastic marrow. This marrow is packed with megaloblastic red cell precursors. The megaloblast can be identified by the large cell size and the immature-looking nucleus with its characteristically open chromatin. (**B**) Normal marrow, for comparison.

stripped nuclear maturation, so that the nucleus appears younger than it should for the stage of development of the cell. The nucleus is larger than it ought to be, and its chromatin meshwork is more open. Furthermore, the entire cell is larger than normal, because it undergoes fewer divisions before reaching maturity than does the normal cell. All these features are most readily seen in the final stages of red cell differentiation, but they can be detected at all stages (Fig. 6-2). Greatly enlarged late-stage white cell precursors (giant metamyelocytes and bands) may also be seen in megaloblastic bone marrow.

The foregoing features are common to all megaloblastic anemias. They are summarized in the box at left. Other clinical manifestations, not common to megaloblastic anemias in general, but seen in only specific types, are described in the sections dealing with the anemias in which they occur.

FOLATE AND MEGALOBLASTIC ANEMIA

Folate is required for the synthesis of three of the four bases found in DNA. Deficiency of this vitamin is probably the most common cause of megaloblastic anemia.

Clinical Features of Megaloblastic Anemia

Blood cells
  Reticulocytes decreased
  Mean cell volume increased
  Macroovalocytes and hypersegmented
    polymorphonuclear leukocytes on
    smear
Blood chemistries
  Iron increased
  Bilirubin increased
  Lactate dehydrogenase increased
Marrow
  Packed with red cell precursors
  Megaloblasts present

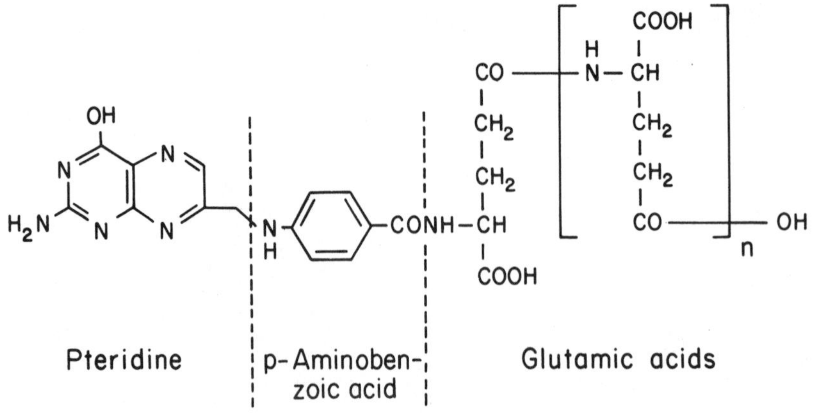

Fig. 6-3. Folic acid. The three parts of the molecule are indicated in the figure. For the sake of clarity, some of the hydrogens have been omitted.

Normal Function

METABOLIC ROLE

An understanding of the basis for the megaloblastic anemia in folate deficiency requires knowledge of the role played by folate in normal metabolism. Folate (Fig. 6-3) consists of three parts: a nitrogen-containing ring system known as the *pteridine*, a second ring consisting of *p*-aminobenzoic acid, and a chain of glutamic acid residues that prevent the vitamin from leaking out of cells. The vitamin itself is metabolically inert; the active form is produced by reduction of the right-hand half of the pteridine to give tetrahydrofolate (THF). This reduction is accomplished by an enzyme called *dihydrofolate reductase*.

The function of THF is to transfer one-carbon fragments from various donors—mostly the amino acid serine—to various acceptors, primarily intermediates of nucleotide biosynthesis. These one-carbon fragments are transferred to and from a very small region of the complex THF molecule. This region, which in a sense is the business end of THF, is a simple chain of four atoms with the so-called N^5 nitrogen at one end and the N^{10} nitrogen at the other (Fig. 6-4).

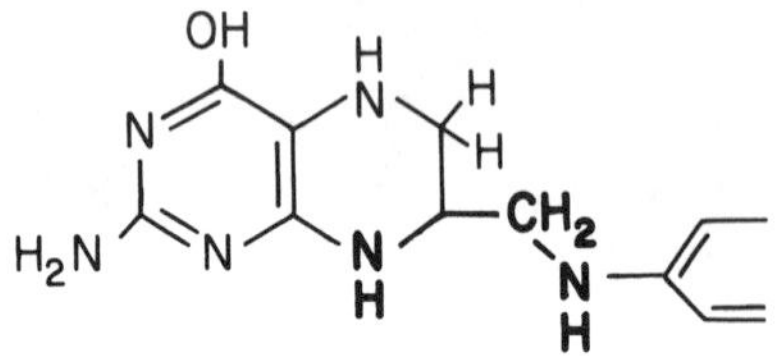

Fig. 6-4. A portion of the tetrahydrofolate (THF) molecule, showing the "business end" (**boldface**) and the partly reduced pteridine.

The main reaction that loads folate with one-carbon fragments is the transfer of the one-carbon side chain from serine to THF. This yields glycine together with a form of THF in which N^5 and N^{10} are linked by a —CH2— bridge: $N^{5,10}$-methylene THF. This bridge may be oxidized to produce the forms of THF that function in purine production; it may be reduced to produce N^5-methyl THF, the major circulating form; or it may be transferred as such to the uracil of dUMP to form dTMP. These interconversions are summarized in Figure 6-5.

The conversion of dUMP to dTMP is unique among folate one-carbon transfers in that the pteridine is oxidized during the course of the reaction and must be re-reduced before it can participate further in one-carbon metabolism (Fig. 6-6). The product of the thymidylate

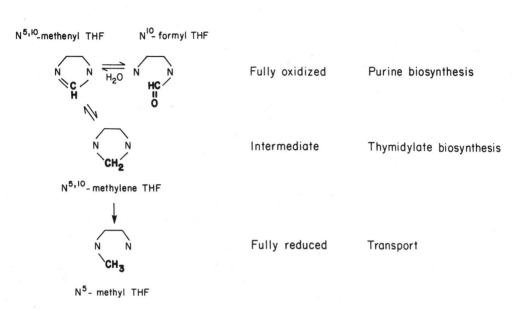

Fig. 6-5. Interconversions of folate-bound one-carbon fragments. *(Top)* Fully oxidized forms; carbons from the oxidized form are incorporated into the purine ring during purine nucleotide biosynthesis. *(Bottom)* Fully reduced form, the major circulating folate. For the sake of clarity, THF is represented by its "business end" only, and the one-carbon fragments are shown in boldface.

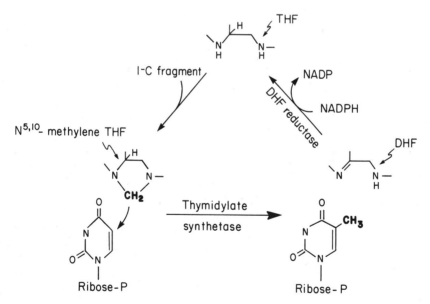

Fig. 6-6. Folate and the synthesis of thymidylic acid (dTMP). Thymidylic acid is synthesized by the transfer of a one-carbon fragment from $N^{5,10}$-methylene tetrahydrofolate (THF) to deoxyuridine monophospate (dUMP). During this transfer, the folate is oxidized from the tetrahydro- to the dihydro- form. This dihydrofolate, a metabolically inert compound, is reduced back to the metabolically active tetrahydrofolate by the enzyme *dihydrofolate reductase.*

synthetase reaction is dihydrofolate (DHF); it is reduced back to THF by dihydrofolate reductase. Certain highly effective chemotherapeutic agents act by inhibiting dihydrofolate reductase, thereby killing dividing cells by gradually diverting all their metabolically active folates into an inert pool of DHF (see below).

ASSIMILATION

Folate is present in most foods; it is especially abundant in vegetables, where its presence in leafy parts gave it its name. Almost all of this folate contains a polyglutamate chain, a structural feature described by the term *conjugated*. During absorption (Fig. 6-7), which can take place throughout the length of the small intestine, the polyglutamate chain is split off by an enzyme known as *deconjugase*, which is present on the brush border of the intestinal epithelial cell. The deconjugated folate moves into this cell, where it is converted to N^5-methyl THF and is then released into the bloodstream. Almost all the circulating folate is in the form of unconjugated (i.e., containing only a single glutamate residue) N^5-methyl THF.

The circulating N^5-methyl THF is taken up into cells by means of a specific THF carrier. Here it rapidly transfers its methyl group to homocysteine to form THF and methionine in a cobalamin-requiring reaction that is catalyzed by an enzyme known in short form as *methyltransferase*. The demethylated THF is then reconjugated by the addition of a chain of glutamate residues (5 to 7 is the normal number) to produce the tissue form of THF, ready to play its role in one-carbon metabolism.

There are two points of interest in regard to the reconjugation reaction: (1) the glutamates are attached to each other by peptide bonds, but these bonds involve the "wrong" carboxyl group and are therefore resistant to hydrolysis by ordinary proteases: and (2) the methyltransferase reaction is an essential preliminary to reconjugation, because N^5-methyl THF is a poor substrate for the conjugating enzyme and must be converted to THF before conjugation can take place.

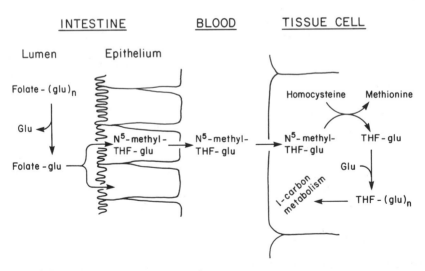

Fig. 6-7. Absorption of folate. Folate is deconjugated in the intestinal lumen, and then converted by the intestinal cell to N^5-methyl THF and released into the bloodstream. In this form, it is actively transported into cells. The methyl group is then removed by transfer to homocysteine, and the resulting THF is reconjugated, entering into one-carbon metabolism.

Folate Deficiency

CAUSES

Folate deficiency usually occurs because folate intake fails to meet needs. Occasionally it is the result of a defect in intestinal absorption.

Folate-Poor Diet

The most common cause of folate deficiency is a folate-poor diet. This is seen in alcoholics, whose customary diet of ethanol and congeners is lacking in folate and many other vitamins, and in the poor, especially the elderly poor, who for financial and other reasons are unable to obtain enough food to stave off malnutrition.

Increased Folate Requirements

Under certain circumstances, folate requirements may increase to the point at which an ordinary diet cannot meet the augmented needs of the patient. This occurs in patients in whom for one reason or another cell replication is greatly increased. Folate deficiency resulting from increased requirements is most frequently seen in pregnancy, in which the growing products of conception impose a severe stress on folate supplies. In pregnant women, the macro-cytosis typical of folate-deficient megaloblastic anemia may be offset by microcytosis caused by iron deficiency, so that folate deficiency may be easily overlooked in this circumstance. Routine supplementation of pregnant women with folate as well as iron is a good idea. Other conditions in which increased folate requirements may lead to vitamin deficiency are severe hemolytic anemias and exfoliative dermatitis, with greatly augmented erythropoiesis and epidermal cell production, respectively. Like pregnant women, patients with these conditions may require folate supplementation.

Malabsorption

Certain intestinal diseases are characterized by a reduction in nutrient absorption by the affected bowel. Occasionally, folate absorption is sufficiently impaired in these conditions to lead to folate deficiency. The disease most commonly associated with clinically significant folate malabsorption is tropical sprue.

MANIFESTATIONS

Megaloblastic Anemia

The most typical manifestation of folate deficiency is megaloblastic anemia, a hematopoietic disorder whose features have already been discussed. The salient molecular abnormality in folate deficiency is a marked slowing of DNA synthesis, a defect expressed not only in the characteristic morphological abnormalities of the megaloblastic cells, but also in a marked prolongation of the S (DNA synthetic) phase in replicating cells and in a disruption in chromatin structure detectable as chromosomal tangles and breaks. Despite extensive study, a biochemical explanation for the slowing of DNA synthesis in folate deficiency is not yet available, although it appears to be somehow related to the defect in dTMP formation seen in folate-deficient cells.

**Causes of
Folate Deficiency**

Folate-poor diet
   Alcoholism
   Poverty
Increased folate requirements
   Pregnancy
   Severe hemolytic anemia
Malabsorption

Other Manifestations

Folate deficiency affects other rapidly dividing tissues. A stomatitis characterized by a sore mouth and a smooth, beefy red tongue occurs frequently. It probably results from impaired proliferation of the oral mucosa, which is worn away during eating and must be constantly renewed. The gastric and intestinal mucosa acquire megaloblastic characteristics that can lead to confusion on cytological examination, although functional impairment due to these changes is slight.

MANAGEMENT

The diagnosis of folate deficiency is made by demonstrating reduced levels of folate in the serum. Serum folate responds rapidly to alterations in dietary folate status; hence a reduced serum folate level means that a state of folate deficiency has existed over the previous few days. Red blood cells, on the other hand, contain roughly the quantity of folate they held when they were released from the marrow, so measurement of red cell folate provides an indication of folate status over the preceding weeks. It is sometimes useful to measure the red cell folate in a treated patient if it is desirable to establish the existence of a prior state of folate deficiency.

Folate deficiency is treated simply by giving the vitamin. The response to treatment is striking. The megaloblastic morphology of cells in the bone marrow is gone within 24 to 48 hours. The reticulocyte count begins to rise by 3 to 5 days and rapidly reaches a peak that in severe cases may exceed 50 percent reticulocytes. Concomitantly, there is healing of the stomatitis. The reticulocyte count then begins to fall, and returns to normal with a complete resolution of the anemia. The whole process takes 3 to 6 weeks depending on the severity of the initial disease. A typical treatment response is shown in Figure 6-8.

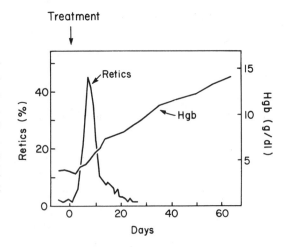

Fig. 6-8. Response of anemia of folate deficiency to treatment. (Data from Erslev A, Gabuzda TG [1975] Pathophysiology of Blood. WB Saunders, Philadelphia.)

COBALAMIN AND MEGA-LOBLASTIC ANEMIA

Cobalamin has two metabolic functions: (1) It participates in folate metabolism, and (2) it is required for the degradation of certain fatty acids. Megaloblastic anemia and neurological abnormalities are the typical manifestations of cobalamin deficiency. Both appear to be caused by disturbances involving the cobalamin–folate connection.

This vitamin is currently undergoing a change in nomenclature. It was originally called vitamin B12, but cobalamin is now the preferred terminology, the term *vitamin* B12 being reserved for the cyanide-containing form of the vitamin (see below). The old terminology, however, is still used from time to time.

Normal Function of Cobalamin

METABOLIC ROLE

Like folate, cobalamin consists of three basic parts: the corrin ring, a hemelike struc-

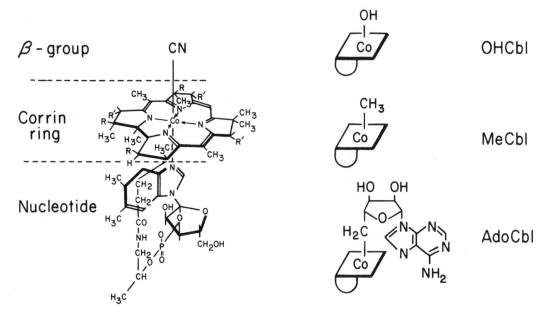

Fig. 6-9. Cobalamin. The full structure is cyanocobalamin, one of the four types of cobalamin found in tissues. The three parts of the molecule are indicated in this structure. The partial structures are hydroxocobalamin, methylcobalamin, and adenosylcobalamin, the other cobalamins found in tissues. The nucleoside base in these cobalamins is not the usual purine or pyrimidine, but instead is the rare base, 5,6-dimethylbenzimidazole. Cobalamin is the only biological compound in which this base occurs.

ture that contains cobalt at its center; the nucleotide, attached to the ring by a side chain and bonded to the cobalt through one of the nitrogens of its base; and the β-group, attached to the cobalt on the opposite side of the ring from the nucleoside (Fig. 6-9). Tissue cobalamins contain four different kinds of β-groups: methyl, adenosyl, OH⁻, and CN⁻ (Fig. 6-9). The methyl- and adenosylcobalamins serve as coenzymes, each working in a different reaction (see below). Hydroxo- and cyanocobalamin have no coenzymatic activity of their own, but are readily converted to the coenzymatically active forms by tissue enzymes. Cyanocobalamin is the form of the vitamin that is usually sold commercially.

Methylcobalamin is necessary for only one reaction in mammalian systems: the conversion of N^5-methyltetrahydrofolate to tetrahydrofo-

late (Fig. 6-10). This reaction serves two purposes: (1) to produce methionine by the transfer of a methyl group to homocysteine; and (2) to convert newly acquired cellular folate to a form that can be conjugated to a polyglutamate chain.

Adenosylcobalamin also serves as the cofactor for a single mammalian reaction (Fig. 6-10). This is the rearrangement of methylmalonyl CoA to succinyl CoA, catalyzed by the adenosylcobalamin-dependent enzyme methylmalonyl CoA mutase. Methylmalonyl CoA is generated by the addition of CO_2 to propionyl CoA, a compound produced in large quantities by the combustion of valine and isoleucine, amino acids that serve as important fuels for muscle. The product of the methylmalonyl CoA mutase reaction is a Krebs cycle intermediate that can be burned in the mitochondria to yield energy.

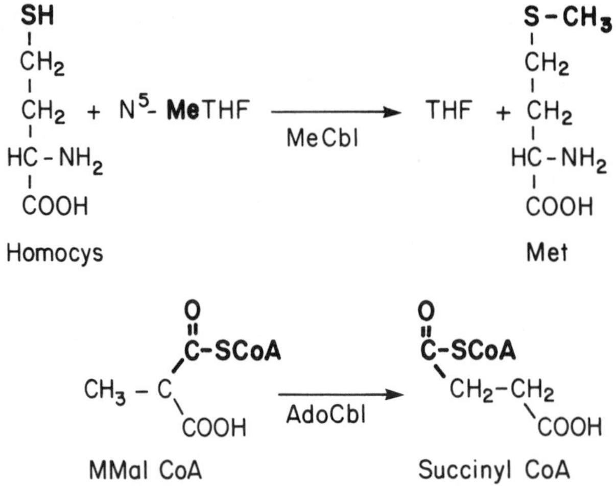

Fig. 6-10. Cobalamin-dependent reactions.

ASSIMILATION

The assimilation of cobalamin is a complex process involving several carrier proteins as well as a series of specialized cellular transport systems (Fig. 6-11 and Table 6-1). As will be seen, defects in one or another of the elements of this process are responsible for most cases of cobalamin deficiency.

The process of assimilation of cobalamin begins in the duodenum. Here the vitamin becomes attached to intrinsic factor (IF), a glycoprotein that is secreted by the parietal cells of the stomach. The cobalamin–IF complex does not form in the stomach because at the low pH of the working stomach, cobalamin is preferentially bound to R binder, a cobalamin-binding protein of unknown function present in all secretions, including saliva and gastric juice. The change in pH that occurs when the gastric contents pass into the duodenum causes the cobalamin to shift from the R binder to intrinsic factor. The R binder is digested, but the cobalamin–IF complex remains intact, because intrinsic factor is highly resistant to proteolysis.

The cobalamin–IF complex passes through the small intestine until it reaches the ileum. Here it attaches to specific receptors and is taken up into the ileal mucosal cells, where the IF is degraded and the cobalamin released. After several hours, the cobalamin passes from the ileal mucosal cell into the portal circulation, now complexed to transcobalamin II (TC II), a protein synthesized by the intestinal epithelium and probably most other tissues.

It is as this complex that cobalamin is taken up into cells. Cells contain surface receptors that bind the TC II–cobalamin complex. Once bound, the complex and its receptor are rapidly carried into the cell by pinocytosis. The internalized cobalamin is released from TC II, which is degraded. The cobalamin is then converted to its coenzymatically active forms.

Although newly absorbed cobalamin circulates in the form of a TC II complex, most of the cobalamin in the bloodstream is complexed to transcobalamin I (TC I) a circulating member of the R-binder family. Unlike the cobalamin–TC II complex, which circulates

Table 6-1. Cobalamin-Binding Proteins

Protein	Source	Required for
Intrinsic factor	Gastric parietal cells	Absorption of cobalamin by intestine
Transcobalamin II	Liver, intestinal mucosa, other	Uptake of cobalamin into cells
R binders	All secretions	Unknown

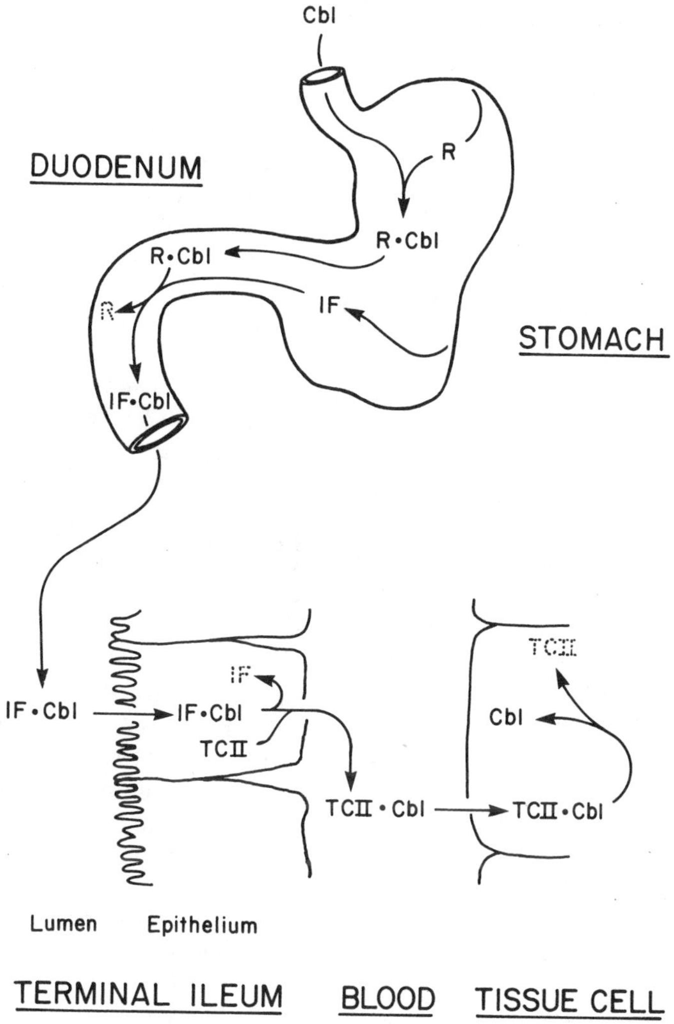

Fig. 6-11. Assimilation of cobalamin. The stomach secretes two cobalamin-binding proteins: intrinsic factor, which is essential for the absorption of cobalamin, and R binder, whose function is unknown. On entering the stomach, cobalamin forms a complex with R binder. This complex enters the duodenum, where cobalamin is transferred from R binder to intrinsic factor. The intrinsic factor–cobalamin complex passes through the intestine until it reaches the ileum, where the complex attaches to receptors on the ileal mucosal cells. These cells take up the intrinsic factor-cobalamin complex, then release the cobalamin and transport it into the bloodstream, some complexed to a new carrier, transcobalamin II, and the rest as the free vitamin. Once in the bloodstream, the free cobalamin rapidly binds to circulating TC II. The TC II–cobalamin complex then attaches to receptors on the surfaces of cells throughout the body. These cells take up the complex and release the cobalamin for use in their metabolism.

for less than an hour before being taken up by the tissues, the cobalamin-TC I complex has a very long survival, with a half-time measured in days. Because of the relative rates of turnover of the TC I and TC II complexes, most of the cobalamin in blood drawn at random is found to be associated with TC I. It is not known how the cobalamin–TC I complex is formed, but it is thought to be eliminated by excretion in the bile.

Cobalamin Deficiency

CAUSES

Cobalamin deficiency is almost invariably caused by a derangement in absorption. This derangement may result from a failure of IF secretion by the stomach, from disease or absence of terminal ileum, or from the presence in the small intestine of organisms that trap cobalamin on its way from the stomach to the terminal ileum.

Gastric Failure

The most common cause of cobalamin deficiency is a failure of IF secretion caused by atrophy of the gastric mucosa. This atrophy, currently thought to result from autoimmune destruction, leads to the condition known as *pernicious anemia*. The term pernicious anemia is sometimes used as a synonym for anemia caused by cobalamin deficiency from any cause, but it should be reserved for this one specific condition.

Other conditions that lead to the destruction or elimination of the gastric mucosa will also cause cobalamin deficiency of gastric origin.

Causes of Cobalamin Deficiency

Gastric
    Gastric atrophy (pernicious anemia)
    Total gastrectomy
Ileal
    Disease of terminal ileum (regional
        enteritis, tropical sprue)
    Ileal resection
Competing organisms
    Bacterial overgrowth (blind loops,
        intestinal strictures)
    Fish tapeworm

The most common of these conditions is total gastrectomy.

Disease or Absence of the Terminal Ileum

Cobalamin deficiency can result from the destruction or elimination of the terminal ileum, the portion of the small intestine that possesses the capacity to absorb IF–cobalamin. Diseases that can affect the terminal ileum so as to cause cobalamin deficiency include regional enteritis (Crohn's disease), tropical sprue, and others. Absence of the terminal ileum is invariably the result of surgical resection.

Competing Organisms in the Small Intestine

Normally the small intestine is relatively free of bacteria. However, abnormalities that impede the free flow of material through the organ may permit the accumulation of bacteria in the small intestine in numbers sufficient to cause cobalamin deficiency by taking up the vitamin from the gut before it can reach the terminal ileum. Conditions such as intestinal diverticula or surgically created blind loops contain masses of bacteria that are constantly overflowing into the intestinal lumen, where they can take up the vitamin. Similarly, cobalamin-trapping bacteria will accumulate behind intestinal strictures. Clinically significant cobalamin deficiency is a common complication of these conditions.

The fish tapeworm, *Diphyllobothrium latum*, accumulates cobalamin avidly. Infestation with this worm can result in cobalamin deficiency.

MANIFESTATIONS

Megaloblastic Anemia

The megaloblastic anemia of cobalamin deficiency is identical to that seen in folate deficiency and in fact arises because of a deficiency in tissue folate that develops in cobalamin-deficient patients (Fig. 6-12). The basis of this anemia is an impairment in the activity of the cobalamin-requiring methyltransferase that occurs in cobalamin deficiency. After entering the cell, N^5-methyl THF, the circulating form of folate, is demethylated to THF by methyltransferase. The THF is then conjugated to a polyglutamate side chain, converting it to a form that can be retained by the cell. In cobalamin deficiency, conjugation is compromised because of an impairment in the conversion of the poorly conjugable N^5-methyl THF to the readily conjugable demethylated form. With the failure of conjugation, there is leakage of folate out of the cell, leading to a deficiency of tissue folate. In this connection it should be pointed out that the megaloblastic anemia of cobalamin deficiency can be fully corrected by the administration of folic acid, though the dose required is several times larger than that necessary to correct the anemia of folate deficiency.

Stomatitis and gastrointestinal mucosal alterations similar to those seen in folate deficiency are also observed in cobalamin deficiency, probably for the same reason.

Neurological Manifestations

A critically important feature of cobalamin deficiency not seen in folate deficiency is neurological disease. The disease is a demyelinating condition that most frequently affects peripheral nerves, presenting as a symmetrical mixed motor and sensory neuropathy, but it may involve the brain and spinal cord as well (Fig. 6-13). Involvement of the brain leads to dementia, psychological disturbances, or both, while cord involvement in its most severe form leads to demyelination of the posterior and lateral columns, with spastic paralysis and absent proprioception. The spinal cord disease is known as *combined system disease*, because demyelination affects both the proprioception and motor conducting systems of the cord.

Demyelination is currently thought to be caused by a defect in methylation that arises because of diminished methyltransferase activity (Fig. 6-14). The principal biological methy-

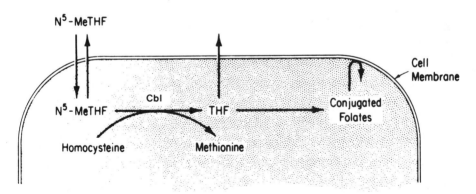

Fig. 6-12. Cobalamin deficiency leading to tissue folate depletion. Folate is taken up by cells as N^5-methyl-THF, an unconjugated form of the vitamin. Once in the cells, the folate must be conjugated (i.e., supplied with a polyglutamate chain) to keep it from leaking out again. Before the folate can be conjugated, however, it must first be demethylated. Cobalamin is required in order for this demethylation reaction to occur. When cobalamin is in short supply, demethylation is impaired. As a result, conjugation is defective, and the cells are unable to retain their folate. (Adapted from Babior BM, Bunn HF [1987] Megaloblastic anemias. In Braunwald E et al [eds]: Harrison's Principles of Internal Medicine. 11th Ed. McGraw-Hill, New York, with permission.)

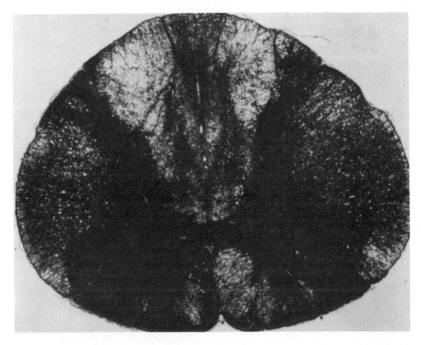

Fig. 6-13. Spinal cord demyelination in cobalamin deficiency. The myelin stains dark in this section; demyelinated areas appear as white patches. (From Robbins SL [1974] Pathologic Basis of Disease. WB Saunders, Philadelphia, with permission.)

lating agent is S-adenosylmethionine, formed from methionine and ATP. The reduction in methyltransferase activity that occurs in cobalamin deficiency leads to a decrease in methionine production, with an accompanying fall in S-adenosylmethionine formation. The result is an impairment in S-adenosylmethionine-dependent methylations—in particular, the methylation of phosphatidylethanolamine to phosphatidylcholine, and the methylation of a critical histidine in myelin basic protein. Demyelination is presumably a consequence of this impairment in methylation.

A crucial feature of this demyelinating condition is that it may be seen in the absence of megaloblastic anemia and under these circumstances is easy to misdiagnose. This is a tragic error, because, unlike the anemia, the neurological disease may not be completely reversed by vitamin replacement therapy. Indeed, neurological disease has been reported to occur after the erroneous treatment of cobalamin-deficient

megaloblastic anemia with folate, which will correct the anemia, but will obviously have no effect on the neurological abnormalities of cobalamin deficiency.

Pernicious anemia

Pernicious anemia has clinical features not seen in other forms of cobalamin deficiency.

Epidemiological. Pernicious anemia is typically a disease of late middle age, although onset in late childhood or adolescence occurs very occasionally. It is seen most frequently in northern Europeans and American blacks. There is a tendency for the disease to run in families.

Gastric. Because of the atrophy of parietal cells, total achlorhydria is a universal feature of pernicious anemia. The frequency of gastric cancer is increased in pernicious anemia, although malignancy generally develops only after many years of disease.

NORMAL

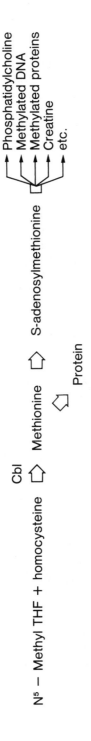

COBALAMIN DEFICIENCY

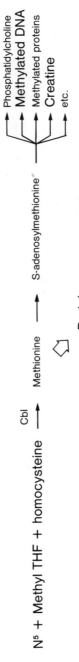

Fig. 6-14. Deficient methylation in cobalamin deficiency. In cobalamin deficiency, the production of methionine from homocysteine and N^5-methyltetrahydrofolic acid is decreased. As a result, there is an impairment in the biosynthesis of S-adenosylmethionine, the principal biological methylating agent. This leads in turn to a drop in the rates of reactions in which S-adenosylmethionine participates. These reactions include the methylation of DNA, important in the regulation of gene expression, and the production of a large number of essential biochemical materials, including among others phosphatidylcholine, creatine, and methylated proteins.

cause of the cobalamin deficiency, however, requires further testing.

A useful test for this purpose is the Schilling test, which measures cobalamin absorption by determining the fraction of an orally administered dose of radioactive cobalamin excreted in the urine over 24 to 48 hours (Fig. 6-15). To carry out this test, radioactive cobalamin is given by mouth. TC I and TC II are then saturated by means of a large parenteral dose of nonradioactive cobalamin. Because of the saturation of the transcobalamins, any labeled cobalamin absorbed from the intestine is carried in the blood in the unbound form and is rapidly cleared by the kidney. Decreased excretion of label in the urine therefore indicates decreased intestinal absorption of the vitamin (assuming normal renal function). This can arise from any of the causes noted above. To distinguish among these causes, the Schilling test is repeated with the modification that intrinsic factor is given by mouth along with the labeled vitamin. Cobalamin malabsorption of gastric origin is corrected by this procedure, whereas cobalamin malabsorption caused by ileal disease is not; cobalamin malabsorption resulting from competition by intestinal organisms may or may not be corrected by oral intrinsic factor.

Other investigations that may be carried out will depend on the whole clinical story. They should be directed toward ascertaining the cause of the condition in the most efficient way.

Cobalamin deficiency is treated by parenteral administration of the vitamin. Depending on whether the cause of the deficiency is reversible, parenteral vitamin therapy may be necessary for the duration of the patient's life. Treatable conditions such as bacterial overgrowth, anatomical abnormalities of the intestine, or fish tapeworm infestation should be corrected where possible by appropriate medical or surgical therapy.

The response of the anemia to treatment is similar to that seen in folate-deficient anemia: reversal of the marrow abnormalities in 1 to 2 days and a reticulocytosis peaking within about 1 week after the start of therapy (Fig. 6-8). Neurological manifestations, however, may correct themselves only partially, or not at all.

SPECIAL FEATURES OF PERNICIOUS ANEMIA

Epidemiological
    Most frequent in northern Europeans, American blacks
    Tends to run in families
Gastric
    Achlorhydria
    Increased incidence of gastric cancer
Immunological
    Antibodies against parietal cells and intrinsic factor
    Associated with other autoimmune diseases (e.g., Hashimoto's thyroiditis)

Immunological. Almost all patients with pernicious anemia have a serum antibody against parietal cells, and most show antibodies against intrinsic factor. The antiparietal cell antibodies are currently thought to play a role in the pathogenesis of the condition. Other autoimmune diseases, particularly Hashimoto's thyroiditis, are increased in frequency in pernicious anemia.

Other Manifestations

Manifestations specific for the cause of the vitamin deficiency may be seen. Ileal disease is associated with characteristic gastroenterological signs and symptoms. Bacterial overgrowth may be associated with fat malabsorption, and an anatomical lesion of the small intestine (e.g., intestinal diverticula) may be seen on the radiograph. *Diphyllobothrium latum* infestation may be indicated by eggs or macroscopically visible proglottids in the stools.

MANAGEMENT

The existence of a state of cobalamin deficiency can be established by measurements of serum cobalamin levels. To determine the

Other Causes of Megaloblastic Anemia

Drugs that interfere with DNA synthesis can cause megaloblastic anemia (see also Ch. 30). These drugs fall into two categories: those that interfere with DNA synthesis per se (examples are hydroxyurea, which inhibits ribonucleotide reductase, and cytosine arabinoside, an analog of cytosine) and those that antagonize folate (examples are the antiprotozoal drugs pentamidine and pyrimethamine, the diuretic triamterine, and the antibiotic trimethoprim). Megaloblastic anemia induced by these drugs is usually mild, occurring as a rather harmless concomitant of their therapeutic action, and generally needs no treatment. If treatment is required, the most effective measure is to eliminate the drug or lower its dose, and give supplemental folic acid. Correction of the anemia occurs promptly.

With one drug, however, megaloblastic anemia can represent a very serious problem. This drug is methotrexate, a commonly used chemotherapeutic agent (Fig. 6-16).

NON-NUTRITIONAL CAUSES OF MEGALOBLASTIC ANEMIA

Drugs
  Inhibitors of DNA synthesis
  Folate antagonists
    Methotrexate
    Other
Idiopathic
  Refractory megaloblastic anemia
  Di Guglielmo syndrome
  Congenital dyserythropoietic anemia

Methotrexate is an exceedingly powerful inhibitor of dihydrofolate reductase, the enzyme necessary for the regeneration of tetrahydrofolate from the dihydrofolate produced in the thymidylate synthetase reaction. In the presence of toxic concentrations of the drug, this reaction is almost totally blocked, with the result that most of the tissue folate becomes trapped in a metabolically inert pool

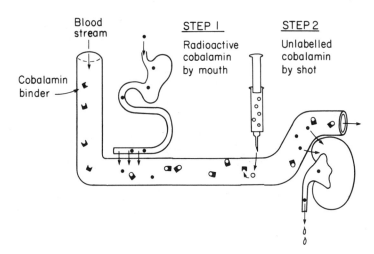

Fig. 6-15. Schilling test. A dose of radioactive cobalamin is first given by mouth. The circulating cobalamin binders are then saturated by giving a large dose of unlabeled cobalamin by injection. Because the binders are saturated with unlabeled cobalamin, any free radioactive cobalamin absorbed from the intestine will find nothing to bind to and will have to circulate as the free vitamin, which is rapidly excreted into the urine. The amount of radioactivity appearing in the urine thus indicates how well the vitamin is absorbed from the intestine.

Methotrexate

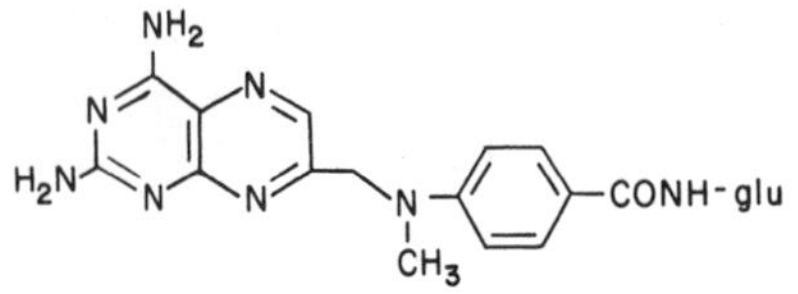

N^5-formyl THF

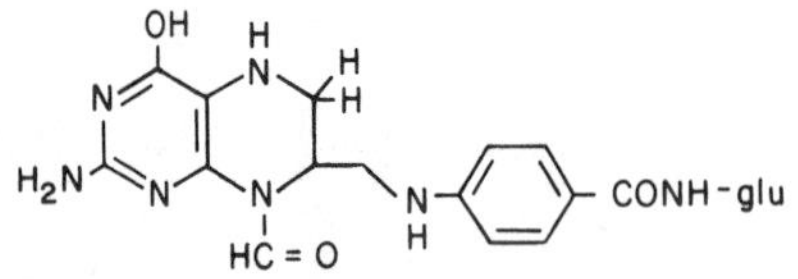

Fig. 6-16. Methotrexate and its antidote. Methotrexate is a powerful inhibitor of dihydrofolate reductase, blocking the regeneration of THF and bringing to a halt all folate-requiring reactions. Methotrexate blockade can be circumvented by giving N^5-formyl-THF, a metabolically functional form of THF that can be given as a drug.

of dihydrofolate. Folate-requiring processes such as the biosynthesis of purines and dTMP are thereby brought to a halt, with serious clinical consequences affecting rapidly replicating tissues. A florid megaloblastic anemia quickly develops. A severe and agonizingly painful stomatitis also ensues. The most serious consequence, however, is necrosis of the mucosa of the gastrointestinal tract, with severe nausea and vomiting and fulminant diarrhea that may be grossly bloody. A fatal outcome can be expected in severe methotrexate poisoning.

Fortunately, there exists a specific antidote for methotrexate poisoning: citrovorum factor, or N^5-formyltetrahydrofolate. This compound, unlike other tetrahydrofolate derivatives, is stable in air and consequently can be used to provide an exogenous supply of fully reduced folate. After administration, it is converted in an ATP-requiring reaction to N^{10}-formyl THF, which is freely interconvertible with the other forms of THF that are normally present in tissues. In this manner, the pool of metabolically active folates is replenished, and the clinical manifestations of methotrexate poisoning are rapidly corrected.

Idiopathic Conditions

REFRACTORY MEGALOBLASTIC ANEMIA

A form of bone marrow failure of unknown etiology, refractory megaloblastic anemia occurs generally in patients of late middle age or older. It is characterized clinically by reduced numbers of any or all of the formed elements of the blood, a variable incidence of morphological peculiarities especially among cells of the granulocyte series (e.g., hypogranularity, abnormal nuclear segmentation), and a marrow that is hypocellular and shows megaloblastic changes in the red cell series only (i.e., no giant bands of metamyelocytes). The condition is a form of myelodysplasia (Ch. 27), with a similarly bad prognosis and a similar tendency to evolve into a particularly intractible form of acute myelogenous leukemia. Treatment is generally supportive, although an occasional patient may respond to pharmacological doses of pyridoxine.

DI GUGLIELMO SYNDROME

Di Guglielmo Syndrome is a form of leukemia in which malignant red cell precursors are particularly evident. It is mentioned here because megaloblastic red cell precursors are almost invariably seen in the marrow in this condition.

CONGENITAL DYSERYTHROPOIETIC ANEMIAS

Congenital dyserythropoietic anemias are rare and poorly understood inherited disorders that present as an isolated anemia with no other hematological abnormalities. Anemia is present from birth, but may not be picked up for years. The diseases (there are three types) are characterized by ineffective erythropoiesis together with abnormalities in the nuclei of red cell precursors, the most obvious of which is multiple nuclei. Megaloblastic changes are seen in the most common type, which seems to be due to a defect in the synthesis of a particular class of cell surface carbohydrates. Life expectancy in the congenital dyserythropoietic anemias is normal, and treatment is generally not required.

SUGGESTED READINGS

Allen RH (1976) The plasma transport of vitamin B12. Br J Haematol 36:153

Babior BM (ed) (1975) Cobalamin: Biochemistry and Pathophysiology. Wiley, New York

Beck WS (1991) Diagnosis of megaloblastic anemia. Annu Rev Med 42:311

Beck WS (1991) Neuropsychiatric consequences of cobalamin deficiency. Adv Intern Med 36:33

Besa EC (1992) Myelodysplastic syndromes (refractory anemia). A perspective of the biologic, clinical, and therapeutic issues. Med Clin North Am 76:599

Chanarin I (1979) The Megaloblastic Anemias. 2nd Ed. Blackwell, Oxford

Chanarin I, Deacon R, Perry J, Lumb M (1981) How vitamin B12 acts. Br J Haematol 47:487

Chanarin I, Deacon R, Lumb M, Perry J (1992) Cobalamin and folate: recent developments. J Clin Pathol 45:277

Hoffbrand AV (ed) (1976) Megaloblastic anaemia. Clin Haematol 5, no. 3.

Herbert V (1985) Megaloblastic anemias. Lab Invest 52:3

Kapadia CR, Donaldson RM, Jr (1985) Disorders of cobalamin (vitamin B12) absorption and transport. Annu Rev Med 36:93

Lindenbaum J (1979) Aspects of vitamin B_{12} and folate metabolism in malabsorption syndromes. Am J Med 67:1037

Lindenbaum J, Roman MJ (1980) Nutritional anemia in alcoholism. Am J Clin Nutr 33:2727

Rosenblatt DS, Cooper BA (1987) Inherited disorders of vitamin B12 metabolism. Blood Rev 1:177

Scott JM, Weir DG (1980) Drug-induced megaloblastic change. Clin Haematol 9:587

Shane B, Stokstad EL (1985) Vitamin B_{12}-folate interrelationships. Annu Rev Nutr 5:115

Shojania AM (1984) Folic acid and vitamin B_{12} deficiency in pregnancy and in the neonatal period. Clin Perinatol 11:433

Shojania AM (1980) Problems in diagnosis and investigation of megaloblastic anemia. Can Med Assoc J 122:999

7

Hypoproliferative Anemia

In a few conditions anemia develops because of an isolated suppression of erythropoiesis. White cell and platelet production are normal, but red cell production is sluggish and feeble. The clinical picture is almost invariably that of a normochromic, normocytic anemia. The reticulocyte count may be low, normal, or high, but it is always less than expected for the observed hematocrit, and the bone marrow shows a reduction in red cell precursors (Fig. 7-1).

RENAL FAILURE

The most frequent cause of an isolated hypoproliferative anemia is chronic renal failure. Patients with severe chronic renal failure may have hematocrits as low as 20 solely on the basis of their underlying disease (Fig. 7-2). Other anemia-producing factors are also at work in these patients (e.g., red cell survival is often somewhat decreased, the tendency to bleed from the gastrointestinal tract may lead to iron deficiency, and complications caused by dialysis may also contribute to the anemia), but diminished red cell production caused by renal insufficiency is the baseline on which all these other factors are superimposed.

The anemia of chronic renal failure is generally attributed to the decrease in erythropoietin production that results from the reduced mass of the failing kidney (Ch. 2). This is clearly part of the story, because erythropoietin levels in patients with chronic renal failure are defi-nitely lower than in patients with equally severe anemias from other causes. Erythropoietin, however, does not disappear from the blood; in fact in some patients, erythropoietin levels are substantially higher than normal, although not as high as would be expected from the degree of anemia. This indicates that the patient with chronic renal failure exhibits not only a deficiency of erythropoietin, but also a deficiency in the response of the bone marrow to such erythropoietin as is present. Apparently a second factor plays a role in the anemia of renal failure, acting directly on the marrow to suppress red cell production. The identity of this second factor is unknown.

Clinically, the anemia is normochromic and normocytic, with a reduction in reticulocytes, just as expected for a hypoproliferative anemia. Under the microscope, the red cells may be normal in shape, or they may show knobs distributed in a regular pattern over the red cell surface—the so-called burr cells (Fig. 7-3). Functionally, the red cells may show a reduction in oxygen affinity caused by an elevation in red cell 2,3-diphosphoglyceric acid (2,3-DPG), a consequence of the elevation in serum phosphate typical of chronic renal failure. The marrow shows a decreased number of red cell precursors. The spleen is normal in size. Other manifestations are primarily those of chronic renal failure, including elevations of the BUN and creatinine, characteristic electrolyte abnormalities, and abnormal findings on renal roentgenograms, as well as such clinical abnormalities as nausea and vomiting, polyuria,

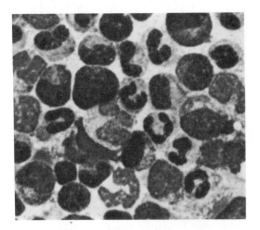

Fig. 7-1. Bone marrow in hypoproliferative anemia. This is a particulary striking example, showing no red cell precursors. (From Marmont AM, Damasio E [1981] Aplastic, hypoplastic, and metaplastic myelopathies. pp. 243. In Zucker-Franklin D et al [eds]: Atlas of Blood Cells: Function and Pathology. Edi. Ermes s.r.l., Milan, with permission.)

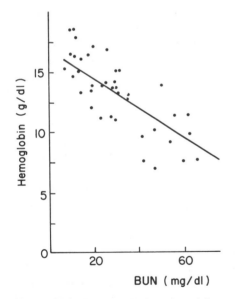

Fig. 7-2. Relationship between creatinine and hematocrit levels in chronic renal failure. (Modified from Kaye M [1958] The anemia associated with renal disease. J Lab Clin Med 52:83, with permission.)

HYPOPROLIFERATIVE ANEMIAS

Renal failure
Endocrine disorders
  Hypothyroidism
  Hypopituitarism
Pure red cell aplasia

hypertension, eye-ground abnormalities, cardiac signs and symptoms, and many others.

The anemia is treated with erythropoietin, which in adequate doses will restore hemoglobin levels to normal. The major complication of erythropoietin treatment is hypertension, which probably results from an increase in blood volume and is easily corrected by lowering the dose. Factors that aggravate the anemia (e.g., folate deficiency) should also be corrected. Dialysis is of little benefit—indeed, it can impose problems of its own—but the anemia is cured by renal transplantation.

Dialysis has added a number of types of anemia to the standard assortment seen in undialyzed renal failure patients:

1. *Iron deficiency.* This problem arises with hemodialysis because a certain amount of

FACTORS CONTRIBUTING TO THE ANEMIA IN CHRONIC RENAL FAILURE

Diminished red cell production
  Decreased erythropoietin
  Circulating inhibitor(s) of erythropoiesis
Shortened red cell life span
Chronic gastrointestinal bleeding
Dialysis
  Iron deficiency
  Folate deficiency
  Other

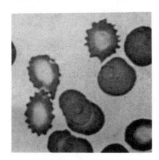

Fig. 7-3. Burr cells in renal failure. (From Erslev AJ, Gabuzda TG [1975] Pathophysiology of Blood. WB Saunders, Philadelphia, with permission.)

blood is lost through priming every time the patient is put on a hemodialysis machine. Iron deficiency may result from this recurrent loss of blood into the machine.

2. *Folate deficiency.* Folate is fully dialyzable, so folate deficiency can easily arise in patients on either hemodialysis or peritoneal dialysis as a result of losses of this vitamin into the dialysis fluid. Patients on chronic dialysis should be routinely placed on folate supplements.

3. *Other dialysis-associated anemias.* Aluminum poisoning may be the cause of a microcytic anemia in dialysis patients with normal iron stores. Very occasionally, peculiar anemias have developed in patients because of dialysis against fluids that have been defective in one way or another (e.g., too hot, deficient in a trace element required for hematopoiesis, contaminated with a hemolytic chemical). Identifying the culprit in this sort of situation can require imaginative detective work.

ENDOCRINE DISEASE

Endocrine disorders involving the thyroid and the pituitary can cause isolated hypoproliferative anemias.

Hypothyroidism

An isolated anemia is often seen in hypothyroidism. The anemia may be either normocytic or slightly macrocytic. Other clinical manifestations are those of the underlying disorder, and the anemia remits when the thyroid status is corrected.

The anemia of hypothyroidism is interesting in physiological terms, because in a sense it is not an anemia at all. It represents an appropriate response on the part of the bone marrow to the decreased tissue oxygen consumption in the hypothyroid patient. It is slow to develop and slow to remit; 3 or 4 months may be required from the onset of replacement therapy before the hematocrit returns to normal.

Aside from anemia caused by thyroid disease per se, the possibility of anemia due to cobalamin deficiency must be kept in mind in this situation. The incidence of cobalamin deficiency is increased in patients with thyroid disease because of the association between pernicious anemia and autoimmune diseases, of which both hypothyroidism (Hashimoto's) and hyperthyroidism (Graves') are examples.

Hypopituitarism

Anemia is seen in patients with panhypopituitarism. This anemia has several causes. The decrease in thyroid function that occurs in hypopituitary states accounts for some of the anemia. In men, a decrease in androgen production also accounts for some of the anemia, since androgens stimulate erythropoiesis, exerting their effect by promoting erythropoietin formation as well as by a direct effect on the marrow. (It is this action of androgens that explains why men have higher hematocrits than women.) Finally, pituitary deficiency itself has an effect on erythropoiesis over and above that caused by thyroid and gonad hypofunction. This effect is thought to be caused by a deficiency of growth hormone, which has a trophic effect on the bone marrow similar to its effect on other tissues.

The anemia of panhypopituitarism is normochromic and normocytic, with a reduction in reticulocytes and a somewhat hypocellular marrow. It is a minor component of the constellation of manifestations that make up clinical pituitary insufficiency. Treatment of the endocrine disorder is the only therapy required.

PURE RED CELL APLASIA

Pure red cell aplasia is a typical hypoproliferative anemia, with a normochromic, normocytic smear, reticulocytopenia, and a selective reduction in marrow normoblasts. It is usually caused by the immunological destruction of marrow red cell precursors. This anemia is discussed fully in the chapter on immunologically mediated blood cell disorders (Ch. 30).

Two forms of pure red cell aplasia are seen in very young children: Diamond-Blackfan syndrome and transient erythroblastopenia.

Diamond-Blackfan Syndrome

Diamond-Blackfan syndrome is a serious disorder that begins in infancy. Red cell precursors show a decreased sensitivity to erythropoietin, and the red cells themselves are fetal in character, with a high mean cell volume and elevated fetal hemoglobin (Ch. 10). The anemia, which responds variably to steroids, may last for life.

Transient Erythroblastopenia of Childhood

Transient erythroblastopenia of childhood is a typical pure red cell aplasia of immune origin. The red cells are qualitatively normal. The disorder lasts a few weeks to a few months, and then resolves spontaneously.

SUGGESTED READINGS

Ammus SS, Yunis AA (1987) Acquired pure red cell aplasia. Am J Hematol 24:311

Bailey RO, Dunn HG, Rubin AM, Ritaccio AL (1988) Myasthenia gravis with thymoma and pure red blood cell aplasia. Am J Clin Pathol 89:687

Desforges JF (1975) The role of hemodialysis in the hematological disorders of uremia. Kidney Int, suppl. 2:5123

Mansell M, Grimes AJ (1979) Red and white cell abnormalities in chronic renal failure. Br J Haematol 42:169

Dessypris EN (1991) The biology of pure red cell aplasia. Semin Hematol 28:275

Glader BE (1990) Red blood cell aplasias in children. Pediatr Ann 19:168

Hocking WG (1987) Hematologic abnormalities in patients with renal diseases. Hematol Oncol Clin North Am 1:229

Humphries JE (1992) Anemia of renal failure. Use of erythropoietin. Med Clin North Am 76:711

Nissenson AR, Nimer SD, Wolcott DL (1991) Recombinant human erythropoietin and renal anemia: molecular biology, clinical efficacy, and nervous system effects. Ann Intern Med 114:402

Raine AE (1988) Hypertension, blood viscosity, and cardiovascular morbidity in renal failure: implications of erythropoietin therapy. Lancet 1:97

8

Hemolytic Anemias: Extravascular Destruction of Red Cells

The accelerated destruction of red cells is referred to as *hemolysis*. A degree of hemolysis is seen in many diseases (e.g., renal failure, cirrhosis of the liver, megaloblastic anemias), contributing to a greater or lesser extent to the clinical manifestations that occur in these disorders. In certain conditions, however, hemolysis is the predominant pathogenetic mechanism. These conditions are known as hemolytic anemias.

The hemolytic anemias can be divided into two groups, depending on the predominant site of red cell destruction. In *extravascular* hemolysis, red cells are destroyed primarily by tissue macrophages, especially those in the spleen. In these anemias, red cell destruction can be seen as an exaggeration of the normal mechanisms of red cell disposal. In *intravascular* hemolysis, red cells are destroyed primarily by lysis in the bloodstream (see Ch. 9).

EXTRAVASCULAR HEMOLYSIS: GENERAL CONSIDERATIONS

Normal Disposal of Red Cells

Red cells normally live for 4 months, and then die of old age. The disposal of senile red cells is thought to be handled mainly by the spleen.

To understand how such disposal is accomplished requires some feeling for the anatomy of this complex organ (Fig. 8-1). The spleen contains two regions, the red pulp and the white pulp, surrounded by a fibrous capsule and fed by a vasculature having an unusually complicated organization. By tracing the splenic blood supply from the arterial side to the venous side, the relationship between anatomy and function can be understood.

Arteries enter the spleen from the capsule and from fibrous extensions of the capsule into the splenic pulp. These arteries are surrounded for much of their length by a sheath of lymphoid cells known as the white pulp. The arteries give off branches along their length, some passing through the white pulp and other more remote branches entering the red pulp directly. These branches terminate in two ways:

1. Some expand to form thin-walled sinuses that eventually join to form veins that carry blood out of the spleen. Blood cells can pass through the relatively open structure of the sinus walls, although it is a tight squeeze (Fig. 8-2).

2. Others empty directly into the cords. The cords, so called because of their appearance under the microscope, actually represent a continuous mass of loosely organized tissue

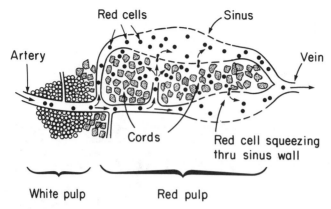

Fig. 8-1. Anatomy of the spleen, bird's eye-view. To understand how the spleen is organized, trace the artery shown by the arrow. It tunnels through a sheath of lymphoid cells, then penetrates into a loosely organized mass of phagocytes and reticular cells known as the splenic cords. All along its course it sends out branches. Some of these branches widen into sinuses that meander through the cords and eventually join to form the splenic veins. Others end as open pipes that empty directly into the splenic cords. The sheath of lymphoid cells is called the white pulp, and the region of cords and sinuses is called the red pulp. Blood flowing through the spleen follows one of two routes. In one route, known as the closed circulation, the blood flows directly from an arterial branch into a sinus. In the other route, known as the open circulation, the blood is first delivered into the splenic cords, where it percolates through the mass of cordal cells. Only then does it enter the sinus, penetrating the sinus wall from the outside. It is while in the cords that the blood is worked on by the spleen.

composed largely of reticular cells and mononuclear phagocytes, through which the sinuses ramify.

The mass of cordal tissue and associated vasculature constitute the red pulp of the spleen.

Of the blood that enters the spleen, a fraction is delivered directly into the sinuses, where flow is brisk. The remainder is delivered into the cords. Plasma delivered into the cords is able to enter the sinuses freely, but the entry of cells into the sinuses is impeded because of the resistance to passage offered by the sinus wall. The local hematocrit in the splenic cords therefore rises sharply, and the continuing metabolic activity combined with sluggish flow causes the local oxygen tension, pH, and glucose concentration to drop. Normal red cells can resist these metabolic assaults and will eventually make their way into the sinuses and out into the general circulation. Senile or defective cells have impaired resistance to

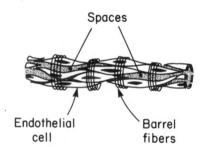

Fig. 8-2. The sinus wall. The sinus is a flattened tube with a wall consisting of a single layer of endothelial cells laid down with their long axes parallel to the direction of blood flow. Along their lateral edges the endothelial cells are only loosely attached to each other, so they are able to separate to form an opening through with blood cells can pass. Wrapped around the sinuses are the barrel fibers, thin strands of collagen that serve to shape and strengthen the sinus wall. The barrel fibers occur only at intervals along the sinus wall; between them, the endothelial cells are in direct contact with the splenic cords. Blood cells squeeze into the sinuses through spaces bounded on the top and bottom by the edges of the separated endothelial cells and on the sides by the barrel fibers.

these stresses and sooner or later are destroyed in the splenic cords with the aid of the resident mononuclear phagocyte system.

It is not known how the mononuclear phagocytes recognize susceptible red cells. Once recognition occurs, however, the phagocytes appear to dispose of each defective red cell piecemeal, like a school of hungry piranhas. Fragments of the red cell are ingested and degraded in a characteristic way. Most of the components, including the globin portion of the ingested hemoglobin, are degraded to their constitutent building blocks (e.g., amino acids), which can then be used for other purposes.

Heme, however, is lost almost completely, only the iron being saved for reuse.

The disposal of heme is of clinical significance, since the accumulation of the products of heme degradation is responsible for some important signs of hemolysis. The following are the steps in heme degradation (Fig. 8-3):

1. *Cleavage of porphyrin ring.* The porphyrin ring is opened by the oxidation of the a–methene bridge (the one-carbon bridge between the two vinyl-bearing pyrrole rings). This oxidation is catalyzed by the microsomal enzyme heme oxygenase. The products of this reaction are iron, the linear tetrapyrrole

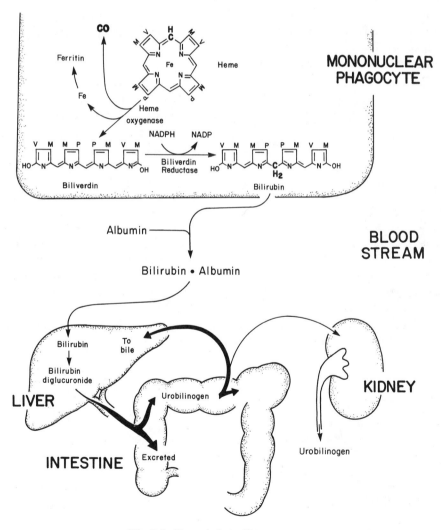

Fig. 8-3. Degradation of heme.

biliverdin, and a molecule of carbon monoxide that represents the oxidized a–methene bridge. Heme degradation is virtually the only endogenous source of carbon monoxide in humans.

2. *Disposal of cleavage products.* The liberated iron is incorporated into ferritin, while the biliverdin is reduced to bilirubin, and then released into the bloodstream. Here it binds tightly to albumin and is carried in this form to the liver for final elimination.

3. *Bilirubin in the liver.* On reaching the liver, bilirubin dissociates from its albumin carrier and enters the hepatocyte. In this cell it is converted to a highly water-soluble derivative, bilirubin diglucuronide, through a reaction known as conjugation. Finally, the conjugated bilirubin is excreted through the bile into the intestine.

4. *Urobilinogen.* On reaching the intestine, a portion of the bilirubin is acted on by bacteria, which further reduce it to urobilinogen. The urobilinogen is absorbed into the bloodstream but is then rapidly re-excreted, most by the liver but some by the kidneys.

Phagocytes are messy eaters. As a result, extravascular hemolysis, whether normal or pathological, is always accompanied by the spillage of some hemoglobin into the plasma. This free hemoglobin is not handled by the mononuclear phagocytes, but is dealt with instead by the hepatocytes, which take it up with the aid of a circulating protein known as haptoglobin (Fig. 8-4). This protein is avid for hemoglobin, forming a very tight 1:1 complex with the hemoglobin tetramer. The release of hemoglobin into the plasma is followed almost instantly by the formation of the hemoglobin–haptoglobin complex. This complex is rapidly transported into the hepatocytes (the half-life for the disappearance of the circulating complex is about 10 minutes). Once there, the hemoglobin is degraded just as it would be in the mononuclear phagocytes, that is, the protein is digested, the iron is deposited as ferritin, and the porphyrin ring is converted to bilirubin and excreted.

Asplenia (Absence of the Spleen)

In the absence of the spleen, screening for defective erythrocytes is impaired, and red cells with characteristic morphological abnormalities appear in the circulation. Many of the cells are misshapen, whereas others may contain nuclear remnants, such as Howell-Jolly bodies and Cabot rings (Fig. 8-5), or precipitates of denatured hemoglobin (not seen on routine smears, but visible as Heinz bodies when the blood is stained with crystal violet). These abnormal red cells are not seen in normal blood, presumably because they are rapidly recognized and destroyed by the spleen after release into the bloodstream. Howell-Jolly bodies and Cabot rings are so typical of asplenia that their presence in a blood smear strongly suggests that the spleen is either absent or nonfunctional.

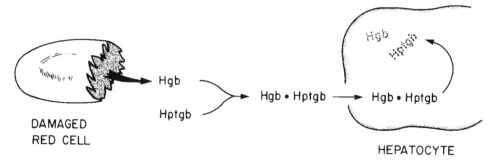

Fig. 8-4. Haptoglobin removal of free hemoglobin from the bloodstream.

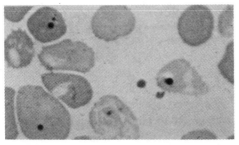
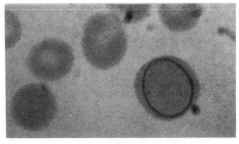

A   B

Fig. 8-5. Howell-Jolly bodies and a Cabot ring. (**A**) Howell-Jolly bodies are small, round, darkly-stained nuclear fragments. (**B**) The Cabot ring is a thin, darkly-stained ring that follows the margin of the red cell. (From Castoldi GL [1981] Erythrocytes. In Zucker-Franklin D et al [eds]: Atlas of Blood Cells: Function and Pathology. Edi. Ermes s.r.l., Milan, with permission.)

Asplenia also causes a rise in both the white count and the platelet count (especially the latter), and induces an unusual susceptibility to certain types of infections. The red cell lifespan is not altered by the absence of the spleen, probably because the liver and other mononuclear phagocyte-containing organs are able to take over the spleen's job of destroying senile red cells.

Manifestations

Accelerated extravascular hemolysis, of whatever origin, always leads to (1) hypertrophy of the spleen, to handle the increased red cell load; (2) a compensatory increase in red cell production on the part of the marrow; and (3) increased hemoglobin breakdown, associated with a rise in the consumption of haptoglobin and an increased bilirubin load for the liver to excrete (Table 8-1). Many of the signs and symptoms of hemolysis reflect these secondary consequences of red cell destruction. Others,

caused by the anemia itself, are ordinarily not prominent unless the condition is severe in degree or abrupt in development.

SPLENIC HYPERTROPHY

Enlargement of the spleen is one of the most constant clinical findings in extravascular hemolysis.

INCREASED RED CELL PRODUCTION

Signs include the release of young erythrocytes into the peripheral blood and an increase in marrow cellularity as red cell precursors expand in response to need. A reticulocytosis is therefore an almost invariable consequence of hemolysis. The release of younger forms is unusual, but if hemolysis is both severe and acute, normoblasts may appear. With increased red cell production comes an increased need for iron by the marrow, leading to a rise in the plasma iron turnover (PIT).

Table 8-1. Principal Manifestations of Extravascular Hemolysis

Mechanism	Clinical	Laboratory
Splenic hypertrophy	Splenomegaly	
Increased red cell production		Reticulocytosis Marrow red cell hyperplasia
Increased hemoglobin breakdown	Jaundice Gallstones	Indirect bilirubinemia Decreased serum haptoglobin
Red cell destruction	Pallor and faintness Cardiac symptoms Aggravation of underlying vascular disease	Anemia

Normal marrow can increase its red cell production as much as eightfold. Anemia occurs when the marrow's ability to manufacture red cells is outstripped by the hemolytic process. In some cases the marrow can keep up; under such circumstances anemia does not develop, although other signs of hemolysis (e.g., reticulocytosis) are still evident.

INCREASED HEMOGLOBIN BREAKDOWN

The rise in bilirubin production leads to an increase in serum bilirubin concentration. This condition can be detected at the bedside as well as in the laboratory, because excess bilirubin is deposited in the skin and sclerae, where it gives rise to jaundice. In uncomplicated hemolytic anemia, the bilirubin that accumulates in the bloodstream is in the unconjugated form, because a normal liver can conjugate and excrete bilirubin as fast as it can be taken up. Unconjugated bilirubinemia is reported by the laboratory as an increase in "indirect bilirubin," a term referring to a method for measuring bilirubin that detects mostly the unconjugated form. If there is liver damage along with hemolytic anemia, both unconjugated and conjugated bilirubin appear in the blood, the latter leaking into the bloodstream from the damaged liver cell before it can be excreted in the bile.

Conjugated bilirubinemia is reported as an increase in direct bilirubin.

Products of bilirubin metabolism can also be detected in the urine. The increase in bilirubin delivered to the intestine leads to an increase in urobilinogen production and consequently to the delivery of more urobilinogen into the urine, where it is detected both as such and as its product of oxidation, urobilin. Conjugated bilirubin will also be excreted in the urine if it is present in the blood in significant concentrations; unconjugated bilirubin is insoluble in water, and never appears in the urine.

Another sign of increased hemoglobin breakdown is an alteration in iron kinetics (Fig. 8-6). Red cell iron leaves the bloodstream with unusual speed and accumulates in the spleen in greater than normal amounts as the short-lived red cells are trapped and destroyed in the splenic pulp. There is also an increase in haptoglobin consumption, as haptoglobin molecules capture the hemoglobin spilled into the plasma during hemolysis and carry it to the liver. The result is a fall in serum haptoglobin levels.

ANEMIA

Pallor, faintness, signs of cardiac dysfunction, and signs and symptoms localized to areas in which the blood supply has previously been compromised by vascular disease are indicators of anemia.

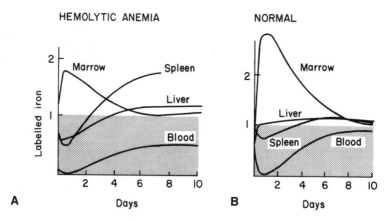

Fig. 8-6. Ferrokinetics of hemolytic anemia. (**A**) Hemolysis. (**B**) Normal. (**B:** From Finch CA et al [1970] Ferrokinetics in man. Medicine 49:17, with permission.)

Special Problems

Adding to all the foregoing are three special problems that can cause trouble in patients with extravascular hemolysis, especially if their condition is chronic and severe:

GALLSTONES

The increased load of excreted bilirubin may lead to the precipitation of bilirubin stones in the gallbladder. These stones tend to be multiple and small and are sometimes radiopaque because of their calcium content. Gallstones in an adolescent or young adult should suggest a hemolytic anemia of long duration.

APLASTIC CRISES

These episodes are characterized by the disappearance of reticulocytes from the blood and a plummeting hematocrit. Aplastic crises are usually caused by acute marrow suppression secondary to a parvovirus infection. Parvovirus-related marrow suppression also occurs in persons with normal red cell survival, but it usually goes unnoticed because marrow function returns before the uncompensated loss of senile red cells from the circulation has had a chance to produce a significant degree of anemia. When the red cell lifespan is short, however, a cutoff of red cell production can cause an abrupt drop in the hematocrit as a result of uncompensated hemolysis. Despite their transiency, aplastic crises may result in life-threatening degrees of anemia.

ICTERUS NEONATORUM

In newborns and especially in premature infants with extravascular hemolysis, unconjugated bilirubin can rise to very high levels in the serum, because the bilirubin-conjugating system in the liver is not mature enough to handle all the bilirubin that is delivered to it. The result is neonatal jaundice (so-called *icterus neonatorum*). This is very dangerous, because bilirubin at high concentrations is a potent central nervous system toxin that can rapidly cripple or kill a jaundiced infant. Jaundice develops within a day or so after birth, and CNS toxicity appears shortly thereafter unless steps are taken immediately to reduce bilirubin levels.

Measuring Red Cell Survival

It is possible to establish the diagnosis of a hemolytic state by measuring the red cell lifespan. This measurement is generally made by labeling red cells with radioactive chromium and following the disappearance of the tagged cells from the blood over a period of time. Labeling is accomplished by withdrawing whole blood from the patient and incubating it with $Na^{51}CrO_4$. The label is taken up by the red cells, reduced to $^{51}Cr^{3+}$, and fixed to protein. Cells are then reinfused, and blood samples are obtained at intervals for measurements of ^{51}Cr levels.

A normal survival curve is shown in Figure 8-7. Since red cells of all ages are labeled by the ^{51}Cr tagging procedure, and since red cells die at about age 120 days, it would be expected that the survival curve of ^{51}Cr-tagged red cells would be a straight line, reaching zero at 120 days. What is seen, however, is a nonlinear disappearance curve with the 50 percent survival point at about 25 days, not the 60 days expect-

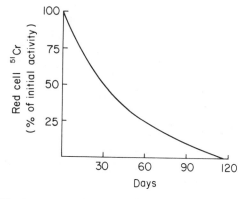

Fig. 8-7. Survival of ^{51}Cr-tagged red cells. (Adapted from Wintrobe MM et al [1974] Clinical Hematology. 7th Ed. Lea & Febiger, Philadelphia, with permission.)

ed from what is known about red cell kinetics. This deviation from expected results occurs because ^{51}Cr is lost from the blood through leaching from the cells as well as through destruction of the cells, making absolute red cell survival difficult to measure by this method. Red cell survival relative to normal, however, can be measured reliably with this technique and has proved useful for demonstrating accelerated red cell destruction in anemic patients.

The site of red cell destruction (i.e., spleen versus other mononuclear phagocyte-containing organs, particularly the liver) can also be determined using ^{51}Cr-tagged red cells. For this determination, the amount of radioactivity taken up by the organ in question is measured by scanning. This method has been used to try to predict the usefulness of splenectomy in patients with extravascular hemolysis, but without much success.

EXTRAVASCULAR HEMOLYTIC ANEMIAS

Hemolytic anemias in which red cell destruction is accomplished primarily by the mononuclear phagocyte system are listed below.

EXTRAVASCULAR HEMOLYTIC ANEMIAS

Autoimmune hemolytic anemia
Diseases of the red cell membrane
    Hereditary spherocytosis
    Others
Spur cell anemia
    Liver disease
    Abetalipoproteinemia (very rare)
Congenital nonspherocytic hemolytic
  anemia
    Pyruvate kinase deficiency
    Others
Unstable hemoglobin disease

Autoimmune Hemolytic Anemia

The commonest cause of extravascular hemolysis is autoimmune hemolytic anemia. This disease results from the presence of an antibody that binds to autologous red cells, marking them for destruction by phagocytes. See Chapter 30 for a full discussion of this anemia.

Hereditary Spherocytosis and Other Diseases of the Red Cell Membrane

Certain inherited red cell disorders result in a characteristic abnormality of red cell shape. These disorders are thought to be caused by an abnormality of one or another of the constituent proteins of the red cell membrane. In all but one of these disorders, extravascular hemolysis is an invariable feature.

THE RED CELL MEMBRANE

Like all cells, the red cell is enclosed within a plasma membrane composed of lipids and proteins. The lipids, which consist principally of cholesterol and phospholipids, are arranged in a bilayer in which the membrane proteins are embedded. The plasma membrane can thus be characterized as a sort of two-dimensional solution of proteins in lipid. Some of the proteins are free to move, floating about in the bilayer like icebergs in the sea; others are anchored more or less firmly in place.

Lying immediately beneath the plasma membrane is the cytoskeleton, a network of structural proteins that confers on the red cell its unique discoid shape. The most characteristic protein of the cytoskeleton is *spectrin,* a large (MW $\sim 10^6$) tetramer unique to red cells. The spectrin tetramers are long and flexible and form a fibrous network that lines the inner surface of the membrane (Fig. 8-8). The flexibility of the spectrin strands give the network a rubberlike elasticity. This elasticity is what makes the red cell able to deform reversibly

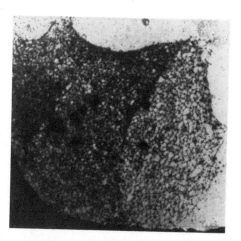

Fig. 8-8. The red cell cytoskeleton. The red cell membrane has been stretched to show the network of supporting proteins that lies beneath the lipid bilayer. The links that connect the nodes of the network are spectrin tetramers, each composed of a pair of long, thin spectrin dimers attached end to end. The spectrin dimers in turn are made up of a pair of threadlike spectrin monomers twisted around each other like the strands of a rope. (From Palek J, Sahr KE [1992] Mutations of the red blood cell membrane proteins: from clinical evaluation to detection of the underlying genetic defect. Blood 80:308, with permission.)

when passing through narrow spaces in capillaries and the spleen.

Other cytoskeletal components include actin, adducin, ankyrin (sometimes called band 2.1), and band 4.1. *Ankyrin* and *band 4.1* anchor the cytoskeleton to the plasma membrane, ankyrin attaching to band 3, the anion exchanger that resides in the red cell membrane, and band 4.1 to a membrane glycoprotein called glycophorin C. (Band 3 and glycophorin C are examples of plasma membrane proteins that are unable to move freely in the plane of the bilayer.) The way these proteins are assembled to form the cytoskeleton is shown in Figure 8-9.

The red cell plasma membrane contains many different proteins, but few have been assigned a function. Of those few, the most important in clinical terms is the Na^+/K^+ ATPase, the ion pump that maintains the Na^+ and K^+ gradients across the red cell membrane.

In the normal erythrocyte, the intracellular Na^+ concentration is about 15 mEq/L, and the K^+ concentration 85 mEq/L. By contrast, in the plasma, the Na^+ and K^+ concentrations are 140 and 5 mEq/L, respectively. This disparity between the intracellular and extracellular ion concentrations passively drives Na^+ into the red cell and K^+ out. Though these passive ionic movements are very slow because of the low permeability of the plasma membrane, there is nevertheless a steady trickle of ions that has to be counteracted if the difference between the intracellular and extracellular ion concentrations is to be maintained. The agent responsible for counteracting this slow tendency to ionic equilibration is the membrane Na^+/K^+ ATPase. This enzyme, a multisubunit protein that completely traverses the plasma membrane, catalyzes an ion exchange reaction in which Na^+ is pumped out of the red cell in exchange for K^+ or H^+, which is pumped in. In this uphill process, energy is obtained from the hydrolysis of ATP, one molecule for each exchange reaction. This is thought to be the major ATP-consuming reaction of the red cell.

Much of the information on red cell membrane proteins has been obtained through gel electrophoresis of purified red cell membrane preparations. Protein patterns obtained by this technique are shown in Figure 8-10. The protein bands, which are highly reproducible from sample to sample, are numbered according to molecular weight, the bands of highest molecular weight (those migrating the smallest distance into the gel) being given the lowest numbers. This numbering pattern provides the basis for the numerical terminology referred to above. Names and functions have been assigned to several of the numbered proteins (Table 8-2).

HEREDITARY SPHEROCYTOSIS

Hereditary spherocytosis (HS) is the commonest of the inherited disorders of red cell shape. In this disorder, cells have a smaller surface-to-volume ratio than normal; they are thicker than the normal red cell, and on the

Table 8-2. Names and Functions of Some Red Cell Membrane Proteins

Band	Name	Function
1.2	Spectrin monomers	Network-forming component of the cytoskeleton
2.1	Ankyrin	Couples spectrin to band 3
3	Anion channel	Facilitates passage of Cl⁻ in and out of the cell
4.1		Couples spectrin to actin
5	Actin	A component of the cytoskeleton
6	Glyceraldehyde 3-phosphate dehydrogenase	Glycolytic enzyme
PAS-1, PAS-2[a]	Glycophorin	Function unknown; carries the MN antigen system

[a]These proteins are designated PAS-1 and PAS-2 because they are stained by periodic acid-Schiff, indicating that they are glycoproteins.

peripheral smear they lack the normal area of central pallor, resulting in the spherical appearance that has given the disease its name (Fig. 8-11). The abnormality in cell shape in HS strongly suggests that the condition is caused by a defect in the cytoskeleton. Recent studies have borne this out, showing that in most HS patients, the disease results from an abnormally low level of red cell spectrin, though the underlying molecular defect may involve any of several cytoskeletal proteins: spectrin itself, ankyrin, or band 3. Moreover, clinical severity correlates with the red cell spectrin content: the lower the spectrin, the worse the disease. This correlation between the red cell spectrin levels and the severity of the disease explains the peculiar genetics of HS, which in milder forms is transmitted as an autosomal recessive trait but in severe forms becomes autosomal dominant. It is likely that in mild HS, the genetic defect causes only a modest decline in spectrin production, so that a double dose of the defective gene is necessary to reduce red cell spectrin to a clinically significant level (autosomal

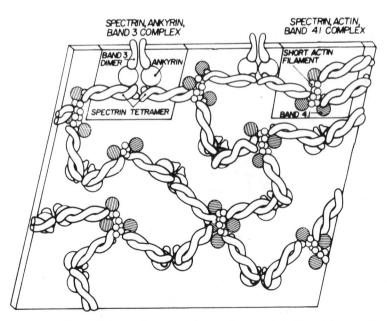

Fig. 8-9. The red cell cytoskeleton. Shown are four major cytoskeletal proteins: spectrin, actin, and the coupling proteins ankyrin and band 4,1. Ankyrin (the anchor) attaches the cytoskeleton to the plasma membrane by coupling spectrin to band 3, a plasma membrane protein. Band 4.1 couples spectrin to actin. (From Lux SE [1979] Dissecting the red cell membrane skeleton. Nature 281:426, with permission.)

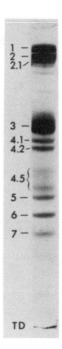

Fig. 8-10. Gel electrophoresis of red cell membrane proteins. (From Steck TL [1974] The organization of proteins in the human red blood cell membrane. J Cell Biol 62:1, with permission.)

recessive transmission); but in severe HS, spectrin production is so seriously impaired by the genetic defect that only a single defective gene is needed to produce clinically significant spectrin deficiency (i.e., autosomal dominant transmission).

The other important problem with the HS cell is its abnormal permeability to Na^+. This ion leaks into the HS cell at about 10 times the normal rate. The leak is compensated for by a proportionate increase in the activity of the membrane Na^+/K^+ ATPase, but this requires an increase in energy production to supply the ATP necessary for ion pumping. Glucose metabolism is therefore substantially accelerated in HS cells.

The combination of abnormal shape and the permeability defect account for the increase in the destruction of HS cells by the spleen. Because of their spherical shape, these cells lack the flexibility of normal cells, causing them to become trapped in the cords of the spleen because of the difficulty they have squeezing into the sinuses. The increased ion pumping caused by their Na^+ leak forces them to burn more glucose; this accelerated rate of glucose metabolism works against them, and they quickly run out of fuel in the glucose-poor environment of the splenic cords. Energy production ceases, and the cells are destroyed.

The manifestations of HS are attributable to the destruction of the defective cells in the spleen. These manifestations are often detected in childhood, but sometimes are not picked up until later in life. Presenting findings include an anemia of variable severity, plus the big three of extravascular hemolysis: splenomegaly, reticulocytosis, and indirect bilirubinemia. In addition, gallstones and aplastic crises are particularly common in HS.

HS should be suspected in a patient with a hemolytic anemia and an appropriate family history whose blood smear contains spherocytes (Fig. 8-11). The presence of spherocytes and reticulocytosis on smears from family members provides even stronger evidence of HS. The diagnosis of HS is usually made by the *osmotic fragility* test, which depends on the fact that the thicker shape of HS cells makes it difficult for them to increase their volume to the same extent as normal cells. In this test, red cells are incubated in hypotonic saline at various concentrations. The cells imbibe water and increase their volume until their internal osmolarity is reduced to that of the saline, or until they burst. Because of their shape, normal cells are able to tolerate much lower osmolarities than HS cells (Fig. 8-12); the latter are therefore said to exhibit increased osmotic fragility. Incubation for a day at 37°C greatly increases the susceptibility of HS cells to osmotic stress and can be used to bring out the defect if the osmotic fragility of fresh red cells from a suspected HS patient is ambiguous.

As to therapy, the anemia virtually always responds to splenectomy, making it the treatment of choice. In considering splenectomy, however, three points should be borne in mind: (1) splenectomy should not be done unless warranted by the degree of anemia; (2) in patients with gallstones, the spleen should be

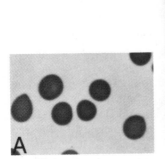
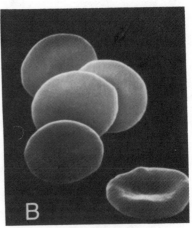

Fig. 8-11. Red cells in hereditary spherocytosis. (**A**) Blood smear, showing the typical sphero-cytes. (**B**) Spherocytes as seen by scanning electron microscopy. (**A:** From Lessin LF, Bessis M [1972] Morphology of the erythron. In Williams WJ et al [eds]: Hematology. McGraw-Hill, New York, 1982, with permission. **B:** From Castoldi GL [1981] Erythrocytes. In Zucker-Franklin D et al (eds): Atlas of Blood Cells: Function and Pathology. Edi. Ermes s.r.l., Milan, with permission.)

removed along with the gallbladder, to prevent stone formation in the bile ducts caused by the continued excretion of excessive amounts of bilirubin by the liver; (3) splenectomy should be avoided if possible in children below the age of 5 or 6, because of the high risk of fulmi-nant septicemia, often pneumococcal, in splenectomized children. Even in adults,

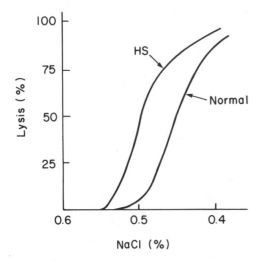

Fig. 8-12. Osmotic fragility in HS.

splenectomy increases the risk of fulminant pneumococcal septicemia, so splenectomized patients should be routinely vaccinated against pneumococcus. Folate supplements should be given to meet the increased folic acid require-ments associated with chronic hemolysis. *Aplastic crisis* is managed by supportive thera-py, primarily transfusions as necessary. *Icterus neonatorum* is treated by (1) exchange transfu-sions, to decrease bilirubin production by replacing the defective red cells with normal cells, and (2) exposure of the skin to very bright light, to convert bilirubin in the skin and surface blood vessels to nontoxic breakdown products that are excreted in the urine.

RELATED DISORDERS

Other disorders of red cell shape that result from defective proteins in the cytoskeleton or plasma membrane are hereditary elliptocytosis (HE) and (probably) hereditary stomatocytosis. Most cases of HE are caused by mutations in spectrin or band 4.1 that weaken protein–pro-tein interactions involving the ends of the spec-trin molecules. The red cell morphology in

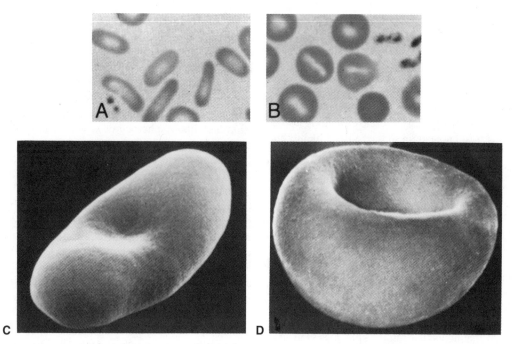

Fig. 8-13. Red cell morphology in two other disorders of the red cell membrane. Hereditary ellipto-cytosis: (**A**) blood smear; (**C**) scanning electron micrograph. Hereditary stomatocytosis: (**B**) blood smear; (**D**) scanning electron micrograph. The diseases are named for the morphology of the red cells. The origin of "elliptocyte" is obvious. "Stomatocyte" is a fanciful term derived from the mouth (*stoma*)-like appearance of the cells on the smear. (**A, B:** From Lessin LF, Bessis M [1972] Morphology of the erythron. In Williams WJ et al [eds]: Hematology. McGraw-Hill, New York, 1982, with permission. **C, D:** From Bessis M [1973] Living Blood Cells and Their Ultrastructure. Springer-Verlag, New York, with permission.)

these two conditions is shown in Figure 8-13. The important points to remember are that (1) they are quite rare; (2) in HE, the more common of these conditions, the red cell lifespan is usually normal or only modestly decreased; and (3) an acquired form of stomatocytosis is seen in alcoholics.

Spur Cell Anemia

Spur cells are red cells whose shape is altered because of an increase in the area of the red cell membrane without an accompanying increase in red cell volume. This increase usually results from the uptake of cholesterol by the cell membrane. The cholesterol in red cell membrane exchanges freely with the cholesterol in plasma lipoproteins; when the concentration of these proteins changes, so does the amount of cholesterol in the red cell membrane. Under normal circumstances, the variations in lipoprotein concentration are small enough that the accompanying fluctuations in red cell membrane cholesterol do not cause a detectable change in red cell shape. At sufficiently high lipoprotein concentrations, however, enough cholesterol is transferred to the red cell membrane that changes in shape become evident. Modest increases lead to flattened red cells that appear on blood smears as target cells. Sufficiently large increments of cholesterol cause the membrane to be thrown up into spikes, forming spur cells (Fig. 8-14).

LIVER DISEASE WITH HYPERCHOLESTEROLEMIA

By far the commonest cause of spur cell anemia is severe liver disease, especially alcoholic cirrhosis. In this condition, serum lipoproteins typically increase, leading to the transfer of cholesterol to the red cell membrane and the appearance of target cells and spur cells in the blood smear. The spur cells are subject to destruction in the spleen. Here phagocytes first nip off some of the projecting spurs, accounting for the irregular shape of most of the spur cells. (The nibbling away of defective parts of red cells by splenic phagocytes is termed *pitting* or *conditioning*. It is also seen in autoimmune hemolytic anemias and in diseases associated with intracellular precipitation of denatured hemoglobin). This process is soon followed by the elimination of the cells, an event that takes place in the spleen as well. It is obvious that the spleen is important in the pathogenesis of the anemia, though not the spurs, in spur cell disease. The fact that this organ is enlarged in liver disease makes its role in spur cell anemia all the more important.

Splenectomy has in fact been shown to ameliorate hemolysis in this condition and to regularize the appearance of the spur cells on the smear (Fig. 8-14). Nevertheless, this operation is hazardous in liver disease and should therefore be undertaken only after the most careful evaluation. Fortunately, it is rarely necessary in this condition.

HEREDITARY ABETALIPOPROTEINEMIA

Spur cells are also seen in abetalipoproteinemia, a very rare inherited abnormality of lipid metabolism. Sphingomyelin accumulation seems to be the culprit in this condition; red cell cholesterol levels are normal. Hemolysis is negligible in abetalipoproteinemia.

Disorders of Red Cell ATP Production

PYRUVATE KINASE DEFICIENCY

Pyruvate kinase deficiency is one of the group of inherited conditions known as the congenital nonspherocytic hemolytic anemias (CNSHAs). These conditions are characterized by the presence from birth of hemolytic anemia; a smear showing variable numbers of irregularly shaped cells but few spherocytes (the absence of spherocytes distinguishes them from hereditary spherocytosis, which they otherwise closely resemble); and typical manifestations of extravascular red cell destruction (reticulocytosis, marrow hyperplasia, splenomegaly, and indirect bilirubinemia). The CNSHAs described to date are all caused by inherited deficiencies of enzymes involved in either glycolysis or the protection of the red cell against oxidative damage. The CNSHAs are very rare; pyruvate kinase deficiency, although an unusual disease, is observed with greater frequency than the others.

The problem in pyruvate kinase deficiency is a defect in energy production. This defect is less of a problem in reticulocytes than in older cells, because reticulocytes still contain mitochondria and can therefore make much more ATP than older cells can produce from the trickle of pyruvate that seeps past the block. The defect in energy production leads to a marked shortening of red cell survival. A minor but interesting abnormality in pyruvate kinase deficiency is an increase in red cell 2,3-diphophoglyceric acid (2,3-DPG), leading to a reduction in oxygen affinity of uncertain clinical significance.

The diagnosis of pyruvate kinase deficiency is made by measuring the level of pyruvate kinase in the red cell. The mainstay of therapy is folic acid supplements and transfusion as necessary. Splenectomy generally leads to some improvement and reduces the transfusion requirement, but it does not completely correct the anemia. This is surprising in view of the fact that most of the red cell destruction in this condition occurs extravascularly; it probably reflects the fact that in pyruvate kinase deficiency, the liver and other organs containing large numbers of mononuclear phagocytes can take up the slack when the spleen is removed. Another unexpected feature of pyruvate kinase deficiency is that after splenectomy, the reticulocyte count rises, even though the improvement in the anemia that follows the operation

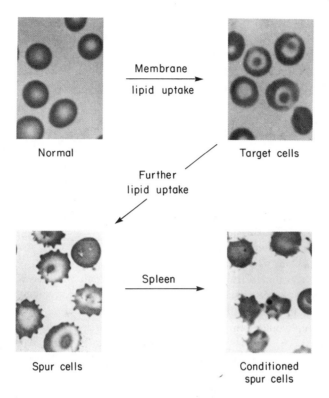

Normal

Membrane
lipid uptake

Target cells

Further
lipid uptake

Spleen

Spur cells

Conditioned
spur cells

Fig. 8-14. Formation of spur cells. Spur cells develop when the area of the red cell membrane increases without an increase in the red cell volume. With a modest increase in membrane area, the erythrocyte appears on the smear as a target cell. As the area increases further, the erythrocyte becomes a spur cell, with long spikes projecting uniformly in all directions. Finally, some of the spikes are amputated in the spleen, causing the spur cell to acquire an irregular, asymmetric appearance. Spur cells are sometimes called acanthocytes (*acantho-*, "thorn"). They are distinguished from the knob-covered burr cells of renal failure by the length and shape of the spikes. (**Bottom:** From Cooper RA [1980] Hemolytic syndrome and red cell membrane abnormalities in liver disease. Semin Hematol 17:103, with permission. **Top:** From Lessin LF, Bessis M [1972] The morphology of the erythron. In Williams WJ et al [eds]: Hematology. McGraw-Hill, New York, 1972, with permisssion.)

would be expected to result in decreased red cell production by the marrow. It would appear that pyruvate kinase-deficient reticulocytes, although metabolically healthier than mature red cells, are nevertheless subject to destruction by the spleen, accounting for their improved survival once this organ is removed. No one knows why this is so.

OTHER DISORDERS OF ATP PRODUCTION

In *severe hypophosphatemia,* red cell glycolysis may be impeded by very low intracellular phosphate levels, leading to a hemolytic anemia with acquired spherocytosis and very low erythrocyte ATP levels. Levels of 2,3-DPG also fall sharply, resulting in impaired oxygen release by these cells. The anemia is cured by correcting the serum phosphate.

Inherited *pyrimidine-5′-nucleotidase deficiency* causes a hemolytic anemia associated with prominent basophilic stippling of the affected red cells. The hemolysis is thought to result from abnormal ATP generation, while basophilic stippling reflects impaired RNA degradation. Both have been attributed to the inhibition of red cell enzymes by undegraded pyrimidine nucleotides.

Unstable Hemoglobin Diseases

Unstable mutant hemoglobins that denature and precipitate in the circulating red cell are another cause of extravascular hemolysis. These are almost always the result of amino acid alterations that weaken the interaction between the heme and the globin chain.

More than 75 unstable hemoglobins have been identified to date. In most instances these hemoglobins have been found in only one family, but hemoglobin Köln ($\beta^{98 \text{ val} \rightarrow \text{met}}$), by far the most common of the unstable hemoglobins, has been found in more than 10 kindreds. Unstable hemoglobin disease is inherited as an autosomal dominant trait—not surprising, because the unstable variant will amount to roughly one-half the hemoglobin in the red cell of a heterozygote, and the denaturation of this fraction of the cell's hemoglobin would definitely cause symptoms.

The sequence of events involved in the pathogenesis of unstable hemoglobin disease is straightforward (Fig. 8-15). The key event is the denaturation of the unstable hemoglobin by some sort of oxidative process. The denatured hemoglobin forms an intracellular precipitate that causes the red cell to be held up and destroyed in the spleen (in severe cases, the liver and other macrophage-containing organs participate in red cell destruction as well). In most patients with unstable hemoglobin disease, the red cells are destroyed in a perfectly conventional manner, their heme going to bilirubin and storage iron. In a few patients, however, only part of the heme goes to bilirubin; the rest is converted by a poorly understood series of reactions to highly colored dipyrroles (Fig. 8-15), which are for the most part excreted in the urine.

The clinical manifestations of unstable hemoglobin disease are those of an extravascular hemolytic anemia. The hematocrit may be normal or reduced, depending on the severity of the disease, but a reticulocytosis is generally present. Jaundice or splenomegaly may be seen, and gallstones may appear at an early age. In a small minority of patients the urine is intermittently dark, sometimes nearly black, a very unusual feature in extravascular hemolysis. The urinary pigment in these patients is not bilirubin, which in any case would not be expected to appear in the urine of a patient with uncomplicated hemolysis because it would be in the unconjugated form; rather, the pigment consists of the dipyrroles referred to above (Fig. 8-15). The anemia is typically episodic, with acute attacks precipitated primarily by infections and by certain drugs that impose an oxidant stress on red cells.

The severity of the disease varies widely from patient to patient, depending on the nature

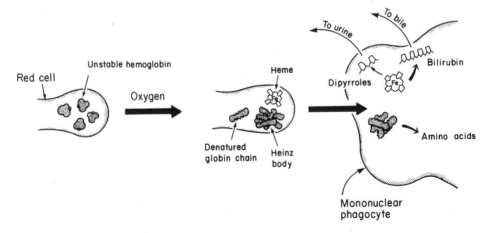

Fig. 8-15. Pathogenesis of unstable hemoglobin disease.

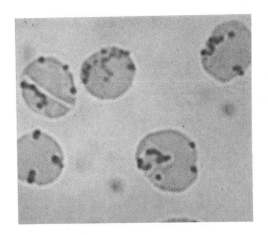

Fig. 8-16. Heinz bodies in crystal violet-stained red cells. (From Kapff CT, Jandl JH [1981] Blood: Atlas and Sourcebook of Hematology. Little, Brown, Boston, with permission.)

of the unstable hemoglobin. In the most severe cases, a profound anemia is present from early childhood. The mildest forms have no clinical manifestations whatsoever. Most patients have a disease of intermediate severity, displaying a modest reticulocytosis with or without anemia. These patients are usually picked up in adolescence or early adulthood, although the disease was present since birth.

There are two characteristic tests for unstable hemoglobin disease:

1. *Heinz bodies.* When red cells containing precipitates of denatured hemoglobin are stained with crystal violet, the denatured protein, undetectable on a routine smear, takes up the dye and becomes visible as a small, round, purple-staining mass. This precipitate is the Heinz body (Fig. 8-16). It appears in the three varieties of red cells disease in which hemoglobin denaturation is a prominent feature: unstable hemoglobin disease, oxidant hemolysis, and thalassemia. Since red cells containing precipitates of denatured hemoglobin (i.e., Heinz body-positive cells) are ordinarily removed from the circulation by the spleen, Heinz bodies are particularly prominent in splenec-

tomized patients with unstable hemoglobin diseases.

2. *Hemoglobin precipitation.* Because of the ease with which unstable hemoglobins undergo denaturation, they will precipitate in response to stresses that have no effect on normal hemoglobin. The formation of a precipitate when a hemolysate is gently heated (50°C for a few minutes) or mixed with dilute isopropyl alcohol is so characteristic of an unstable hemoglobin that either one of these tests can be used to make the diagnosis of unstable hemoglobin disease.

It may be possible to detect the presence of an abnormal hemoglobin by electrophoresis, but this test cannot always be done, and in any case hemoglobin electrophoresis can offer no conclusive evidence as to whether the abnormal hemoglobin is unstable. Once an unstable hemoglobin is detected, it can be characterized further to determine the precise nature of the molecular defect, but this is a complicated undertaking generally carried out for research purposes only.

The treatment of unstable hemoglobin disease is similar to that of other hemolytic diseases: folate supplements and transfusions as required. Oxidant drugs should be avoided. Splenectomy has been useful in some cases.

SUGGESTED READINGS

Berlin NI, Berk PD (1981) Quantitative aspects of bilirubin metabolism for hematologists. Blood 57:983

Beutler E (1979) Red cell enzyme defects as diseases and non-diseases. Blood 54:1

Cashore WJ (1990) the neurotoxicity of bilirubin. Clin Perinatol 17:437

Cohen CM, Branton D (1981) The normal and abnormal red cell cytoskeleton: A renewed search for molecular defects. Trends Biochem Sci 6:266

Cooper RA (1980) Hemolytic syndromes and red cell membrane abnormalities in liver disease. Semin Hematol 17:103

Glader BF, Nathan DG (1975) Hemolysis due to pyruvate kinase deficiency and other glycolytic enzymopathies. Clin Hematol 4:123

Lestas AN, Bellingham AJ (1990) A logical approach to the investigation of red cell enzymopathies. Blood Rev 4:148

Lux SE, Wolfe LC (1980) Inherited disorders of the red cell membrane skeleton. Pediatr Clin North Am 27:463

Miwa S (1981) Pyruvate kinase deficiency and other enzymopathies of the Embden-Myerhoff pathway. Clin Haematol 10:57

Ohba Y (1990) Unstable hemoglobins. Hemoglobin 14:353

Paglia DE, Valentine WN (1981) Haemolytic anaemia associated with disorders of the purine and pyrimidine salvage pathways. Clin Haematol 10:81

Palek J (1987) Hereditary elliptocytosis, spherocytosis and related disorders: consequences of a deficiency or a mutation of membrane skeletal proteins. Blood Rev 1:147

Palek J, Sahr KE (1992) Mutations of the red blood cell membrane proteins: from clinical evaluation to detection of the underlying genetic defect. Blood 80:308

Pankard TAJ, Bellingham AJ (1975) Haematolytic anemias. Clin Haematol 4 No. 1

Schacter BA (1988) Heme catabolism by heme oxygenase: physiology, regulation and mechanism of action. Semin Hematol 25:249

Schmid R et al (1972) Physiology and disorders of hemoglobin degradation. Semin Hematol 9: nos. 1 and 2

Sills RH (1987) Splenic function: physiology and splenic hypofunction. CRC Crit Rev Oncol Hematol 7:1

Smith MA, Ryan MA (1988) Parvovirus infections. From benign to life-threatening. Postgrad Med 84:124

Stuart J, Nash GB (1990) Red cell deformability and haematological disorders. Blood Rev 4:141

Tabbara IA (1992) Hemolytic anemias. Diagnosis and management. Med Clin North Am 76:649

Tan KL (1991) Phototherapy for neonatal jaundice. Clin Perinatol 18:423

Tanaka KR, Zerez CR (1990) Red cell enzymopathies of the glycolytic pathway. Semin Hematol 27:165

Valentine WN, Tanaka KR, Paglia DE (1985) Hemolytic anemias and erythrocyte enzymopathies. Ann Intern Med 103:245

Winterbourn CC (1990) Oxidative denaturation in congenital hemolytic anemias: the unstable hemoglobins. Semin Hematol 27:41

9

Hemolytic Anemias: Intravascular Destruction of Red Cells

The second mechanism for the pathological destruction of erythrocytes is intravascular hemolysis, a process in which the cells rupture during circulation, spilling their hemoglobin into the plasma. Some hemoglobin is normally released into the plasma during the course of extravascular red cell destruction (both normal and pathological), simply because mononuclear phagocytes are messy eaters. In diseases associated with major intravascular hemolysis, however, almost all the hemoglobin in the lysed red cell is released into the plasma. The presence of this hemoglobin aids in the detection of these conditions, although their diagnosis usually depends on more specific investigations.

INTRAVASCULAR HEMOLYSIS: GENERAL CONSIDERATIONS

Disposal of Plasma Hemoglobin

Mechanisms for clearing hemoglobin from the plasma can be divided into two classes: (1) a haptoglobin-dependent mechanism (recall that haptoglobin is the hemoglobin-scavenging protein of the plasma) and (2) a group of haptoglobin-independent mechanisms. Normally the haptoglobin mechanism is the only one in operation, because free hemoglobin is cleared so rapidly that nothing is left behind to be disposed of by the other mechanisms. The haptoglobin mechanism, however, can only handle a limited amount of hemoglobin at a time, because there is only a small quantity of haptoglobin in the blood to begin with (equivalent to about 1 mg hemoglobin/ml whole blood), and this haptoglobin is used up in the hemoglobin-clearing reaction. In clinically significant intravascular hemolysis, the limited capacity of the haptoglobin mechanism is almost always exceeded, either because of the sudden release of large amounts of hemoglobin by a major hemolytic event or because ongoing intravascular hemolysis consumes haptoglobin faster than it can be replaced. Under these circumstances, haptoglobin vanishes from the bloodstream, and free hemoglobin appears. The second class of mechanisms now takes over the disposal of the hemoglobin.

MECHANISMS FOR CLEARING HEMOGLOBIN FROM THE PLASMA

Haptoglobin dependent
Haptoglobin independent
    Clearance by the kidney
    Destruction in the plasma

One of these mechanisms involves the kidney (Fig. 9-1). In the plasma, free hemoglobin will dissociate to a limited extent into $\alpha\beta$-dimers. These dimers are small enough to pass freely into the glomerular filtrate. In the nephron, the hemoglobin dimers are rapidly resorbed by the proximal tubular cells, where they are degraded in the usual way; the protein is destroyed, the iron is deposited as hemosiderin, and the heme is converted to bilirubin, which is released into the bloodstream and eventually excreted in the bile. The proximal tubular cell, however, has only a limited capacity to take up hemoglobin dimers; if this capacity is exceeded, hemoglobin appears in the urine.

The other mechanism involves the oxidation of the iron of the circulating hemoglobin (Fig. 9-2). This is a fairly rapid reaction that may take place before the hemoglobin is lost through the kidney. The product is methemoglobin, which quickly dissociates into ferriheme (heme in which the iron is trivalent) and the apoproteins. Some of the ferriheme is taken up by the heme-binding protein hemopexin, which carries it to the liver for the usual processing to iron and bilirubin. The rest is taken up by albumin to form methemalbumin; this ferriheme eventually ends up in the liver as well, where it suffers the same fate. What happens to the apoproteins is not known.

Signs of Hemoglobinemia

There are many ways to demonstrate that hemoglobin has been released into the plasma (Table 9-1), all of which depend on measuring hemoglobin itself or the traces it leaves behind as it is degraded.

1. *Fall in haptoglobin.* The most sensitive indicator of hemoglobin release into the plasma is a fall in haptoglobin. In extravascular hemolysis, haptoglobin levels will vary from near normal to zero, depending on the severity of the condition. With intravascular red cell destruction, however, haptoglobin almost always disappears completely. A point to remember is that haptoglobin levels rise during illness, so that a "normal" level in a sick patient in whom hemolysis is suspected might actually be the result of the offsetting effects of the hemolytic process (causing a fall) and the illness (causing a rise).

2. *Free hemoglobin in the plasma or urine; hemosiderinuria.* Straightforward evidence of intravascular hemolysis is provided by the finding of free hemoglobin itself, either in the plasma or the urine. Hemoglobinemia leads to red plasma, a bedside indicator of intravascular hemolysis, although the clinical

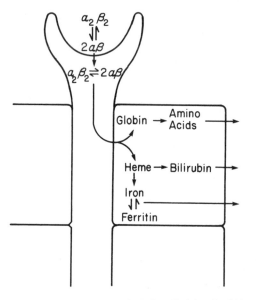

Fig. 9-1. How hemoglobin is handled by the kidney. (From Bunn HF, Jandl JH [1969] The renal handling of hemoglobin. II. Catabolism. J Exp Med 129:925, with permission.)

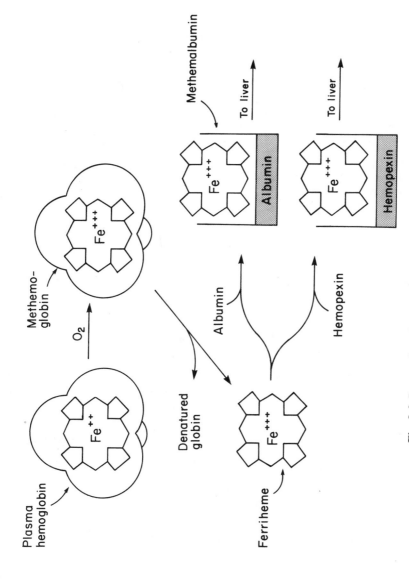

Fig. 9-2. Destruction of hemoglobin in the plasma.

Table 9-1. Detecting the Release of Hemoglobin in the Plasma

Sign	Remarks
Haptoglobin absent	Most sensitive test: occurs in all intravascular hemolysis, as well as in brisk extravascular hemolysis (e.g., sickle cell disease, immune hemolytic anemia)
Hemoglobinemia and hemoglobinuria	Red plasma, red urine: indicates active release of hemoglobin into plasma and disappears a few hours after cessation of hemolysis
Methemoglobinemia	Brown plasma: disappears 2 to 3 days after cessation of hemolysis
Hemosiderinuria	Lasts a few weeks after hemolysis ends: a good sign of prior or chronic release of hemoglobin into the plasma

impression must be confirmed by a laboratory measurement. Because of the rate at which hemoglobin is cleared from the plasma, the red color disappears within a few hours after the cessation of hemolysis. Sometimes, but not always, the red is replaced by the brown of methemalbumin, which persists for a day or two after the episode of hemolysis. Hemoglobinuria results in dark urine that gives a positive test for blood. Laboratory confirmation is essential here too, because myoglobin and red blood cells also produce dark urine that tests positive for blood. Free hemoglobin also gives rise to hemosiderinuria. The proximal tubule cells that have taken up hemoglobin dimers converts the iron to hemosiderin. These cells are shed over the course of a few weeks and are excreted in the urine, carrying their load of hemosiderin with them. The presence of these hemosiderin-containing cells in the urine is therefore a strong indication of intravascular hemolysis.

In applying these findings to the diagnosis of intravascular hemolysis, their transitory nature must be kept in mind. After a bout of intravascular hemolysis, hemoglobin can be detected in the blood and urine for only a few hours, haptoglobin is depressed for a couple of days, and hemosiderin is detected in the urine for at most a few weeks. It is easy to see how a single episode of acute intravascular hemolysis could be missed by these tests. Chronic intravascular hemolysis, however, is another story. Hemoglobinemia and hemoglobinuria may be hard to detect in chronic intravascular

hemolysis because they are intermittent and low grade, but the haptoglobin is usually low, and hemosiderinuria is virtually always present because of the steady processing of free hemoglobin dimers by the kidney. Persistent hemosiderinuria is probably the best single clue to the diagnosis of chronic intravascular hemolysis.

Clinical Features of Intravascular Hemolysis

The general clinical features of intravascular hemolysis are identical to those of extravascular hemolysis, except for two points: splenomegaly does not occur, and plasma hemoglobin is seen. The features are summarized in Table 9-2.

INTRAVASCULAR HEMOLYTIC ANEMIAS

Traumatic Hemolysis ("Waring Blender" Syndrome)

Traumatic hemolytic anemia, also known as *microangiopathic hemolytic anemia*, is a form of intravascular hemolysis caused by the mechanical destruction of red cells in the circulation. It occurs under three types of circumstances:

1. *When red cells pass at high velocity through regions of turbulent flow.* The cells break under these conditions by smashing against rigid obstructions in their path or by stretching past their limit of deformability, tearing themselves apart. Such flows are produced

Table 9-2. Principal Manifestations of Intravascular Hemolysis

Mechanism	Clinical Findings	Laboratory Findings
Increased red cell production		Reticulocytosis Marrow red cell hyperplasia
Plasma hemoglobin	Dark urine Red plasma	Absent serum haptoglobin Hemoglobinemia and hemoglobinuria Hemosiderin in urine
Increased hemoglobin breakdown	Jaundice Gallstones	Indirect bilirubinemia
Red cell destruction	Pallor and faintness Cardiac symptoms Aggravation of underlying vascular disease	Anemia

(1) in malignant tumors, in which the blood vessels tend to be highly tortuous and irregular; (2) in malignant hypertension, because of rapid flow produced by the extreme degree of vasoconstriction characteristic of this condition; and (3) in tight aortic stenosis and prosthetic valve leaks, in which blood flows with great velocity through a narrow opening past rigid walls. The anemia in giant hemangioma of childhood (Kasabach-Merritt syndrome) is caused by red cell damage that occurs as blood passes through the deformed vessels of the tumor.

2. *When red cells pass through regions of intravascular coagulation.* Although blood normally does not clot in the vascular tree, there are conditions in which coagulation takes place within blood vessels. In two of these conditions, disseminated intravascular coagulation and thrombotic thrombocytopenia purpura, clotting occurs within capillaries, which may fill with a mesh of fibrin strands through which the blood must flow (fibrin is the protein, generated at sites of coagulation, whose polymerization produces the solid clot). Red cells rupture as they are clotheslined by the fibrin strands (Fig. 9-3). Traumatic hemolytic anemia is therefore characteristic of these two clotting disorders.

3. *When red cells pass through vessels in the soles of the feet.* Some people have red cells that are unusually susceptible to mechanical damage. Every time such persons take a step, a few of the red cells in the soles of their feet are broken. With sufficient vigorous activity, this sort of red cell damage may increase to the point at which it becomes clinically evident as a traumatic hemolytic anemia.

CONDITIONS PRODUCING TRAUMATIC HEMOLYSIS

Rapid turbulent blood flow
    Malignant tumors
    Malignant hypertension
    Tight aortic stenosis
    Prosthetic valve leaks
Intravascular coagulation
"March hemoglobinuria"

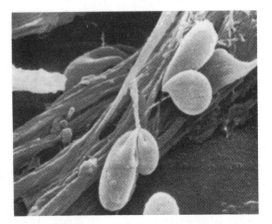

Fig. 9-3. Red cell clotheslined by a fibrin strand. (From Bull BS, Kuhn IN [1970] The production of schistocytes by fibrin strands [a scanning electron microscope study]. Blood 35:104, with permission.)

This condition tends to be seen in athletes and in soldiers after a long march, hence the name march hemoglobinuria. It has also been reported in bongo drummers and martial artists, in whom the damage is inflicted as the blood passes through the palms of the hands.

The clinical manifestations of traumatic hemolytic anemia are those of intravascular hemolysis together with the signs and symptoms of the underlying disorder. Anemia, reticulocytosis, and indirect bilirubinemia are seen, the hallmarks of hemolysis, but the spleen tends not to be palpable in this and other intravascular hemolytic anemias. If the hemolysis is mild, the haptoglobin is low, but evidence of free plasma hemoglobin is lacking. More severe hemolysis results in hemoglobinemia. This is most likely to be detected only through hemosiderinuria, but there may be enough hemoglobin in the plasma to be found by laboratory tests. Frank hemoglobinemia and hemoglobinuria, detectable at the bedside in the form of red plasma and dark urine, are unusual in traumatic hemolysis and are seen only in the most severe cases.

In a patient with chronic traumatic hemolytic anemia, enough iron may be lost through hemosiderinuria to lead to a superimposed iron deficiency anemia. In such patients, the morphological abnormalities resulting from the iron deficiency may mask the characteristic changes seen in the underlying hemolytic condition, so that they are missed unless looked for after the iron-deficient state is corrected. In patients with iron deficiency unexplained by menses, pregnancy, or gastrointestinal bleeding, the urine should not be overlooked as a source of iron loss.

The diagnostic feature of traumatic hemolytic anemia is found in the blood smear (Fig. 9-4). Here, red cell fragments are seen in the form of helmet cells, triangles, and other oddly shaped pieces of erythrocyte. These shapes are produced when the membrane of a red cell fragment reseals before all the hemoglobin is lost. Such fragments are not seen in

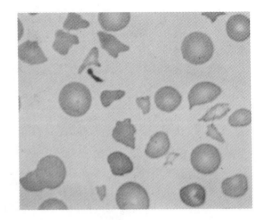

Fig. 9-4. Blood smear in traumatic hemolysis. Red cell fragments are abundant. (From Kapff CT, Jandl JH [1981] The anemias. In Blood: Atlas and Sourcebook of Hematology. Little, Brown, Boston, with permission.)

every case of traumatic hemolysis—they are generally absent, for instance, in march hemoglobinuria, a condition in which only a small number of red cells are damaged—but in severe traumatic hemolytic anemia, these fragments may represent more than 10 percent of the cells on the smear.

Treatment is aimed primarily at the underlying disease. The anemia itself may be treated with transfusions if sufficiently severe. If the condition is chronic, folate should be given to prevent a deficiency that might otherwise result because of the increased erythropoiesis. Iron supplements may also be needed to offset iron losses in the urine.

Glucose-6-Phosphate Dehydrogenase Deficiency and Oxidant Hemolysis

OXIDANT DEFENSE IN THE RED CELL

The function of the red cell is to transport oxygen from the lungs to the tissues. Ordinarily, oxygen is picked up and released by the red cell without undergoing any chemical changes; it is transported as inert cargo. Occasionally, however, an oxygen molecule

OXIDANT DEFENSES IN THE RED CELL

Glutathione-dependent system
    Glutathione peroxidase/reductase
    Hexosemonophosphate shunt
Superoxide dismutase
Catalase

will be converted to a more reactive oxidizing species such as superoxide (O_2^-) or hydrogen peroxide (H_2O_2). O_2^- is produced when oxyhemoglobin is converted to methemoglobin:

$$Hb(Fe^{2+}) - O_2 \rightarrow Hb(Fe^{3+}) + O_2^-$$

H_2O_2 is also produced from the aberrant dissociation of oxyhemoglobin; it arises as well from additional sources, the latter not well characterized. These two compounds represent a potent oxidizing threat and must be destroyed, or they will destroy the red cell.

The red cell has several ways of dealing with these oxidizing species. It contains superoxide dismutase, an enzyme that represents the major defense against O_2^-, converting it to H_2O_2 and oxygen. It also contains catalase, which eliminates H_2O_2 by converting it to oxygen and water. The most important defense against H_2O_2, however, is a glutathione-requiring system. Defects in this system cause clinically important intravascular hemolytic conditions.

The glutathione antioxidant system consists of glutathione itself; two enzymes, namely, glutathione peroxidase and glutathione reductase; and a source of reducing power. The destruction of H_2O_2 is accomplished by glutathione peroxidase, which catalyzes its reduction to water by glutathione:

$$2GSH + H_2O_2 \rightarrow GSSG + 2H_2O$$

The oxidized glutathione formed in this reaction is converted back to the reduced state by NADPH in a reaction catalyzed by glutathione reductase:

$$GSSG + NADPH \rightarrow 2GSH + NADP$$

Thus in the glutathione antioxidant system, glutathione cycles between its reduced and oxidized form, converting one molecule of H_2O_2 to water with each turn of the cycle. Because NADPH is consumed by this system, this reducing agent has to be regenerated to maintain the system's capacity to destroy H_2O_2.

In the red cell, the sole source of NADPH is the hexosemonophosphate shunt. The NADPH-producing reactions in this metabolic path are the glucose-6-phosphate dehydrogenase (G6PD) reaction:

$$Glucose\ 6\text{-}phosphate + NADP$$
$$\rightarrow 6\text{-}phosphogluconate + NADPH$$

and the 6-phosphogluconate dehydrogenase reaction:

$$6\text{-}Phosphogluconate + NADP$$
$$\rightarrow ribulose\ 5\text{-}phosphate + CO_2 + NADPH$$

It is clear that the normal operation of the hemosemonophosphate shunt, particularly its first reaction, is essential if the antioxidant defenses of the red cell are to retain their effectiveness.

GLUCOSE-6-PHOSPHATE DEHYDROGENASE DEFICIENCY

G6PD deficiency is the most common inherited enzyme deficiency affecting red cells. The gene that encodes G6PD is on the X chromosome, so the deficiency is inherited as an X-linked trait. From the foregoing discussion, it is apparent that G6PD is critical for the antioxidant defenses of the red cell. It is therefore not surprising that G6PD deficiency leads to an anemia associated with an increase in the susceptibility of the cell to injury by oxidants.

Oxidants cause two kinds of damage to red cells: damage to hemoglobin and damage to the membrane (Fig. 9-5). The attack of oxidants on hemoglobin may result first in the production

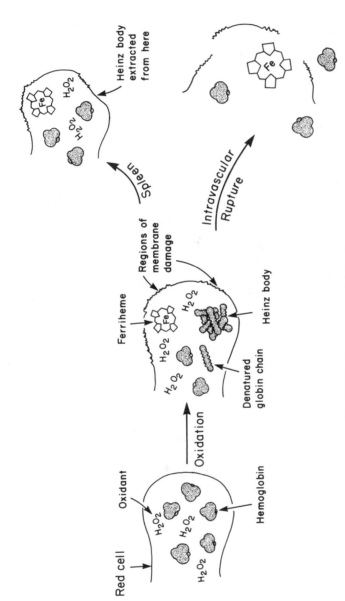

Fig. 9-5. Oxidant damage of red cells.

of methemoglobin, which accumulates because it is generated faster than it can be reconverted to hemoglobin. From the methemoglobin, the oxidized heme dissociates, leaving behind the free globin, which is destroyed by further oxidation. Alternatively, the initial damage may be sustained by the globin protein, which is destroyed without losing its heme. In either case, the denatured hemoglobin eventually precipitates as an intracellular mass of agglutinated protein. These masses are extracted when damaged red cells pass through the spleen, another version of splenic "conditioning" or "pitting" of defective erythrocytes (cf. the amputation of projections from spur cells by splenic macrophages). The extraction of the hemoglobin precipitate results in a reduction in the size of the red cell and an alteration in its shape, which becomes more spherical than before. At the same time, the oxidants attack the red cell membrane, destroying its integrity. It is probably membrane damage, rather than hemoglobin denaturation, that is responsible for the intravascular hemolysis characteristic of G6PD deficiency.

Hemolysis in G6PD deficiency is precipitated when the red cells are exposed to an oxidant stress. The two most common stress-inciting agents are infections and oxidant drugs. Just how infections impose an oxidant stress on red cells is unclear, but it is certain that they do,

---

CLINICAL MANIFESTATIONS OF G6PD DEFICIENCY

X-linked inheritance
Most common in blacks
Precipitated by
    Infections
    Drugs
Signs and symptoms
    Hemolysis
        Primarily intravascular
        Usually episodic, occasionally chronic
    Enlarged spleen
    Gallstones

---

because hemolysis is a common occurrence in infected patients with G6PD deficiency. With oxidant drugs, the mechanism is better understood: these drugs enter the red cell and then function as artificial electron carriers, passing electrons from endogenous reductants (e.g., NADH) to oxygen to produce H_2O_2. A number of drugs are able to precipitate oxidant hemolysis in G6PD-deficient red cells; those most commonly associated with this problem are certain sulfonamides and some antimalarials. Finally, a particularly serious hemolytic event that has led to a number of fatalities will occur when certain patients with an unusually severe form of G6PD deficiency eat broad beans (fava beans), which contain pyrimidine derivatives having potent oxidant properties.

The clinical manifestations of G6PD deficiency are primarily those of intravascular hemolysis. There is an acute fall in the hematocrit, accompanied by a reticulocytosis and an increase in indirect bilirubin. Haptoglobin falls sharply, and signs of hemoglobin release into plasma are often seen (i.e., hemoglobinemia, hemoglobinuria, hemosiderinuria). Some extravascular red cell destruction also takes place because of the presence of hemoglobin precipitates in cells that have not been damaged enough to rupture in the bloodstream. This occurs in the spleen, which enlarges

---

OXIDANT DRUGS

Acetanilid
Antimalarials
    Quinacrine
    Primaquine
    (Chloroquine is safe)
Dapsone
Doxorubicin
Nitrofurantoin
Nitrofurazone
Para-aminosalicylic acid
Sulfonamides

through a sort of work hypertrophy as it conditions the red cells by extracting the precipitated hemoglobin. Evidence of conditioning may be seen in the smear as misshapen red cells and microspherocytes (the latter to be distinguished from spherocytes of normal size, which are seen in hereditary spherocytosis [HS]). Often, however, the smear shows no abnormalities. As with all congenital hemolytic anemias, there is a tendency to gallstone formation.

This bare listing of signs and symptoms gives a qualitative idea of the clinical picture in G6PD deficiency. What cannot be gathered from this list is a feel for the quantitative aspects of the disease. As it happens, G6PD deficiency is one of the most variable of the inherited red cell disorders. The anemia in this condition can range from a form so mild as to be apparent only during the most rigorous oxidant stress to a form so severe that it has caused death from massive acute hemolysis. What accounts for this variability is the difference from patient to patient in the proportion of red cells destroyed during a hemolytic event. This in turn is directly related to the properties of the defective enzyme.

More than 100 different forms of the human enzyme have been described to date. Two of these forms are found in normal subjects: the B form, present in normal whites and in most normal blacks, and the A (or A⁺) form, present in about 30 percent of normal black men and 55 percent of normal black women, most of whom are AB heterozygotes. These normal forms are easy to distinguish by electrophoresis (Fig. 9-6.) Virtually all the other forms of the enzyme have been isolated from patients with clinical G6PD deficiency.

These different forms of G6PD have been found to vary widely in their properties. Of particular importance is the variation in stability among these enzymes, because it is this as

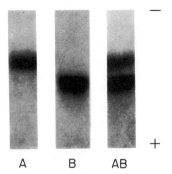

A B AB

Fig. 9-6. Electrophoresis of G6PD, showing three patterns. (*Left*) Black subject with the A type. (*Center*) White subject with the B type. (*Right*) Black subject with both types. The enzyme is detected by an activity stain. (From Giblett ER [1969] *Genetic Markers in Human Blood.* Blackwell Scientific Publishers, Oxford, with permission.)

much as anything that determines the clinical severity of the disease. The relationship between stability and clinical severity is best explained by considering the two extreme forms of G6PD deficiency: the very common mild form seen in blacks, and the rare severe form found in people from the Mediterranean basin (Table 9-3).

1. *G6PD Type A⁻ form.* By far the most common form of G6PD deficiency is caused by G6PD type A⁻, a low-activity variant of the type A enzyme (G6PD A$^{202\ val\ \rightarrow\ met}$). The condition is seen almost exclusively in blacks. The gene for the A⁻ enzyme is carried by about 20 percent of black women, so roughly 10 percent of black males have the disease. The important property of the A⁻ enzyme is its reduced stability compared with the normal enzyme. Red cells containing the A⁻ enzyme have adequate levels of G6PD when they are released from the marrow, but activity declines as the enzyme decays, so that by the time the cells are 1

Table 9-3. Two Extremes of G6PD Deficiency

	G6PD$_{A^-}$	G6PD$_{Mediterranean}$
Instability of enzyme	Mild	Severe
Deficiency seen in	Old red cells	All red cells
Clinical severity	2+	4+
G6PD levels immediately after attack	May be normal	Always low

month old they no longer contain any G6PD. When these cells are stressed, as by the ingestion of an oxidant drug, cells old enough to have lost their G6PD will be lysed, but the younger cells will survive; only a fraction of the red cell population is therefore lost, and the resulting anemia is mild. It is important to remember that a second oxidant challenge will have little effect if it occurs shortly after the initial exposure, because the cells that survived the first oxidant exposure and the new cells released from the marrow in response to the initial hemolytic event will contain enough G6PD to fend off the second challenge. Furthermore, the diagnosis of G6PD deficiency may be difficult to make immediately after a hemolytic event, because the deficient cells will have been swept from the bloodstream; it may not be possible to diagnose the disease until several weeks have elapsed, during which the deficient population will reaccumulate as the surviving cells age and lose their G6PD.

2. *G6PD Type B$_{Mediterranean}$ form.* A much more severe hemolytic disease is caused by G6PD type B$_{Mediterranean}$ (G6PD B$^{188\ ser\ \to\ phe}$). This rare variety occurs mostly in whites from the Mediterranean basin: Italians, Greeks, persons from the Near East and North Africa, and those from the Mediterranean islands (e.g., Sicily, Sardinia). The enzyme is extremely unstable, so G6PD activity is greatly diminished in all red cells, even those newly released from the marrow. As a result, virtually all red cells are susceptible to oxidant hemolysis, and an oxidative challenge of sufficient magnitude will cause hemolysis of the most severe degree, with gross hemoglobinemia and hemoglobinuria and a sudden fall in the hematocrit to life-threatening levels. Lesser degrees of hemolysis can cause fatal icterus neonatorum in infants with G6PD type B$_{Mediterranean}$. In this form of the disease there is no resistance to a subsequent oxidative challenge, and the diagnosis can always be made because G6PD-deficient red cells are always present in the bloodstream.

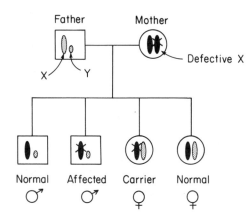

Fig. 9-7. X-linked transmission. X-linked diseases are transmitted primarily by female carriers. In such carriers, one X chromosome has a defective gene and the other X chromosome is normal. The child of a carrier mother has a 50:50 chance of inheriting the defective X chromosome. If a male child inherits the defective chromosome, he will have the disease in its full-blown form, because the only X chromosome in his cells is the defective one received from his mother. In contrast, a female who inherits the defective chromosome will be clinically normal, or at worst will have a milder form of the disease, because she will have inherited a second X chromosome from her father that can compensate for the defect in her maternal X chromosome; she will herself, however, be a carrier of the disease.

A feature of G6PD and other X-linked diseases (Fig. 9-7) is that female heterozygotes (i.e., females who inherited a defective X chromosome from one parent and a normal one from the other) always contain two populations of cells: one that is completely normal, and another that expresses the inherited defect in its full-blown form. Affected males, however, contain only a single population of cells, all defective. The duality of population in female heterozygotes is known as mosaicism. As a result of this mosaicism, female heterozygotes show much less hemolysis than do affected males, simply because female heterozygotes always have some normal red cells in their circulation. In the rare female homozygote (one who has inherited G6PD deficiency from both her patients), hemolysis is just as severe as in the male.

Mosaicism results from the fact that early in female embryogenesis, one of the two X chromosomes loses its capacity to code for protein synthesis. The loss of function is referred to as X-chromosome inactivation (Fig. 9-8). Inactivation is a random process in that each of the two X chromosomes in a given cell is equally likely to become inactivated. In the case in which one of the X chromosomes contains a defective gene, the effect of random inactivation will be to create a fetus containing some cells in which the functioning X chromosome is normal and others in which the functioning X chromosome is defective. The cells will breed true thereafter with respect to the functioning X chromosome, accounting for the mosaicism in adult female carriers of X-linked diseases.

The diagnosis of G6PD deficiency is made by measuring the level of G6PD in the red cell. It will be very low in patients having severe disease and a badly defective enzyme (e.g., G6PD type B$_{Mediterranean}$), but it may be only moderately decreased in patients with enzymes whose properties are closer to normal (e.g., G6PD type A⁻), especially if the measurement is made shortly after an episode of hemolysis. The disease can also be diagnosed by staining a blood smear for G6PD (Fig. 9-9); a population of cells that lacks the enzyme is seen in G6PD-deficient patients. The enzyme can be characterized by electrophoresis of hemolysates followed by an activity stain (Fig. 9-6) and by genetic analysis to identify the responsible mutation, although genetic analysis is usually carried out only in research laboratories.

Although the definitive diagnosis requires measurements of G6PD levels, the presence of Heinz bodies can furnish a valuable clue to the existence of the disease in a patient with an undiagnosed acute hemolytic anemia. Heinz bodies are intracellular precipitates of denatured hemoglobin that become visible when the cell is stained with crystal violet. Heinz bodies are typically seen in oxidant hemolysis, unstable hemoglobin disease, and thalassemia. In oxidant hemolysis, they are present only transiently, appearing at the onset of an attack and disappearing with the elimination of the last damaged red cells. If they are seen in the blood of a patient with an acute hemolytic anemia, G6PD deficiency should be strongly suspected, and drugs that precipitate hemolysis in this condition should be scrupulously avoided until the diagnosis is confirmed or refuted by direct measurement of the enzyme.

G6PD deficiency is managed primarily through the avoidance of agents known to provoke hemolysis. Antimalarials are particularly hazardous in this regard. Other drugs represent

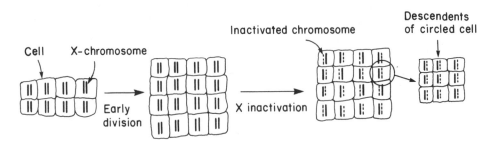

Fig. 9-8. X-chromosome inactivation. When the founder cell that gives rise to the blood-forming tissues starts to differentiate in a female embryo, both X chromosomes are active. After the newly established blood-forming tissue has reached the 16- or 32-cell stage, however, one of the two X chromosomes in each cell undergoes inactivation, losing its capacity to code for proteins, but retaining its ability to duplicate itself when the cell divides. In a given cell, the choice as to which of the two X chromosomes will undergo inactivation is completely random. Once that cell has made its choice, however, all its descendents will inherit the same pattern of X-chromosome inactivation.

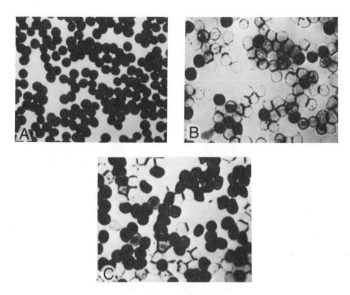

Fig. 9-9. Blood smears stained for G6PD. (**A**) Normal. (**B**) Affected male. (**C**) Female heterozygote, showing mosaicism. (From Gall JC, Jr, Brewer GJ, Dern RT [1965] Studies of glucose-6-phosphate dehydrogenase activity of individual erythrocytes: the methemoglobin elution test for identification of females heterozygous for G6PD deficiency. Am J Hum Genet 17:359, with permission.)

less potent oxidant challenges and can be used in patients with mild G6PD deficiency if given with great care, but it is best to avoid all oxidant drugs in G6PD deficiency if at all possible. The eating of fava beans by a person with severe G6PD deficiency can be catastrophic. An acute attack is treated supportively with fluids to maintain urine flow and transfusions as required. A few patients with severe G6PD deficiency may have congenital nonspherocytic hemolytic anemia (CNSHA); in these, splenectomy may be of some help, although it is usually of little value in this condition. Icterus neonatorum is treated with exchange transfusions and phototherapy as described in Chapter 8.

OTHER ENZYME DEFICIENCIES

Deficiencies of enzymes involved in glutathione metabolism may lead to oxidant hemolysis. Deficiency of 6-phosphogluconate dehydrogenase, the second enzyme of the hexosemonophosphate shunt, does not cause anemia.

OTHER ENZYME DEFICIENCIES
THAT CAUSE OXIDANT
HEMOLYSIS

Glutathione reductase
γ - Glutamylcysteine synthetase

Immune Hemolytic Anemias

Intravascular hemolysis is characteristic of certain types of immune hemolytic anemias. Intravascular hemolysis is typically seen in transfusion reactions caused by ABO incompatibility. A very rare but potentially fatal cause of intravascular hemolysis is the so-called Donath-Landsteiner antibody, which causes red cells to lyse when they are transiently cooled below body temperature and is responsible for the condition known as paroxysmal cold hemoglobinuria. These conditions are discussed in full in Chapters 30 and 31.

Infections

Intravascular hemolysis is a prominent feature of a few infectious diseases, some rare and some not so rare. *Clostridium perfrigens* secretes a toxin that can cause intravascular hemolysis by breaking down phospholipids in the red cell membrane. *Bartonella bacilliformis* is the cause of the rare Andean disease known as Oroya fever, one of whose manifestations is an intravascular hemolytic process of a few weeks' duration. The most common infections causing intravascular hemolysis, however, are those caused by *Plasmodia*; malaria is one of the most prevalent infections in the world and is responsible for hundreds of thousands of deaths yearly.

Paroxysmal Nocturnal Hemoglobinuria

Paroxysmal nocturnal hemoglobinuria is a stem cell disease of unknown etiology in which the abnormal marrow cell line produces, among other things, a population of red cells that are unusually susceptible to lysis by complement. Chronic recurrent intravascular hemolysis is one of the hallmarks of this disease. Paroxysmal nocturnal hemoglobinuria is discussed in more detail in Chapter 22.

SUGGESTED READINGS

Arese P, De Flora A (1990) Pathophysiology of hemolysis in glucose-6-phosphate dehydrogenase deficiency. Semin Hematol 27:1

Beutler E (1971) Abnormalities of the hexose-monophosphate shunt. Semin Hematol 8:311

Beutler E (1991) Glucose-6-phosphate dehydrogenase deficiency. N Engl J Med 324:169

Beutler E (1992) The molecular biology of G6PD variants and other red cell enzyme defects. Annu Rev Med 43:47

Bunn HF, Forget BD (1984) Human Hemoglobins. 2nd Ed. WB Saunders, Philadelphia

Gaetani GF (1988) Recent developments on Mediterranean G6PD. Br J Haematol 68:1

Gordon-Smith EC (1980) Drug-induced oxidative haemolysis. Clin Haematol 9:557

McClung JA, Stein JH, Ambrose JA et al (1983) Prosthetic heart valves: a review. Prog Cardiovasc Dis 26:237

Miwa S (1990) Pyruvate kinase deficiency. Prog Clin Biol Res 344:843

Morgan EH, Baker E (1986) Iron uptake and metabolism by hepatocytes. Fed Proc 45:2810

Morse EE (1988) Toxic effects of drugs on erythrocytes. Ann Clin Lab Sci 18:13

Müller-Eberhard U (1970) Hemopexin. N Engl J Med 283:1090

Murgo AJ (1987) Thrombotic microangiopathy in the cancer patient including those induced by chemotherapeutic agents. Semin Hematol 24:161

Prankerd TAJ, Bellingham AJ (1975) Haemolytic anaemias. Clin Haematol 4, no. 1

Reider RF (1974) Human hemoglobin stability and instability: molecular mechanisms and some clinical correlations. Semin Hematol 11:423

Schmid R (1972) Physiology and disorders of hemoglobin degradation. Semin Hematol 9, nos. 1 and 2

Schulman JD, Mudd SH, Schneider JL et al (1980) Genetic disorders of glutathione and sulfur amino acid metabolism. Ann Intern Med 93:330

Tabbara IA (1992) Hemolytic anemias. Diagnosis and management. Med Clin North Am 76:649

Valentine WN, Paglia DE (1990) Erythroenzymopathies and hemolytic anemia: the many faces of inherited variant enzymes. J Lab Clin Med 115:12

Weatherall DJ, Abdalla S (1982) The anaemia of *Plasmodium falciparum* malaria. Br Med Bull 38:147

10

Hemoglobin Biosynthesis: Thalassemia and Hemoglobin E

At first glance, it would appear that hemoglobin biosynthesis should be a straightforward, uncomplicated matter. Hemoglobin A is by far the predominant protein in the red cell, and its production should proceed smoothly along the path defined by the so-called central dogma of molecular biology:

$$gene \rightarrow messenger \rightarrow protein$$

In fact, though, many hemoglobins besides hemoglobin A occur normally in red cells. These are particularly prominent in the very young, and their proportions change extensively during fetal development and the first 6 months or so of postnatal life. The biosynthesis of these hemoglobins involves (1) the activation and inactivation of more than a dozen genes distributed between two pairs of chromosomes, (2) the production of highly complex messenger RNA precursors that undergo extensive post-transcriptional processing to yield the templates on which the hemoglobin chains are assembled, and (3) the synthesis of different types of hemoglobin chains at rates that are somehow balanced so that they are all used up in the assembly of the final hemoglobin tetramers.

Thalassemia results when there is an impairment in the biosynthesis of one of the two constituent chains of hemoglobin A, the major

adult hemoglobin. Because of what has been learned about hemoglobin biosynthesis, it is probably fair to say that thalassemia is as well understood at a molecular level as any human disease.

NORMAL HEMOGLOBIN PRODUCTION

Normal Hemoglobin Species: The Ontogeny of Hemoglobin

During the course of our lifetime, we manufacture six different normal hemoglobins (Table 10-1). These hemoglobins are assembled from two families of chains: the α-family, containing the α chain itself and the ζ-chain, and the β-family, containing the β-, γ-, δ-, and ε-chains. The prototype hemoglobin, hemoglobin A, is a tetrameric protein composed of two α-chains and two β-chains (Ch. 3). Each of the other five normal hemoglobins is also a tetramer containing a pair of α-family chains and a pair of β-family chains.

The amount of a given chain that occurs in the red cells is not constant throughout life, but varies with age in a manner that is characteristic for each type of chain (Fig. 10-1). As a consequence, different hemoglobins are found in

Table 10-1. Normal Human Hemoglobins[a]

Hemoglobin	Chain Composition
Embryonic	
Gower I	$\zeta_2\varepsilon_2$
Gower II	$\alpha_2\varepsilon_2$
Portland	$\zeta_2\gamma_2$
Fetal	
Hemoglobin F	$\alpha_2\gamma_2$
Adult	
Hemoglobin A	$\alpha_2\beta_2$
Hemoglobin A$_2$	$\alpha_2\delta_2$

[a]There are two families of globin chains: the α-family and the β-family. The α-family contains the α- and ζ-globin chains; these are coded for by genes on chromosome 16. The β-family contains the β-, γ-, δ-, and ε- chains; the genes for these are on chromosome 11. Each normal hemoglobin species contains a pair of chains from each family.

the human at different ages. Three of the six hemoglobins are normally found only in the embryo, while the other three are present at birth and remain present throughout the lifetime of the individual. This will all become clear as the individual hemoglobins are discussed.

EMBRYONIC HEMOGLOBINS

The first red cells that appear during fetal development arise from the blood vessels of the embryo. These vessels begin as clusters of mesodermal cells known as blood islands that appear on the yolk sac during the first week of development. These blood islands send out cords that join and hollow out to form the primitive vascular network. The cells at the periphery of these cords differentiate into the blood vessel walls, while those in the center form the large, nucleated, hemoglobin-filled cells that constitute the embryonic erythrocytes. Yolk sac erythrocytes appear in the embryo about the third week of gestation and remain for about 10 weeks. They then disappear, never to return.

The major hemoglobins of these primitive erythrocytes are the Gower hemoglobins, of which there are two, both containing ε, the embryonic β-family chain. One, Gower I, also contains ζ, the embryonic member of the α-family; its complete composition is $\zeta_2\varepsilon_2$. The other, Gower II, contains the adult α-chain ($\alpha_2\varepsilon_2$). The Gower hemoglobins, the first that can be detected in the developing embryo, decline as yolk sac erythropoiesis is overtaken by hepatosplenic erythropoiesis and are gone by 10 weeks.

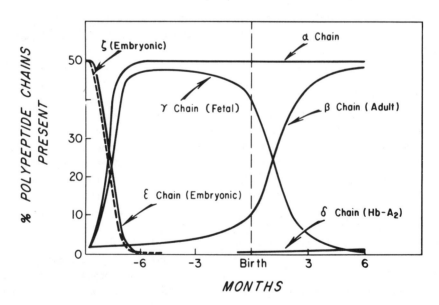

Fig. 10-1. Hemoglobin composition of red cells during fetal development and the first year after birth. (From Bunn HF, Forget BG, Ranney HM [1977] Hemoglobin biosynthesis. In: Human Hemoglobins. WB Saunders, Philadelphia, with permission.)

The third embryonic hemoglobin, hemoglobin Portland, is present only in traces. It resembles Gower I in containing the embryonic α-family chain ζ, but instead of the very primitive β-family chain ϵ, it contains its ontogenic successor, the γ-chain. Accordingly, the composition of hemoglobin Portland is $\zeta_2\gamma_2$. This hemoglobin can be detected in tiny amounts throughout fetal life.

HEMOGLOBIN F

At about 6 weeks, a new population of hematopoietic cells begins to express itself. These cells will be responsible for hematopoiesis during the rest of the individual's life. They appear first in the liver and spleen, which rapidly become the major source of blood cells in the developing fetus. After about the fourth month, blood formation begins in the bone marrow, and the liver and spleen decline in importance as hematopoietic organs until by the time of birth they no longer make blood. However, they retain the memory of their former hematopoietic role and in certain pathological states will once again make blood cells, an activity known as *extramedullary hematopoiesis*.

From the time the permanent hematopoietic line takes over until several weeks past birth, the major hemoglobin in the red cell is hemoglobin F, or fetal hemoglobin. The β-class chain of this hemoglobin is the γ-chain; its composition is $\alpha_2\gamma_2$. Hemoglobin F actually consists of several closely related species:

1. There are two types of g-chains in hemoglobin F, one containing a glycine at position 136 (^{G}g) and the other alanine (^{A}g); all hemoglobin F-containing red cells have some of each.
2. About one-half of the hemoglobin F is acetylated at the N-terminus of the g-chain.

All these species behave similarly, however, so that in functional terms there is only one kind of hemoglobin F.

As the predominant hemoglobin in fetal red cells, hemoglobin F bears the major responsi-

---

PROPERTIES OF HEMOGLOBIN F

Structure
$\alpha_2\gamma_2$
Two types of γ-chains: $^G\gamma$ (γ^{136gly}) and $^A\gamma(\gamma^{136ala})$
Partly acetylated
Function
Oxygen affinity similar to hemoglobin A
2,3-DPG has little effect on oxygen binding

---

bility for delivering oxygen to the fetal tissues. To obtain this oxygen, it must steal from the maternal bloodstream. This act of theft is made easier by the difference in the way the oxygen affinities of fetal (F) and maternal (A) hemoglobin are regulated by 2,3-diphosphoglyceric acid (2,3-DPG). Although the inherent oxygen affinities of these two hemoglobins are about equal, hemoglobin A is much more sensitive than hemoglobin F to the oxygen unloading effect of 2,3-DPG. The effect of this difference is to lower the oxygen affinity of the hemoglobin A-containing maternal red cells with respect to the hemoglobin F-containing fetal red cells, since 2,3-DPG is a major regulator of oxygen affinity in intact erythrocytes. As a result, it is easy for the fetal red cells to strip oxygen from the maternal red cells as these two red cell populations flow past each other in the placenta.

Hemoglobin F begins to decline about the 30th week of gestation and is nearly gone by 6 months of age (Fig. 10-1). Unlike the case of the embryonic hemoglobins, however, a small amount of hemoglobin F persists in the circulation throughout life. This trace of hemoglobin F is not uniformly distributed among the red cells, but is found mainly in a minor population known as F cells, each of which contains some 10 percent or so of hemoglobin F. These F cells can be detected by a special procedure in which blood smears are treated with acid before staining (Fig. 10-2). The acid pretreatment leaches hemoglobin A from the red cells,

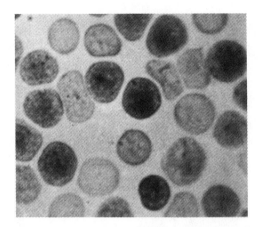

Fig. 10-2. F cells in a blood smear. The F cells take up stain because of their hemoglobin F, which stays behind during the staining procedure while hemoglobin A is washed away. The F cells stain darkly. The F-cell stain is sometimes called the Betke-Kleihauer stain. (From Castoldi GL [1981] Erythrocytes. In Zucker-Franklin D et al [eds]: Atlas of Blood Cells: Function and Pathology. Edi. Ermes s.r.l., Milan, with permission.)

but hemoglobin F, which is relatively acid resistant, remains behind and is visualized by the subsequent staining procedure.

HEMOGLOBIN A AND A$_2$

The hemoglobins of the adult red cell are hemoglobin A ($\alpha_2\beta_2$) and hemoglobin A$_2$ ($\alpha_2\delta_2$). Hemoglobin A replaces hemoglobin F during late gestation and infancy, reaching adult levels by 6 months of age or so (Fig. 10-1). In the adult, hemoglobin A constitutes more than 95 percent of the hemoglobin in the red cell. Hemoglobin A$_2$ begins to appear at birth and increases over the first year or two of life. It never amounts to much more than 1 percent of the total hemoglobin in normal red cells. Because it is present in such low concentrations, it is of no practical use as an oxygen-carrying protein. It does, however, provide physicians with a useful diagnostic tool for evaluating patients with thalassemia.

Genetics of Hemoglobin Production

The genes that code for the hemoglobin chains have been identified on chromosomes 11 and 16 (Fig. 10-3). Chromosome 16 carries the α-family genes, two coding for the α-chain and one for the ζ-chain. Between the ζ-gene and the two α-genes is a long stretch of DNA of unknown function. Reading from 5′ to 3′, the direction of DNA transcription, the genes are lined up as follows: ζ, space, α, α.

The β-family genes are on chromosome 11. These are arranged in three groups with two long stretches of DNA between them. The order is as follows: ε, space, $^G\gamma$, $^A\gamma$, space, δ, β. It is curious that the order of the genes on the chromosomes is the same as the order in which the chains appear during fetal development. Upstream from the ε gene is the *locus control region*, which contains DNA sequences that cause the β-family genes to be expressed exclusively in red cell progenitors. The locus control region is also involved in some way in the changes that take place in red cell hemoglobin composition during the course of fetal development.

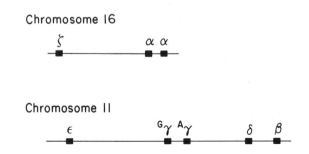

Fig. 10-3. Arrangement of globin genes on chromosomes 11 and 16.

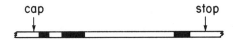

Fig. 10-4. Diagram of a globin gene. Exons are shown in black. The *arrow* shows the location of the "cap" site, the point at which messenger RNA transcription begins. Rates of messenger transcription are controlled by untranslated stretches on both sides of the exon/intron portion of the gene.

The globin genes themselves have a complex structure (Fig. 10-4). The template for the globin chain is present in the gene as a sequence of nucleotides arranged in a particular order. The template sequence, however, is not present as a continuous stretch of nucleotides; instead, it is present in segments interrupted by stretches of DNA whose nucleotide sequences are never translated into protein. The segments of template are known as *exons*, because they are *ex*pressed in the final globin product, while the untranslated stretches are known as *introns*, because they are *inter*vening sequences that separate the template segments from each other. Finally, there are untranslated regions on both 5′ (left)

and 3′ (right) sides of the exon/intron portion of the gene that are involved in the regulation of gene expression.

From this gene, the messenger RNA is produced (Fig. 10-5). Transcription begins at the "cap" site in the 5′ untranslated region, continues straight through the exon/intron region, and terminates somewhere in the 3′ untranslated region. The initial RNA product is thus a faithful copy of a stretch of an entire gene sequence, containing introns, exons, and all. This product is not translated directly, but is first converted to the true messenger RNA by post-transcriptional modifications. These modifications include (1) the excision of the introns to fuse the exons into a continuous stretch of message for translation, a process known as splicing; (2) the attachment of a 7-methyl G cap to the 5′ end of the messenger (this is why the transcription initiation site is called the "cap" site); and (3) the addition of a poly-A chain to the 3′ end of the messenger. This mature messenger RNA is then used as the final template for globin chain synthesis.

Evaluating Hemoglobin Biosynthesis

With current techniques, it is possible to evaluate hemoglobin biosynthesis from the finished product back to the level of the gene.

HEMOGLOBIN ELECTROPHORESIS

Abnormalities in hemoglobin biosynthesis often alter hemoglobin proportions or cause the appearance of a hemoglobin not normally found in red cells. Accordingly, the simplest way to evaluate hemoglobin biosynthesis is to measure the proportions of the various hemoglobins in the circulating red cells. This is most often done by hemoglobin electrophoresis.

Hemoglobin electrophoresis is usually carried out at pH 8.6 on cellulose acetate strips or starch gels. Under these conditions, hemoglobin A, A_2, and F are separated, and abnormal hemoglobins whose electrophoretic mobilities

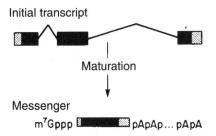

Fig. 10-5. Production of the globin messenger. The initial transcription product is a complete copy of the globin DNA gene from the "cap" site to the termination site. It includes exons (*thick black*), introns (*thin*), and flanking sequences, the portions of the transcript lying outside the exon/intron region (*stippled*). The initial transcript is converted to mature globin messenger RNA by splicing out the introns, adding a 7-methyl G cap to the end of the 5′ flanking sequence, and adding a poly-A chain to the end of the 3′ flanking sequence.

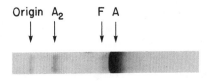

Fig. 10-6. Normal hemoglobin electrophoresis. The major band is hemoglobin A. Running slightly behind this is the faint band of hemoglobin F. Much slower than either of these is hemoglobin A_2.

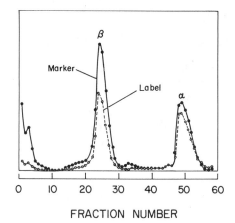

Fig. 10-7. Globin chain synthesis in normal reticulocytes. Whole blood is first incubated with radioactive leucine. Labeled globin chains are then separated by column chromatography, and the amount of radioactivity in each of the chains is determined by counting the fractions from the column, using authentic α- and β-globin chains to mark the locations of the labeled chains. The α- and β-chain peaks are seen to contain about the same number of counts, indicating that in these reticulocytes the two chains were synthesized at equal rates. (It is not necessary to correct for difference in the leucine content of the two chains, because they contain the same number of leucines.) (From Bunn HF, Forget BG, Ranney HM [1977] The thalassemias. In: Human Hemoglobins. WB Saunders, Philadelphia, with permission.)

differ from those of the normal species appear as bands distinct from the normal hemoglobins. The separated hemoglobins are quantified by staining and measuring the intensity of color. A normal hemoglobin electrophoresis pattern is shown in Figure 10-6.

GLOBIN CHAIN SYNTHESIS

Reticulocytes newly released from the marrow retain their ability to synthesize protein for 24 to 48 hours. The protein manufactured by these cells is almost entirely hemoglobin. Reticulocytes thus provide an easily obtained system in which to examine globin chain synthetic rates.

These rates are measured as follows. Radioactive leucine is incubated for a short time (1 to 2 hours) with whole blood, which serves as the source of the reticulocytes. During the incubation, the labeled amino acid becomes incorporated into the globin chains. These chains are then isolated, separated chromatographically into the individual species, and counted. The number of counts incorporated into a given chain is directly proportional to the rate at which that chain was synthesized in the reticulocytes.

The results from a typical study of normal blood are shown in Figure 10-7. It can be seen that the ratio of counts incorporated into the α- and β-chains is close to 1.0. A deviation from this value suggests the diagnosis of thalassemia.

SOUTHERN BLOTTING

The human genome consists of 3 billion pairs of nucleotides lined up in a precisely ordered sequence. Somewhere in this chain of nucleotides are the stretches corresponding to the globin genes. To map these genes in the sense of defining their precise locations within the entire genome has not yet been accomplished. It has been possible, however, to break up the genome into fragments of sharply defined length and then determine which of these fragments contain the globin genes. This procedure, known as *Southern blotting*, has yielded important information concerning the pathogenesis of the thalassemias.

To perform Southern blotting, the DNA is split into fragments of defined length by a restriction endonuclease, an enzyme that recognizes a particular short sequence of nucleotide pairs and cuts double-stranded DNA wherever this sequence occurs (Fig. 10-8). The resulting restriction fragments are separated according to size by gel electrophoresis, and the sized frag-

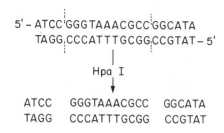

5' – ATCC'GGGTAAACGCC'GGCATA
  TAGG,CCCATTTGCGG,CCGTAT – 5'

Hpa I

ATCC   GGGTAAACGCC   GGCATA
TAGG   CCCATTTGCGG   CCGTAT

Fig. 10-8. Mechanics of a restriction enzyme. The restriction enzyme Hpa I, which is specific for the C—G bond in CCGG, will split a stretch of double-standard DNA into fragments of precisely defined size.

ments are blotted onto a nitrocellulose sheet. The fragments (one or more) containing the globin gene are located on the blot by soaking it in a solution containing a radioactively labeled probe consisting of a short length of DNA that includes part of the globin gene sequence. This probe will hybridize to any DNA that contains a complementary sequence; in particular, it will hybridize to those fragments on the blot that contain regions of globin gene corresponding to those in the probe. Finally, the globin gene-containing fragments are visualized by autoradiography of the blot,

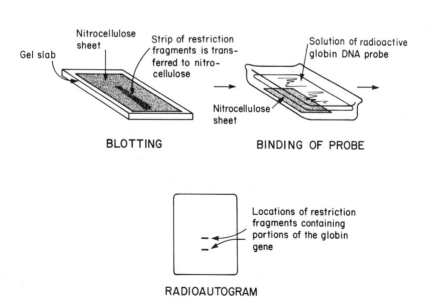

DIGESTION   ELECTROPHORESIS

BLOTTING   BINDING OF PROBE

RADIOAUTOGRAM

Fig. 10-9. Restriction mapping. DNA is chopped up into fragments of defined size by a restriction enzyme. These fragments are separated according to molecular weight by gel electrophoresis. The separated fragments are blotted onto a nitrocellulose sheet, which is then soaked in a solution of radioactive globin DNA probe. This probe will bind to the blot whenever it meets a fragment of DNA containing a sufficiently large part of the globin gene. The locations of the fragments are then determined by autoradiography.

and their size determined by comparison with standards. The steps involved in producing a restriction map are shown in Figure 10-9.

Any cell in the body can be used as a source of DNA for mapping the globin genes, because every gene is present in the DNA of every cell; in contrast, tests that assay globin proteins (hemoglobin electrophoresis and measurements of globin chain synthesis) can only be carried out on erythroid cells, because only those cells make those proteins. Typical restriction maps of the α- and β-globin genes in the normal genome are shown in Figure 10-10. A map obtained with the restriction endonuclease EcoRI shows a single α-globin gene-containing fragment 23 kilobases (kb) in size. Using other restriction enzymes, this fragment has been shown to contain both α-globin genes. These two genes therefore lie within 23 kb of each other. The map of the β-globin gene was also obtained with EcoRI. This enzyme splits the β-globin gene such that part of it is found in one fragment (5.2 kb) and part in another (3.6 kb). The 2.2-kb band is a δ-gene containing fragment picked up by a stretch of δ-gene sequence present in this particular β-globin probe.

GENE SEQUENCING

It is possible not only to map a patient's globin genes, but to determine their nucleotide sequence as well. The sequencing of globin genes has made it possible to pinpoint the mutations responsible for the defects in hemoglobin production in many patients with thalassemia.

POLYMERASE CHAIN REACTION

The polymerase chain reaction, familiarly known as "PCR," is a technique for amplifying selected DNA sequences more than a billion-fold by repeated cycles of DNA replication. The technique employs primers consisting of two oligonucleotides: one (the Watson primer) exactly complementary to a short DNA sequence on the Crick strand of the double helix, and the other (the Crick primer) exactly complementary to a short stretch of DNA on the opposite (Watson) strand of the double helix, a little distance downstream from the first primer (Fig. 10-11). The reaction mixture for the PCR starts with the DNA to be amplified, together with large excesses of these two primers. The reaction then proceeds as follows:

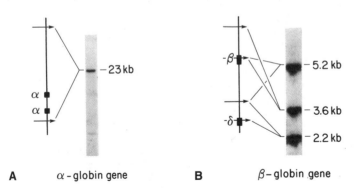

A   α - globin gene   **B**   β - globin gene

Fig. 10-10. Restriction maps of the α- and β-globin genes. (**A**) α-Globin genes mapped using EcoRI. Both genes are found in a single 23-kb fragment. (**B**) The β-globin gene mapped using EcoRI. This enzyme cuts the β-globin gene in two, so part is found in one fragment (5.2 kb) and part in another (3.6 kb). The 2.2-kb fragment contains part of the δ-globin gene. The *arrows* show the locations of the EcoRI cuts. (**A:** Modified from Kan YW et al [1979] Molecular basis of hemoglobin-H diseases in the Mediterranean population. Blood 54:1434, with permission. **B:** Modified from Orkin SH et al [1980] Cloning and direct examination of a structurally abnormal human β⁰-thalassemia globin gene. Proc Natl Acad Sci 77:3558, with permission.)

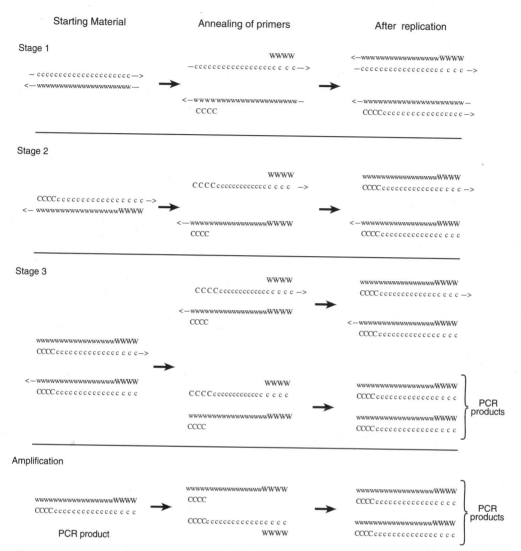

Fig. 10-11. The polymerase chain reaction. In this figure, the complementary DNA strands are arbitrarily referred to as the Watson (...www...) and Crick (...ccc...) strands. Primers are represented by uppercase letters, and other DNA by lower case letters. *Stage 1: The original DNA is the template.* The reaction mixture initially contains the DNA to be amplified plus a very large excess of two primers, one (CCCC, the Crick primer) hybridizing to the Watson strand and the other (WWWW, the Watson primer) to the Crick strand. The products of stage 1 are the original DNA molecules and a pair of "half-strands" of variable length, one beginning with the Watson primer and the other with the Crick primer. *Stage 2: Half-strand templates.* The products of stage 2 consist of the original half-strand templates and a pair of DNA strands of defined length (PCR strands). If for a particular reaction the half-strand template is, for example, a Crick strand, the 5' end of the new PCR strand will consist of the Watson primer, which will have hybridized to the half-strand to start the reaction, while the 3' end will consist of a stretch of DNA complementary to the Crick primer that was incorporated into the far end of the half-strand template during an earlier stage 1 reaction. *Stage 3: Half-strand and PCR strand templates.* The products of a stage 3 reaction consist of a new pair of PCR strands, which anneal to form a new PCR product, and the original half-strand template (i.e., the PCR product duplicates itself). The stage 3 reaction is repeated 30 to 35 times during a typical PCR run. *Amplification* occurs because each successive stage 3 reaction produces two PCR products for every PCR product present at its start.

1. *The first stage of DNA replication.* In the first stage of DNA replication, two new strands are synthesized from each DNA molecule to be amplified. The strands synthesized in the first stage of replication (hereafter referred to as "half-strands") are of variable lengths, but one strand begins with the Watson primer and the other with the Crick primer. The DNA duplexes are then separated by heat and allowed to reanneal. Because of the large excess of primers initially added to the reaction mixture, this annealing process results in primer uptake by the newly synthesized half-strands: the Watson primers join the Crick strands, and the Crick primers join the Watson strands.

2. *The second stage of DNA replication; synthesis of the first "PCR products."* During the second stage of DNA replication, the half-strands are copied. These half-strand copies consist of DNA segments of precisely defined length—the "PCR products." Each starts with the primer (say, the Watson primer) that annealed to the half-strand, which is now the template; and each terminates opposite the half-strand's 3′ end, which (in the example under discussion) actually consists of the Crick primer that was incorporated into the half-strand during the first stage of DNA synthesis. Heating and cooling then causes new primers to hybridize to these short but precisely defined PCR products. It is these that are amplified exponentially in the key event of the PCR.

3. *The third stage of DNA replication: amplification of the PCR products.* During the third stage of DNA replication, the first set of PCR products is copied, yielding new PCR products, each running from the Watson primer to the Crick primer and each paired to its template. Heating and cooling then melts these short double helixes to produce single strands of the defined DNA, each now annealed to its complementary primer (these primers are still present in vast excess). Each new cycle of DNA replication now doubles the number of PCR products, all of identical length and sequence. After 30 to 35 cycles of DNA synthesis, melting, and annealing, the DNA segment between the two primers has been amplified to the point where it can be seen on gel electrophoresis even without a radioactive probe, and can be sequenced and otherwise manipulated with ease.

Many genetic questions can be answered by PCR in just a fraction of the time taken by classical cloning methods. To identify a new β-thalassemia mutation by classical cloning technology, for example, it would be necessary to isolate DNA from the thalassemic patient and fragment that DNA with an appropriate restriction endonuclease; to insert the DNA fragments into an appropriate bacteriophage (the bacteriophages that contain these DNA fragments are known collectively as a genomic library); to grow the recombinant bacteriophage library on a lawn of bacteria, and then screen tens of thousands of individual bacteriophage plaques by hybridization with a suitable probe to find one that contains β-globin gene sequences; and finally, to purify and amplify the β-globin gene-containing recombinant bacteriophage and sequence its DNA insert. In contrast, it is possible through PCR to amplify the genomic region of interest without ever isolating it. Amplification by PCR followed by the sequencing of the amplified products then gives the desired information in just a few days, instead of the months that might be required using traditional methods. Other situations in which this technique could be of use are easy to imagine.

THE β-THALASSEMIAS

The β-thalassemias are a group of inherited disorders in which the synthesis of the β-globin chain is impaired for one reason or another. Anemia is the rule in all but one of these conditions. In the homozygous state, the anemia is so severe that affected patients commonly die in their teens or early twenties.

Pathogenesis

The fundamental problem in β-thalassemias is the uncoupling of α- and β-chain synthesis. Normally, these chains are made in almost equal quantities. In β-thalassemias, however, β-chain production is depressed—moderately in the heterozygous form (β-thalassemia minor or trait), and very severely in the homozygous state (β-thalassemia major). The depression in β-chain synthesis has two adverse consequences. First, there is a reduction in total red cell hemoglobin. This is partly offset by increases in hemoglobins containing other β-class chains (hemoglobins F and A_2), but these do not compensate fully for the decreased quantity of hemoglobin A in thalassemia cells. Second, and more importantly, there is an accumulation of free α-chains in the red cells.

It is the free α-chains that do most of the damage. The free α-chains are very unstable and denature rapidly to form precipitates within the red cells. In β-thalassemia minor, in which a relatively small proportion of the red cell hemoglobin is lost as denatured α-chain, these precipitates are pitted out by mononuclear phagocytes, leaving behind oddly shaped red cells of diminished size. In β-thalassemia major, however, denatured α-chains represent the bulk of the hemoglobin in the red cell. Most of these precipitate-filled red cells are destroyed in the marrow before they are ever released into the bloodstream; this ineffective erythropoiesis is the major factor responsible for the anemia of β-thalassemias. A fraction of the cells released from the marrow are destroyed prematurely in the spleen, but this hemolytic process is relatively low grade and contributes in only a small way to the anemia

of β-thalassemia. Finally, there is a phenomenal increase in erythropoiesis, represented not only by a vast expansion of marrow red cell production, but also by the persistence of erythropoiesis in the spleen and liver (extramedullary hematopoiesis).

In molecular terms, there are several varieties of β-thalassemia. All are characterized by sharp reductions in β-chain synthetic rates in the homozygote. They differ in the extent to which β-chain synthesis is blocked, in the amounts of other hemoglobins present in the affected red cells, and, most fundamentally, in the nature of the genetic defect responsible for the disease. These varieties are listed in Table 10-2. Two deserve special comment.

HEMOGLOBIN LEPORE DISEASE

Hemoglobin Lepore disease is a form of β-thalassemia in which an abnormal β-family chain is produced. This chain is a hybrid in

---

> **PATHOGENESIS OF β-THALASSEMIA**[a]
>
> Ineffective erythropoiesis
> Hemolysis
> Increased red cell production
>   In the bone marrow
>   In the liver and spleen (extramedullary hematopoiesis)
>
> ---
> [a]Diminished production of β-globin chains leads to a surplus of α-globin chains, which denature and precipitate, causing the manifestations listed.

Table 10-2. Varieties of β-Thalassemia

Variety	Defect in Globin Chain Production
β+-Thalassemia	Diminished β-chain
β0-Thalassemia	No β-chain
δβ-Thalassemia	No β- or δ-chain
Hemoglobin Lepore	No β-chain; δ-chain replaced by δβ hybrid
Hereditary persistence of fetal hemoglobin (HPFH)	No β- or δ-chain; defect fully compensated by increased γ-chain production

which the amino end of a normal δ-chain has been fused to the carboxy-terminal end of a β-chain. Hemoglobin Lepore is hemoglobin A in which the two β-chains have been replaced by the hybrids.

The fused chains appear to have arisen through a defect in chromosome recombination during meiosis. It may be recalled that before the division that reduces the number of chromosomes in a sperm or ovum to 23, an active exchange of material takes place between the two members of the chromosome pair. What seems to happen is that homologous portions of the two chromosomes pair up, break at equivalent sites, and then exchange partners (Fig. 10-12). These homologous portions usually represent corresponding regions in each of the two chromosomes (e.g., the β-globin gene regions). Occasionally, however, a mismatch will occur, so that exchange takes place not between corresponding regions, but between noncorresponding regions having sufficiently similar molecular structures. The β-globin and δ-globin genes represent such structurally similar noncongruent regions. It is thought that the hemoglobin Lepore gene is the product of an aberrant recombination event between these two regions, the event resulting in a shortened chromosome in which the upstream portion of the δ-gene has been fused to the downstream portion of the β-gene, with a deletion of the remaining portions of the two genes together with the intergenic region.

HEREDITARY PERSISTENCE OF FETAL HEMOGLOBIN

Although technically a form of β-thalassemia, hereditary persistence of fetal hemoglobin (HPFH) is clinically very different from the classical forms of the disease, because it involves an increase in γ-chain production sufficient to compensate almost fully for the defects in β- and δ-chain synthesis, defects that are total

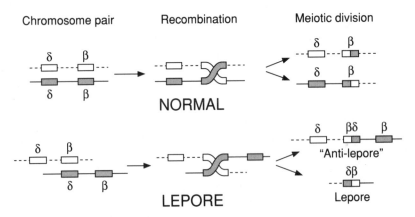

Fig. 10-12. Origin of hemoglobin Lepore. Hemoglobin Lepore is thought to arise through a chromosomal deletion that occurs during meiosis. In meiosis, a cell divides without duplicating its chromosomes. During this division, the pairs of chromosomes in the parent cell are split up, one member of each pair going to each of the two daughter cells. Just before this division takes place, the pairs of chromosomes exchange pieces, an event known as recombination. The pieces exchanged are almost always from chromosomal regions that correspond exactly to each other (e.g., the β-globin gene regions might exchange places). Occasionally, however, the pieces will be from noncorresponding regions having similar structures. The effect will be to delete material from one chromosome of the pair and give it to the other. Hemoglobin Lepore results when the β-chain region of one chromosome exchanges material with the δ-chain region of the other; the deletion resulting from this abnormal exchange gives rise to a new gene that codes for a hybrid globin chain that is δ at the amino end and β at the carboxyl end. Other thalassemia-causing gene deletions are thought to occur in the same way.

in homozygous HPFH. As a result, there is no accumulation of denatured α-chain precipitates in affected red cells, and anemia is mild in the homozygote and absent in the heterozygote. Red cells from homozygotes contain 100 percent hemoglobin F, while heterozygote red cells contain 10 to 30 percent hemoglobin F, which is distributed uniformly throughout the population of cells, not concentrated preferentially in F cells as in the normal state.

HPFH represents an important but as yet undeciphered message about red cell development. Whereas γ-chain production in other forms of thalassemias occurs only at a low rate (the adult pattern), rates of production of α- and γ-chains are almost equivalent in HPFH (the fetal pattern). The genetic lesion in HPFH has somehow inactivated the "switch" responsible for the change in the pattern of hemoglobin synthesis around the time of birth. The nature of this switch remains to be elucidated.

Clinical Manifestations

The clinical manifestations of all the various forms of β-thalassemia are similar (except for HPFH). The disease occurs primarily in persons of Mediterranean European descent (e.g., Italian, Greek, Sardinian), in Arabs, and in blacks. In the heterozygote (thalassemia minor or thalassemia trait) it presents as a mild to moderate anemia associated with splenomegaly (Fig. 10-13). The red cells are very small, the mean cell volume (MCV) averaging 65 femtoliters (fl) compared with a normal of about 95 fl (it is important to recognize that thalassemia and iron deficiency anemia are the two major causes of microcytic anemia). The microcytosis is confirmed on the smear (Fig. 10-14), which shows small red cells that vary widely in size and shape, with many target cells, occasional basophilic stippling, and a reticulocytosis whose severity depends on the

MAJOR

Severe anemia and retarded growth, plus –

MINOR

Mild anemia, plus –

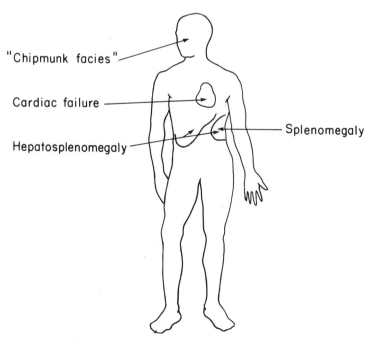

"Chipmunk facies"

Cardiac failure

Hepatosplenomegaly

Splenomegaly

Fig. 10-13. Clinical manifestations of thalassemia.

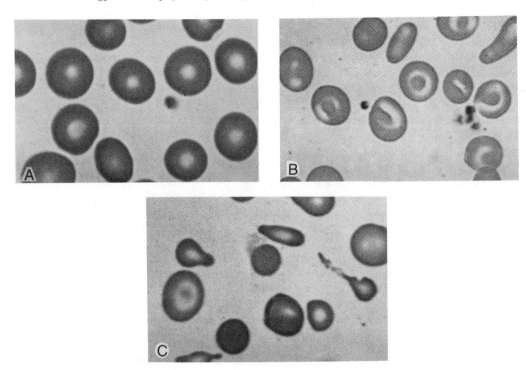

Fig. 10-14. Blood smear in thalassemia. (**A**) Normal. (**B**) Thalassemia minor. (**C**) Thalassemia major. Thalassemia shows microcytosis, target cells, deformed red cells, basophilic stippling, and (in thalassemia major) nucleated red cells. (From Kapff CT, Jandl JH [1981] The anemias. In: Blood: Atlas and Sourcebook. Little, Brown, Boston, with permission.)

degree of anemia. Other manifestations are those of ineffective erythropoiesis: a serum iron on the high side, slight indirect bilirubinemia, and a juicy hypercellular marrow with hyperplasia of the red cell precursors and an increase in iron. Perhaps the most important point about β-thalassemia heterozygotes is that they are for the most part clinically well, but their children are at risk for homozygous β-thalassemia.

Patients with homozygous β-thalassemia (β-thalassemia major) are generally quite ill (Fig. 10-13). At the root of their problems is an exceedingly severe anemia. The degree of anemia in these patients places such a heavy burden on the cardiovascular system that death in childhood from high-output congestive failure used to be the typical outcome in β-thalassemia major; most patients now receive chronic transfusion therapy, so life expectancy has increased

by a decade or two, and the mode of death has changed from high-output failure to hemochromatosis. Growth and maturation in these patients is retarded, and they develop a greatly enlarged liver and spleen along with a characteristic facial deformity ("chipmunk facies," Fig. 10-15) caused by bones that have expanded to accommodate the greatly increased amount of hematopoietic tissue that fills their marrow cavities.

The blood and marrow picture is similar to that seen in thalassemia trait, but much more severe (Fig. 10-14). Microcytosis and gross deformities of the red cells are seen on the smear, together with a marked reticulocytosis and prominent basophilic stippling. Nucleated red cells are common. The exceedingly hyperplastic marrow, which is packed with red cell precursors and loaded with iron, fills and expands the marrow cavity of every bone; this

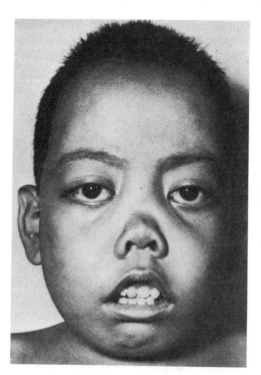

Fig. 10-15. "Chipmunk facies" of thalassemia major. Gross marrow hyperplasia has expanded the facial bones. (From Weatherall DJ, Clegg JB [1972] Disorders resulting from defective β- or δ-chain synthesis: the β- and δβ-thalassemias. In: The Thalassemia Syndromes. Blackwell Scientific Publishers, Oxford, with permission.)

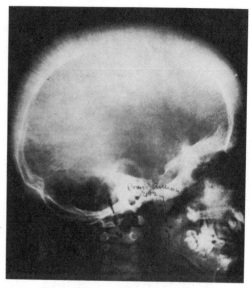

Fig. 10-16. "Hair-on-end" skull of thalassemia major. (From Weatherall DJ, Clegg JB [1972] Disorders resulting from defective β- or δ-chain synthesis. The β- and δβ-thalassemias. In: The Thalassemia Syndromes. Blackwell Scientific Publishers, Oxford, with permission.)

is strikingly evident on radiographs, which show distended bones criss-crossed with hyperplastic trabeculae (the remarkable "hair-on-end" picture of the skull (Fig. 10-16). Extramedullary hematopoiesis is prominent in the liver and spleen.

The diagnosis of thalassemia is established by showing the typical quantitative abnormalities in the hemoglobin content of the red cells. This is usually accomplished by hemoglobin electrophoresis. The usual finding in β-thalassemia trait is a modest increase in the minor hemoglobins whose pattern is a logical consequence of the genetic defect (e.g., in δβ-thalassemia, hemoglobin F is elevated, but hemoglobin A_2 is normal or decreased, because the genetic lesion in this condition involves the δ-

chain as well as the β-chain). Hemoglobin A remains the predominant hemoglobin in β-thalassemia trait, despite the impairment in β-chain production in this condition. In thalassemia major, however, hemoglobin A is greatly decreased (β^+-thalassemia) or absent (β^0-thalassemia). The major hemoglobin in the red cell is hemoglobin F, while the amounts of other hemoglobins in the cell depend on the nature of the genetic defect. The red cell hemoglobin patterns in the three classical varieties of β-thalassemia (i.e., all but HPFH) are shown in Table 10-3.

Hemoglobin electrophoresis is usually all that is necessary to establish a diagnosis of β-thalassemia. The only situation in which hemoglobin electrophoresis fails is when it is necessary to make the diagnosis in a fetus at risk for β-thalassemia major (a fetus is at risk if both parents have some form of β-thalassemia). This problem is discussed below.

CONSEQUENCES OF DECREASED α-CHAIN PRODUCTION IN α-THALASSEMIA

Reduced concentrations of all normal hemoglobins (A, A_2, and F)

Assembly of excess β-class chains into abnormal hemoglobin tetramers

Hemoglobin H ($β_4$)

Hemoglobin Bart's ($γ_4$)

Hemoglobin Portland ($ζ_2γ_2$) in cells that completely lack α-chains

---

THE α-THALASSEMIAS

Inherited impairment of α-chain synthesis leads to the group of diseases known as the α-thalassemias. This group contains four clinical forms of α-thalassemia. They range from a form that is totally asymptomatic to one that is invariably fatal during gestation or early infancy.

Pathogenesis

α-Thalassemia is caused by a functional abnormality in one or more of the four α-globin genes on the chromosome 16 pair. In most cases, the disease results because the affected genes are no longer able to code for the globin chain, so their contribution to total α-chain production is lost altogether. In the Far East, however, there is a common form of α-thalassemia caused by a mutant gene that codes

for the production of an abnormal α-chain known as α Constant Spring. For some reason, α Constant Spring cannot be synthesized except at exceedingly low rates, so that patients carrying the Constant Spring gene show a deficit in α-chain production nearly as severe as that in patients with a total failure of α-gene function. (The analogy is clear between hemoglobin Constant Spring versus classical α-thalassemia as compared with $β^+$- versus $β^0$-thalassemia.)

The decrease in the rate of α-chain synthesis has three consequences. First, there is a reduction in the concentration of all α-chain containing hemoglobins in the α-thalassemic red cell. This includes all three hemoglobins normally present in the adult erythrocyte. Second, there is an accumulation of free β-family chains, resulting from the imbalance between α- and β-chain production in α-thalassemia. These associate to form hemoglobins consisting of four identical β-class chains; hemoglobin H, from the β-chains ($β_4$), and hemoglobin Bart's (discovered in St. Bartholomew's Hospital in London), from the γ-chains ($γ_4$). In the α-thalassemic patient, hemoglobins Bart's and H show the same pattern of changes with age that hemoglobins F and A show in the normal, and for the same reason: the changes in the rates of production of the γ- and β-chains as fetal and infant development proceeds. The changes in the concentrations of these hemoglobins in the α-thalassemic patient are of considerable clinical importance, as will be seen. Finally, if α-chain synthesis is lacking altogether, the ζ-globin gene, which codes for the production of the embryonic α-class ζ-chain, retains its activity,

Table 10-3. Hemoglobins A and A_2 in β-Thalassemia[a]

Variety	Major		Minor	
	Hb A	Hb A_2	Hb A	Hb A_2
$β^+$-Thalassemia	Sharply ↓	↑	Slightly ↓	↑
$β^0$-Thalassemia	Absent	↑	Slightly ↓	↑
δβ-Thalassemia (and Hemoglobin Lepore)	Absent	Absent	Slightly ↓	Not ↑

[a]All β-thalassemia patients have elevated hemoglobin F. The different kinds of β-thalassemia can be distinguished by looking at the percentages of hemoglobins A and A_2.

so hemoglobin Portland ($\zeta_2\gamma_2$) remains a component of the red cell throughout fetal life.

α-Thalassemia occurs in four degrees of severity, depending on the number of malfunctioning genes in the patient. These forms are listed in Table 10-4. Varieties in which one or two genes are defective are mild or asymptomatic. Characteristic diseases, however, are caused by the lack of three or four of the α-globin genes. The problems associated with these diseases are attributable more to the behavior of the hemoglobins formed from the surplus β-class chains than to the deficit in total hemoglobin production (Table 10-5).

The dysfunction of three of the α-globin genes causes hemoglobin H disease. As the name implies, this disease features the accumulation of substantial quantities of hemoglobin H in the erythrocyte—never the majority of the hemoglobin, but always enough to cause serious damage to the red cells. The full-blown disease is not seen until the patient is a few months of age, the time it takes for the concentration of hemoglobin H to rise to adult levels. Problems arise because this hemoglobin is unstable, forming precipitates of denatured protein in affected red cells. These precipitates are pitted out, leading to small, malformed red cells. Ineffective erythropoiesis results because of the destruction of the abnormal cells in the bone marrow; it is never as severe as in β-thalassemia, however, because enough normal hemoglobin is present as a result of the single functioning α-globin gene to moderate the destruction of red cells in the marrow. On the other hand, hemolysis is brisk and contributes substantially to the anemia in patients with hemoglobin H disease.

Table 10-4. Varieties of α-Thalassemia

Variety	α-Globin Genes Out of Commission (no.)
α_2-Thalassemia trait ("silent carrier")	1
α_1-Thalassemia trait (α-thalassemia minor)	2
Hemoglobin H disease	3
Hydrops fetalis	4

Table 10-5. Properties of the Abnormal Hemoglobins in α-Thalassemia

Hemoglobin	Property
Hemoglobin H (β_4)	Unstable
Hemoglobin Bart's (γ_4)	Very high oxygen affinity

When all the α-globin genes are out of commission, no α-chains can be made. This situation leads to a fatal clinical syndrome called *hydrops fetalis*. The total absence of α-chain synthesis means that in the fetus, the red cells contain no hemoglobin F. They are filled instead with hemoglobin Bart's (γ_4), a hemoglobin whose oxygen affinity is so high that for practical purposes it is unable to release oxygen to tissues. Death from tissue anoxia is the inevitable outcome in hydrops fetalis.

Clinical Manifestations

α-Thalassemia is primarily a disease of the Far Eastern and black populations, although it occurs to a slight extent among Mediterranean Europeans. The severe forms occur almost exclusively among Orientals, because chromosomes carrying two defective α-globin genes are restricted almost entirely to that population (Fig. 10-17). In other populations subject to α-thalassemia, the genetic lesion almost always involves only one of the two α-globin genes, accounting for the generally mild form of the disease in these populations.

MILD α-THALASSEMIA

The mild forms of α-thalassemia result from the malfunction of one or two genes. The condition in which a single gene is defective is called α_2-thalassemia trait, or silent carrier α-thalassemia. The term "silent carrier" is highly appropriate, because most of these patients are completely asymptomatic; slight microcytosis is all that is seen, and even this subtle manifestation is often missing. The major clue to the silent carrier state is the presence of more severe forms of α-thalassemia in family members.

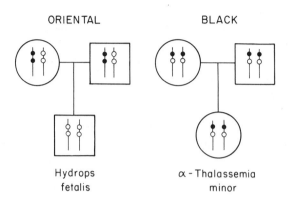

Fig. 10-17. Example showing why α-thalassemia is worse in Orientals than in blacks. Each parent has α-thalassemia minor because of two defective α-globin genes. In blacks, the defective genes are on different chromosomes, so their offspring have at worst α-thalassemia minor. In Orientals, the defective genes are on the same chromosome, so an unfortunate pairing can produce a fetus with hydrops fetalis.

When two genes are out of commission, α_1-thalassemia trait, or α-thalassemia minor, is the disease that results. The signs and symptoms are virtually identical to those of β-thalassemia minor: (1) anemia, generally mild, with very small red cells; (2) a blood smear showing small, misshapen red cells, target cells, basophilic stippling, and reticulocytosis; (3) a marrow showing hyperplasia of the red cell series and increased iron; and (4) modest splenomegaly.

In adults, it is difficult to make the diagnosis of α-thalassemia trait (either variety). Hemoglobin electrophoresis, the mainstay of the workup in β-thalassemia trait, is always normal in α_2-thalassemia trait and is often normal in α_1-thalassemia trait, although the presence of some hemoglobin H in the latter may permit the diagnosis to be made (Table 10-6). In newborns, the diagnosis is somewhat easier, since slight elevations in hemoglobin Bart's are seen in cord blood in both forms of α-thalassemia trait. If necessary, the diagnosis can be established by measuring globin chain production to look for a decrease in the α:β synthetic ratio, or by performing Southern blotting with an α-gene probe, looking for patterns previously found in patients known to have α-thalassemia.

Measurements of globin chain production and analysis of DNA are expensive to perform; these tests are carried out only in a few institutions, usually in connection with research on the molecular biology of thalassemia. When should these tests be done? They are indispensable for prenatal diagnosis in pregnant women with either α- or β-thalassemia trait and cannot be replaced by any other procedure. They are unnecessary in adults with β-thalassemia trait, because this diagnosis can always be established by hemoglobin electrophoresis. What about adults suspected of having α-thalassemia trait in whom hemoglobin electrophoresis is normal? Family studies can sometimes estab-

Table 10-6. Manifestations of a α-Thalassemia

	Findings	
Disorder	Clinical	Hemoglobin Electrophoresis
α_2-Thalassemia trait	None	Normal
α_1-Thalassemia trait	Like β-thalassemia minor	Normal or a trace of hemoglobin H
Hemoglobin H disease	Like mild β-thalassemia major	Hemoglobin H
Hydrops fetalis	Swollen, pale infant, stillborn or dying shortly after birth	Hemoglobin Bart's and Portland (cord blood); no hemoglobin A

lish a diagnosis with certainty; for instance, the symptomless father of a patient with hemoglobin H disease whose mother has α_1-thalassemia trait would have to be a silent carrier on genetic grounds (Fig. 10-18). When the diagnosis cannot be established by simple means, however, the decision as to whether to carry out these highly specialized tests should be based on whether making the diagnosis will be of sufficient benefit to the patient to warrant the trouble and expense involved in carrying them out.

HEMOGLOBIN H DISEASE

The clinical manifestations of hemoglobin H disease closely resemble those of β-thalassemia major, although the condition tends to be milder than the average case of β-thalassemia major. Anemia is moderate to marked; the smear shows the typical abnormalities of severe thalassemia. The liver and spleen are enlarged, and the marrow undergoes the same expansion in erythropoiesis as seen in β-thalassemia major, leading to the same bony abnormalities.

The diagnosis is made by finding hemoglobin H in the red cells of patients with the clinical picture of thalassemia. This can be done by staining a blood smear with cresyl violet, a procedure that causes the unstable hemoglobin H to precipitate as small clumps of uniform size that fill all the red cells and are easily seen under the microscope (Fig. 10-19). Hemoglobin H may also be demonstrated by electrophoresis, where it is easily detected as a rapidly moving band that migrates well ahead of hemoglobin A (Fig. 10-19). Electrophoresis also illustrates the point that most of the hemoglobin in hemoglobin H disease erythrocytes is hemoglobin A, not hemoglobin H. Indeed, in newborns with hemoglobin H disease, the red cells may contain little hemoglobin H, because of the low β-chain synthetic rate at this time of life; the tip-off to hemoglobin H disease in these patients is a major elevation of hemoglobin Bart's in cord blood.

More sophisticated tests, such as globin chain synthetic measurements and Southern blotting, are not necessary for the diagnosis of hemoglobin H disease in a patient with clinical thalassemia. They are required, however, for prenatal diagnosis.

HYDROPS FETALIS

Hydrops fetalis is the clinical picture caused by fulminant intrauterine congestive heart failure. The affected fetus has a grossly enlarged heart and liver together with edema and massive ascites. In the most severe form of α-tha-

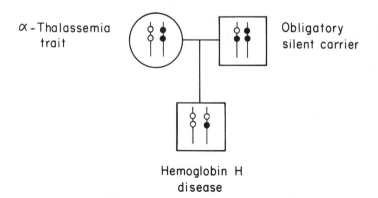

α-Thalassemia trait

Obligatory silent carrier

Hemoglobin H disease

Fig. 10-18. Diagnosing the silent carrier state. The child with hemoglobin H disease has three defective α-globin genes. Two were inherited from his mother, who has α-thalassemia trait. The third must have come from his symptomless father, who has to be a silent carrier.

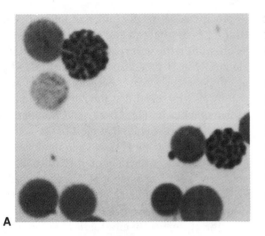

A

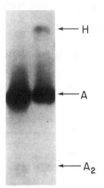

B

Fig. 10-19. The diagnosis of hemoglobin H disease. (**A**) Hemoglobin H stain. The red cells contain small uniform clumps of hemoglobin H. (**B**) Hemoglobin electrophoresis. Hemoglobin H moves ahead of hemoglobin A. Hemoglobin A is the major hemoglobin in these red cells. (**A**: From Castoldi GL [1981] Erythrocytes. In Zucker-Franklin D et al [eds]: Atlas of Blood Cells: Function and Pathology. Edi. Ermes s.r.l., Milan, with permission. **B**: Modified from Pressley L et al [1980] Gene deletions in thalassemia prove that the 5'ζ locus is functional. Proc Natl Acad Sci 77:3586, with permission.)

lassemia, in which there is total absence of α-chain synthesis, hydrops is the result. Red cells in this condition contain primarily hemoglobin Bart's, which releases its oxygen only with great difficulty, leading to oxygen-starved tissues. In an attempt to compensate for this tissue anoxia, cardiac output increases to the point of congestive heart failure, which also has highly deleterious effects on fetal develop-

ment. The consequences are so serious that this form of hydrops is always fatal, either in utero or shortly after birth.

The diagnosis, usually post-mortem, is made by electrophoresis of cord blood. The only hemoglobins present on electrophoresis are hemoglobin Bart's and a small amount of hemoglobin Portland ($\zeta_2\gamma_2$). Because of the seriousness of the disease, prenatal diagnosis should be strongly considered in any pregnant woman whose fetus is at risk for this form of α-thalassemia.

MOLECULAR GENETICS OF THALASSEMIA

The thalassemias are all caused by mutations in the region of the globin genes. The study of these disorders by molecular genetic techniques has made it clear that the mutations responsible for the thalassemias are highly diverse, involving all regions of the α- and β-globin gene clusters and ranging from simple nucleotide substitutions to huge deletions affecting thousands of bases. A great many of these mutations have been characterized at a molecular level (Fig. 10-20), and their effects on messenger RNA formation and catabolism have been analyzed.

The effect of a mutation depends in part on which region of the gene is involved. Mutations in an intron can slow or stop messenger RNA production by disrupting the splicing process. Mutations in the 3' or 5' untranslated regions can decrease messenger RNA production by (1) delaying or preventing the transcription of the messenger RNA from the DNA template; (2) altering post-transcriptional processing of the message (splicing, polyadenylation, export from the nucleus); or (3) decreasing the life of the message in the cytoplasm. Mutations in an exon may (1) impair messenger RNA production; (2) produce a messenger RNA that codes for an abnormal globin (a chain with amino acid substitutions, or one that is shortened or lengthened because of abnormal termination); or (3) produce a messenger RNA

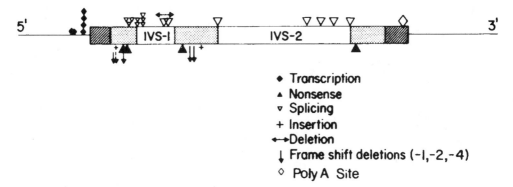

Fig. 10-20. Types and locations of mutations that cause β-thalassemia. IVS, intervening sequence (= intron). (From Orkin SH [1987] Disorders of hemoglobin synthesis. p. 108. In Stamatoyannopoulos G, Nienhuis AW, Leder P, Majerus PW [eds]: The Molecular Basis of Blood Diseases. WB Saunders, Philadelphia, with permission.)

that uses a slightly altered code to make a perfectly normal globin. Among the dozens of mutations responsible for the thalassemia phenotype, examples of all these effects have been found.

There is a rough relationship between thalassemia types and the nature of the responsible mutations. Many of the α-thalassemias, the δβ-thalassemias and HPFH are due to gene deletions of major size. On the other hand, most β⁰- and β⁺-thalassemias seem to be caused by genetic defects that are much more localized: substitutions or small deletions. Large deletions routinely cause abnormalities in Southern blots because of the changes in restriction fragment size that result from the loss of major quantities of DNA from the globin gene region (Fig. 10-21). Localized mutations, however, will cause changes in the Southern blot only if they accidentally generate or eliminate a restriction enzyme recognition site. This is rather unlikely, so in most instances, Southern blots from patients with thalassemia caused by a localized mutation have been perfectly normal.

Prenatal Diagnosis

When a pregnant mother and the father both come from thalassemic families, their fetus is at risk for high-grade thalassemia. In such cases, prenatal testing is often used to determine whether or not the fetus actually has the disease. The prenatal diagnosis is usually made by molecular genetic techniques.

In families with β-*thalassemia*, prenatal diagnosis is usually accomplished by an approach in which the sequences of the defective parental β-globin genes are used to design pairs of short DNA oligomers (one pair for each parent), one of which will bind selectively to the normal gene and the other to the abnormal gene. DNA is then isolated from amniotic fluid cells, which are of fetal origin and are safely and easily obtained by amniocentesis. The amniocyte DNA is probed with the oligomers to find out which of the parental genes are carried by the fetus. From this the fetal phenotype (normal, carrier, thalassemic) can be predicted.

The serious forms of α-*thalassemia* (hemoglobin H disease and hydrops fetalis) can also be diagnosed prenatally in a fetus at risk. This diagnosis is usually made by Southern blotting, since α-thalassemia often results from major gene deletions that cause obvious abnormalities in α-globin gene Southern blots. The first step is to make a Southern blot of DNA from the parents, using α-globin DNA as the probe. If the analysis of these Southern blots confirms

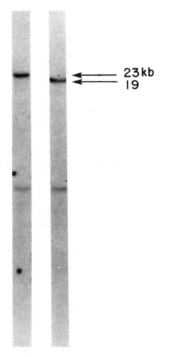

← 23kb
← 19

Fig. 10-21. Restriction mapping in α-thalassemia caused by deletion of a major gene. The patient has hemoglobin H disease as a result of the deletion of three of the four α-globin genes. The restriction map of the remaining α-globin gene region (*right*) is different from normal (*left*) because the deletion of a 3-kb portion containing one of the two α-globin genes has changed the size of the α-globin restriction fragments obtained from his DNA. (Modified from Kan YW et al [1979] Molecular basis of hemoglobin diseases in the Mediterranean population. Blood 54:1434, with permission.)

that the fetus is at risk (i.e., if one parent is missing two α-globin genes from a single chromosome and the other lacks at least one α-globin gene), the fetal DNA is mapped. A comparison of the fetal map with maps from the parents will make the diagnosis by establishing the number of α-globin genes the fetus inherited from each parent.

Often the Southern blot of a defective gene is normal, and an oligomer probe to identify the defective gene is unavailable. Under these circumstances, a prenatal diagnosis may still be achieved by taking advantage of *restriction*

fragment length polymorphisms (RFLPs, sometimes pronounced "ruflups"). RFLPs are detected by Southern blotting, and consist of subject to subject differences in the size of a restriction fragment that carries a given piece of genetic material (e.g., the β-globin gene). RFLPs arise because of small differences in the DNA sequence of different individuals (among humans, DNA sequences vary by 1 base in several hundred). The origin of an RFLP is illustrated by the following example. Consider a sequence difference involving a restriction site (say, a HincII site) near the β-globin gene, so that DNA from some individuals contains that HincII site while DNA from others does not. An RFLP will be seen on a Southern blot of HincII-digested DNA when probed for the β-globin gene (Fig. 10-22). The globin gene-containing fragments obtained from DNA samples isolated from different individuals will be of two different sizes, a shorter fragment generated from DNA that contains the variable HincII site and a longer fragment from DNA that does not. DNA from a single individual may show both fragments, if one of his chromosomes contains the variable restriction site and the other does not.

In a family carrying both β-thalassemia and an RFLP linked to the defective globin gene, analysis of Southern blots from enough family members may reveal that the size of the fragment carrying the defective globin gene is different from that of the fragment carrying the normal gene. If so, the RFLP may be used as a marker to establish the presence or absence of the thalassemic gene in a fetus. Consider, for example, two parents, both with β-thalassemia trait (Fig. 10-22). Suppose that the HincII restriction map of DNA from the father showed a single β-globin band at 7.6 kb, indicating that both the normal and defective gene are on 7.6-kb fragments; but that the HincII map of DNA from the pregnant mother showed two β-globin bands, a 7.6-kb band from one allele and a 6.0-kb band from the other; and suppose further that through family studies it was determined that the thalassemia gene was associated with (say) the 6.0-kb band. If the Southern blot of

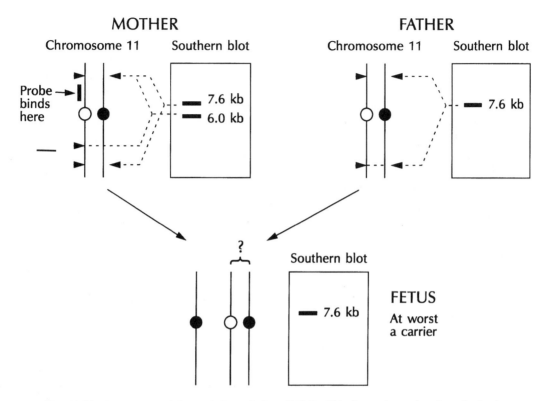

Fig. 10-22. How a prenatal diagnosis is made from RFLPs. This figure shows data from the family described in the text: the father and the pregnant mother, both with β-thalassemia trait, and the fetus, who is at risk for β-thalassemia major. For each family member, the figure shows (1) a map of the HincII restriction sites near the β-globin genes on the two alleles for chromosome 11 (*arrowheads*), and (2) a diagram of the corresponding Southern blot, which was prepared with DNA cut at the hypothetical restriction sites and examined with a probe containing β-globin DNA sequences. In the map, the normal β-globin gene is shown as •, and the thalassemic β-globin gene as o. In both of the father's alleles, the β-globin gene is flanked by identical HincII restriction sites 7.6 kb apart, so that after digestion with HincII the normal and thalassemic β-globin genes will be on fragments of the same size. The Southern blot of the paternal DNA therefore shows only a single β-globin band at 7.6 kb. The mother's alleles, however, show a polymorphism. The HincII restriction sites on the normal maternal allele are the same as in the father, but the thalassemic allele has an extra restriction site (*arrow*). Consequently, when the mother's DNA is cut, the thalassemic β-globin gene will be on a short fragment, and the Southern blot of her DNA will show two β-globin bands: a 7.6-kb band containing the normal gene, and a 6.0-kb band containing the thalassemia gene. What about the fetus? Her Southern blot shows only a 7.6-kb band. This provides no information as to which of the father's β-globin genes was inherited by the fetus, because both the normal and the thalassemic paternal β-globin genes are found on a 7.6-kb fragment. From the mother, however, the fetus had to have inherited the normal β-globin gene, because the maternal β-thalassemia gene would have been found in a 6.0-kb fragment, and no such fragment appeared on the fetus' Southern blot. At worst, then, the fetus will only have β-thalassemia trait.

the fetal DNA shows only a 7.6-kb band but no 6.0-kb band, it can be concluded that the fetus has inherited the normal gene from its mother, and is therefore not at risk for β-thalassemia major. If suitable RFLPs occur in both parents' families, it may be possible by this approach to make a complete and accurate prenatal diagnosis of β-thalassemia. Furthermore, it is clear that this type of analysis may be used for prenatal diagnosis of any disease in which the defective gene is linked to a particular RFLP.

MANAGEMENT OF THALASSEMIA

Thalassemia major is usually a fatal disease. The child with untreated thalassemia major is weak and wasted, showing stunted growth, poor development, and the characteristic bony deformities of the disease. The most serious problems involve the cardiovascular system. The chronic high-output state resulting from this anemia causes the heart to fail after only a few years, so that by the time the child is 5 or 6 years old, he has all the signs and symptoms of congestive heart failure and is usually dead from this cause before reaching his teens.

The solution to all these problems should be blood transfusion. In principle, transfusion to a normal hematocrit should lift the burden from the cardiovascular system and cause the hyperplastic marrow to return to its normal state, fully correcting the functional disorders of thalassemia. Unfortunately, however, blood transfusion has proved a two-edged sword, inducing iron overload and hemochromatosis at the same time that it corrects the anemia. So the management of thalassemia has become a balancing act in which the benefits of transfusion are weighed against the costs, the goal being to optimize the life expectancy of the patient.

The major approach to achieving this goal has been to give patients enough blood to reduce the strain on their hearts to a tolerable level and to suppress their own marrow's production of red cells. This is generally accomplished by transfusing to a hematocrit of 35. Transfusions are obviously unnecessary in patients with thalassemia trait, whose degree of anemia poses no threat to their life expectancy.

Transfusion, the mainstay of therapy in thalassemia major, can be supplemented by two measures designed to minimize its risks:

1. *Splenectomy.* Splenectomy is often carried out in thalassemic patients to reduce the transfusion requirement. To the extent that thalassemic red cells are damaged by the spleen, splenectomy will increase their survival, thereby decreasing the need for transfusions. It is a useful procedure in treating this condition, yet it generally results in only a modest reduction in the transfusion requirement and puts the patient at increased risk for certain bacterial infections.

2. *Iron chelation therapy.* Because of the iron burden imposed by chronic transfusion therapy, hemochromatosis leading to fatal congestive failure with death in the teens has until recently been the usual outcome of thalassemic patients on this form of treatment. This complication has been ameliorated through the concurrent use of the iron chelator desferrioxamine (Ch. 4). By binding the excess iron and allowing it to be excreted by the kidneys, desferrioxamine has been able to prevent the hemochromatosis that was formerly such a difficult problem for these patients.

A few patients with very severe thalassemia major have been cured by *bone marrow transplantation.* This risky form of treatment should be considered only as a last resort.

MANAGEMENT OF THALASSEMIA

Blood transfusions
Iron chelation therapy
Splenectomy
Bone marrow transplantation
Prenatal diagnosis

The other major aspect of management in thalassemia is prenatal diagnosis (see above). Safe and effective techniques are now available for making the diagnosis of thalassemia major in a fetus at risk for the disease. Thalassemic families should be told about the availability of these techniques.

HEMOGLOBIN E

Hemoglobin E disease is a form of β-thalassemia in which the underproduced β-chain (designated $β^E$) contains the amino acid substitution $β^{26:glu \rightarrow lys}$. It is caused by a β-globin gene mutation that has a remarkable dual effect. The first and most obvious effect is the alteration in the amino acid sequence of the β-globin chain at position 26. The second effect—much more subtle—is a disturbance in the processing of the β-globin messenger RNA. It is the second effect that explains why hemoglobin E disease is a form of thalassemia.

What the mutation does to RNA processing is to create a false splicing site within an exon of the $β^E$ messenger RNA transcript (Fig. 10-23). This false splicing site leads to defective post-transcriptional modification of the messenger transcripts. Some of the transcripts are processed normally, but others are processed in such a way that exon fusion takes place, not

after the coding triplet for amino acid 30, the normal splicing site, but in the middle of the mutated coding triplet for amino acid 26, some dozen nucleotides upstream from the normal splicing site. From this abnormally processed messenger no β-chain is synthesized. The result is an underproduction of β-chain, the hallmark of β-thalassemia.

Hemoglobin E is second only to sickle cell hemoglobin in its worldwide prevalence. It occurs primarily in Asia, where it is exceedingly common in certain population groups. Among Southeast Asians in particular, it is present in more than 10 percent of the population.

Persons with hemoglobin E have no symptoms, no anemia, and little or no shortening of the red cell lifespan. Blood smears from both heterozygotes (A/E) and homozygotes (E/E) show microcytosis, but target cells are only seen in the homozygote. The diagnosis is made by hemoglobin electrophoresis, in which hemoglobin E is seen to run well behind hemoglobin A. The difference between the electrophoretic mobilities of the two hemoglobins can be explained by the reduction in the overall negative charge of the hemoglobin E molecule that results from the glutamate → lysine substitution.

In contrast to the mildness of A/E and E/E is the severity of the disease caused by combining hemoglobin E with another form of β-tha-

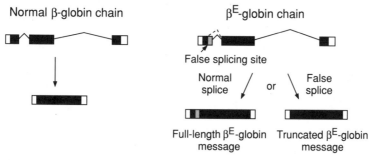

Fig. 10-23. A false splicing site in the hemoglobin E gene. The mutation that gives rise to hemoglobin E is located in the first exon of the gene coding for the β-globin chain. This mutation creates a false splicing site in the $β^E$-chain messenger RNA. As a result, much of the $β^E$-chain message is processed abnormally, with excision of the first intron occuring, not at the normal location, but at the site of the mutation, which lies several nucleotides upstream from the normal splice site. Globin chains cannot be made from this abnormally spliced message.

lassemia. The combination produces thalassemia major, and E/β-thalassemia patients are very sick. It seems that the decrease in β-chain synthesis that occurs when the mildly defective β^E-gene is combined with a grossly defective β^+ -or β^0-gene is large enough to cause serious clinical illness.

SUGGESTED READINGS

Adams JG, 3d, Coleman MB (1990) Structural hemoglobin variants that produce the phenotype of thalassemia. Semin Hematol 27:229

Alter BP (1988) Prenatal diagnosis: general introduction, methodology, and review. Hemoglobin 12:763

Anderson HM, Ranney HM (1990) Southeast Asian immigrants: the new thalassemias in Americans. Semin Hematol 27:239

Bank A (1978) The thalassemia syndromes. Blood 51:369

Bollekens JA, Forget BG (1991) Delta beta thalassemia and hereditary persistence of fetal hemoglobin. Hematol Oncol Clin North Am 5:399

Bunn HF, Forget BD (1984) Human Hemoglobins. 2nd Ed. WB Saunders, Philadelphia

Eisenstein BI (1990) The polymerase chain reaction. A new method of using molecular genetics for medical diagnosis. N Engl J Med 322:178

Fantoni A, Farace MG, Gambari R (1981) Embryonic hemoglobins of man and other mammals. Blood 57:623

Forget BD (1979) Molecular genetics of human hemoglobin synthesis. Ann Intern Med 91:605

Fosburg MT, Nathan DG (1990) Treatment of Cooley's anemia. Blood 76:435

Graham JB, Green PP, McGraw RA, Davis LM (1985) Application of molecular genetics to prenatal diagnosis and carrier detection in the hemophilias: some limitations. Blood 66:759

Gusella JF (1986) Recombinant DNA techniques in the diagnosis of inherited disorders. J Clin Invest 77:1723

Higgs DR, Weatherall DJ (1983) Alpha-thalassemia. Curr Top Hematol 4:37

Kan YW (1992) Development of DNA analysis for human diseases. Sickle cell anemia and thalassemia as a paradigm. JAMA 267:1532

Kazazian HH, Jr (1990) The thalassemia syndromes: molecular basis and prenatal diagnosis in 1990. Semin Hematol 27:209

Kolata GB (1980) Thalassemias: models of genetic diseases. Science 210:300

Lachant NA (1987) Hemoglobin E: an emerging hemoglobinopathy in the United States. Am J Hematol 35:449

Ley TJ (1991) The pharmacology of hemoglobin switching: of mice and men. Blood 77:1146

Nienhuis AW, Benz EJ, Jr (1977) Regulation of hemoglobin synthesis during the development of the red cell. N Engl J Med 297:1319

Orkin SH (1987) Disorders of hemoglobin synthesis. p. 106. In Stamatoyannopoulos G, Nienhuis AW, Leder P, Majerus PW (eds): Molecular Basis of Blood Diseases. WB Saunders, Philadelphia

Steinberg MH (1991) The interactions of alpha-thalassemia with hemoglobinopathies. Hematol Oncol Clin North Am 5:453

Watson JD (1976) Molecular Biology of the Gene. 3rd Ed. WA Benjamin, Menlo Park, CA

Weatherall DJ, Clegg JB (1981) The Thalassemia Syndromes. 3rd Ed. CV Mosby, St. Louis

Wood WG, Clegg JB, Weatherall DJ (1979) Hereditary persistence of fetal hemoglobin (HPHF) and γβ-thalassemia. Br J Haematol 43:509

11

Sickle Cell Anemia and Related Hemoglobinopathies

The functionally abnormal hemoglobins discussed up to now fall into three categories: those with an altered oxygen affinity, those that remain perpetually in the methemoglobin form, and the unstable hemoglobins. Patients with these hemoglobins, however, constitute only a tiny minority of all patients with functional hemoglobinopathy. The majority of patients with symptomatic functional hemoglobinopathy suffer from sickle cell anemia or one of its variants.

THE SICKLE CELL

Sickle cell diseases are caused by the presence in the red cell of a mutant hemoglobin that forms rigid aggregates when in the deoxy form. Red cells containing such aggregates are stiff and cannot change shape as easily as normal cells when forced to pass through blood vessels smaller than their own diameter (i.e., arterioles and capillaries). As a result, the cells tend to plug these blood vessels. Most of the signs and symptoms of the sickle cell diseases are thought to result from this microvascular blockage.

Hemoglobin S

The mutant hemoglobin of sickle cell anemia is known as hemoglobin S. Like hemoglobin A, it is a tetramer composed of two α-chains and two β-chains. The β-chains, however, are abnormal, containing a valine instead of a glutamate at position 6. These abnormal chains are designated β^S, so the subunit composition of hemoglobin S is written $\alpha_2\beta^S_2$.

There is a general tendency for hemoglobin molecules in the deoxy form to polymerize. This tendency is exaggerated in hemoglobin S, presumably because the substitution of an oil-like valine for a charged glutamate residue makes for a very tight fit between the two aggregating hemoglobin molecules (Fig. 11-1). Deoxyhemoglobin S molecules readily assemble into long, stiff bundles composed of 14-strand fibers packed tightly side by side, each strand consisting of thousands of hemoglobin S molecules lined up in single file (Fig. 11-2). The fibers are formed spontaneously within a hemoglobin S-containing red cell when the cell is placed in an environment in which the hemoglobin loses its oxygen. When they pack into bundles, these fibers deform the cell into an elongate irregular rod or crescent (Fig. 11-3).

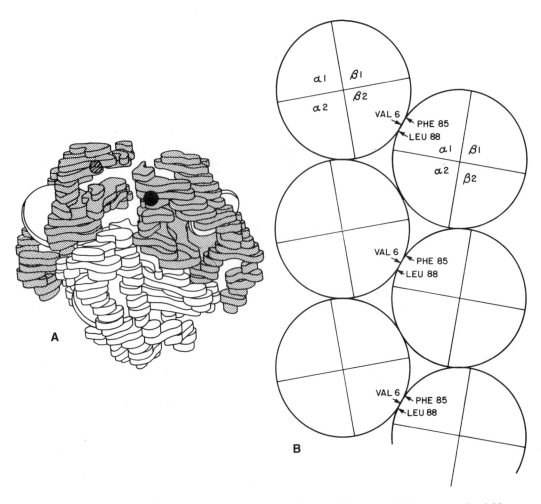

Fig. 11-1. Location of the mutation in sickle hemoglobin. (**A**) The hemoglobin tetramer. In sickle hemoglobin, a valine is substituted for the glutamate normally found in position 6 of the β-subunit. This valine is seen to lie on the outer surface of the mutant subunit. (**B**) Part of a polymerized sickle hemoglobin strand. Because of its exposed location, the β6-valine of sickle hemoglobin is able to interact strongly with the oil-like β85-phenylalanine and β88-leucine residues on the surface of the adjacent hemoglobin tetramer.

Reoxygenation causes the bundles to melt. This ordinarily restores the cell to its disclike form, but a few cells will remain misshapen even under these circumstances, probably because they have gone through so many cycles of deformation that their membranes have become damaged and can no longer spring back to their original shape. It is the crescent shape of many of the deformed cells that gives the name "sickle" to the disease and to the cells themselves.

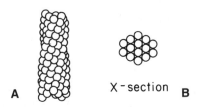

Fig. 11-2. The 14-strand fiber of deoxyhemoglobin S. (**A:** From Dykes G, Crepeau R, Edelstein SJ [1978] Three-dimensional reconstruction of the fibers of sickle-cell haemoglobin. Nature 272:500, with permission.)

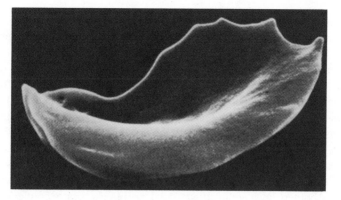

Fig. 11-3. A sickle cell. (From Bessis M [1973] Living Blood Cells and Their Ultrastructure. Springer-Verlag, New York, with permission.)

The polymerization of hemoglobin S takes place in three stages (Fig. 11-4). The first stage is called *nucleation*. It begins with the aggregation of hemoglobin molecules into small clusters. These clusters grow by random collison with molecules in solution until they reach 15 molecules or so in size. At this point they are able to serve as nuclei on which the remaining

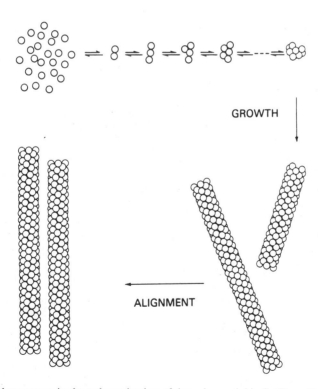

Fig. 11-4. The three stages in the polymerization of deoxyhemoglobin S. (From Dean J, Schechter AN [1978] Sickle-cell anemia: molecular and cellular bases of therapeutic approaches. N Engl J Med 299:752, with permission.)

hemoglobin molecule can assemble. The stage of *polymerization* now begins. Using the nuclei as starting points, the remaining deoxyhemoglobin S molecules rapidly polymerize into thousands of 14-strand fibers. By the end of the polymerization stage, most of the deoxyhemoglobin S molecules will have been incorporated into fibers, with just a few remaining in solution. At this point, the red cell contains what amounts to a saturated solution of deoxyhemoglobin S in contact with the polymerized hemoglobin fibers. Finally comes the stage of *alignment*, when the 14-strand fibers assemble into fiber bundles.

Each of these stages has its counterpart in the intact red cell. The nucleation stage is an interval during which nothing seems to happen; the red cell behaves in an almost completely normal fashion. This interval is known as the *lag period*. It is terminated abruptly by a sudden increase in the viscosity of the red cell contents as the deoxyhemoglobin S polymerizes into 14-strand fibers. It is this sharp rise in viscosity that causes the cell to lose the flexibility it needs to make its way through small blood vessels. Finally, the cell acquires its sickle shape as the 14-strand fibers align into bundles.

The time required for the completion of these stages of polymerization is the key to the clinical severity of sickle cell disease in a given patient. Sickle cells making their circuit through the blood vessels contain significant amounts of deoxyhemoglobin S only during the relatively short interval they spend in the capillaries and veins. For this hemoglobin to polymerize into fibers, the first two stages must be complete before the hemoglobin is reoxygenated in the lungs; for sickling to occur, all three stages must be complete before reoxygenation takes place. The time required for the polymerization and alignment stages is relatively fixed: seconds for polymerization, accounting for the suddenness in the change in viscosity of deoxyhemoglobin S-containing red cells, and minutes for alignment. The time for nucleation, however, is highly variable, ranging from a few milliseconds to more than an hour, depending on local conditions such as pH (which acts through the Bohr effect), oxygen tension, and the intracellular concentration of deoxyhemoglobin S. Because of its variability, the time required for nucleation is probably the most critical factor affecting the degree of severity of sickle cell disease. When conditions are such that nucleation is fast, permitting deoxyhemoglobin S to polymerize in the brief time the red cell is deoxygenated, serious clinical problems result; conversely, slow nucleation means less severe clinical disease.

The polymerization of deoxyhemoglobin S is disturbed by the presence of other types of hemoglobin. This is a matter of great clinical significance, because in the red cell, hemoglobin S is always mixed with other types of hemoglobin, and the extent to which these interfere with polymerization profoundly influences the severity of the clinical disease. Other hemoglobins interfere with polymerization by acting as Trojan horses, in a manner of speaking. Because of their structural resemblance to hemoglobin S, they are incorporated into the hemoglobin S fiber as polymerization takes place. They fit imperfectly into the fiber, however, weakening its structure. Fiber structure is weakened in a particularly effective way by the incorporation of hemoglobin hybrids, asymmetric tetramers containing two different types of β-chains (e.g., $\alpha_2\beta^A\beta^S$). These structural weaknesses disrupt polymerization to a greater or lesser extent. The degree to which polymerization is disrupted will depend of course on how closely the non-S deoxyhemoglobin molecule resembles deoxyhemoglobin S. Certain hemoglobins fit well into the deoxyhemoglobin S polymer, so polymerization is only slightly impaired, while others fit very poorly, causing a substantial reduction in the tendency of hemoglobin S to polymerize. Moreover, the concentration of the non-S hemoglobin will also influence polymerization; the higher the non-S concentration, the less the likelihood that polymerization will occur.

Pathophysiology of Sickle Cell Disease

It is the polymerization of deoxyhemoglobin S within the red cell that is responsible for the clinical manifestations of sickle cell disease. Almost all the hemoglobin polymerizes on complete deoxygenation of the red cell, which then deforms into the typical sickle cell. Polymerization, however, is not an all-or-none phenomenon in which hemoglobin S is either fully polymerized or completely in solution. Rather, it seems that whatever quantity of deoxyhemoglobin is present in the red cell at a given time is incorporated into fibers, so that even normal-appearing red cells contain stiff inclusions of polymerized hemoglobin that grow or shrink as the cell gives up or takes on its load of oxygen. Two effects result from these stiff inclusions of polymerized deoxyhemoglobin:

EXTRAVASCULAR HEMOLYSIS

The hemoglobin S-containing cell is conditioned, and eventually destroyed, by the mononuclear phagocyte system. In the very young, this occurs mainly in the spleen, where the cells are trapped in the cords because the inclusions that grow in the oxygen-depleted splenic environment prevent the cells from squeezing through into the sinuses. By late infancy, the spleen has usually lost its function, and other components of the mononuclear phagocyte system, such as the bone marrow macrophages and the Kupffer cells of the liver, take over the destruction of the red cells. In any case, the result is extravascular hemolysis, the primary cause of the anemia in patients with this condition.

MICROVASCULAR BLOCKAGE

The most important effect of these inclusions is to impede the flow of blood through the microvasculature of the tissues (Fig. 11-5).

This could occur by the following sequence of events, which, though hypothetical, is entirely plausible on the basis of what is known about the behavior of hemoglobin S. As the hemoglobin S-filled red cell passes through the capillary network, it will unload part of its oxygen to the tissues, leaving deoxyhemoglobin S behind. This will polymerize, forming inclusions that will impede the passage of the cell through the capillaries. Passage is further delayed by an unexplained tendency of cells containing hemoglobin S to stick to the endothelium. The continued transfer of oxygen from the retarded red cell to the tissues will cause an additional rise in the intracellular deoxyhemoglobin S concentration, resulting in an increase in the size of the inclusions. They may grow to the point where the cell can no longer move through the capillary at all, and the vessel becomes plugged. More red cells pile up behind the obstructing cell, give up their oxygen, and are themselves incorporated into the growing plug. Meanwhile, the oxygen demand of the small volume of tissue that was originally supplied by the plugged vessel must be satisfied by red cells in nearby capillaries and arterioles. These cells are now obliged to unload more oxygen than usual, because they have to supply a greater volume of tissue than usual. Deoxyhemoglobin inclusions now grow in these cells, and the blockade is extended to adjacent vessels. The ultimate outcome is the complete obliteration of the blood supply to the blockaded region, with necrosis of tissues and symptoms of both an acute and chronic nature.

SICKLE CELL DISEASES

Sickle cell diseases occur primarily in blacks. These diseases are common in the equatorial regions of Africa; natives of this region brought the diseases with them to North America when they were transported to that continent, primarily during the eighteenth and nineteenth centuries. The diseases are also seen

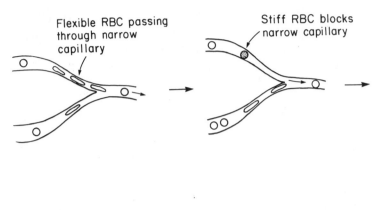

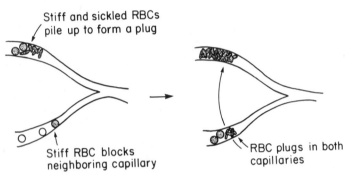

Fig. 11-5. How sickle cells block the microcirculation.

in Arabs and in persons from the Indian subcontinent and are present, although at very low incidence, among Mediterranean Europeans, primarily Greeks, Italians, and Mediterranean islanders (Sicilians and Sardinians).

Sickle Cell Anemia (Homozygous Hemoglobin S Disease)

The worst of the sickle cell diseases is sickle cell anemia. Like other hemoglobinopathies, it is an inherited disease. It is transmitted in an autosomal recessive manner, occurring in persons who have inherited two β^S-globin genes. In these persons, hemoglobin S accounts for more than 90 percent of the hemoglobin in the red cell. Clinical manifestations that are mild or absent in other varieties of sickle cell disease are fully expressed in sickle cell anemia. These clinical manifestations fall into two cate-

gories: those caused by the anemia and those attributable to occlusions of the microvasculature.

ANEMIA AND ITS CONSEQUENCES

A moderate to severe anemia is characteristic of sickle cell anemia. It results primarily from hemolysis, but folate deficiency may occasionally play a part, since folate requirements are increased in sickle cell anemia. In acute infection with parvovirus, suppression of erythropoiesis may lead to an abrupt fall in the hematocrit owing to the now uncompensated hemolytic process; this situation, known as an *aplastic crisis*, is exactly analogous to what happens under similar circumstances in patients with other hemolytic anemias.

Manifestations of hemolysis are also seen. Serum lactate dehydrogenase and indirect bilirubin are elevated. The spleen is initially enlarged, but in four patients out of five it

ANEMIA OF SICKLE CELL DISEASE

Causes
  Extravascular hemolysis
  Aplastic crisis with infections
  Folate deficiency (occasional)
Consequences
  Slowed growth and development
  Chronic congestive heart failure
  Gallstones

shows that they are grossly abnormal in shape. Targets, distorted shapes, and the characteristically deformed sickle cells are easily detected (Fig. 11-6). Reticulocytes are substantially increased (on routine smears, these appear as polychromatophilic cells), and signs of splenic hypofunction such as basophilic stippling, nucleated red cells, Howell-Jolly bodies, and Cabot rings are seen in the smears of almost all patients of sufficient age, even in those in whom the spleen remains enlarged to palpation. The marrow shows marked red cell hyperplasia, and marrow iron is increased. Megaloblastic changes may occasionally be seen in the red and white cell precursors because of a deficiency in folate superimposed on the underlying disease.

MICROVASCULAR OCCLUSIONS

Microvascular occlusions are thought to be responsible for most of the clinical manifestations of sickle cell anemia. They may involve most of the organ systems of the body and are

begins to shrink again after a few years, eventually becoming reduced to an atrophic vestige by repeated microinfarction and scarring; splenic atrophy is so routine that splenomegaly in sickle cell patients over the age of 8 or 10 years is an indication to search carefully for another variety of sickle cell disease. Whether enlarged or atrophied, the spleen loses its function by the time the patient is just a few months of age. Gallstones are exceptionally common in sickle cell anemia, leading to diagnostic complications (see below).

As in thalassemia major, signs and symptoms of cardiac overload are important consequences of the anemia in this condition. The cardiac output is chronically high, leading to hypertrophy, cardiac enlargement, and eventually chronic congestive heart failure. The effects of the anemia on the function of the heart are aggravated by the fact that this organ, like others in sickle cell anemia, is subject to microvascular occlusive disease, with microinfarctions and fibrosis.

Another similarity with thalassemia major is the effect of the anemia on growth and development. Growth may be retarded in patients with severe sickle cell anemia, and resistance to other diseases, particularly infections, is diminished. The high mortality rate in children with sickle cell anemia is largely the result of this impaired ability to resist infection.

The hematocrit in patients with sickle cell anemia is invariably low. The red cells tend to be normal in size, but examination of the smear

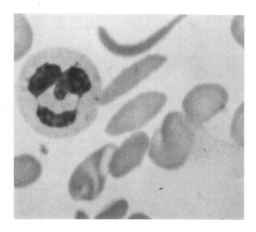

Fig. 11-6. Blood smear in sickle cell anemia. Irreversibly sickled cells are the most characteristic finding. Target cells are also present. The smear may also show nucleated red cells, basophilic stippling, and nuclear remnants (Howell-Jolly bodies and Cabot rings), all of which are indications that the spleen has lost its function. (From Wintrobe MM et al [1974] Clinical Hematology. 7th Ed. Lea & Febiger, Philadelphia, with permission.)

frequently characterized by pain as well as by various signs and symptoms of organ dysfunction (Fig. 11-7).

Sickle Cell Crisis

Perhaps the most characteristic manifestation of sickle cell anemia, and certainly one of the most distressing, is the sickle cell crisis. It consists of an episode of severe pain of 1 to 2 weeks' duration, often accompanied by a relatively low-grade fever and leukocytosis. A crisis may be precipitated by infection, dehydration, or acidosis, but it frequently comes out of a clear blue sky. The pain can involve the extremities, the chest, and either the abdomen or the back, or both; it can be so severe as to mimic an acute surgical emergency. Notable by its absence is any change in the red cell status in sickle cell crisis; the hematocrit holds steady (unless there is a simultaneous aplastic crisis, which may coincide with a sickle cell crisis in infected patients), and the number of irreversibly sickled cells in the blood smear remains unchanged. The crisis will subside spontaneously, only to recur after

> **FEATURES OF A SICKLE CELL CRISIS**
>
> Precipitated by
>   Infection
>   Dehydration
>   Acidosis
>   No special event
>
> Signs and symptoms
>   Severe pain
>   Modest fever and leukocytosis in some cases
>
> No change in hematocrit or in the number of sickle cells in the blood smear

a few weeks or months to afflict the patient once again. Since the pain is severe enough to require narcotics for adequate analgesia, drug addition is not uncommon in patients with sickle cell anemia.

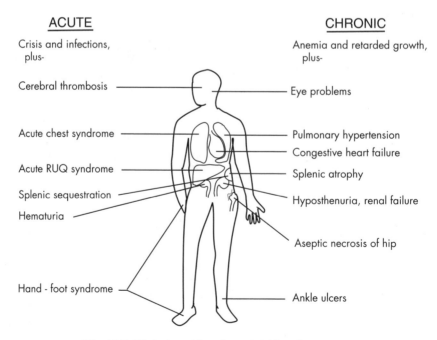

ACUTE

Crisis and infections, plus-

Cerebral thrombosis

Acute chest syndrome

Acute RUQ syndrome

Splenic sequestration

Hematuria

Hand - foot syndrome

CHRONIC

Anemia and retarded growth, plus-

Eye problems

Pulmonary hypertension
Congestive heart failure

Splenic atrophy

Hyposthenuria, renal failure

Aseptic necrosis of hip

Ankle ulcers

Fig. 11-7. Clinical manifestations of sickle cell anemia.

Cardiopulmonary Problems

The cardiac complications of sickle cell disease have been discussed above. Pulmonary problems may be acute or chronic. The acute chest syndrome of sickle cell disease consists of chest pain, fever, cough, and a pulmonary infiltrate, all of relatively abrupt onset. This may be caused by bacterial pneumonia or by a pulmonary infarct resulting from a sickle cell crisis involving the pulmonary circulation; these may be impossible to tell apart, especially since they may occur together, and decisions as to specific treatment may have to be made more or less empirically. In a few patients, pulmonary hypertension with cor pulmonale may develop, the result of recurrent occlusive episodes over many years involving the pulmonary circulation.

Abdominal Organs

The liver is often involved in sickle cell disease. It is usually enlarged, and gallstones are common. Acute right upper quadrant pain is most frequently attributable to a sickle cell crisis, which, if it involves the liver directly, may lead to rapid enlargement of that organ. It may also be attributable to cholelithiasis or to hepatitis of other etiologies. As with the acute chest syndrome, the cause of acute right upper quadrant pain in patients with sickle cell anemia may be exceedingly difficult to determine.

The other abdominal organ routinely involved in sickle cell disease is the spleen. Changes in spleen size and function in sickle cell disease have been discussed above. In children, the spleen can become involved in a very serious complication known as the splenic sequestration syndrome, in which sudden massive intrasplenic sickling leads to acute severe left upper quadrant pain, a rapid increase in the size of the organ, and hypovolemia with an abrupt fall in the hematocrit, rapidly leading to shock. The splenic sequestration syndrome constitutes a medical emergency that can cause death if not quickly treated.

Genitourinary System

Genitourinary manifestations of sickle cell anemia include (1) the excretion of a dilute urine (hyposthenuria), a common problem that appears to result from infarction of the inner portion of the renal medulla, a region of tissue in which the oxygen tension is ordinarily quite low; and (2) hematuria, a rare problem arising from the same cause. There is an increase in the incidence of pyelonephritis in sickle cell anemia. Priapism is a rare but characteristic complication.

Bones, Joints, and Extremities

The bones and joints are often affected in sickle cell disease. Bone films may show sclerotic areas that denote regions of prior bony infarction. On a larger scale, aseptic necrosis of the hip frequently occurs. An acute arthritis can result from a vascular occlusion involving the synovium. The incidence of osteomyelitis is increased.

The hand-foot syndrome is an arthritis-like condition seen in children under 3 years of age with sickle cell anemia. Often the first clinical manifestation of the disorder, it is characterized by transient painful swelling of the hands and feet lasting about 2 weeks and associated with such signs of inflammation as fever and leukocytosis. It may be confused with a number of other diseases affecting the hands and feet of children, especially rheumatic fever.

Chronic nonhealing ankle ulcers are common in sickle cell anemia. They respond poorly to treatment and can be very hard to deal with.

Central Nervous System and Eyes

In sickle cell anemia, strokes may occur at a young age as a result of thrombosis of the cerebral arteries. Recurrent occlusions of retinal arterioles and capillaries may cause blinding eye disease.

Pregnancy

Placental infarctions occur in pregnant women with sickle cell disease, leading to an increase in the incidence of fetal loss and toxemia. Congestive heart failure and thrombophlebitis are more common than usual, and the acute chest syndrome often occurs in the third trimester of pregnancy. In addition, the frequency of crisis is increased throughout the course of the pregnancy. It is evident that the hazards of pregnancy for both the mother and the fetus are considerably increased by sickle cell anemia.

COURSE OF THE DISEASE

The foregoing litany of clinical manifestations shows that sickle cell anemia is a highly generalized disease with acute and chronic effects involving virtually every organ system in the body. Accordingly, it would seem logical to conclude that a short life filled with pain and debility is the fate of patients afflicted with this disease. This is true in many cases, but some patients with sickle cell anemia have surprisingly little trouble with their condition. Crises are mild and infrequent, and complications develop very slowly.

The variation in the severity of sickle cell anemia from patient to patient can be at least partly accounted for by the following:

1. *Fetal hemoglobin.* There is a wide variation in hemoglobin F among patients with sickle cell anemia, with levels ranging from 2 to more than 20 percent (normal, 1 to 3 percent). Patients with a mild clinical course tend to have a high level of hemoglobin F. The high hemoglobin F decreases the incidence of crisis by interfering with deoxyhemoglobin S polymerization through a Trojan horse effect.

2. *Total hemoglobin.* The total red cell hemoglobin concentration is a factor affecting the course of sickle cell anemia. When the hemoglobin concentration is low, nucleation is retarded, reducing the frequency of crises.

3. *Irreversibly sickled cells.* The number of irreversibly sickled cells in the circulation seems to be an index of the severity of the disease, greater numbers predicting a worse course.

Whether the course is mild or severe, however, almost all patients with sickle cell anemia sooner or later die of their disease. Some will die in childhood, carried off by splenic sequestration, or more commonly by an overwhelming bacterial infection, to which they are unusually susceptible because of their general debility and the fact that their splenic function is gone. Most, however, survive into adulthood, the majority eventually succumbing to the complications of their disease: an acute chest syndrome caused by pulmonary embolism or sickling in the lungs, often with an accompanying pneumonia; renal failure, caused by the accumulation of kidney damage over the course of a lifetime of microinfarctions; or stroke.

Other Sickle Cell Diseases

With rare exceptions, patients with sickle cell diseases other than sickle cell anemia are β-globin gene heterozygotes. One of their β-globin genes is the β^S (i.e., sickle) gene, while the other is either a normal β-globin gene or a gene with a mutation different from β^S. Because of this genetic makeup, red cells from these patients (except for sickle/β-thalassemia) contain two major hemoglobins. The presence of the second hemoglobin interferes with the ability of the deoxyhemoglobin S to polymerize in the cell. Consequently, these variant forms of sickle cell disease are almost always milder than sickle cell anemia. Depending on the extent to which polymerization is disrupted, the severity of the variant diseases ranges from virtually asymptomatic to almost as bad as homozygous sickle cell anemia.

OTHER SICKLE CELL DISEASES

Sickle cell trait
S/β-thalassemia
SC
SD$_{Punjab}$
SO$_{Arab}$

SICKLE CELL TRAIT

Patients with one normal β-globin gene and one β^S-gene are said to have sickle cell trait. This condition is by far the most common of the sickle cell variants, occurring in nearly 1 of every 10 African-Americans.

From a clinical standpoint, sickle cell trait is important principally because patients with the trait are carriers of a very serious disease that may appear in their offspring. Statistically, one of every four children born of parents with the trait will have sickle cell anemia (autosomal recessive), while one of two will inherit the trait (autosomal dominant) (Fig. 11-8). Sickle cell trait itself, however, is almost always clinically benign. The hematocrit is normal, blood smears generally show no abnormalities, and the life expectancy is statistically normal. On the other hand, certain problems, some serious, do arise as a result of sickle cell trait. Most patients with the trait eventually develop hyposthenuria because of destruction of the inner portion of the renal medulla, a region so hypoxic and hyperosmolar that even cells with the trait will stiffen there and sickle. Splenic infarcts have occurred in these patients during flights in planes with unpressurized cabins. Of most concern, patients with sickle cell trait are at increased risk of sudden death under circum-stances that combine high tissue oxygen demand with dehydration (e.g., during strenuous military training exercises in hot, muggy climates).

Red cells from patients with sickle cell trait contain major quantities of both hemoglobin S and hemoglobin A, but hemoglobin A exceeds hemoglobin S by a factor of about 3:2. This happens at least in part because α-chains combine more rapidly with normal β-chains than with β^S-chains during the formation of hemoglobin tetramers, so that in the competition for the scarce α-chains, the normal β-chains have the edge. In the relatively common combination of sickle trait and mild α-thalassemia, the A:S imbalance is exaggerated because the free α-chains are even scarcer than normal; A:S ratios of 3:1 are typical of sickle trait/α-thalassemia minor.

SICKLE CELL / β-THALASSEMIA

Certain patients who are sickle cell heterozygotes also carry a gene for β-thalassemia, a disease in which β-globin chain synthesis is greatly slowed or absent (Ch. 10). These patients have a form of sickle cell disease the severity of which depends on the degree of production of normal β-chains permitted by their thalassemia gene. Patients whose cells produce relatively large quantities of normal β-chains will have a very mild form of the disease, because their red cells will contain enough hemoglobin A to prevent symptoms by interfering with the polymerization of deoxyhemoglobin S. In contrast, patients whose cells make few or no normal β-chains can have a disease as severe as homozygous sickle cell anemia.

In patients with S/β-thalassemia, anemia is the rule. Cells are small rather than normal in size, a point of distinction from homozygous sickle cell anemia, and there are more target cells than in sickle cell anemia (Fig. 11-9). Splenomegaly is common, another clinical difference between S/β-thalassemia and the homozygous disease. In other respects, the two conditions are clinically identical.

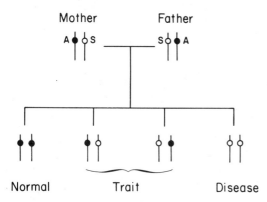

Fig. 11-8. Parents with sickle cell trait can have children with sickle cell anemia.

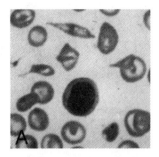
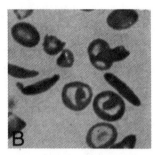

Fig. 11-9. Blood smears in S/β-thalassemia (**A**) and sickle cell anemia (**B**). The S/β-thalassemia cells are microcytic. Target cells are more abundant in S/β-thalassemia than in sickle cell anemia. (From Bunn HF, Forget BG, Ranney HM [1977] Human hemoglobin variants. In: Human Hemoglobin. WB Saunders, Philadelphia, with permission.)

Red cells from patients with S/β-thalassemia may or may not contain hemoglobin A, depending on whether the thalassemic component of the disease is β+ or β⁰. When hemoglobin A is present, its concentration is always lower than that of hemoglobin S, differentiating S/β-thalassemia from sickle cell trait. When hemoglobin A is absent, differentiating this disease from homozygous sickle cell anemia may be difficult, but can usually be accomplished by family studies, which will show some form of thalassemia in one parent and some form of sickle cell disease in the other.

HEMOGLOBIN C AND SC DISEASE

Hemoglobin C is a mutant hemoglobin in which the β6 glutamate is replaced by lysine (it will be recalled that in the βˢ chain, this glutamate is replaced by valine). The gene for hemoglobin C is found exclusively in blacks, in whom its frequency is about one-fourth that of the sickle gene.

Hemoglobin C trait (one normal β-globin gene and one βᶜ gene) is an asymptomatic condition. Homozygous hemoglobin C disease causes a mild hemolytic anemia that is entirely similar to other mild extravascular hemolytic anemias (e.g., reticulocytosis, splenomegaly), except for the characteristic appearance of the red cells on the blood smear. These show a striking degree of targeting (Fig. 11-10), together with an occasional rectangular cell

that appears to be formed by intracellular crystallization of the abnormal hemoglobin during the preparation of the smear. Patients with homozygous hemoglobin C disease are not incapacitated in any way by their disease, and their life expectancy is normal.

Problems with hemoglobin C arise in patients who are doubly heterozygous for hemoglobin C and hemoglobin S. These patients have a form of sickle cell disease that in most respects resembles mild homozygous sickle cell anemia. The principal difference between SC disease and the homozygous disease is the mildness of the anemia, hematocrits

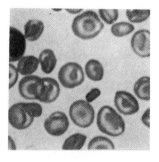

Fig. 11-10. Hemoglobin C disease. Target cells are very prominent. A few deeply stained bricklike rectangular cells are seen; these are characteristic of hemoglobin C disease. (From Bunn HF, Forget BG, Ranney HM [1977] Human hemoglobin variants. In: Human Hemoglobin. WB Saunders, Philadelphia, with permission.)

above 25 being the rule in SC disease. As a result, the cardiac problems so prominent in sickle cell anemia are minimal in patients with SC disease, and their life expectancy is only slightly shorter than normal. As in S/β-thalassemia, but in contrast to SS, splenomegaly is common in SC disease.

Routine laboratory tests in SC disease show a mild to moderate anemia, with normal-size red cells. The smear shows many target cells and a few fat sickle forms (Fig. 11-11). Red cells contain hemoglobin S and hemoglobin C, in equal amounts.

SD AND SO

Hemoglobin D$_{Punjab}$ (β121 glu → gln) and O$_{Arab}$ (β121 glu → lys) are other mutant hemoglobins that cause little disease by themselves, but result in sickle cell disease when present in combination with hemoglobin S. Both are relatively common compared with most mutant hemoglobins, but not nearly as common as hemoglobin S or C. Disease in these double heterozygotes is mild, and splenomegaly is common. The diagnosis is made by demonstrating the presence of the two hemoglobins in the red cells of affected patients.

The features of the most important of the heterozygous sickle cell diseases are listed in Table 11-1.

MANAGEMENT OF SICKLE CELL DISEASES

Diagnosis

Making the diagnosis of a sickle cell disease usually involves two steps: (1) demonstrating that red cells from a patient suspected of having a sickle cell disease actually contain hemoglobin S and (2) identifying all the hemoglobins present in those red cells by electrophoresis. Evidence for the presence of hemoglobin S is usually obtained by one of two screening tests: the solubility test, or the sickle cell preparation. Both are based on the principle that when oxygen is removed from a preparation of hemoglobin S, the hemoglobin will polymerize and precipitate. The agent used to remove the oxygen is usually sodium metabisulfite ($Na_2S_2O_5$), a powerful reducing agent.

1. *Solubility test.* The sodium metabisulfite is added to a solution of hemoglobin in concentrated buffer (usually prepared by releasing the hemoglobin from the suspected red cells with distilled water and then adding buffer as needed); if hemoglobin S is present, a dark red precipitate of deoxyhemoglobin S will appear in the solution.

2. *Sickle cell preparation.* The metabisulfite is added to a suspension of whole red cells in

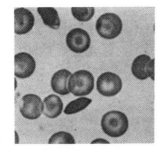
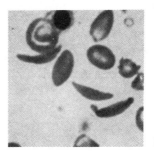

A   **B**

Fig. 11-11. (**A**) SC disease. (**B**) Sickle cell disease. In SC disease, target cells are abundant. The sickle forms are shorter and fatter than in sickle cell anemia, a subtle distinction. (From Bunn HF, Forget BG, Ranney HM [1977] Human hemoglobin variants. In: Human Hemoglobin. WB Saunders, Philadelphia, with permission.)

Table 11-1. Features of the Most Important Heterozygous Sickle Cell Diseases

Disease	Clinical Features	Red Cell Morphology	Hemoglobins
Sickle trait	No crises	Normal	A > S
S/β-thalassemia	Moderate to severe crises Severe anemia Splenomegaly	Small sickle cells Microcytosis 4+ targets	A absent (β⁰) or present but <S (β⁺); A₂ variably ↑
SC disease	Moderate to severe crises Modest anemia Splenomegaly	Fat sickle cells 4+ targets	C equals S

saline. Cells containing any quantity of hemoglobin S—even those from patients with sickle cell trait—will sickle under these conditions. The sickling of these cells is readily seen under the microscope (Fig. 11-12).

As a model of the pathogenetic event in sickle cell diseases, the sickle cell preparation has the appeal of relevance and analogy; screening, however, is usually carried out by the solubility test because it is easier.

Identification of the hemoglobins is accomplished by electrophoresis, which is performed by applying a streak of hemolysate to one end of a solid supporting strip that has been dampened with buffer at the desired pH (usually pH 8.6), and then passing an electrical current along the strip for a given period of time. The hemoglobin molecules march along the strip at rates that depend mainly on their net charge. The various species of hemoglobin in the normal red cell separate nicely, as shown in Figure 11-13, and can be quantitated by their color.

Abnormal hemoglobins characteristic of sickle cell disease differ from hemoglobin A in their net charge. The two most common of these—hemoglobins S and C—differ from hemoglobin A in the loss of one (β^S:glu → val) and two (β^C:glu → lys) negative charges, respectively. These losses of negative charge translate directly into losses in electrophoretic mobility, which decrease in the following order: Hb A > Hb S > Hb C (Fig. 11-14). Accordingly, hemoglobins A, S, and C are easily distinguished by their behavior in an electrical field, and hemoglobin electrophoresis becomes a simple and convenient way to demonstrate their presence in patients with sickle cell disease.

A diagnostic monkey wrench is occasionally thrown into the works in the form of the uncommon abnormal hemoglobins D and O_{Arab}. These forms produce heterozygous sickle cell disease when combined with hemoglobin S. The problem is that each of these hemoglobins moves with one of the more common hemoglobins under the usual conditions of electrophoresis: D migrates with S, and O_{Arab} migrates with C. S/D therefore looks like S/S on the electrophoresis strip, and S/O_{Arab} looks like S/C. If this problem should arise, it can be settled by electrophoresis at pH 6.2, which separates the confusing pairs.

The hemoglobin electrophoretic patterns corresponding to the various sickle cell diseases are shown in Figure 11-14. It is worth repeating that the following pairs of sickle cell

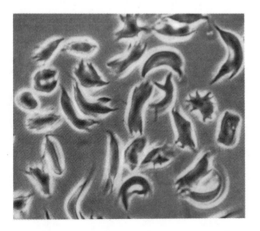

Fig. 11-12. The sickle cell preparation. (From Castoldi GL [1981] Erythrocytes. In Zucker-Franklin D et al [eds]: Atlas of Blood Cells: Function and Pathology. Edi. Ermes s.r.l., Milan, with permission.)

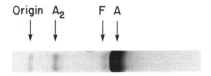

Fig. 11-13. Electrophoresis of the hemoglobins from normal red cells. The most prominent band is hemoglobin A. Hemoglobins A and A_2 are well separated on the strip, whereas hemoglobin F runs just behind hemoglobin A. Hemoglobin A is not homogeneous, but actually consists of a group of closely related species that migrate together in the electrical field. These species represent hemoglobin A tetramers ($\alpha_2\beta_2$) variably substituted with sugars or sugar phosphates on the N-terminal amino group of the β-chain. The major constituent of this group is unsubstituted hemoglobin A. Second is hemoglobin A_{1c}, a molecule in which a glucose has become attached to the β-chain by a nonenzymatic process. The concentration of hemoglobin A_{1c} is an excellent indicator of blood sugar control in diabetics.

diseases give identical electrophoretic patterns: S/S and S/D; S/C and S/O$_{Arab}$; and S/S and S/β^0-thalassemia (although with S/β^0-thalassemia, increases in A_2 similar to those seen in β-thalassemia trait may provide a clue to the true diagnosis). With such pairs of diseases, the decision to look further in order to make a diagnosis is usually based on clinical clues. For example, mild disease in an adult with splenomegaly whose hemoglobin electrophoresis gives an S/S pattern is an indication to look for S/D, because true homozygous sickle cell

anemia is usually a severe disease in which splenomegaly is uncommon. Finally, it should be recalled that hemoglobins A and S are found in both sickle cell trait and S/β^+-thalassemia, but that in sickle cell trait, A > S, while in S/β^+-thalassemia, S > A.

Prenatal Diagnosis

Like thalassemia, sickle cell anemia can sometimes be diagnosed prenatally. The diagnosis can be made by demonstrating the presence of the sickle mutation in the fetal β-globin gene through the use of MstI, a restriction endonuclease whose recognition sequence is altered by the $\beta^A \rightarrow \beta^S$ mutation. It may be more difficult to know what to do with this information than in the case of prenatally diagnosed thalassemia major, because the course of homozygous sickle cell anemia is highly variable, with many patients pursuing a relatively symptom-free course throughout a long and generally healthy life.

Treatment

The treatment of sickle cell diseases generally boils down to the management of the episodes of illness or stress that occur during the course of the disease. The anemia itself usually does not require treatment, although folate supplements should be given routinely to patients with sickle cell disease, just as it is to

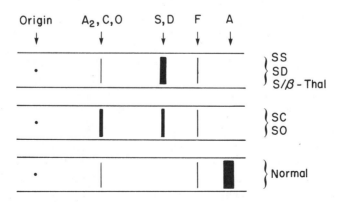

Fig. 11-14. Hemoglobin electrophoresis in the sickle cell diseases.

TREATMENT OF ACUTE PROBLEMS IN SICKLE CELL DISEASES

Treatment of crisis
    Fluids
    Analgesics
    Oxygen and alkali if indicated
Indications for antibiotics
    Infections
    Acute chest syndrome
Indications for partial exchange transfusions
    Acute chest syndrome
    Splenic sequestration syndrome[a]
    General anesthesia
    Acute clinical deterioration in a sickle
       cell patient

---

[a]Splenic sequestration constitutes *an acute emergency.* Shock must be treated immediately. Emergency splenectomy may be neccessary.

patients with other forms of chronic hemolytic anemia.

1. *Crisis.* Despite thousands of man–years of investigation, nothing has been found as yet that can shorten the duration of a sickle cell crisis. Treatment is therefore restricted to supportive measures: analgesics, plenty of fluids, and alkali and oxygen if necessary to correct acidosis or hypoxia, but not on a routine basis. Patients with abdominal crisis must be watched carefully to make sure they do not have an acute surgical abdomen. The *acute chest syndrome* should be treated empirically with antibiotics; partial exchange transfusions should be carried out to replace sickle cells with normal cells; and oxygen should be freely administered to maintain tissue oxygenation and prevent further complications. The *splenic sequestration syndrome* requires immediate fluids, oxygen, and partial exchange transfusions to reverse hypovolemia and shock; emergency splenectomy may be necessary. A program of exchange transfusion, or chronic transfusion to hematocrits of 35 (a level high enough to reduce

levels of hemoglobin S by suppressing endogenous erythropoiesis), is recommended for children with strokes.

2. *Infections.* Bacterial infections are an exceedingly serious problem in patients with sickle cell disease and should be treated aggressively. Pneumococcal infections, which occur frequently in sickle cell disease, can be prevented to some extent by vaccination. Prophylactic antibiotics are recommended for children under age 6.

3. *General anesthesia.* General anesthesia is an indication for partial exchange transfusion therapy to decrease the proportion of hemoglobin S-containing cells in the circulation. This may need to be done on an emergency basis.

A better way to treat sickle cell disease would be to alter the properties of the sickle cell itself so as to decrease its tendency to stiffen in oxygen-poor environments. A treatment that may achieve this goal is currently under development. It is known that red cells from patients on myelosuppressive drugs contain extra hemoglobin F. Based on this knowledge, sickle cell patients are being treated on a trial basis with hydroxyurea, the safest myelosuppressive drug available, in the hope that the extra hemoglobin F in their red cells will decrease stiffening and alleviate symptoms by interfering with the polymerization of deoxygenated hemoglobin S. If this trial is successful, hydroxyurea is likely to become routine therapy for this difficult condition.

LONG-TERM TREATMENT OF SICKLE CELL DISEASES

Folic acid
Prophylactic antibiotics in children under
    age 6
Long-term tranfusion therapy
    Children with stroke
    Pregnant women (?)

SUGGESTED READINGS

Banerjee AK, Layton DM, Rennie JA, Bellingham AJ (1991) Safe surgery in sickle cell disease. Fr J Surg 78:516

Bunn HF (1987) Subunit assembly of hemoglobin: an important determinant of hematologic phenotype. Blood 69:1

Bunn HF, Forget BD (1984) Human Hemoglobins. 2nd Ed. WB Saunders, Philadelphia

Charache S (1981) Treatment of sickle cell anemia. Annu Rev Med 32:195

Charache S (1990) Fetal hemoglobin, sickling, and sickle cell disease. Adv Pediatr 37:1

Charache S (1990) Problems in transfusion therapy. N Engl J Med 322:1666

Dean J, Schechter AN (1978) Sickle-cell anemia: molecular and cellular bases of therapeutic approaches. N Engl J Med 299:752

Eaton WA, Hofrichter J (1990) Sickle cell hemoglobin polymerization. Adv Protein Chem 40:63

Evans JP (1989) Practical management of sickle cell disease. Arch Dis Child 64:1748

Kaul DK, Nagel RL (1993) Sickle cell vasocclusion: many issues and some answers. Experientia 49:5

Koshy M, Burd L (1991) Management of pregnancy in sickle cell syndromes. Hematol Oncol Clin North Am 5:585

Nagel RL (1991) Severity, pathobiology, epistatic effects, and genetic markers in sickle cell anemia. Semin Hematol 28:180

Nathan DG (1990) Pharmacologic manipulation of fetal hemoglobin in the hemoglobinopathies. Ann NY Acad Sci 612:179

Ohene-Frempong K (1991) Stoke in sickle cell disease: demographic, clinical, and therapeutic considerations. Semin Hematol 28:213

Piomelli S (1991) Sickle cell diseases in the 1990s: the need for active and preventive intervention. Semin Hematol 28:227

Platt OS (1988) Is there treatment of sickle cell anemia? [editorial] N Engl J Med 319:1479

Pollack CV, Jr, Sanders DY, Severance HW, Jr (1991) Emergency department analgesia without narcotics for adults with acute sickle cell pain crisis: case reports and review of crisis management. J Emerg Med 9:445

Powars DR (1991) Beta S-gene-cluster haplotypes in sickle cell anemia. Clinical and hematological features. Hematol Oncol Clin North Am 5:475

Powars DR (1991) Sickle cell anemia: beta S-gene-cluster haplotypes as prognostic indicators of vital organ failure. Semin Hematol 28:202

Ranney HM (1992) The spectrum of sickle cell disease. Hosp Pract [Off] 27:133

Smith JA (1991) What do we know about the clinical course of sickle cell disease? Semin Hematol 28:209

Stamatoyannopoulos G, Veith R, al-Khatti A, Papayannopoulou T (1990) Induction of fetal hemoglobin by cell-cycle-specific drugs and recombinant erythropoietin. Am J Pediatr Hematol Oncol 12:21

Steingart R (1992) Management of patients with sickle cell disease. Med Clin North Am 76:669

Thurn J (1988) Human parovirus B19: historical and clinical review. Rev Infect Dis 10:1005

Wayne AS, Kevy SV, Nathan DG (1993) Transfusion management of sickle cell disease. Blood 81:1109

Wayne AS, Kevy SV, Nathan DG (1993) Transfusion management of sickle cell anemia. Blood 81:5

12

Polycythemia

Contrasting with the anemias are the polycythemias, a group of disorders in which the total volume of red cells in the patient is abnormally high. Most forms of polycythemia are caused by the overproduction of erythropoietin, which leads to excessive red cell formation. One variety, however, known as *polycythemia vera*, is caused by an intrinsic abnormality of the stem cell. There is in addition a condition known as *stress erythrocytosis*, which closely resembles the polycythemias but in which the patient's total red cell volume is often in the normal range.

The hallmark of all these conditions is an elevation of the hemoglobin level. A high hemoglobin generally means that the patient has polycythemia, although further testing is sometimes necessary to confirm this impression. Once the existence of polycythemia has been established, its cause must be determined. This determination is based on further clinical and laboratory findings that vary among the different forms of polycythemia.

THE SECONDARY POLYCYTHEMIAS

The secondary polycythemias are caused by the overproduction of erythropoietin. Erythropoietin increases red cell formation by stimulating the growth of the late committed stem cells of the erythrocyte series (Ch. 2). Erythropoietin production is ordinarily regulated by the rate of oxygen delivery to the kidney, a figure that is tied closely to the amount of hemoglobin in the blood. Secondary polycythemia develops when the production of erythropoietin is inappropriately high for the blood hemoglobin level.

Causes

Polycythemia due to inappropriately high erythropoietin production is caused by one of two factors: chronically low tissue oxygenation or an abnormal cell population that produces erythropoietin autonomously.

CHRONICALLY INADEQUATE TISSUE OXYGENATION

As mentioned above, the level of erythropoietin in the blood is normally regulated by the delivery of oxygen to the kidneys. With normal renal oxygen delivery, the kidneys manufacture only small quantities of erythropoietin, and the hemoglobin remains in the normal range. Impaired renal oxygen delivery, however, signals the kidneys to secrete more erythropoietin, which in turn stimulates the bone marrow to increase red cell production in order to correct renal oxygen delivery by providing the blood with additional oxygen-delivering capacity. Polycythemia occurs when even at a normal hemoglobin concentration, the blood cannot deliver oxygen to the kidneys rapidly enough to hold erythropoietin secretion to normal levels. This is seen most commonly in conditions associated with a chronic reduction in arterial oxygen saturation (chronic hypoxemia). Much less frequently, it arises through a failure of fully oxygenated hemoglobin to release its oxygen to the tissues.

The causes of *polycythemia due to chronic hypoxemia* are listed below. The most frequent cause is chronic lung disease, in which hypoxemia occurs because of the mixing of well-oxygenated blood draining from relatively normal regions of the lung with poorly oxygenated blood draining from more diseased regions of the lung, regions that are well-perfused but poorly aerated. Another cause, one that may be subtle and difficult to diagnose, is sleep apnea. In this condition, intermittent obstruction of the upper airway during sleep causes episodes of low arterial oxygen saturation that may be frequent enough to lead to secondary polycythemia. Less common causes include right-to-left shunts secondary to congenital heart disease or other vascular anomalies, and oxygen-poor living environments such as high mountains.

Polycythemia due to impaired oxygen release occurs in patients with high-affinity hemoglobins and with certain rare abnormalities of 2,3-diphosphoglyceric acid (2,3-DPG) metabolism. These are discussed in Chapter 3.

AUTONOMOUS ERYTHROPOIETIN PRODUCTION

Erythropoietin may be secreted autonomously from certain kinds of tumors, and occasionally from tissues involved with other diseases. Polycythemia due to autonomous erythropoietin production is seen most commonly in patients with renal cell carcinoma, 5 percent of whom develop this problem. This form of polycythemia is also seen occasionally in patients with hepatomas, and invariably in patients with the cerebellar hemangioblastomas of von Hippel-Lindau disease. Secondary polycythemia may also be caused by certain benign renal lesions such as polycystic kidney and hydronephrosis, which probably act by interfering with the renal circulation so that critical regions of the organ are underperfused and begin to secrete excess erythropoietin. In patients with autonomous erythropoietin production, polycythemia occurs because the

---

CAUSES OF POLYCYTHEMIA DUE TO CHRONICALLY INADEQUATE TISSUE OXYGENATION

Low arterial oxygen saturation
  Chronic lung disease
  Right-to-left shunts
  High altitude
Normal arterial oxygen saturation
  Sleep apnea
  High-affinity hemoglobin
  Abnormal 2,3-DPG metabolism

CAUSES OF POLYCYTHEMIA DUE TO INAPPROPRIATE ERYTHROPOIETIN SECRETION

Renal
  Renal cell carcinoma
  Renal cysts
  Hydronephrosis
  Renal graft rejection
Extrarenal
  Hepatoma
  Pheochromocytoma
  Cerebellar hemangioblastoma
    (von Hippel-Lindau disease)

secretion of the hormone by the abnormal tissue is unregulated, and fails to shut down even in response to the abnormally large amounts of oxygen that are delivered to the secreting tissue by the hemoglobin-rich polycythemic blood.

Manifestations

GENERAL SIGNS

The characteristic sign of polycythemia of any kind is an elevation in the hemoglobin (and hematocrit). This is usually picked up in the laboratory, although the patient's flushed, ruddy complexion often furnishes an early clue to its presence. The degree of elevation of the hemoglobin and hematocrit varies from patient to patient, ranging from just above normal to twice the normal value or even higher. If the hemoglobin level is sufficiently high, symptoms can result from the associated increase in blood volume and blood viscosity (Fig. 12-1). These symptoms may include fatigue, headaches, a feeling of engorgement in the head, and shortness of breath, as well as aggravation of congestive heart failure. The blood pressure may be elevated, and the veins in the eyegrounds are distended.

Certain features are especially important in helping to make the very important distinction between secondary polycythemia and polycythemia vera (Table 12-1). The spleen is almost never felt on physical examination in a patient with uncomplicated secondary polycythemia, but is palpable in the majority of patients with polycythemia vera. The white cell count, platelet count, and uric acid levels are generally normal in secondary polycythemia, but are likely to be high in polycythemia vera. Finally, erythropoietin levels are high in secondary polycythemia, but are low to nil in polycythemia vera. For a fuller discussion of polycythemia vera, see the discussion of myeloproliferative disorders in Chapter 22.

DECREASED VERSUS NORMAL ARTERIAL OXYGEN SATURATION

In evaluating patients with polycythemia, one of the most useful measurements is the oxygen saturation of the arterial blood. From the results of this measurement, patients with polycythemia can be divided into two groups: those who show a decrease in arterial oxygen saturation and those who do not. The diseases responsible for the polycythemia are very different in these two groups.

Decreased Arterial Oxygen Saturation

If the oxygen saturation of the arterial hemoglobin is 89 percent or less, the polycythemia is probably due to one of the conditions that cause chronic hypoxemia. In persons living at very high altitudes and in patients with congenital heart disease with a right-to-left shunt, the hematocrit and hemoglobin can rise to remarkably high levels; hematocrits of 80 or more may be seen in such individuals. By contrast, hematocrits rarely exceed the high 50s in patients with chronic lung disease, probably because the smoldering pulmonary infection present in most of these patients

Table 12-1. The Differential Diagnosis of Polycythemia

Finding	Secondary Polycythemia	Polycythemia Vera	Stress Erythrocytosis
Arterial oxygen tension	Normal or low	Normal	Normal
Splenomegaly	Absent	Present	Absent
White cell count and platelet count	Normal	Usually high	Normal
Uric acid	Normal	Often high	Normal
Red cell mass	High	High	High normal
Serum erythropoietin	High	Low	High

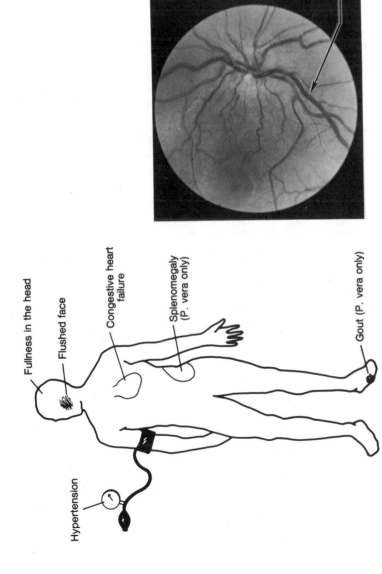

Fig. 12-1. Signs and symptoms of polycythemia. Most of them are caused by the combination of increased total blood volume and increased blood viscosity. Splenomegaly occurs only in polycythemia vera.

gives rise to an anemia of chronic disease that partly offsets their hypoxia-driven increase in red cell production.

Normal Arterial Oxygen Saturation

Polycythemia combined with a normal arterial oxygen saturation is most frequently due to "stress erythrocytosis" (see below) or to polycythemia vera (Ch. 22). On occasion, however, this combination may betray the presence of certain forms of secondary polycythemia. These include polycythemias caused by erythropoietin-producing lesions (e.g., a renal cell carcinoma) and by sleep apnea, and the rare cases of polycythemia due to a high-affinity hemoglobin or an abnormality in 2,3-DPG metabolism.

Among the causes of secondary polycythemia, sleep apnea is unique because, even though polycythemia in this disorder results from chronic hypoxemia, random arterial oxygen saturations are almost always normal. This is because random arterial oxygen saturations are usually drawn during the day, when the patient's breathing is normal and the blood fully oxygenated, while desaturation occurs only in sleep, during episodes of apnea, which in severe cases may number hundreds in the course of a night. The diagnosis of sleep apnea is generally made in a sleep laboratory, although its presence is suggested by overwhelming daytime drowsiness and a history of violent snoring (the latter elicited, of course, from the patient's spouse or other nocturnal companion).

Borderline Arterial Oxygen Saturation

Arterial oxygen saturations of 89 to 92 percent are on the borderline between normal and decreased. This oxygen saturation, although low enough to give rise to polycythemia as a secondary response, also occurs in forms of polycythemia more typically associated with a normal arterial oxygen saturation (for example, polycythemia vera). A borderline oxygen satu-

ration is seen with exasperating frequency in polycythemias of all kinds, and offers little help in diagnosis.

POLYCYTHEMIA VERSUS HIGH HEMATOCRIT

In thinking about diseases characterized by overproduction of red cells, it is important to keep in mind the distinction between polycythemia and a high hematocrit. Polycythemia refers to the elevation in red cell mass that is the hallmark of these diseases, while a high hematocrit represents only an abnormally high red cell mass/plasma volume ratio. (The term "red cell mass" refers to the total quantity of red cells in the patient. Despite this terminology, the red cell "mass" is always expressed as a volume—usually as milliliters of red cells.) An elevated hematocrit, although highly suggestive of polycythemia, may not be enough to make the diagnosis, because there are circumstances under which the hematocrit can be as high as 60 in the face of a normal red cell mass. To diagnose polycythemia, it is often necessary to measure the red cell mass directly. This is accomplished by labeling a known quantity of the patient's red cells with ^{51}Cr, reinjecting them, and after allowing sufficient time for complete mixing, determining by what factor the tagged cells were diluted by the patient's own circulating red cells. Patients with clinically significant secondary polycythemia will almost invariably show an increase in the red cell mass (Fig. 12-2).

Management

The secondary polycythemias are ideally managed by treating the underlying disease. This may not be possible, however, or even if possible may yield only a partial response. The question then remains as to what to do about the elevated hemoglobin. Often, the answer to this question is, "Nothing." If, however, the hemoglobin level is sufficiently high, symp-

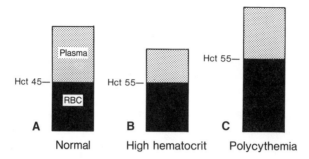

Fig. 12-2. Determination of the red cell mass helps establish whether a patient with a moderately elevated hematocrit has true polycythemia or not. (**A**) The normal situation: the hematocrit, red cell mass, and plasma volume are all normal. (**B**) An elevated hematocrit but no polycythemia; the red cell mass is normal and the plasma volume is low. (**C**) An elevated hematocrit with true polycythemia; the red cell mass and the plasma volume are both high.

toms may occur because the high viscosity of the polycythemic blood reduces tissue oxygen delivery and imposes a strain on the heart (Ch. 2). In this situation, phlebotomy can be used to lower the hemoglobin and relieve symptoms.

In patients with polycythemia due to chronic hypoxemia, treatment by phlebotomy appears contrary to logic, because the elevation in red cell volume would seem to be needed to compensate for the reduction in arterial oxygen saturation. In severe chronic lung disease, however, it has been found that patients do best when their hemoglobins are in the range of 18 g/100 ml. Thus even in chronic hypoxemia, more hemoglobin is not necessarily better, and a symptomatic patient with a very high hemoglobin will often benefit from phlebotomy.

POLYCYTHEMIA VERA

In polycythemia vera, normal marrow stem cells are replaced by an abnormal stem cell population whose response to growth regulators (e.g., erythropoietin) is disturbed. As discussed above, the high hemoglobin in polycythemia vera is usually accompanied by findings that are very unusual in the secondary polycythemias, including splenomegaly and high white cell and platelet counts. Polycythemia vera is covered in more detail in Chapter 22.

STRESS ERYTHROCYTOSIS

The combination of a modest elevation in the hematocrit and a normal red cell mass is common. Known as Gaisböck syndrome or stress erythrocytosis, this combination is typically seen in hard-driving middle-aged males, usually smokers, who in addition tend to be

---

TYPICAL PATIENT WITH STRESS ERYTHROCYTOSIS

Middle-aged man

Intense personality

Smoker

Overweight

Hypertensive

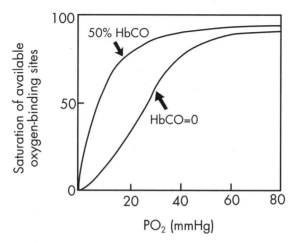

Fig. 12-3. The effect of carbon monoxide on the oxygen saturation curve of whole blood. When some of the four oxygen-binding sites on a hemoglobin molecule are occupied by CO, the remaining oxygen-binding sites lose much of their cooperativity. The result is a high-affinity hemoglobin that carries fewer oxygens than normal and is reluctant to release any of its oxygen to the tissues.

overweight and hypertensive. The red cell mass in these patients is generally on the high side of normal, while plasma volumes are in the low-normal range, leading to a high hemoglobin without an increase in red cell mass. Stress erythrocytosis is important to diagnose, because patients with this condition are at risk of heart attacks and other vascular occlusive disease.

In the pathogenesis of stress erythrocytosis, the carbon monoxide inhaled with the tobacco smoke plays a special role. When a CO molecule is taken up by hemoglobin, the CO both prevents the binding of oxygen to the occupied site and eliminates cooperativity at the remaining three sites (Ch. 3), so that a hemoglobin carrying a molecule of CO behaves like a high-affinity hemoglobin (Fig. 12-3). Furthermore, CO inhalation causes an abrupt drop in plasma volume, for reasons that are not clear. It is easy to see how CO, producing both a "high-affinity"-like hemoglobin and a low plasma volume, can give rise to the syndrome of stress erythrocytosis.

SUGGESTED READINGS

Berlin NI (1986) Polycythemia vera. Semin Hematol 23:131

Doll DC, Weiss RB (1985) Neoplasia and the erythron. J Clin Oncol 3:429

Erslev AJ, Caro J (1983) Pathophysiology and classification of polycythaemia. Scand J Haematol 31:287

Flenley DC (1982) Oxygen transport in chronic hypoxic lung disease. J Clin Pathol 35:797

Harrison BD, Stokes TC (1982) Secondary polycythaemia: its causes, effects and treatment. Br J Dis Chest 76:313

Murphy S (1992) Polycythemia vera. Dis Mon 38:153

Pearson TC (1991) Apparent polycythaemia. Blood Rev 5:205

Strandling JR, Lane DJ (1981) Development of secondary polycythaemia in chronic airways obstruction. Thorax 36:321

Territo MC, Rosove MH (1991) Cyanotic congenital heart disease: hematologic management. J Am Coll Cardiol 18:320

Section II

Coagulation

Blood clotting involves two components of the circulation: the clotting factors, a group of circulating proteins most of which are made in the liver; and the platelets, which are manufactured in the bone marrow. These are the elements of a highly complex system that is elaborately regulated so as to permit clotting to take place only at precisely dified times and locations. Clotting disorders occur when the function of one or more of these elements is disturbed. Patients with clotting disorders usually present with abnormal bleeding; occasionally, they may present because of the occurrence of spontaneous coagulation under inappropriate circumstances.

13

The Clotting Cascade and Its Regulation: Congenital and Acquired Clotting Factor Disorders

At the simplest level, the formation of a clot involves the gelation of a protein known as fibrin. This protein is not normally present as such in the circulation, but is produced in large quantities at the site of coagulation from a circulating precursor, fibrinogen. The production of fibrin from fibrinogen involves a sequence of reactions the effect of which is to amplify the tiny biochemical signal produced by a damaged blood vessel into a fibrin-generating reaction vigorous enough to form a clot capable of stopping the bleeding from the damaged vessel. Because this process of amplification occurs in a series of stages, the sequence of reactions by which the initial signal is transmuted into a fibrin clot is known as the clotting cascade.

THE CLOTTING CASCADE

The proteins involved in the formation of a clot are all present in the plasma, but they circulate as precursors with little or no activity. When blood vessels and surrounding tissues are damaged, two of these clotting factors, factor VII and factor XII (contact or Hageman factor), are converted from an inactive to an active form. In their active form, these two

clotting factors activate the next factors down the line. These in turn activate the succeeding factors, the final outcome being the production of a fibrin clot. In every case, the inactive clotting factor is converted to the active form by the cleavage of one or two particular peptide bonds, a process known as *activation by limited proteolysis*.

Stages and Factors

The clotting cascade can be divided into three stages: the initial stage, the intermediate stage, and the stage of clot formation. These stages and the clotting factors activated during each are listed in Table 13-1.

INITIAL STAGE

The clotting cascade can be initiated by the activation of either factor VII or factor XI.

Activation of Factor VII

Most cells contain tissue factor, a membrane-associated protein that binds factor VII. When these cells are damaged, their tissue fac-

189

Table 13-1. Stages of the Clotting Cascade

Stage	Factors Activated
Initial	VII, or contact factors (XII, prekallikrein, XI)
Intermediate	IX, X, prothrombin
Clot formation	Fibrinogen, XIII

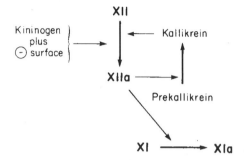

Fig. 13-2. The contact phase.

tor is exposed to factor VII in the blood, and the tissue factor–VII complex forms (Fig. 13-1).This complex is a feeble protease that slowly converts factor X, the next clotting factor down the line, to its active form Xa. The newly formed Xa transforms the tissue factor–VII complex to the much more potent tissue factor-VIIa complex, which now converts X to Xa much faster than it did before activation. By activating factor X, factor VII accelerates its own activation and vice versa, a clear case of positive feedback. The self-amplifying character of this process makes it a highly efficient mechanism for generating factor VIIa.

The Contact Phase and the Activation of Factor XI

The activation of factor XI is the end result of a set of mutually reinforcing reactions known as the *contact phase* of coagulation (Fig. 13-2). The contact phase begins when blood comes into contact with a negatively charged surface (in vivo, a site of blood vessel injury; in vitro, glass or clay). The negative surface charge attracts from the bloodstream the four proteins of the contact phase: *factor XII* and *high molecular weight kininogen*,

which attach directly to the charged surface, and *factor XI* and *prekallikrein*, which are bound to the high molecular weight kininogen and travel with it to the surface.

On the negatively charged surface, factor XII, acquiring a weak but highly specific proteolytic activity, begins to act on its two substrates, converting factor XI to XIa and prekallikrein to kallikrein. Reinforcement results from the prekallikrein → kallikrein conversion, because kallikrein, itself a very specific protease, feeds back to convert circulating factor XII into XIIa (i.e., activated XII), which then generates more kallikrein from prekallikrein. Therefore the production of factor XIa, like the production of factor VIIa, is a self-amplifying process.

An Unsolved Mystery

Clotting is initiated by two pathways: the *tissue factor/VII* pathway and the *contact factor/XI* pathway. The importance of these pathways in vivo can be judged by the severity of the bleeding in patients with very low levels of one of the initiating factors (less than 1 percent of normal). On the average, deficiencies of this magnitude cause the following: factor VII deficiency, severe bleeding; factor XI deficiency, moderate bleeding; contact factor deficiency, no bleeding. This suggests that under normal conditions, the clotting cascade is initiated chiefly by the tissue factor/VII pathway, with relatively little participation by the contact factor/XI pathway (although the contact factor/XI

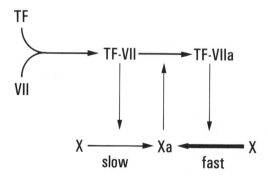

Fig. 13-1. Activation of factor VII. TF, tissue factor.

pathway may be important for clot formation in certain disease states such as gram-negative septicemia; Ch. 15). What remains unexplained is why patients with a deficiency of factor XI have a bleeding disorder, while patients with contact factor deficiency (i.e., a deficiency of the factor XI activating system) are perfectly normal. This suggests that in addition to the contact pathway, there must be a second way to activate factor XI. Despite an intensive search, however, a second way to activate factor XI has not yet been defined.* This paradox remains an unsolved mystery of coagulation.

INTERMEDIATE STAGE

In the intermediate stage, factors IX, X, and II (prothrombin) are activated. Activated factor II (thrombin) is the enzyme that converts fibrinogen to fibrin, initiating the formation of the clot per se. Its production is the final step in the intermediate stage.

Activation of Factor IX

Both of the products of the initial stage—factors XIa and VIIa—are able to activate factor IX (Fig. 13-3). Activation is accomplished as usual by limited proteolysis. Calcium is necessary for activation by factor XIa, while calcium, phospholipid, and tissue factor are all required for factor VIIa-mediated activation.

Factor IXa can do nothing further by itself. In association with Ca^{2+}, phospholipid, and factor VIII, however, it becomes a potent activator of factor X, the next factor in line. This complex of factor IXa, factor VIII, Ca^{2+}, and phospholipid is called *tenase*, because it is an enzyme that acts on factor X. In this complex, factor IXa functions as a protease, while factor VIII plays a purely accessory role as an accelerator of the reaction, having no proteolytic activity of its own. The importance of this accessory role must not be underestimated,

*It has recently been found that factor XI is activated by thrombin, a factor generated at a later stage in the clotting cascade. If this finding is confirmed by further work, it could solve the mystery.

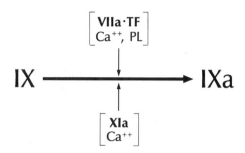

Fig. 13-3. Activation of factor IX. Factor IX can be activated by either of the two complexes shown in brackets. TF, tissue factor; PL, phospholipid.

however; the most severe coagulation disorders in clinical medicine are attributable to the deficiency of factor VIII.

Activation of Factor X

Like factor IX, factor X can be activated in two ways (Fig. 13-4). It can be activated by tenase, the factor IXa- and VIII-containing species described in the preceding paragraph, or it can be activated by factor VIIa in the presence of Ca^{2+}, phospholipid, and tissue factor. Activation again involves limited proteolysis.

Activated factor X (Xa) now associates with factor V plus Ca^{2+} and phospholipid to form *prothrombinase*, the species that catalyzes the activation of prothrombin to thrombin. Factor Xa is the protease, carrying out the peptide-splitting reactions by which the prothrombin activation reaction is accomplished, while factor V serves as accelerator. The resemblance between prothrombinase and tenase is evident.

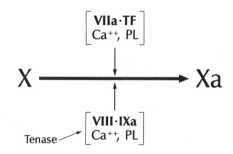

Fig. 13-4. Activation of factor X. Factor X can be activated by either of the two complexes shown in brackets. TF, tissue factor; PL, phospholipid.

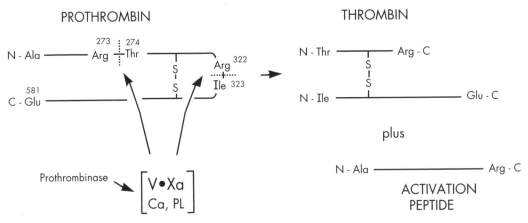

Fig. 13-5. Conversion of prothrombin to thrombin. Prothrombin is converted to thrombin by limited proteolysis—that is, by the cleavage of a few specific peptide bonds (*arrows*). When a prothrombin molecule binds to the prothrombin converting complex, these bonds are exposed to the action of factor Xa, the proteolytic component of the converting complex. The factor Xa converts prothrombin to thrombin by (1) splitting off the activation peptide and (2) cutting the loop made by the disulfide bridge.

Activation of Prothrombin (Factor II)

The conversion of prothrombin to thrombin is carried out solely by the prothrombin converting complex. No other activated clotting factor of the clotting factor complex is able to carry out this reaction. Limited proteolysis is once again the mechanism of activation. Figure 13-5 shows that active thrombin is generated from prothrombin by two proteolytic cleavages: one that removes the amino-terminal half of the prothrombin molecule, a piece known as prothrombin fragment 1·2, and one that splits the remaining peptide chain into two pieces held together by a disulfide bridge. Because the removal of fragment 1·2 is necessary for the activation of prothrombin to thrombin, this fragment is sometimes referred to as an activation peptide. The activation of factors VII, IX, and X follows a very similar pattern.

Thrombin too is a protease, the final one produced in the clotting cascade. It has several actions. It may be able to activate factor XI, as discussed above. It can convert factors V and VIII into forms that are much more potent than the native circulating factors, thereby promoting its own production—another example of positive feedback in the clotting cascade. How thrombin acts on platelets is discussed in Chapter 14. Its most obvious effect, however, is to convert fibrinogen into a clot.

FINAL STAGE: CLOT FORMATION

Clot formation begins with the thrombin-catalyzed conversion of fibrinogen to monomeric fibrin (Fig. 13-6). This conversion transforms a molecule of solitary habits into one that is driven to polymerize. The rapid spontaneous polymerization of these fibrin monomers is what forms the clot, a gelatinous mass consisting of tangled strands of polymerized fibrin molecules. Initially, the clot is held together by the weak noncovalent forces

---

ACTIONS OF THROMBIN

Fibrinogen → fibrin
Activation of factors V and VIII
XIII → XIIIa
Activation of protein C
Effects on platelets

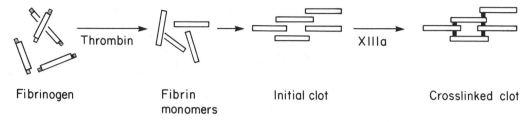

Fig. 13-6. Formation of the fibrin clot.

responsible for the polymerization of the fibrin monomers. Within minutes, however, the strands are joined covalently through the action of a cross-linking enzyme, factor XIIIa. This cross-linking causes the clot to reach maturity and achieve its maximum strength.

The conversion of fibrinogen to fibrin monomer occurs by limited proteolysis, the recurrent theme of coagulation. Fibrinogen is a long, thin molecule composed of three pairs of chains—Aα, Bβ, and γ—tied together at their C-terminal ends by a group of disulfide bonds known as the *disulfide knot*. Thrombin acts on fibrinogen by splitting pieces off the N-terminal ends of the Aα- and Bβ-chains (Fig. 13-7). With the release of these pieces, known as *fibrinopeptide A* and *fibrinopeptide B*, the fibrinogen is converted to fibrin monomer, which polymerizes spontaneously to form the initial clot.

The cross-linking enzyme also circulates as an inactive precursor. This precursor, factor XIII, is converted to factor XIIIa by thrombin. Factor XIIIa forms cross-links between the outer ends of the fibrin molecules by replacing the —NH_2 of a glutamine in one of its constituent chains with the ε-amino group of a lysine in an adjacent chain (Fig. 13-8). The γ-chains are cross-linked first, and then later the α-chains. The exchange of glutamine amino groups is known as *transglutamination*; factor XIIIa is referred to as a *transglutaminase*.

THE CLOTTING CASCADE IN SUMMARY

The clotting cascade is clearly a complex subject that may be hard to grasp in toto on the first or even second reading. The process can

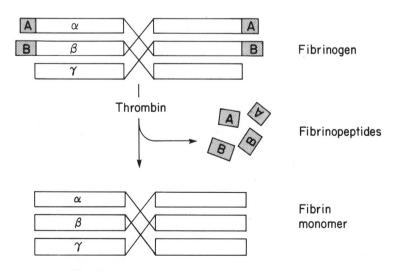

Fig. 13-7. Cleavage of fibrinogen by thrombin.

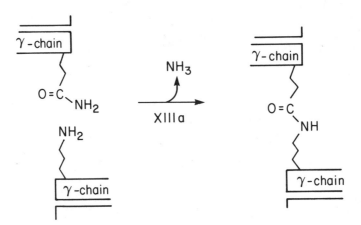

Fig. 13-8. Transglutamination.

be summarized, however, by the following two statements, which may serve as guides through the labyrinth and may assist in explaining the basis for the various tests used in evaluating the clotting cascade:

1. Up through the activation of factor X, the clotting cascade actually consists of a pair of activation sequences that run in parallel. One comprises the sequence

$$\text{Tissue factor} \rightarrow \text{VIIa} \rightarrow \text{Xa}$$

This sequence is referred to as the extrinsic pathway, because it is triggered by tissue factor, which is extrinsic to the plasma. The other consists of the sequence

$$(\text{XIIa, kallikrein}) \rightarrow \text{XIa} \rightarrow \text{IXa} \rightarrow \text{Xa}$$

This sequence is called the intrinsic pathway, because it is triggered by factors intrinsic to (i.e., present in) the plasma. Apart from the single crossover reaction

$$\text{VIIa} \rightarrow \text{IXa}$$

the extrinsic and intrinsic pathways represent completely separate activating tracks. From factor X on, of course, there is only the single common track:

$$\text{Xa} \rightarrow \text{IIa} \rightarrow \text{clot}$$

These sequences are summarized in Figure 13-9.

2. Calcium and phospholipid are necessary for almost all the steps in the initial and intermediate stages. The only exceptions are the

activation of factor IX by factor XIa, which requires only Ca^{2+}, and the reactions of the contact phase, which require neither.

Testing The Cascade

The methods for testing the cascade are summarized in Table 13-2.

SCREENING TESTS

Screening tests for the clotting cascade are carried out on plasma in which clotting has been prevented by a calcium-sequestering agent—citrate or oxalate. The cascade is initiated by adding calcium plus an activating agent, and the time required for the formation of a clot is measured. There are three such tests, each using a different activating agent and each examining a different portion of the cascade:

1. *Partial thromboplastin time.* For the PTT test, activation is accomplished by a negatively charged surface: the glass wall of a test tube, or (for the so-called activated PTT) a contact activator such as finely divided kaolin, a form of clay. Phospholipid is also added. In this test, clotting is started by the activation of factor XII. The test measures the intrinsic system and the common path.

2. *Prothrombin time.* For the PT test, tissue thromboplastin, which contains phospholipid plus tissue factor, is used as the activat-

Intrinsic pathway Extrinsic pathway

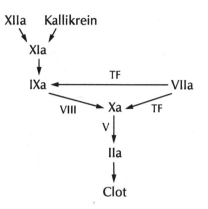

Fig. 13-9. Clotting cascade. The cascade consists of two separate activating pathways—the intrinsic pathway and the extrinsic pathway—which converge to a common pathway at factor X. Except for tissue factor (TF) and factors V and VIII, all the clotting factors named in this diagram are proteases.

ing agent. In this test, clotting is started by the activation of factor VII. The test measures factor VII and the common path.

3. *Thrombin time.* In the TT test, thrombin is the activating agent. This test measures the sequence: fibrinogen → fibrin monomer → initial clot.

The end point for each of these tests is the production of the initial clot. Therefore, none of these tests measures factor XIII, although among them they measure every other factor in the clotting cascade.

SPECIFIC FACTORS

Fibrinogen

Fibrinogen is usually measured as thrombin-clottable protein. Enough thrombin is added to convert all the fibrinogen to fibrin, and the amount of protein in the resulting fibrin clot is determined by one of a variety of techniques. Fibrinogen can also be determined by immunological and precipitation methods; these measure the factor by its structure, not its function.

Factor XIII

The initial clot, held together only by weak noncovalent forces, is soluble in mild denaturing agents, while a clot cross-linked by factor XIIIa is not. The solubility of a clot in a solution of a mild denaturant (urea or monochloroacetic acid) is therefore used to measure factor XIII.

Other Factors

A PT or PTT may be prolonged because of a deficiency in a specific clotting factor. Such a test would be fully corrected by mixing the deficient plasma with an equal volume of normal plasma, or of a second plasma lacking a different clotting factor, but would remain uncorrected if the second plasma were lacking the same clotting factor that was missing from the first plasma. A clotting factor deficiency can therefore be diagnosed by showing that an abnormal PT or PTT is corrected by all but one

Table 13-2. Testing the Clotting Cascade

Method	Component Tested	Test
Screening tests	Intrinsic and common pathways	Partial thromboplastin time (PTT)
	Factor VII and the common pathway	Prothrombin time (PT)
	Fibrinogen → clot	Thrombin time (TT)
Specific factors	Fibrinogen	Thrombin-clottable protein
	Factor XIII	Solubility of clot in urea or $ClCH_2COOH$
	Other factors	PT or PTT of test plasma mixed with plasmas deficient in known factors
		Immunoassay
Inhibitors		PT or PTT of test plasma mixed with normal plasma

of a panel of plasmas with known deficiencies: the unknown plasma and the plasma that fails to correct the test are missing the same clotting factor.

The concentration of the deficient clotting factor, an important consideration in the treatment of clotting factor deficiencies, can be determined from the PT or PTT using a standard curve obtained with mixtures of normal plasma and plasma with a known deficiency. The concentration of a clotting factor can also be determined by immunological testing. Clotting factor concentrations as measured by immunological testing often agree with concentrations as measured functionally (i.e., by the PT or PTT), but sometimes there is a discrepancy, with the immunological concentration exceeding the functional concentration. Such a discrepancy indicates the presence of an abnormal clotting factor that is antigenically close to normal but functionally defective.

INHIBITORS

When an abnormal screening test fails to be corrected by mixing the defective plasma with an equal volume of normal plasma, the presence of an inhibitor is indicated. The potency of the inhibitor can be determined by measuring the effect of various concentrations of the inhibitor-containing plasma on the clotting properties of normal plasma. Identifying which factor(s) the inhibitor acts against may be difficult, however, because both the PT and the PTT depend on the activation of many factors, and an inhibitor acting against any one of them will prolong the test. Fortunately, it is rarely necessary to know precisely which factor is blocked in order to treat the patient.

BLEEDING TIME

The bleeding time, a crude but valuable screening test, is performed by measuring how long it takes for bleeding to stop from a fresh cut of defined size. The cut is ordinarily made on the inner surface of the forearm, its length and depth being fixed by means of a template. A prolonged bleeding time usually indicates a platelet disorder (qualitative or quantitative); very occasionally, it may be caused by an abnormality of small blood vessels (e.g., scurvy). In pure disorders of the clotting cascade, the bleeding time is almost invariably normal.

BIOSYNTHESIS OF CLOTTING FACTORS

All the clotting factors except a portion of factor VIII are synthesized in the liver. Factor VIII is synthesized in two parts, one part coming from endothelium and megakaryocytes and the other being produced in many kinds of cells, including hepatocytes. The part made by the endothelium and megakaryocytes, usually known as the *von Willebrand factor* but sometimes called *factor VIII antigen*, does not participate directly in the clotting cascade. The other part, known as *factor VIII* or *factor VIII coagulant protein*, is the active clotting factor. Unfortunately, the term factor VIII is also used to refer to the combination of the two parts. For a full explanation of the makeup of factor VIII, and the confusing dual use of the term factor VIII, see the discussion of von Willebrand's disease in Chapter 14. In the present chapter, the term factor VIII refers exclusively to the factor VIII coagulant protein.

VITAMIN K-DEPENDENT PROTEINS

Clotting factors
  II (prothrombin)
  VII
  IX
  X
Anticoagulant proteins
  Protein C
  Protein S

A lipid-soluble vitamin, vitamin K (Fig. 13-10), is required for the production of four of the clotting factors made in the liver: factors II (prothrombin), VII, IX, and X. The N-terminal (activation peptide) portions of all four of these clotting factors contain a series of γ-carboxy-glutamyl (gla) residues that appear to function in calcium binding. The gla residues are not incorporated into the proteins during translation, but rather are produced by the post-translational addition of CO_2 to selected glutamate residues in the protein chain (Fig. 13-11). It is this carboxylation reaction that requires vitamin K. It will be seen that the drugs most commonly used for long-term therapeutic anticoagulation act by interfering with this reaction.

Vitamin K is also required for the production of two anticoagulant proteins: protein C and protein S.

REGULATION OF CLOTTING

The clotting process is regulated by two general mechanisms: the elimination of activated clotting factors and the destruction of the fibrin clot.

Elimination of Activated Clotting Factors

Activated clotting factors are rapidly removed from the circulation by the liver. They may also be directly inactivated in the plasma by three circulating anticoagulant systems: the antithrombin III (AT III)/proteoglycan

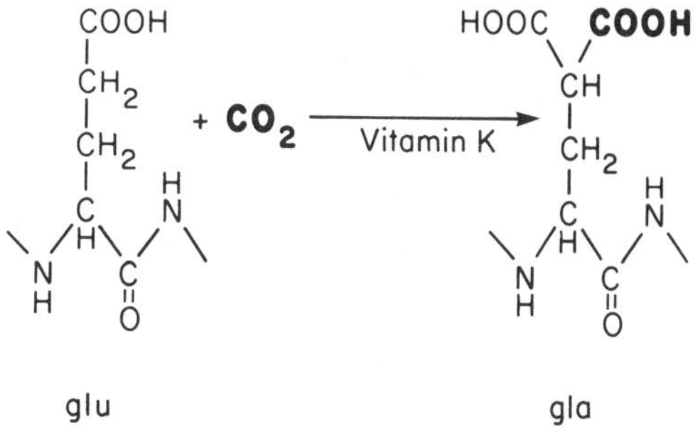

Fig. 13-11. Formation of gla from a glutamic acid residue.

system, the tissue factor pathway inhibitor (TFPI)/phospholipid system, and the protein C/protein S system.

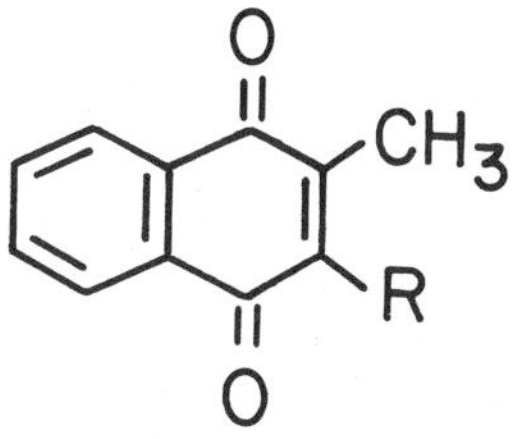

ANTITHROMBIN III

AT III is a member of a family of protease inhibitors known as the *serpins* (*ser*ine *pro*tease *in*hibitor). These protease inhibitors work by combining with their targets to form extremely stable, inactive 1:1 complexes (Fig. 13-12). AT III is the serpin that inactivates clotting factors that have proteolytic activity. It acts against all the proteolytic clotting factors except factor VIIa (Fig. 13-9). Its importance in vivo is shown by the fact that persons with an inherited deficiency of AT III are highly susceptible to thrombosis on the venous side of the circulation.

Fig. 13-10. Vitamin K. R, a long hydrocarbon side chain.

ELIMINATION OF CLOTTING FACTORS FROM THE BLOOD

Clearance by the liver
Inactivation by
  Antithrombin II (proteases except factor VIIa)
  Tissue factor pathway inhibitor (factor VIIa)
  Protein C (factors V and VIII)

The action of AT III is greatly potentiated by binding to certain proteoglycans. These include *endothelial cell proteoglycans*, which bind AT III to line the inner surfaces of blood vessels with a layer of anticoagulant, and *heparin*, an anticoagulant drug that works through its interaction with AT III.

TISSUE FACTOR
PATHWAY INHIBITOR

Factor VIIa is neutralized by its own unique protein antagonist, tissue factor pathway inhibitor (TFPI). This antagonist acts in two steps. In step one, TFPI forms a complex with phospholipid and factor Xa, inhibiting Xa as it does so. In the second step, this complex binds to the tissue factor–VIIa complex (Fig. 13-13), eliminating the activity of VIIa. The result is a blockade of both factors VIIa and Xa.

PROTEIN C AND PROTEIN S

Protein C is a vitamin K-dependent protein that neutralizes factors V and VIII by limited proteolysis. Like the clotting factors, protein C circulates as an inert precursor, and must itself be activated before it can function as an anticoagulant. Activation is accomplished by a limited proteolytic reaction in which thrombin is the active protease. Before it can act on protein C, however, thrombin has to be modulated in such a way as to alter its substrate specificity. Modulation is accomplished by thrombomodulin, an endothelial cell protein that forms a complex with thrombin, eliminating its coagulant activity and at the same time endowing it with a protein C-converting activity that it lacks when free. Because protein C can only function after being activated by thrombin, its effect tends to be limited to regions where active clotting is taking place.

Activated protein C then destroys the activity of factors V and VIII. To carry out this task, the activated protein C combines with Ca^{2+}, phospholipid, and another vitamin K-dependent protein known as protein S to form what might be termed a "factor V/VIII inactivating complex" (Fig. 13-14). This complex, contain-

ing a protease (activated protein C) and an accelerator (protein S), plus Ca^{2+} and phospholipid, is completely analogous to the factor X- and prothrombin-converting complexes described above. The "factor V/VIII inactivating complex" inactivates these factors by limited proteolysis.

Protein C is complementary to AT III, working on nonproteolytic clotting factors against which AT III has no effect. Patients deficient in either protein C or protein S have a greatly increased risk of venous thrombosis. In infants homozygous for protein C or protein S deficiency, this is expressed as *purpura fulminans*, a rapidly spreading hemorrhagic necrosis of the skin that is often fatal. This indicates that, like AT III, protein C and protein S have important roles in the prevention of coagulation in vivo.

Fibrinolysis

As important as the formation of a clot at a site of injury is its removal when its usefulness is over. The clot is removed by enzymatic digestion, a process referred to as *fibrinolysis*.

PLASMIN AND FIBRIN-SPLIT
PRODUCTS

Fibrinolysis is accomplished by a fibrin-splitting protease called *plasmin*. This enzyme is produced in the vicinity of a clot by limited proteolysis of plasminogen, its circulating precursor. Plasminogen is converted to plasmin by two activators: tissue plasminogen activator, which initiates clot lysis by activating plasminogen bound to the fibrin in the clot (it has little effect on circulating plasminogen); and urokinase, which keeps hollow organs (e.g., the ureter) free from clots. Both are secreted in active form by appropriately stimulated endothelial cells and mononuclear phagocytes, and urokinase is secreted by epithelial cells as well. The route of plasmin formation is shown in Figure 13-15.

The digestion of a fibrin molecule by plasmin takes place in an orderly manner (Fig. 13-16). Plasmin first releases the outer portions of

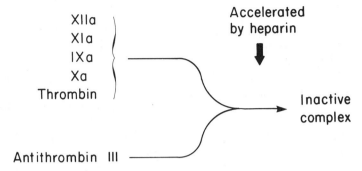

Fig. 13-12. The mechanism of action of antithrombin III.

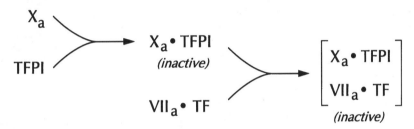

Fig. 13-13. Inactivation of factors Xa and VIIa by tissue factor pathway inhibitor (TFPI). TFPI first binds to factor Xa plus phospholipid, abolishing the activity of Xa. The TFPI-Xa-phospholipid complex then binds to the factor VIIa–tissue factor complex, abolishing the activity of factor VIIa.

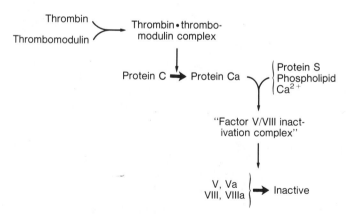

Fig. 13-14. Inactivation of factors V and VIII by protein C. Thrombin liberated in the vicinity of a clot attaches to thrombomodulin on the surface of an endothelial cell. When it binds to thrombomodulin, thrombin acquires the ability to activate protein C. The activated protein C combines with protein S, Ca^{2+} and phospholipid to form a "factor V/VIII inactivating complex" that destroys the activities of factors V and VIII by proteolysis.

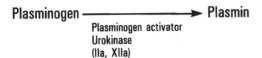

Fig. 13-15. Formation of plasmin.

the α-chains, producing the so-called X fragment. This fragment is then split on one side of the disulfide knot into a D (small) and a Y (large) fragment. A similar cleavage on the other side of the disulfide knot releases a second D fragment, leaving behind a small piece known as the E fragment.

When digesting a clot, plasmin cuts the covalently linked fibrin polymers in the same places: at the outer portions of the α-chains, and next to the disulfide knots. The fragments of polymer cut away by the plasmin are released from the clot as fibrin-degradation products (FDPs) (or fibrin-split products [FSPs]). Some of these fragments are identical to those produced by the digestion of an individual fibrin molecule. Many, however, are larger, containing portions of two or more fibrin molecules. These are produced when fragments are released from the polymer by cuts in two separate fibrin units (Fig. 13-16).

Fibrin-split products are potent inhibitors of clotting. They impair coagulation through two mechanisms, both based on their close similarity to fibrin and fibrinogen:

1. They interfere with the action of thrombin by binding to thrombin at its fibrinogen-binding site.

2. They interfere with the polymerization of fibrin monomers by forming monomer–split product complexes. Some of these complexes remain in solution, while others bind abnormally to the growing clot, weakening its structure.

Normally, the quantities of fibrin-split products in the blood are too small to affect coagulation. In certain conditions, however, they can increase sufficiently to cause clinical bleeding through their anticoagulant action.

Plasmin also degrades other proteins of the clotting cascade. The most important of these

is fibrinogen, but plasmin also acts to destroy factors V and VIII.

REGULATION OF FIBRINOLYSIS

The principal regulators of fibrinolysis are two antiproteases: α_2-*plasmin inhibitor*, which inactivates plasmin itself, and *plasminogen activator inhibitor type 1 (PAI-1)*, which slows the formation of plasmin from plasminogen by inactivating the two plasminogen activators (Fig. 13-17). Both α_2-antiplasmin and PAI-1 are members of the serpin family. A deficiency of either of these regulators results in a severe bleeding disorder, testifying to their importance in the control of fibrinolysis in vivo.

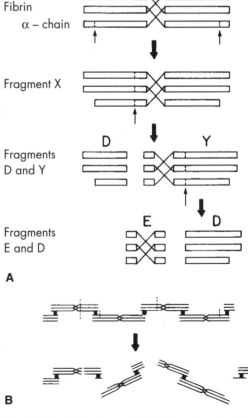

Fig. 13-16. Digestion of fibrin by plasmin. (A) Digestion of a single molecule. (B) Digestion of a cross-linked clot.

MEASURING FIBRINOLYSIS

Although fibrinolysis in the normal person is so slow as to be undetectable, there are diseases in which it is greatly accelerated. Accelerated fibrinolysis can be diagnosed by demonstrating the presence of fibrin-split products in the serum or by finding increased plasminogen activation in the circulation.

Fibrin-Split Products

Like other anticoagulants, fibrin-split products cause abnormalities in the screening assays (PT, PTT, and especially TT); their presence may be suspected on that basis. To confirm their presence, two types of tests are used: direct measurements and paracoagulation.

Direct Measurements. The best test for fibrin-split products is the *plasma D-D dimer* level. D-D dimers are fragments released from *cross-linked* fibrin when it is cut by plasmin. The dimer consists of a D fragment from each of two adjacent fibrin molecules, held together by the cross-links that originally joined the two fibrin molecules (Fig. 13-18). Unlike some other fibrin-split products, a D-D dimer cannot be produced from circulating fibrinogen, but only from a clot, because cross-linked fibrin is only found in clots. An elevated D-D dimer

level is therefore strong evidence that a previously formed clot is undergoing dissolution—that is, that fibrinolysis is taking place.

There are other direct ways to measure the levels of fibrin-split products in serum. The most widely used is the *Staphylococcus* clumping assay, which is based on the ability of fibrin-split products to agglutinate *Staphylococcus aureus*. These other assays are slowly being replaced by the D-D dimer test.

Paracoagulation. Ethanol or protamine gelation paracoagulation tests depend on the fact that fibrin-split products can form soluble complexes with fibrin monomers, preventing the bound monomers from polymerizing into a fibrin clot. When ethanol or protamine is added to serum containing such complexes, the complexes fall apart, releasing their fibrin monomers. The liberated monomers polymerize in a normal fashion, forming a visible clot. This is known as paracoagulation. It is a quick but indirect way of demonstrating that fibrin-split products are present in a serum sample.

Euglobulin Lysis Time

The euglobulin lysis time test determines whether the plasma contains any circulating activators of the fibrinolytic system (i.e., plasminogen activators) (Fig. 13-19). It takes advantage of the fact that when plasma is treat-

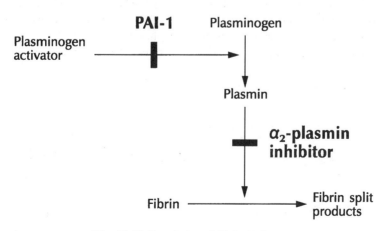

Fig. 13-17. Regulation of fibrinolysis.

ed with dilute acid, fibrinogen precipitates out, carrying with it (1) other clotting factors and (2) the components of the fibrinolytic system (plasmin, plasminogen, and any circulating plasminogen activators) but leaving behind (3) circulating inhibitors of the fibrinolytic system. This precipitate, known as the *euglobulin fraction*, can be isolated and redissolved in neutral buffer containing a calcium-binding anticoagulant. When excess calcium is added to this solution of euglobulin fraction, the clotting factors act on fibrinogen to produce a fibrin clot. This clot will dissolve over the next few hours if plasminogen activators are present, because of the unopposed action of the plasmin newly generated by the activators during the period of incubation. The rate at which the clot dissolves is closely related to the quantity of circulating plasminogen activators pre-

sent in the original plasma. The time required for the euglobulin precipitate to dissolve, a period referred to as the *euglobulin lysis time*, is thus a measure of the fibrinolytic activity of the plasma; the shorter the euglobulin lysis time, the greater the fibrinolytic activity.

DISORDERS OF THE CLOTTING CASCADE

Inherited Disorders

HEMOPHILIA

Hemophilia A (hereinafter referred to as hemophilia) is a clotting disorder caused by an inherited deficiency of factor VIII. In some instances, the factor VIII deficiency is caused by an absolute reduction in the amount of circulating factor VIII, while in others it is caused by the production of normal quantities of a defective clotting factor. Hemophilia is both the most common and the most serious of the inherited disorders of the clotting cascade.

Hemophilia is transmitted in an X-linked manner. This means that the disease is seen almost exclusively in males, although it is transmitted by both carrier mothers and affected fathers. The pattern of transmission (Fig. 13-20) guarantees that the sons of a carrier mother have a 50:50 chance of being carriers. A hemophiliac male can only transmit the condition to his daughters, all of whom will be carriers. Carriers of hemophilia are usually rec-

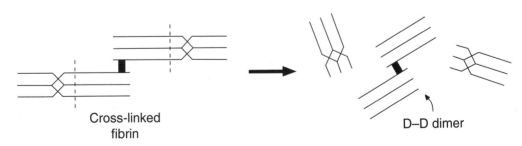

Cross-linked
fibrin

D–D dimer

Fig. 13-18. The D-D dimer. D-D dimers are formed when plasmin degrades crosslinked fibrin.

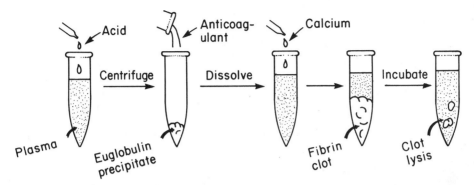

Fig. 13-19. Euglobulin lysis time.

ognized by virtue of the fact that they have had a hemophiliac child, but it is sometimes possible to identify them before this occurs.

Clinical Manifestations

Intractable bleeding is the problem in hemophilia. It is seen after injury, of course, but it can occur spontaneously in otherwise healthy patients. The sites affected by spontaneous bleeding are characteristic (Fig. 13-21).

Joints. The large joints—especially the hip, knee, and ankle—are the sites most commonly involved in a spontaneous bleed. The affected joint swells and becomes extremely painful over the course of a few hours. Because the joint is a closed space, the bleeding eventually stops, so signs and symptoms regress over several days. Recurrent bleeding is the rule, however, eventually leading to a crippling arthritis caused by repeated joint injury.

Soft Tissues. Spontaneous bleeding into soft tissues may take place. Seepage of blood may continue for hours or days, with the gradual development of a massive hematoma. The diagnosis is made on the basis of the presence of a growing mass (demonstrated by physical examination or scan) along with signs of blood loss (falling hematocrit and shock). Symptoms of compression may also occur, depending on the site of the bleed. Hemorrhage into the iliopsoas muscle, for example, can cause an entrapment syndrome affecting the nerves of the lumbar plexus. One of the most dangerous places for a soft tissue bleed is the base of the tongue, because of the possibility of death from asphyxia due to closure of the pharynx.

Other Problems. Nosebleeds and urinary bleeding are common, although not especially dangerous, in patients with hemophilia. Gastrointestinal (GI) bleeding, either spontaneous or from a lesion in the GI tract, is a moderately frequent complication. A particularly dangerous problem is bleeding into the brain, a frequent cause of death in hemophilia. *Headaches and head injuries, however mild they may seem, have to be taken extremely seriously in these patients.*

Bleeding after trauma is also a problem. A major injury such as that resulting from an automobile accident causes massive bleeding that must be stopped to prevent death from exsanguination. Minor injuries, however, may also result in extensive blood loss. For example, a small cut in a hemophiliac will typically stop bleeding after a few minutes as a result of arteriolar constriction and the formation of a platelet plug, but will then begin to bleed again a few hours later and continue to leak blood in a slow, steady trickle for days. The amount of blood that can be lost from a slow leak should not be underestimated; unstanched bleeding at the seemingly trivial rate of 0.5 ml/min represents a loss of 3 units/day.

The clinical severity of the disease varies from patient to patient depending on the factor VIII level, which tends to remain constant in a given hemophiliac. Patients whose factor VIII level is greater than 5 percent of normal have few problems with spontaneous

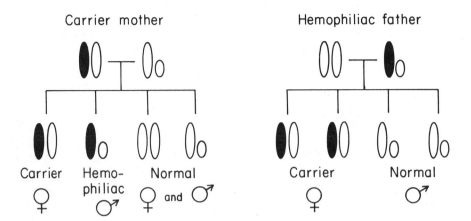

Carrier mother

Hemophiliac father

Carrier
♀

Hemo-
philiac
♂

Normal
♀ and ♂

Carrier
♀

Normal
♂

Fig. 13-20. Transmission of hemophilia. X and Y chromosomes of the parents and children are shown. Defective X chromosomes are black.

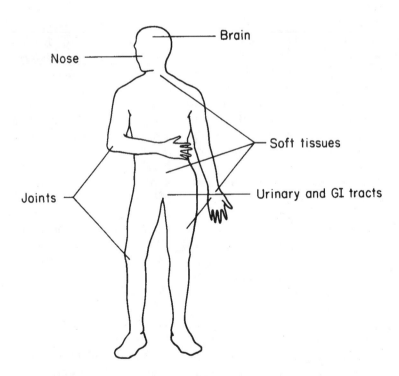

Brain

Nose

Soft tissues

Urinary and GI tracts

Joints

Fig. 13-21. Sites of spontaneous bleeding in hemophilia.

bleeds or minor injuries. As the factor VIII level drops, the severity of the disease increases. The worst problems are seen in patients whose factor VIII level is less than 1 percent of normal.

A complication that poses great difficulties for the management of the disease is the appearance of a so-called inducible inhibitor. Inhibitors are factor VIII-neutralizing antibodies that develop in about 10 percent of patients with hemophilia. One-half of these are "stable" inhibitors whose levels remain constant over time. The other half are referred to as "inducible" inhibitors because their levels respond anamnestically to factor VIII treatment, rising sharply within a few days after replacement therapy is started and remaining at elevated levels for weeks or months thereafter. The problems of treating hemophiliacs with inducible inhibitors are discussed below.

Management

Hemophilia is suspected in a patient with a history of bleeding, especially spontaneous bleeding and most especially spontaneous bleeding into a joint. Male sex and a family history are of course highly suggestive, although hemophilia is seen from time to time in females, and will occasionally occur sporadically, the result, it is thought, of a spontaneous mutation.

In the laboratory, the only abnormal screening test is a prolonged PTT. The bleeding time is normal, but bleeding from the cut is likely to resume after an hour or so. The diagnosis is made by showing that factor VIII is decreased. In making the diagnosis, it is important not simply to demonstrate the deficiency, but to determine the level of the clotting factor as well, since the severity of the disease depends critically on the degree of the deficiency.

Laboratory data are also needed for the genetic counseling of hemophilia families. Using restriction fragment length polymorphisms* (RFLPs) in and around the factor VIII

gene, carriers can be identified, and most cases of hemophilia can be diagnosed prenatally. In the few cases in which RFLPs are not helpful, a carrier can sometimes be identified by measuring the ratio of factor VIII clotting activity to the "factor VIII antigen" level. Unfortunately, the term "factor VIII antigen" does not refer to the factor VIII coagulant protein, but to another circulating protein, the von Willebrand factor, one of whose functions seems to be to stabilize the real factor VIII in the blood (which is how it got the name "factor VIII antigen"). This confusing state of affairs is discussed more fully in Chapter 14. In terms of detecting the carrier state, the important point is that the factor VIII clotting activity/factor VIII antigen ratio tends to be constant from person to person and can therefore be a fairly reliable indicator of carrier status. When measurements are made with care, the activity:antigen ratio can detect five carriers out of six.

The treatment of hemophilia involves replacement therapy with factor VIII concentrates; it is generally based on the principle that factor VIII is given when, and only when, bleeding occurs. Two types of concentrates are currently in use: cryoprecipitate, which in addition to factor VIII contains fibrinogen and von Willebrand factor, and purified factor VIII, which contains little of either. Minor bleeds may be treated at home by the patient, who has been taught how to adminster the concentrate and keeps a supply in his refrigerator. Home therapy has resulted in much better control of minor bleeds, because patients are instructed to treat themselves at the first sign of bleeding. As a result, severe hemarthroses are much less common than they used to be, and crippling arthritis is no longer an inevitable outcome of hemophilia. In patients with mild hemophilia, minor bleeds can also be treated with desmopressin (DDAVP), a vasopressin analogue that increases plasma factor VIII levels by stimulating the secretion of "factor VIII antigen" (see above) by the endothelium.

Major bleeds usually require hospitalization. The approach to therapy is to administer enough factor VIII concentrate so that the plas-

---

*For a discussion of RFLPs, see Chapter 10.

DIAGNOSING HEMOPHILIA IN THE LABORATORY

Patient
- PTT usually prolonged
- Factor VIII activity greatly reduced

Carrier
- Normal clotting screen
- Factor VIII activity normal or moderately reduced
- Factor VIII activity/factor VIII antigen about half normal
- Diagnostic restriction fragment length polymorphisms

ma factor VIII always remains above a fixed level, the exact value of which depends on the severity of the bleed. To do this it is necessary to know how rapidly factor VIII disappears from the circulation. The half-life of factor VIII averages about 12 hours, but it is generally a good idea to measure the half-life in the patient by giving an infusion of concentrate and measuring factor VIII levels before and at various times after the infusion is administered. From this measured half-life and the patient's plasma volume (estimated at 40 ml/kg), the daily dose of factor VIII can be calculated. The dose is checked and adjusted if necessary by measuring factor VIII levels during the course of therapy. Factor VIII is generally given two to three times a day; treatment for a major bleed may need to be continued for 10 days to 2 weeks. These same principles apply to factor VIII coverage for surgery.

A recent complication of replacement therapy is the occurrence of acquired immunodeficiency syndrome (AIDS) in patients with hemophilia. With the spread of AIDS (which became epidemic in the middle 1970s), the factor VIII supply, produced from thousands of units of pooled plasma, became widely contaminated with human immunodeficiency virus, (HIV, the cause of AIDS). As a result, most patients with hemophilia are now infected with HIV. The factor VIII supply is now much safer than before, because ways have been developed to eliminate HIV from factor VIII preparations without destroying the clotting factor, but the years of HIV contamination have left a tragic legacy.

Certain strict caveats apply to the management of hemophilia. Drugs that inhibit platelet function (e.g., aspirin) are strictly contraindicated. Venipuncture is usually not a problem, but biopsies, including bone marrow aspiration, must not be performed without factor VIII coverage.

What about the patient who has an inhibitor? If the inhibitor is stable, treatment is the same, except that the dose of concentrate must be high enough to overcome the inhibitor and provide therapeutic levels of factor VIII. If the inhibitor is inducible, the whole approach to treatment changes. With a high level of inhibitor, the best chance for hemostasis is offered by porcine factor VIII, because the activity of the porcine clotting factor is unaffected by most factor VIII inhibitors. If this fails or is unavailable, patients can be treated with recombinant factor IX. Alternatively, very large doses of factor VIII concentrate may be tried; neutralization of factor VIII by the antibody requires a certain amount of time, so the rapid administration of large doses of concentrate may permit a small amount of active factor VIII to reach the bleeding site and exert its effect. If the inhibitor level is low, treatment with more or less standard doses of concentrate is likely to be effective, at least until the inhibitor level begins to rise, at which time treatment will have to be changed unless the bleeding has stopped. Hemarthrosis is treated by immobilization, ice packs, and analgesics. Factor VIII is avoided if at all possible, because the induction of the inhibitor poses worse problems than does a blood-filled joint. The ideal treatment, of course, would be the elimination of the inhibitor. This has not been possible by plasmapheresis or immunosuppressive therapy; one current approach, still experimental, is to attempt to eliminate the antibody by inducing tolerance through the chronic administration of factor VIII. The treatment of hemophilia is summarized below.

Factor IX Deficiency (Hemophilia B; Christmas Disease)

Factor IX deficiency is about one-fifth as common as factor VIII deficiency. Clinically, the two diseases are virtually identical; both are X-linked, and both show the same patterns of bleeding. The disease is treated with recombinant factor IX.

Contact Factor Deficiencies

The contact factors are Hageman factor (XII), prekallikrein, and high molecular weight kininogen. Deficiencies of each of these factors have been described; factor XII deficiency is the most common. These deficiencies are laboratory diseases, presenting as an isolated prolongation of the PTT and a reduction in the level of the deficient factor. There is no clinical bleeding tendency whatsoever. Indeed, Mr. Hageman, the patient who lent his name to the clotting factor that was missing from his blood, died of pulmonary embolism at a ripe old age.

Dysfibrinogenemias

The hereditary dysfibrinogenemias are diseases in which normal quantities of a defective fibrinogen circulate in the bloodstream. The defect is expressed functionally as an abnormality involving one or another of the steps leading from circulating fibrinogen to the cross-linked fibrin clot. Patients with a dysfibrinogenemia may be clinically normal, or they may show a mild tendency toward either bleeding or venous thrombosis. The typical laboratory findings are a prolonged TT and a disparity between the fibrinogen levels as determined by different techniques, those measuring thrombin-clottable protein giving lower values than those measuring fibrinogen itself (immunological or precipitation methods).

Others

The inherited clotting factor deficiencies are listed in Table 13-3. The mode of transmission

---

TREATMENT OF HEMOPHILIA

No inhibitor
  Purified factor VIII
  Home therapy for minor bleeds
  DDAVP for mild hemophilia
Inhibitor present
  Stable
      Replacement at doses sufficient
        to overcome the inhibitor
  Inducible
      Low level: standard doses of purified
        factor VIII
      High level (initial, or after induction):
        porcine factor VIII, or factor IX,
        or very high doses of purified factor VIII
      Hemarthrosis: no replacement;
        immobilization and local measures
Contraindicated
  Aspirin and other antiplatelet drugs
  Biopsy or other invasive procedures
    without factor VIII coverage

---

and features unique to each disorder are also given. A point worth noting is that the screening tests (PTT, PT, TT, and bleeding time) are invariably normal in factor XIII deficiency, α_2-antiplasmin deficiency, and PAI deficiency, and are sometimes normal in prothrombin deficiency.

ACQUIRED DISORDERS

Vitamin K Deficiency

Vitamin K deficiency causes a bleeding disorder that results from impaired production of the vitamin K-dependent clotting factors: II (prothrombin), VII, IX, and X. The causes of vitamin K deficiency are listed below. The deficiency is most often seen in conditions associated with the malabsorption of fat (e.g., chronic pancreatitis, biliary cirrhosis, sprue), but it may occasionally result from malnutrition, especially in the elderly or in patients on

Table 13-3. Inherited Clotting Factor Disorders

Deficiency	Transmission[a]	Special Features	Treatment
Fibrinogen	A	Bleeding from umbilical stump; poor wound healing	Cryoprecipitate or purified fibrinogen
Prothrombin	A	Screening tests may be normal	Plasma or prothrombin concentrate
Factor V	A	Bleeding time may be prolonged	Fresh frozen plasma
Factor VII	A	PTT normal, PT prolonged	Plasma or prothrombin concentrate
Factor VIII	X		Purified factor VIII
Factor IX	X		Recombinant factor IX
Factor XI	A	Usually mild	Plasma
Contact factors	A	No clinical manifestations	None needed
Factor XIII	A	Bleeding from umbilical stump; poor wound healing; screening tests always normal	Plasma
α_2-Plasmin inhibitor	A	Screening tests always normal	Tranexamic acid (a plasmin inhibitor; see Ch. 15)
PAI-1	A	Screening tests always normal	Tranexamic acid

[a]A, Autosomal recessive; X, X-linked.

oral antibiotics whose alternative source of the vitamin (intestinal bacteria, which provide small amounts of vitamin K to all of us) has been destroyed. In the newborn, vitamin K levels are marginal, and any factors that impose an additional stress on vitamin K metabolism (e.g., postpartum malnutrition, or hypoxia during delivery with damage to an already immature liver) can lead to frank vitamin K deficiency and hemorrhagic disease of the newborn. Finally, certain anticoagulants are antagonists of vitamin K and give rise to a clotting disorder identical to that of vitamin K deficiency.

The outstanding abnormality on laboratory testing is a prolonged PT. The PTT may also be prolonged, although it is generally not as abnormal as the PT. Other tests are normal except for decreased levels of the vitamin K-dependent clotting factors. It is usually not necessary to measure these, however; a PT that corrects within 2 days after vitamin K treatment confirms the diagnosis.

The deficiency is treated by giving vitamin K. Oral treatment is usually good enough, but parenteral therapy is occasionally necessary in patients with malabsorption. Hemorrhagic disease of the newborn is prevented by the routine

CAUSES OF VITAMIN K DEFICIENCY

Malabsorption of fat
Malnutrition
    In the elderly
    In patients receiving oral antibiotics
Newborn
Anticoagulation with vitamin K antagonists

MANAGEMENT OF VITAMIN K DEFICIENCY

Diagnosis
    Prolonged prothrombin time corrected by vitamin K
Treatment
    Replacement with vitamin K

administration of the vitamin to all newborn infants. The response to treatment is exceedingly rapid; in the absence of other diseases, the clotting defect will be fully corrected within 2 days. Management of vitamin K deficiency is summarized on page 208.

Liver Disease

Liver disease causes a highly complex acquired coagulopathy affecting virtually every segment of the clotting cascade. The coagulopathy results mainly from a failure of clotting factor production by the diseased liver, but it also reflects the release of an abnormal clotting factor, as well as the failure of the liver to clear certain coagulation-related proteins from the blood. Specifically:

1. Failure of clotting factor production leads to falls in factors II (prothrombin), V, VII, IX, and X, as well as a fall in prekallikrein. Fibrinogen falls as well, but this appears to be caused primarily by increased fibrinolysis (see point 3).
2. A functionally abnormal fibrinogen is produced that contains insufficient quantities of sialic acid. This amounts to an acquired dysfibrinogenemia.
3. Clearance of activated clotting factors (IXa, Xa, and XIa) is impaired, as is the clearance of plasminogen activator. The latter is the cause of the increased fibrinolysis so typical of liver disease. In addition to these, platelets are decreased, mainly because of the splenomegaly that is a common concomitant of liver disease.

Because of the comprehensive nature of the clotting disorder, virtually every test of coagulation is abnormal. The specific abnormalities and their probable causes are listed in Table 13-4. It will be seen that these abnormalities are virtually indistinguishable from those caused by disseminated intravascular coagulation (DIC), a condition common in seriously ill patients. Attempts to make the diagnosis of DIC in the presence of severe liver disease are usually in vain.

As to treatment, any patient with liver disease should be given a single large dose of vitamin K on the chance that vitamin K deficiency is a contributing factor, but improvement after a dose of vitamin K is rare. The mainstay of treatment is replacement therapy. This is only used in patients who are actively bleeding. Fresh frozen plasma is given because it contains all the clotting factors deficient in liver disease. *Cryoprecipitate*, a plasma protein fraction containing fibrinogen, factor VIII, and von Willebrand factor, is given if necessary to supply extra fibrinogen, and platelets are administered if the patient is sufficiently thrombocytopenic. Replacement is only a stopgap measure; improvement, although frequent, is transient, often lasting only a few hours before additional replacement is needed. The only definitive treatment of the coagulopathy is cure of the underlying liver disease.

Acquired Anticoagulants (Circulating Inhibitors)

The acquired anticoagulants of clinical significance are listed below. Their presence is suspected from mixing studies.

Table 13-4. Clotting Disorder in Liver Failure

Abnormality	Explanation
Long prothrombin time	Deficiency of vitamin K-dependent clotting factors; presence of fibrin-split products
Long partial thromboplastin time	Deficiency of factors II, V, IX, prekallikrein; presence of fibrin-split products
Long thrombin time	Presence of fibrin-split products; abnormal fibrinogen
Long bleeding time	Decreased platelets
Low fibrinogen Increased fibrin-split products Shortened euglobulin lysis time }	Increased fibrinolysis

ACQUIRED ANTICOAGULANTS

Lupus anticoagulant
Fibrin-split products
Antibodies against clotting factors
    Anti-factor VIII (in hemophilia or
      spontaneous)
    Anti-factor V
    Anti-factor XIII (during INH therapy
      for tuberculosis)
Abnormal immunoglobulins in multiple
myeloma and related diseases
Anticoagulant drugs

The lupus anticoagulant is an antibody that recognizes certain phospholipids. This anticoagulant is sometimes seen in patients with lupus erythematosus, the prototypical autoimmune disease. It also appears from time to time in the elderly, and occasionally in pregnant women, in whom it can cause repeated spontaneous abortions. The lupus anticoagulant rarely causes clinical problems, and those it causes are related to thrombosis, not hemorrhage. Most often it is solely a laboratory disease, presenting as a prolonged PTT not corrected by normal plasma. An inhibitor found by accident in a patient with no clinical bleeding disorder is usually the lupus anticoagulant.

Other acquired anticoagulants are discussed in Chapters 15 and 16.

SUGGESTED READINGS

Antonarakis SE (1988) The molecular genetics of hemophilia A and B in man. Factor VIII and factor IX deficiency. Adv Hum Genet 17:27

Bauer KA, Rosenberg RD (1991) Role of antithrombin III as a regulator of in vivo coagulatioin. Semin Hematol 28:10

Bennett B (1977) Coagulation pathways: interrelationships and control mechanisms. Semin Hematol 14:301

Bick RL, Ucar K (1992) Hypercoagulability and thrombosis. Hematol Oncol Clin North Am 6:1421

Bloom AL (1980) The von Willebrand syndrome. Semin Hematol 17:215

Bloom AL (1981) Factor VIII inhibitors revisited. Br J Haematol 49:319

Boisclair MD, Ireland H, Lane DA (1990) Assessment of hypercoagulable states by measurement of activation fragments and peptides. Blood Rev 4:25

Clouse LH, Comp PC (1986) The regulation of hemostasis: the protein C system. N Engl J Med 314:1298

Cochrane CG, Griffin JH (1979) Molecular assembly in the control phase of the Hageman factor system. Am J Med 67:657

Cooper DN (1991) The molecular genetics of familial venous thrombosis. Blood Rev 5:55

Creagh MD, Greaves M (1991) Lupus anticoagulant. Blood Rev 5:162

Davie EW, Fujikawa K (1975) Basic mechanisms in blood coagulation. Annu Rev Biochem 44:799

Davie EW, Fujikawa K, Kisiel W (1991) The coagulation cascade: initiation, maintenance, and regulation. Biochemistry 30:10363

Esmon CT (1992) The protein C anticoagulant pathway. Arterioscler Thromb 12:135

Furie B, Furie BC (1992) Molecular and cellular biology of blood coagulation. N Engl J Med 326:800

Gralnick HR, Coller BS, Shulman NR et al (1977) Factor VIII. Ann Intern Med 86:598

Hoyer LW (1981) The factor VIII complex: Structure and function. Blood 58:1

Jackson CM, Nemerson Y (1980) Blood coagulation. Annu Rev Biochem 49:767

Jones P (1977) Developments and problems in the management of hemophilia. Semin Hematol 14:375

Kane WH, Davie EW (1988) Blood coagulation factors V and VIII: structural and functional similarities and their relationship to hemorrhagic and thrombotic disorders. Blood 71:539

Kaplan AP (1978) Initiation of the intrinsic coagulation and fibrinolytic pathways of man. Prog Hemost Thromb 4:127

Kaplan AP, Silverberg M (1987) The coagulation-kinin pathway of human plasma. Blood 70:1

Kasper CK (1981) Management of inhibitors of factor VIII. Prog Hematol 12:143

Kasper CK (1991) Complications of hemophilia A treatment: factor VIII inhibitors. Ann NY Acad Sci 614:97

Kasper CK, Mannucci PM, Bulyzhenkov V et al (1992) Hemophilia in the 1990s: principles of management and improved access to care. Semin Thromb Hemost 18:1

Lane DA (1981) Fibrinogen derivatives in plasma. Br J Haematol 47:329

Lusher JM, Warrier I (1992) Hemophilia A. Hematol Oncol Clin North Am 6:1021

Mammen EF (1992) Coagulation abnormalities in liver disease. Hematol Oncol Clin North Am 6:1247

Mann KG (1987) The assembly of blood clotting complexes on membranes. Trends Biochem Sci 12:229

Mann KG, Nesheim ME, Church WR et al (1990) Surface-dependent reactions of the vitamin K-dependent enzyme complexes. Blood 76:1

Markwardt F (1991) Past, present and future of hirudin. Haemostasis 21 (suppl. 1):11

Marlar RA, Neumann A (1990) Neonatal purpura fulminans due to homozygous protein C or protein S deficiencies. Semin Thromb Hemost 16:299

Moake JL (1990) Hypercoagulable states. Adv Intern Med 35:235

Mosesson MW (1992) The roles of fibrinogen and fibrin in hemostasis and thrombosis. Semin Hematol 29:177

Nemerson Y (1988) Tissue factor and hemostasis. Blood 71:1

Nemerson Y (1992) The tissue factor pathway of blood coagulation. Semin Hematol 29:170

Rapaport SI (1991) The extrinsic pathway inhibitor: a regulator of tissue factor-dependent blood coagulation. Thromb Haemost 66:6

Ratnoff OD, Jones PK (1978) The art of betting: which of a bleeder's female relatives is a carrier. Ann Intern Med 89:281

Ratnoff OD (1978) Antihemophiliac factor (factor VIII). Ann Intern Med 88:403

Rizza CR (1979) Congenital coagulation disorders. Clin Haematol 8, no. 1

Schick P, Stormorken H (1985) Platelets and megakaryocytes. Semin Hematol 22:123

Schick P, Stormorken H (1986) Platelets and megakaryocytes. Semin Hematol 23:1

Shearer MJ (1990) Vitamin K and vitamin K-dependent proteins. Br J Haematol 75:156

Stump DC, Taylor FB, Jr, Nesheim ME et al (1990) Pathologic fibrinolysis as a cause of clinical bleeding. Semin Thromb Hemost 16:260

Vassalli JD, Sappino AP, Belin D (1991) The plasminogen activator/plasmin system. J Clin Invest 88:1067

White GC, Shoemaker CB (1989) Factor VIII gene and hemophilia A. Blood 73:1

Wu KK (1992) Endothelial cells in hemostasis, thrombosis, and inflammation. Hosp Pract [Off] 27:145

14

Platelets

Platelets are small cell fragments that circulate in the bloodstream. They are produced by the disintegration of megakaryocytes, the large precursor cells found in the bone marrow. Platelets play an indispensable role in coagulation, plugging breaches in small blood vessels and helping initiate the processes of repair in injured tissues.

NORMAL PLATELETS

Platelet Structure

Platelets in the circulation are disc-shaped objects about one-fifth the diameter of a red cell (Fig. 14-1). Their shape is maintained by a ring of microtubules at the margin of the disc. Of special importance to their hemostatic function are the following structures:

THE PLASMA MEMBRANE

The plasma membrane contains a number of glycoproteins that function in the interactions of platelets with external surfaces, as well as receptors for exogenous activators (including thrombin) and for the von Willebrand factor. On stimulation of the platelet, receptors for fibrinogen and factors V and VIII appear in the membrane; a stimulated platelet moves in a cloud of clotting factors.

GRANULES

The platelet contains three types of granules: the α-granules, the δ- (dense) granules, and the lysosomes. Each granule consists of a packet of materials wrapped in a single layer of membrane. The contents differ by granule class. On activation of the platelet, the α- and δ-granules release their contents into the external environment. This degranulation event is of great importance for the control of bleeding by platelets.

THE CANALICULAR SYSTEM

A system of tubules extends inward from the outer surface of the platelet and ramifies through its cytoplasm. Granule contents are thought to be discharged into this canalicular system, from which they make their way into the external environment.

Platelet Production

Platelets are produced from distinctive cells called megakaryocytes (*mega-*, "large"; *karyo-*, "nucleus"). These very large cells have multiform nuclei easily seen in the marrow even under low power (Fig. 14-2). They arise from stem cells that commit themselves to the megakaryocyte line. These committed stem

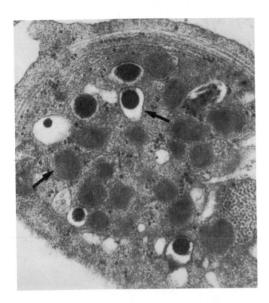

CONTENTS OF THE PLATELET GRANULES

Dense granules
 ADP
 Serotonin
 Calcium
α-Granules
 Clotting factors (fibrinogen and factor V)
 von Willebrand factor
 Thrombospondin
 Platelet factor 4
 β-Thromboglobulin
 Platelet-derived growth factor
Lysomes
 Hydrolytic enzymes active at low pH

Fig. 14-1. Platelet viewed through an electron microscope. A bullseye-like dense granule and a uniformly gray α-granule are indicated by the *arrows*. Small empty spaces representing sections through the canalicular tubules can be seen, and the marginal ring of microtubules is clearly apparent. (From White JG (1974) Electron microscopic studies of platelet secretion. Progr Hemost 2:49, with permission.)

cells grow into megakaryocytes by a unique process known as *endomitosis*. In this process, the DNA of the cell is repeatedly duplicated, but the nucleus does not divide. Instead, it grows bigger and more bizarre in shape, its

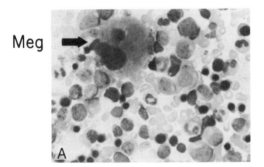

Meg

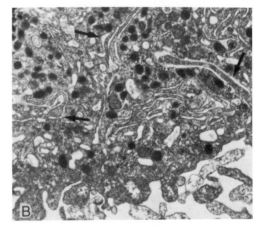

Fig. 14-2. Megakaryocytes. (**A**) Viewed under low power. (**B**) Electron micrograph, showing demarcation membranes (*arrows*) and granules. (**A:** From Lessin LF, Bessis M (1972) Morphology of the erythron. In Williams WJ et al (eds): Hematology. McGraw-Hill New York, with permission. **B:** From Zucker-Franklin D (1981) Megakaryocytes and platelets. In Zucker-Franklin D et al (eds): Atlas of Blood Cells: Function and Pathology. Edi. Ermes s.r.l., Milan, with permission.)

DNA content doubling with each cycle of DNA replication. At the same time, the cytoplasm grows, roughly doubling its mass each time the DNA is replicated. As the cell grows, it differentiates, acquiring the structures and functions of mature platelets—for example, the three classes of granules and the ability to secrete von Willebrand factor. The cell also acquires an intricate network of internal channels, the demarcation membranes, that divide it into platelet-size domains. Finally, after two to five cycles of DNA replication, the cell disintegrates: Its cytoplasm folds into pseudopods that work their way through the wall of a marrow sinusoid into the stream of flowing blood and then break apart along the demarcation membranes into individual platelets, while its huge shapeless nucleus remains behind to be destroyed by the mononuclear phagocytes. The production of platelets is summarized in Figure 14-3.

It takes roughly 5 days for a committed stem cell to give birth to a mass of new platelets. The new platelets then circulate for about 10 days before disappearing from the bloodstream. Aging as they circulate, the platelets shrink in size and steadily lose functional capacity, until they finally become senile and are swept from the blood. What finally happens to these outdated, expendable fragments is not known.

Platelet production is stimulated by three growth factors: granulocyte-macrophage colony-stimulating factor (GM-CSF), interleukin 3 (IL-3), and interleukin 6 (IL-6). It also appears to be under the influence of a hormone called *thrombopoietin*, about which almost nothing is known except that it can be detected in the blood of patients with thrombocytopenia. In response to these growth factors, and certainly others yet to be identified, the marrow can increase platelet production by as much as

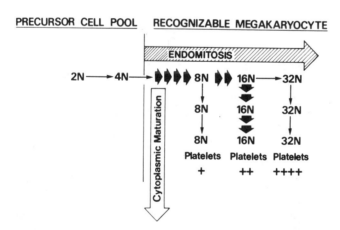

Fig. 14-3. How platelets are made. The megakaryocyte grows by endomitosis (DNA replication without nuclear division), doubling in size with each endomitotic cycle. After two to four cycles (ploidy 8N to 32N, where 2N is the amount of DNA in a normal diploid cell), the cell stops growing and begins to differentiate, acquiring platelet-specific granules and a network of demarcation membranes as it matures. Maturation reaches completion with the disintegration of the magakaryocyte, which breaks apart along the demarcation membrane network into thousands of platelets. (Based on the work of Odell TT, Anderson HR (1959) Production and life span of platelets. In Stohlman F (ed): The Kinetics of Cellular Proliferation. Grune & Stratton, Orlando, FL, and Odell TT, McDonald TP (1961) Life span of mouse blood platelets. Proc Soc Exp Biol Med 106:107. Modified from Hirsh J, Doery JCG (1972) Platelet function in health and disease. Prog Hematol 7:185 Wintrobe MM (1981) Platelets and megakaryocytes. In Clinical Hematology. 8th Ed. Lea & Febiger, Philadelphia, with permission.)

six- or sevenfold. Increased production results from increases in (1) the number of megakaryocytes in the marrow and (2) the number of platelets per megakaryocyte, as each cell doubles its size by an extra cycle of DNA replication before it breaks up.

Platelet Function

In the circulation, platelets normally travel separately, showing little tendency to interact with each other or with the endothelial cells that form the capillaries and line the walls of larger blood vessels. When blood vessels are damaged, however, the platelets adhere to the injured surfaces, where they are exposed to activating agents that appear at the site of injury. This contact with activating agents initiates an integrated series of events the final outcome of which is the formation of a hemostatic plug composed of thousands of platelets fused into a single mass.

ADHESION

Platelets do not stick to intact endothelium, but they bind very strongly to surfaces exposed when endothelium is damaged. Attachment takes place through several glycoprotein receptors on the platelet membrane (Table 14-1).

GP Ib/IX and von Willebrand Factor

GP Ib and GP IX are platelet membrane glycoproteins. When combined they form a receptor, GP Ib/IX, that binds to a protein known as von Willebrand factor. von Willebrand factor, which is secreted by megakaryocytes and endothelial cells, circulates as a series of immense multimers of regularly increasing

molecular weight, some as large as 15 to 20 million (Fig. 14-4). These very large multimers are deposited on surfaces that are exposed when endothelium is injured. From these surfaces the von Willebrand multimers reach into the flowing blood, seize resting platelets by their GP Ib/IX, and pull them out of the circulation and onto the damaged tissue (Fig. 14-5).

GP IIb/IIIa and von Willebrand Factor

GP IIb/IIIa is a surface receptor that appears when platelets are activated (see below). Its most important ligand is fibrinogen, but it also binds von Willebrand factor, helping platelets to stick to von Willebrand factor-coated surfaces.

Collagen Receptors

Collagen is exposed when the endothelium is disrupted. Platelets adhere to this collagen by means of their collagen receptors, GP IVa and GP Ia/IIa.

ACTIVATION OF THE PLATELET

The encounter of a platelet with an activating agent provokes major changes in the platelet's shape and properties (Fig. 14-6). A disc at rest, the stimulated platelet rapidly assumes the shape of a sphere. Its granules retreat to the center, and from its surface sprout

Table 14-1. Platelet Adhesion Proteins

Receptor	Ligand
GP Ib/IX	von Willebrand factor
GP IIb/IIIa	Fibrinogen
	von Willebrand factor
GP IVa	Collagen
GP Ia/IIa	Collagen

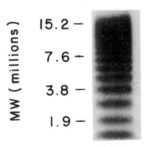

Fig. 14-4. Multimers of von Willebrand factor. (Modified from Ruggeri ZM et al (1982) Multimeric composition of factor VIII/von Willebrand factor following administration of DDAVP: implications for pathophysiology and therapy of von Willebrand's disease subtypes. Blood 59:1271, with permission.)

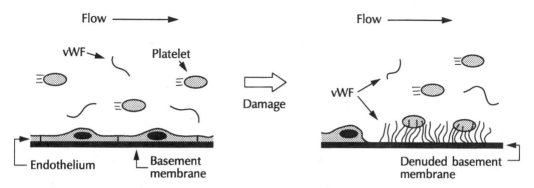

Fig. 14-5. Attachment of platelets to an injured surface by von Willebrand factor (vWF). The vWF molecule is only 250K in size, but it circulates in the form of huge linear polymers whose length may exceed the diameter of a platelet. These polymers are not taken up by circulating platelets, however, because the vWF receptors on the platelet membrane are in a resting state and can not bind vWF. When a blood vessel is damaged, circulating vWF polymers are deposited onto the newly exposed subendothelial surfaces to form a forest of flexible molecules that extend into the flowing stream of blood. At the same time, the vWF receptors on the platelet are activated as the platelets encounter thrombin, collagen, or other stimuli released at the site of injury. The stimulated platelets stick to the vWF-coated surface through interactions between the now activated vWF receptors and the vWF polymer forest.

a number of long hairlike projections known as *filipodia*. It then undergoes the *release reaction*, a complicated series of events during which (1) the α- and δ-granules discharge their contents to the outside; (2) an exceedingly potent lipid mediator is secreted; and (3) the ability of the platelet to promote the activation of the clotting cascade is greatly augmented.

During activation, platelets grow very sticky and begin to adhere to each other in a process known as *aggregation*. Simultaneously, the release reaction of the freshly activated platelets liberates substances that are able to activate other platelets. Like the first crop of activated platelets, these newly activated platelets become sticky, adhering to each other

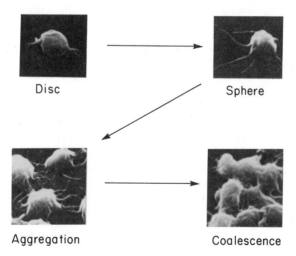

Fig. 14-6. Activation of platelet. (From Barnhart MI, Walsh RT, Robinson JA (1972) A three-dimensional view of platelet responses to chemical stimuli. Ann NY Acad Sci 201:360, with permission.)

as well as to the original platelet aggregate. The newly activated platelets also undergo the release reaction, activating still more platelets and recruiting them into the growing aggregate. It can be seen how this sequence of events will lead to the formation of a large platelet mass at a site of blood vessel injury. Eventually, this mass will grow large enough to plug the injured vessel, and bleeding will stop. (Obviously, this mechanism will only work for vessels below a certain size; there is no way that bleeding from a major vessel can be stopped by a platelet plug.) It appears that the platelet plug is responsible for initial hemostasis in minor injuries, the fibrin clot forming later to reinforce the hemostatic occlusion. During the course of a few hours, the platelets in this mass coalesce and lose their identity. The final plug is a homogeneous, featureless gel, nearly indistinguishable from the fibrin clot in which it will have become enmeshed.

The Release Reaction

In the release reaction, a stimulated platelet makes available various substances that affect clotting, inflammation, and repair at a site of injury (Table 14-2). The substances made available in the release reaction include the α- and δ-granule contents, the lipid mediator thromboxane A_2, and a procoagulant on the platelet surface that stimulates the formation of a fibrin clot.

Degranulation. The release of α- and δ-granule contents occurs within a few seconds after an encounter between platelets and an activating agent. A glance at Table 14-2 shows that the δ-granule contents discharged during the release reaction are low molecular weight substances, while the α-granule contents are proteins. Functions for several of these substances are recognized.

Of the substances released from the δ-granules, serotonin and adenosine diphosphate (ADP) are platelet-activating agents, representing two of the three endogenous activators liberated during the release reaction (the other is thromboxane A_2; see below). Serotonin may also work through its vasoconstrictive effect. Finally, δ-granule release supplies Ca^{2+}, which is required for the binding of fibrinogen to GP IIb/IIIa.

As for the α-granules, roles have been proposed for a number of the proteins liberated from these granules during the release reaction, as summarized in the box. Factor V promotes the formation of a fibrin clot at sites of platelet release. The α-granule fibrinogen, however, probably has little to do with fibrin clot formation, as it is released in such small quantities; this fibrinogen may have a role in platelet aggregation. The von Willebrand factor helps the platelets adhere to surfaces and to each other, and thrombospondin promotes platelet aggregation by binding simultaneously to fibrinogen and the platelet surface. Platelet factor 4 neutralizes the anticoagulant heparin in vitro and possibly exerts a similar effect in vivo, perhaps countering antithrombin (AT) III activation by endothelial proteoglycans (Ch. 13). Platelet-derived growth factor stimulates the growth of fibroblasts and smooth muscle cells

Table 14-2. Functions of the α-Granule Contents

Component	Function
Factor V	Promotes formation of fibrin clot
Fibrinogen	Required for platelet aggregation
von Willebrand factor	Required for platelet adherence
Thrombospondin	Enhances platelet aggregation
Platelet factor 4	Neutralizes heparin: ?acts against a heparinlike molecule in blood vessels or tissues
β-Thromboglobulin	?
Platelet-derived growth factor	Stimulates growth of fibroblasts and smooth muscle cells; probably promotes tissue repair; may promote atherosclerosis

in culture; it has been postulated to function in the repair of damaged tissue (as well as in the formation of the atherosclerotic plaque, perhaps an example of overrepair).

Lipid Mediators. Lipid mediators are low molecular weight lipid-soluble compounds that exert potent biological effects on a wide variety of cell types at very low concentrations. These mediators can be classified according to their structures into several groups. Among these groups are the phospholipid mediators, which are closely related to phosphatidylcholine; the leukotrienes, which are straight-chain compounds derived from arachidonic acid; and the prostaglandin/thromboxane group, also derived from arachidonic acid, but containing a ring.

Of these, the group most directly involved with platelets is the prostaglandin/thromboxane group. The members of this group can be divided into two categories: stable (prostaglandins of the E and F classes), and unstable (thromboxane A$_2$ and prostacyclin). The unstable members play the major role in platelet function.

The first of these, thromboxane A$_2$, is an exceedingly potent platelet activator that is produced by the platelets themselves during the release reaction. Its route of metabolism is shown in Figure 14-7. This can be divided into three steps:

1. *Production of arachidonic acid.* Arachidonic acid is produced in platelets by the hydrolysis of membrane phospholipids. Phosphatidylinositol in particular is a major source. This phospholipid contains almost

100 percent arachidonic acid at its 2- (i.e., middle) position. When platelets are stimulated, a phospholipase is activated that is highly specific for this phosphatidylinositol, splitting it into inositol phosphate and diglyceride. Arachidonic acid is then released from this diglyceride by the action of another enzyme, diglyceride lipase. Arachidonic acid can also be released in a one-step reaction. Release by this direct route results from the activation of a second phospholipase, one that splits the fatty acid from the 2-position of several classes of phospholipids. The products of this reaction are arachidonic acid and a lysophospholipid (Fig. 14-7).

2. *Production of thromboxane A2.* Arachidonic acid is converted to thromboxane A$_2$ by an oxidation reaction followed by rearrangement. The oxidation is catalyzed by cyclo-oxygenase and takes arachidonic acid to an intermediate product known as prostaglandin H$_2$. This is converted by thromboxane A$_2$ through a rearrangement of the ring, which is catalyzed by thromboxane synthetase.

3. *Destruction of thromboxane A2.* The duration of action of thromboxane A$_2$ is very brief because it is extremely unstable, hydrolyzing in seconds to the stable but biologically inert thromboxane B$_2$. Because of its stability, thromboxane B$_2$ is a useful footprint of its precursor, its presence indicating that thromboxane A$_2$ was produced at some earlier time.

Prostacyclin, the other unstable member of the prostaglandin/thromboxane group, is a powerful antagonist of platelet activation. It is produced by the vascular endothelium and is thought to aid in preventing activation of platelets in the bloodstream. Like thromboxane A$_2$, it is made from arachidonic acid via the cyclo-oxygenase product, prostaglandin H$_2$. In the endothelial cell, however, the rearrangement of prostaglandin H$_2$ is catalyzed by prostacyclin synthetase, not thromboxane syn-

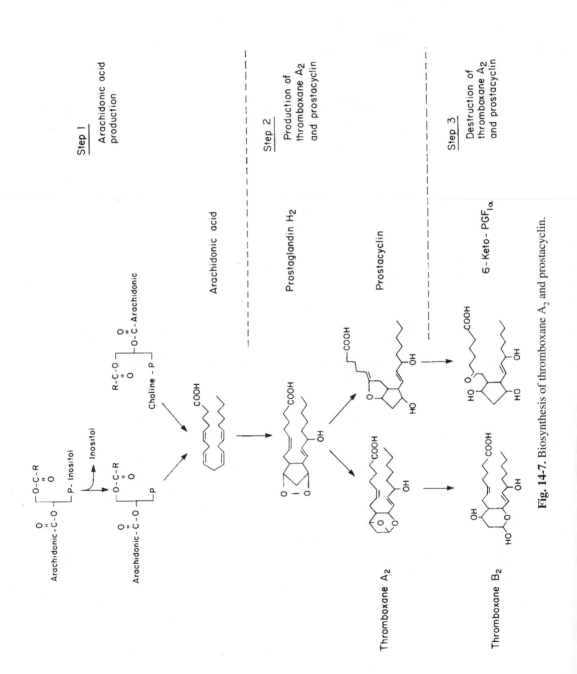

Fig. 14-7. Biosynthesis of thromboxane A₂ and prostacyclin.

thetase, and the product is prostacyclin (Fig. 14-7). The lifespan of prostacyclin is as short as that of thromboxane A_2; it is hydrolyzed in seconds to 6-keto $PGF_{1\alpha}$, a stable, inert compound whose presence signifies the prior release of prostacyclin.

Procoagulant. Activated platelets participate directly in the clotting cascade by serving as constituents of tenase and prothrombinase (Ch. 13). Their ability to participate in this way results from a large increase in the concentration of clotting factor receptors that takes place during the release reaction. These clotting factor receptors appear first on the surface of the platelet itself, but then are locally disseminated in the form of receptor-rich microvesicles of high procoagulant power that are shed from the platelet surface.

Three receptors are known to appear during release: the fibrinogen receptor and receptors for factors V and VIII. The fibrinogen receptor probably participates in platelet aggregation, rather than the clotting cascade. The factors V and VIII receptors, however, could well be involved in the clotting cascade. In particular, it is not unreasonable to imagine that prothrombinase is put together by the Ca^{2+}-dependent binding of a factor Xa molecule to a factor Va molecule sitting in its receptor on the surface of an activated platelet, and that tenase is similarly created on the platelet surface from factors VIIIa and IXa and Ca^{2+}. Such events would explain the increased effectiveness of activated platelets as promoters of fibrin clot formation.

Aggregation

Platelet aggregation is easily seen when an activating agent is added to a well-stirred suspension of resting platelets (Fig. 14-8). It begins about 30 seconds after the stimulus is added and normally reaches completion in 5 to 10 minutes. Fibrinogen must be present in the medium or the platelets will not aggregate; this has clinical ramifications, notably in Glanzmann's thrombasthenia.

From the way they elicit aggregation, platelet-activating agents can be divided into two categories: (1) *direct activators*, which cause platelets to aggregate as a primary effect of the platelet-activator interaction; and (2) *indirect activators*, which work entirely through platelet release, the platelets aggregating solely because of the endogenous aggregating agents (ADP, serotonin, thromboxane A_2) liberated during the release reaction. Almost all platelet-activating agents are direct activators; collagen, however, is an indirect activator.

With direct activators, platelets typically aggregate in two successive waves, known as the *primary* and *secondary* waves of aggregation. The primary wave is caused directly by the interaction of the activator with the platelets. The secondary wave results from further stimulation of the platelets by endogenous aggregating agents (ADP and thromboxane A_2) liberated in the associated release reaction. In such a dual-wave event, platelet aggregation during the primary wave is imperfect; complete aggregation is achieved only during the secondary wave. In certain platelet disorders, or with very low concentrations of an activator that ordinarily causes dual-wave aggregation (for example, ADP; see Fig. 14-8A), platelets will fail to undergo a secondary wave because the release reaction is inadequate. Under these circumstances, the weak aggregates formed during the primary wave will disperse. Conversely, platelets aggregating in response to very high concentrations of such an activator will show only a primary wave. Why a secondary wave is not seen under these conditions is not known; perhaps the number of platelets remaining dispersed after the primary response is complete is too small to produce a secondary wave.

With collagen, an indirect activator, only a secondary wave of aggregation is seen (Fig. 14-8B). This wave of aggregation is provoked by the activators released from the platelets when they interact with collagen. Platelets with a defective release reaction cannot be aggregated by collagen.

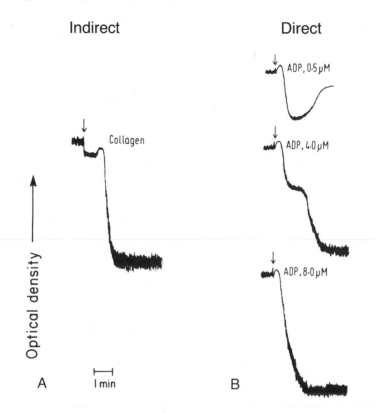

Fig. 14-8. Platelet aggregation. Platelet aggregation is measured by following the change in light transmission after adding an aggregating agent to a stirred sample of platelet-rich plasma, prepared by centrifuging heparinized blood at low speed to remove red cells and white cells. Before aggregation, the platelets form turbid suspension through which light passes with difficulty. The suspension clears up as platelets cluster into aggregates, increasing light transmission. The magnitude of change in light transmission gives a rough indication of the degree to which platelets have aggregated in response to the stimulus. (**A**) One-phase aggregation: response to indirect aggregating agent. (**B**) Two-phase aggregation: response to direct aggregating agent. (Modified from Holmsen H, Salganicoff L, Fukami MH (1977) Platelet behavior in biochemistry. In Ogston D, Bennett JS (eds): Hemostasis: Biochemistry, Physiology, Pathology. John Wiley & Sons, Chichester, England, with permission.)

Platelet Activators

At sites of tissue injury, the principal platelet activators are thrombin and collagen. Activation of the clotting cascade steeps the platelets in thrombin, whereas damage to blood vessels and underlying tissues brings the platelets into contact with collagen, a ubiquitous tissue component from which they are ordinarily separated by the thin vascular endothelium. Thrombin is an aggregating agent, causing platelets in the circulation to aggregate and release, while collagen brings

the platelets to the injured surface. Stimulated by the collagen, the attached platelets undergo the release reaction, attracting additional platelets to form an aggregate in response to released ADP and thromboxane A_2.

Other platelet activators include epinephrine, serotonin, ADP, and thromboxane A_2. As discussed above, the last three are platelet constituents that are secreted during the release reaction. Epinephrine and (at low concentrations) ADP cause platelets to aggregate in a classical dual-wave manner. The list on page

Table 14-3. Platelet Function Tests

Test	Function Tested
Bleeding time	General
Aggregation	
Indirect stimuli	Aggregation
Direct stimuli	Aggregation; release of ADP and thromboxane
Ristocetin	Adhesion
Granule content release	
Serotinin or ATP	Discharge of dense granules
Platelet factor 4 and β-thromboglobulin	Discharge of α-granules
Thromboxane B$_2$	Thromboxane secretion

223 classifies platelet-activating agents into those typically provoking single-wave and dual-wave aggregation.

Platelets are also agglutinated by the antibiotic ristocetin in a process that depends on the von Willebrand factor. Unlike the agents discussed above, ristocetin acts on dead (formalin-fixed) as well as live platelets. It is therefore clear that the response of platelets to ristocetin can have little physiological significance. Nevertheless, ristocetin-mediated platelet agglutination has proved extremely useful in diagnosing platelet function disorders.

Testing Platelet Function
(Table 14-3)

BLEEDING TIME

The bleeding time is the most general test of platelet function. It is usually performed by making a 1 cm x 1 mm incision in the skin of the inner forearm, and then blotting every 30 seconds until the bleeding stops. The time required for the bleeding to stop is the bleeding time.

Any disorder affecting the platelets will prolong the bleeding time, if sufficiently severe. In milder forms of such disorders the bleeding time is often normal, but may be brought into the abnormal range by an aspirin taken a few hours before the test. This is true for both quantitative and qualitative disorders. In conditions associated with reduced numbers of platelets (e.g., thrombocytopenia), there is a nice correlation between platelet count and bleeding time (Fig. 14-9). In conditions associated with defective platelet function, the bleeding time will be prolonged regardless of the platelet count. Because it is so general a test, the bleeding time is exceedingly useful as a screen for platelet function disorders. By the same token, however, it provides little information beyond the fact that a platelet function disorder exists.

PLATELET ADHESION

Experience has unexpectedly shown that ristocetin agglutination can be used to diagnose disorders of platelet adhesion. Ristocetin agglutination is defective in von Willebrand's disease and Bernard-Soulier disease, two inher-

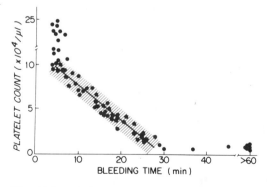

Fig. 14-9. Relationship between platelet count and bleeding time. (From Malpass TW, Harker LA (1980) Acquired disorders of platelet function. Semin Hematol 17:243, with permission.)

ited conditions in which platelet adhesion is impaired. It is generally normal in other platelet disorders.

AGGREGATION AND THE RELEASE REACTION

Platelet aggregation is measured by an optical method using platelet-rich plasma. The technique is described in Figure 14-8, which presents examples of typical single-wave and dual-wave aggregation patterns.

Defects in platelet aggregation fall into two classes: those in which the entire aggregation response is affected, and those in which only the secondary wave is missing. The latter always result from an impairment in the release reaction; endogenous aggregation agents fail to be secreted from the platelets, and the secondary wave does not occur.

The release reaction can be evaluated more completely by directly measuring degranulation and thromboxane production. These can be determined by assaying the quantities of granule components and thromboxane secreted into the medium by stimulated platelets. For this purpose, serotonin is generally used as the δ-granule marker, platelet factor 4 and β-thromboglobin as the α-granule markers, and thromboxane B_2 as the index of thromboxane production. These measurements are seldom needed in the workup of a platelet function disorder, because release can be assessed well enough for most purposes just by examining the secondary wave of aggregation. Their principal use is for research.

By far the most common cause of a defective release reaction is aspirin ingestion. Other nonsteroidal anti-inflammatory agents cause a defect in platelet release as well. Inherited disorders of platelet function are less frequent causes of defective release.

PLATELET FUNCTION DISORDERS

Platelet function is disturbed in a number of conditions, both inherited and acquired. Most of these conditions show a bleeding tendency, but this tendency is surprisingly mild except in a few rare platelet diseases (notably Bernard-Soulier disease and some cases of von Willebrand's disease). The absence of bleeding problems in patients with platelet function defects should be contrasted with their frequency and gravity in patients with severe thrombocytopenia, in whom death from exsanguination or intracranial hemorrhage is a real hazard.

As a rule, bleeding patterns in platelet disorders are distinctly different from bleeding patterns in disorders involving soluble clotting factors (Table 14-4). Patients with clotting factor disorders tend to bleed into joints and soft tissues, sites that are seldom involved in thrombocytopenia or qualitative platelet function defects. The most frequent site of bleeding in platelet disorders is the skin. Patients with severe platelet function disorders or thrombocytopenia will often develop multiple tiny hemorrhagic spots known as petechiae; these are not seen in clotting factor disorders. Larger confluent hemorrhagic areas (purpura) also appear in the skin in platelet function disorders, but these are seen in clotting factor disorders as well. Other sites of bleeding common to both clotting factor and platelet disorders include the orifices (nasal, upper and lower GI, urinary, and vaginal) and the brain.

Inherited Defects of Platelet Adhesion

There are two inherited disorders of platelet adhesion: von Willebrand's disease and Bernard-Soulier disease (Table 14-5). Both are characterized by a defect in the attachment of platelets to collagen. Excessive bleeding occurs because the platelets are unable to adhere normally to the collagen to which they

Table 14-4. Bleeding Sites: Platelet Disorders versus Clotting Factor Disorders

Platelets	Clotting Factors	Both
Petechiae	Joints	Purpura
	Soft tissues	Orifices
		Brain

are exposed when blood vessels are torn at sites of injury.

von WILLEBRAND'S DISEASE

von Willebrand's disease is by far the most common inherited abnormality of platelet function. It is transmitted as an autosomal dominant trait. The bleeding disorder tends to be mild in the heterozygote but is exceedingly severe in the rare homozygote.

von Willebrand Factor

The hallmark of von Willebrand's disease is defective platelet function. The platelets themselves are perfectly normal, however. The actual cause of the platelet function defect is a deficiency of the von Willebrand factor.

As mentioned above, the von Willebrand factor normally circulates in the form of huge multimers. These very large multimers must be present for platelets to (1) adhere to surfaces (e.g., collagen or glass) and (2) aggregate in response to ristocetin. Promotion of adherence is probably the major in vivo function of the von Willebrand factor.

A second function of the von Willebrand factor has to do with its long-recognized relationship to factor VIII, the clotting factor of hemophilia.[*] This relationship is clearly evident in von Willebrand's disease. In most patients with this condition, levels of both factor VIII and von Willebrand factor are reduced to a similar extent (when expressed as percent of normal). By contrast, patients with hemophilia have normal levels of von Willebrand factor, even though their factor VIII levels may be close to zero.

The reason for this relationship between factor VIII and von Willebrand factor is that the von Willebrand factor acts to stabilize factor VIII by forming a complex with it in the circulation (Fig. 14-10). In von Willebrand's disease, the factor VIII level is low because of a deficiency in von Willebrand factor, the factor VIII-stabilizing protein. In hemophilia, though, the factor VIII level is low because factor VIII itself is defective, while the von Willebrand factor is completely normal.

Diagnosis

All patients with inherited platelet disorders have the same clinical picture: a family history of bleeding of a greater or lesser degree of severity. Laboratory investigations are required to make the diagnosis.

Classical von Willebrand's disease is caused by a deficiency of von Willebrand factor. This deficiency can be demonstrated directly in the laboratory by an assay that uses an antibody against the von Willebrand factor. There is in addition a characteristic combination of other laboratory abnormalities: (1) the bleeding time is prolonged as expected in any platelet disor-

Table 14-5. Distinguishing among von Willebrand's Disease, Bernard-Soulier Disease, and Glanzmann's Thrombasthenia

	von Willebrand's Disease	Bernard-Soulier Disease	Glanzmann's Thrombasthenia
Defect	Adhesion	Adhesion	Primary aggregation
Cause	Low plasma vWF	Absent vWF receptors	Absent fibrinogen receptors
Poor aggregation in response to	Ristocetin	Ristocetin, thrombin	Everything except ristocetin (ristocetin aggregation is normal)
Other	Low plasma vWF	Huge platelets	No clot retraction
	Low plasma factor VIII	Absence of GP Ib	Absence of GP IIb and GP IIIa

Abbreviations: GP, glycoprotein; vWF, von Willebrand factor.

[*]A set of three symbols derived from the factor VIII–von Willebrand factor relationship is sometimes used in discussions of von Willebrand's disease. These symbols contain the numeral VIII (for factor VIII) followed by a letter that specifies one or another of the associated activities. The symbols are VIII:C, for factor VIII coagulant activity (that which is missing in hemophilia); VIII:R, for ristocetin cofactor activity (that which promotes platelet aggregation by ristocetin); and VIII:A, for the von Willebrand antigen (that which is detected by an antibody against the von Willebrand factor). In this chapter, von Willebrand factor is named in full, and the term factor VIII always refers to the clotting factor that is missing in hemophilia.

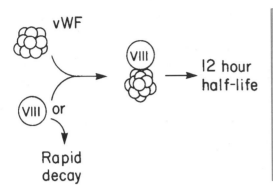

Fig. 14-10. Relationship between factor VIII and von Willebrand factor.

MAKING THE DIAGNOSIS OF
VON WILLEBRAND'S DISEASE

Bleeding time prolonged
Ristocetin aggregation decreased or absent
Factor VIII decreased
von Willebrand antigen decreased

der; (2) the function of platelets (either normal or patient) suspended in von Willebrand factor-deficient plasma is disturbed in a particular way: adhesion is impaired, and the platelets fail to agglutinate with ristocetin, although they aggregate and release in a completely normal fashion with any other aggregating agent; and (3) factor VIII activity is reduced, a consequence of the relationship between this clotting factor and the von Willebrand factor.

Variant forms of von Willebrand's disease also occur (Table 14-6). In some variants, levels of factor VIII and von Willebrand antigen are normal. Two of the variant forms are caused by a functionally defective von Willebrand factor that is unable to form large polymers, while another is due to an intrinsic platelet defect. They are uncommon, but are important to recognize because they are managed somewhat differently than classical von Willebrand's disease.

Management

Like other plasma clotting factor deficiencies, von Willebrand's disease is managed by replacement therapy. The best treatment is with a purified factor VIII preparation that is *rich in von Willebrand factor*. (Some factor VIII preparations can't be used for this purpose, because they contain very little von Willebrand factor.) Cryoprecipitate is an acceptable alternative, if it is obtained from a single donor to minimize the risk of transmitting viral infections such as hepatitis or AIDS. Fresh frozen plasma can also be used, as an inferior third choice. Desmopressin (DDAVP) is useful in mild type I and type IIA von Willebrand's disease, but should not be given in type IIb or pseudo-von Willebrand's disease, because it worsens the thrombocytopenia (see Table 14-6). The effect of treatment should be evaluated by the clinical response and the bleeding time. Other tests are not helpful in managing von Willebrand's disease, because they can show

Table 14-6. Classification of von Willebrand's Disease

Type	Defect	Platelet Count	Ristocetin Aggregation	Response to DDAVP
I	All vWF multimers decreased	Normal	Absent	+
IIa	Large vWF multimers decreased	Normal	Absent	+
IIb	Large vWF multimers decreased, intermediate multimers increased	Low	Increased	Contraindicated
Pseudo-	Like type IIb; platelets show abnormally high affinity for largest vWF multimers	Low	Increased	Contraindicated
III	vWF multimers absent	Normal	Absent	No effect

Abbreviations: DDAVP, desmopressin; vWF, von Willebrand factor.

improvement after replacement therapy without any improvement in the patient's bleeding tendency.

Levels of factor VIII behave in a curious way after a patient with von Willebrand's disease is given a dose of cryoprecipitate or plasma. Factor VIII rises quickly to greater than normal levels, and then stays high for 2 to 3 days before dropping off again. This reaction contrasts with that found in hemophiliacs, whose factor VIII levels begin to fall rapidly immediately after therapy. This behavior is undoubtedly another consequence of the relationship between factor VIII and the von Willebrand factor.

BERNARD-SOULIER DISEASE

Bernard-Soulier disease can be looked at as the platelet counterpart of von Willebrand's disease. In von Willebrand's disease, the problem is with the plasma, which lacks the von Willebrand factor. In Bernard-Soulier disease, the problem is with the platelets, which lack the ability to interact with the von Willebrand factor.

The bleeding problem in Bernard-Soulier disease is extremely severe, although it tends to improve with age. Diagnosis depends on the laboratory results. The platelet count is low, but the individual platelets are huge—the size of the red cells (Fig. 14-11). Platelet function studies are by and large the same as von Willebrand's disease, showing faulty adhesion

and ristocetin agglutination, but a normal response to other aggregating agents (except thrombin; see Table 14-5). The critical defect in Bernard-Soulier disease is the absence of GP Ib/IX, the von Willebrand receptor, from the membrane of the platelet (Fig. 14-12). It is the lack of this receptor that accounts for the abnormalities in hemostasis and platelet function in Bernard-Soulier disease.

Inherited Defect of Platelet Aggregation

GLANZMANN'S THROMBASTHENIA

Glanzmann's thrombasthenia (Table 14-5) appears to result from a defect in the interaction between platelets and fibrinogen. When normal platelets are activated, fibrinogen binding sites appear on their surface. Thrombasthenic platelets lack these fibrinogen

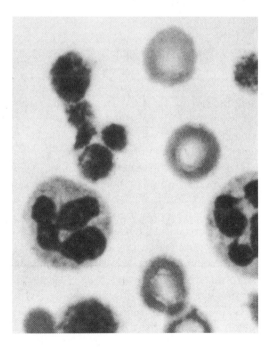

Fig. 14-11. Platelets in Bernard-Soulier disease. (Modified from Bithell TC, Parekh SS, Strong RR (1972) Platelet function in the Bernard-Soulier syndrome. Ann NY Acad Sci 201:145, with permission).

binding sites and show a general defect in aggregation.

Thrombasthenics have a moderately severe bleeding disorder. Unlike Bernard-Soulier disease, platelets are normal in number and size, and adhesion is intact in Glanzmann's thrombasthenia. The aggregation defect is precisely complementary to the von Willebrand defect: These platelets aggregate only in response to ristocetin, and to nothing else. A characteristic feature, somehow related to the platelet defect, is the failure of the thrombasthenic clot to retract (i.e., to shrink and squeeze out serum over the course of a few hours) the way normal clots do.

Like Bernard-Soulier disease, Glanzmann's thrombasthenia is caused by a membrane glycoprotein deficiency. Two glycoproteins are missing in thrombasthenia: GP IIb and GP IIIa (Fig. 14-12). Together, these two glycoproteins form the fibrinogen receptor. Their absence explains the fibrinogen binding defect and other abnormalities in Glanzmann's thrombasthenia.

Disorders of Release

In release disorders, platelets fail to complete the release reaction. In some instances, this is because of a defect in thromboxane production. In other cases, a deficiency of δ-granule ADP is at fault.

Defective thromboxane production almost always results from the administration of anti-inflammatory drugs. Many of these drugs work by blocking the production of prostaglandins and thromboxanes. Such drugs will interfere with the release reaction by preventing the formation of thromboxane A_2. The best example is aspirin, which inactivates cyclo-oxygenase, the first enzyme of the thromboxane A_2 synthetic pathway. One aspirin tablet will completely destroy all the cyclo-oxygenase in whatever megakaryocytes and platelets are present at the time of ingestion. This leads to a defect in platelet release that is corrected only when fresh platelets made from newly differentiated megakaryocytes appear in the blood-

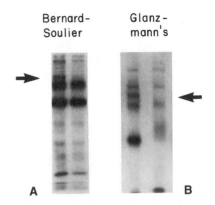

Fig. 14-12. Platelet glycoproteins. (**A**) Bernard-Soulier disease. (Modified from Nurden AT et al (1981) Analysis of the glycoprotein and protein composition of Bernard-Soulier platelets by single- and two-dimensional sodium dodecyl sulfate-polyacrylamide gel electrophoresis. J Clin Invest 67:1431, with permission.) (**B**) Glanzmann's thrombasthenia. (Modified from Phillips DR, Agin PP (1977) Platelet membrane defects in Glanzmann's thrombasthenia. J Clin Invest. 60:535, with permission.)

stream. Other drugs that interfere with thromboxane formation are listed in the box on page 229; unlike aspirin, these agents inhibit thromboxane production reversibly, so their effects last only as long as they are present in the body. In addition to drugs, some inherited abnormalities in thromboxane production cause defective platelet release. Such conditions are very rare.

Steroids, the most potent of the anti-inflammatory drugs, have little effect on normal platelets.

A few patients are found whose platelets contain abnormal δ-granules, or lack these

DISORDERS OF RELEASE

Defective thromboxane production
  Inherited
    Acquired (anti-inflammatory drugs)

Storage pool deficiency

granules altogether. Such patients are said to have *storage pool deficiency.* In their platelets, δ-granule ADP, referred to as "storage pool" ADP to distinguish it from the ADP in the platelet cytoplasm, is greatly decreased. These platelets cannot discharge ADP during the release reaction because they have no storage pool ADP to discharge; release is therefore incomplete.

All release defects produce the same clinical picture. There is usually little in the way of abnormal bleeding unless the defect is superimposed on some other clotting disorder (e.g., thrombocytopenia or hemophilia). The bleeding time may be normal or prolonged. Platelet function studies show an absence of the secondary wave of aggregation (Fig. 14-13); this is the most characteristic finding in platelet release defects and occurs because the abnormal platelets are unable to release their own aggregating agents when exposed to platelet activators. The diagnosis of a release defect can be confirmed by measuring the levels of released products (e.g., thromboxane or ADP), but such studies are ordinarily done only for research purposes.

Acquired Platelet Function Disorders

A number of diseases show disturbances of platelet function. These disturbances may be caused by the disease itself, or they may result from drugs or procedures used in therapy.

DRUGS THAT INTERFERE WITH THROMBOXANE FORMATION

Aspirin

Indomethacin

Phenylbutazone

Ibuprofen and related drugs

Sulfinpyrazone

Clinical bleeding is fairly common in acquired platelet function disorders and occasionally can be quite severe. The diagnosis is suspected in any patient who (1) has one of the associated diseases, or (2) has received a form of treatment known to interfere with platelet function. The laboratory results usually include a long bleeding time and a variety of abnormalities in platelet aggregation.

UREMIA

An acquired platelet function defect is the rule in uremia. The defect is caused by the accumulation in uremic plasma of waste products of unknown identity that interfere with platelet function.

The platelet function defect can be severe, with a very long bleeding time and grossly abnormal platelet function studies. The defect is thought to have a major role in the bleeding associated with uremia: cutaneous, gastrointestinal, and pericardial. It responds to dialysis or kidney transplantation. It has also rather surprisingly been reported to respond to cryopre-

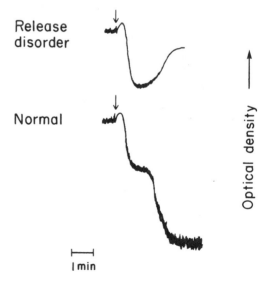

Fig. 14-13. Aggregation defect in release disorders. (From Holmsen H, Salganicoff L, Fukami MH (1977) Platelet behavior in biochemistry. In Ogston D, Bennett JS (eds): Hemostasis: Biochemistry, Physiology, Pathology. John Wiley & Sons, Chichester, England, with permission.)

ACQUIRED PLATELET FUNCTION DISORDERS

Uremia

Drugs
- Anti-inflammatory
- β-Lactam antibiotics (penicillin and cephalothin)
- Alcohol

Postcardiopulmonary bypass

Stem cell disorders
- Polycythemia vera/myelofibrosis
- Myelodysplasia
- Leukemia

Abnormal circulating proteins
- Immunoglobulins in multiple myeloma
- Fibrin-split products
- Antiplatelet antibodies

cipitate, the same material used to treat hemophilia and von Willebrand's disease, as well as to DDAVP. Platelet transfusions are useless, however, because the underlying problem has to do with the plasma, not the platelets.

DRUGS

Several classes of drugs cause platelet function defects. Those of clinical importance are certain anti-inflammatory drugs, the β-lactam antibiotics (e.g., penicillins and cephalothins), and alcohol. The anti-inflammatory drugs have been discussed above. The β-lactum antibiotics cause platelet function disorders when given in high doses; they act by interfering with the binding of stimuli to platelet receptors. The way in which alcohol impairs platelet function is not known.

Drug-induced platelet dysfunction usually requires no treatment. When treatment is necessary, it is generally best to withdraw the drug causing the problem or to cut its dose. Platelet transfusions can be helpful in an emergency.

POSTCARDIOPULMONARY BYPASS

Patients undergoing cardiopulmonary bypass surgery may bleed postoperatively because of an acquired platelet function defect. The platelets acquire the defect as they pass through the pump. The defect is characterized by the discharge of the α-granules and the development of an exceedingly long bleeding time. The long bleeding time does not seem to be related to the loss of α-granules, however, because it returns to normal within a few hours, even though the α-granules are lost permanently. If bleeding occurs as a result of this defect, it may be treated with platelet transfusions.

The second important cause of post-pump bleeding is inadequate ligation of bleeding vessels at the operative site. Other problems include a low platelet count resulting from dilution by transfusions, activation of the clotting cascade within the blood vessels because of disseminated intravascular coagulation (Ch. 15), and under- or overneutralization of the heparin used during surgery to prevent clotting in the pump.

Other Disorders

Other causes of acquired platelet dysfunction include stem cell disorders and the presence of abnormal circulating proteins (see box above).

SUGGESTED READINGS

Ashby B, Daniel JL, Smith JB (1990) Mechanisms of platelet activation and inhibition. Hematol Oncol Clin North Am 4:1

Bellucci S, Caen JP (1988) Congenital platelet disorders. Blood Rev 2:16

Bennett JS (1990) The molecular biology of platelet membrane proteins. Semin Hematol 27:186

Bennett JS, Kolodziej MA (1992) Disorders of platelet function. Dis Mon 38:577

Bevers EM, Comfurius P, Zwaal RF (1991) Platelet procoagulant activity: physiological significance and mechanisms of exposure. Blood Rev 5:146

Bick RL (1992) Acquired platelet function defects. Hematol Oncol Clin North Am 6:1203

Bloom AL (1980) The von Willebrand syndrome. Semin Hematol 17:215

Colman RW (1990) Platelet receptors. Hematol Oncol Clin North Am 4:27

de Groot PG, Sixma JJ (1990) Platelet adhesion. Br J Haematol 75:308

Deranleau DA (1987) Blood platelet shape change ABCs. Trends Biochem Sci 12:439

George JN, Shattil SJ (1991) The clinical importance of acquired abnormalities of platelet function. N Engl J Med 324:27

Gewirtz AM, Hoffman R (1990) Human megakaryocyte production: cell biology and clinical considerations. Hematol Oncol Clin North Am 4:43

Ginsburg D, Bowie EJ (1992) Molecular genetics of von Willebrand disease. Blood 79:2507

Lind SE (1991) The bleeding time does not predict surgical bleeding. Blood 77:2547

Malmsten C (1979) Prostaglandins, thromboxanes and platelets. Br J Haematol 41:453

Malpass TW, Harker LA (1980) Acquired disorders of platelet function. Semin Hematol 17:242

Marcus AJ (1979) The role of prostaglandins in platelet function. Progr Hematol 11:147

McEver RP (1990) The clinical significance of platelet membrane glycoproteins. Hematol Oncol Clin North Am 4:87

Miller JL (1990) von Willebrand disease. Hematol Oncol Clin North Am 4:107

Nurden AT, Caen JP (1978) Membrane glycoproteins and human platelet function. Br J Haematol 38:155

Oates JA, Fitzgerald GA, Branch RA et al (1988) Clinical implications of prostaglandin and thromboxane A_2 formation (first of two parts). N Engl J Med 319:689

Quesenberry P, Levitt L (1979) Hematopoietic stem cells. N Engl J Med 301:755

Remuzzi G (1988) Bleeding in renal failure. Lancet 1:1205

Rodeghiero F, Castaman G, Mannucci PM (1991) Clinical indications for desmopressin (DDAVP) in congenital and acquired von Willebrand disease. Blood Rev 5:155

Ruggeri ZM, Zimmerman TS (1987) von Willebrand factor and von Willebrand disease. Blood 70:895

Tavassoli M (1980) Megakaryocyte-platelet axis and the process of platelet formation and release. Blood 55:537

Vainchenker W, Kieffer N (1988) Human megakaryocytopoiesis: in vitro regulation and characterization of megakaryocytic precursor cells by differentiation markers. Blood Rev 2:102

Weiss HJ (1975) Platelet physiology and abnormalities of platelet function. N Engl J Med 293:531, 580

Weiss HJ (1980) Congenital disorders of platelet function. Semin Hematol 17:228

Weksler BB, Nachman RL (1981) Platelets and atherosclerosis. Am J Med 71:331

Woodman RC, Harker LA (1990) Bleeding complications associated with cardiopulmonary bypass. Blood 76:1680

15

Disseminated Intravascular Coagulation and Thrombotic Thrombocytopenic Purpura

Disseminated intravascular coagulation (DIC) and thrombotic thrombocytopenic purpura (TTP) are highly complex clotting disorders that occur in a setting of serious illness. These disorders are discussed together for convenience because they have certain clinical features in common: complexity, abrupt onset, and a rapid fall in the platelet count. It will be seen, however, that these are two totally different diseases having two entirely different mechanisms.

DISSEMINATED INTRAVASCULAR COAGULATION

DIC is the condition that results when the clotting system is activated in all or a substantial part of the vascular tree. Despite widespread fibrin production, the major problem is usually bleeding, not thrombosis.

Pathogenesis

DIC is caused by the exposure of circulating blood to thromboplastic substances—sub- stances that can trip off the clotting cascade (Fig. 15-1). Small amounts of these substances normally leak into the bloodstream every day—for example, gram-negative bacteria, whose endotoxin coats can activate clotting through several mechanisms, are constantly entering the portal circulation from the intestine—but the usual defenses against runaway coagulation (i.e., antithrombin III, tissue factor pathway inhibitor, protein C, and clearance by the mononuclear phagocyte system) are more than adequate to handle this small thromboplastic load. In certain diseases, however, large quantities of thromboplastic substances are discharged into the circulation. The defenses are swamped, and DIC ensues.

The thromboplastic material thought to be responsible for most cases of DIC is tissue factor itself. Tissue factor occurs normally on most cells outside the bloodstream, and is manufactured by endothelial cells and mononuclear phagocytes in contact with the bloodstream when these cells are exposed to inflammatory cytokines such as interleukin-1 (IL-1) and tumor necrosis factor (TNF).

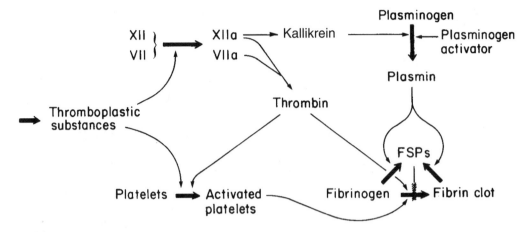

Fig. 15-1. Pathogenesis of DIC. DIC begins when thromboplastic substances are released into the bloodstream in large amounts. These thromboplastic substances activate factors VII and XII, triggering clotting cascade through both extrinsic and intrinsic pathways. Thrombin generated via this cascade then activates circulating platelets (also activated by thromboplastic substances). The combination of thrombin plus activated platelets causes fibrinogen to be converted to fibrin, resulting in formation of clots within the circulatory system. At the same time, plasminogen is converted to plasmin through the actions of kallikrein (activated by factor XIIa) and plasminogen activator (released from endothelial cells and mononuclear phagocytes during the course of the intravascular clotting process). Plasmin digests both fibrinogen and clotted fibrin, dissolving the clot while also releasing fibrin-split products (FSPs), potent anticoagulants that interfere with further conversion of fibrinogen to a fibrin clot. Net effect: the consumption of fibrinogen, platelets, and certain clotting factors and establishment of a confused state in which fibrin clots are perpetually formed and destroyed in circulation, while coagulation at sites of injury is impeded because of depleted platelets and clotting factors and anticoagulant effects of FSPs.

Another thromboplastic material thought to have a role in many cases of DIC is endotoxin. This complex lipid forms the outermost layer of gram-negative organisms and appears in large quantities in the circulation of patients who have serious gram-negative infections. Endotoxin activates factor VII indirectly by inducing the release of inflammatory cytokines, which in turn stimulate tissue factor expression by endothelial cells and mononuclear phagocytes; endotoxin also activates factor XII and platelets directly.

Other substances are also believed capable of triggering DIC. Antigen–antibody complexes are one example, and snake venoms, especially those of the pit vipers, are another.

Aiding the thromboplastic materials in their work are certain factors that affect the properties of the blood itself in patients with DIC.

Tissue acidosis, common in these patients, promotes the activation of the clotting cascade by reducing the local pH of the blood. Stasis of the circulation permits activated clotting factors to accumulate in one region, making it easier for a little thromboplastin to push the clotting system past the point of control and into a state of DIC.

Acting on factor XII, factor VII, and sometimes the platelets, thromboplastic substances trigger every component of the coagulation system. Fibrin is generated through the action of the clotting cascade. Plasmin is generated from plasminogen by kallikrein, which is activated by factor XIIa, and by plasminogen activator, which is manufactured in increased amounts by mononuclear phagocytes and endothelial cells under conditions of stress. The plasmin splits both fibrinogen and the newly generated fibrin, releasing fibrin-split products with their anticoagulant properties. Platelets are activated by newly formed thrombin, by exposed collagen, and sometimes by the thromboplastic substances themselves. Activation exposes the platelet factor Va binding site, which feeds back to accelerate the clotting cascade. The activated platelets are consumed as they aggregate and adhere to damaged tissues. The net effects of all these events are as follows:

1. Loss of plasma fibrinogen as it is consumed by the clotting process and by the action of plasmin.

2. Loss of other clotting factors, notably factors V, VIII, and XIII, as they are used up during the operation of the clotting cascade.

3. Fall in the platelet count, as the platelets aggregate and leave the circulation.

4. Appearance of fibrin-split products, as plasmin acts on its substrates.

The end result is DIC, a complex bleeding disorder caused by these platelet and clotting factor deficiencies and the anticoagulant effects of the fibrin-split products.

Clinical Manifestations

DIC has two forms: acute and chronic. The acute form occurs in a setting of serious illness and is characterized mainly by bleeding. In the chronic form, both bleeding and thrombosis occur.

ACUTE DIC

Acute DIC occurs when a mass of thromboplastic material is introduced into the bloodstream. This occurs in several clinical situations.

Causes

Obstetrical Complications. The fetus, the placenta, and the amniotic fluid are filled with thromboplastic substances. Acute DIC caused by the entry of these thromboplastic substances into the maternal circulation is typical of certain complications of pregnancy: abruptio placenta, in which a portion of the placenta tears away from the uterus; missed abortion, in which a dead fetus is retained in the uterus; and amniotic fluid embolism.

Infections. Infections provide many sources of thromboplastic material. Tissue factor and collagen are exposed to the bloodstream at sites of infection. Endotoxin is also produced if the infection is caused by a gram-negative organism. It is not surprising that acute DIC is a common complication of serious infections, both bacterial and viral.

Injuries and Burns. Acute DIC is often seen with serious injuries and burns, caused by the release of tissue factor from damaged tissues into the bloodstream.

Antigen–Antibody Complexes in the Circulation. Antigen–antibody complexes can trigger DIC, most likely through a primary effect on the platelets. This may account for the DIC sometimes seen in hemolytic transfusion reactions.

Shock and Acidosis. Shock and acidosis are general features of many illnesses once they become sufficiently severe. Illnesses this severe are frequently complicated by acute DIC. Whether the shock and acidosis have an initiating (i.e., thromboplastinlike) role in this DIC is not clear. It is clear, however, that both aggravate the clotting abnormality through stasis and a lowered blood pH, and perhaps through impaired clearance of activated clotting factors by the mononuclear phagocyte system as well.

Symptoms

Bleeding. The prime symptom of acute DIC is bleeding. The bleeding starts all at once and may be very severe. Bleeding from venipuncture sites is highly characteristic and is often the first sign of acute DIC. Areas of purpura, sometimes very large, appear on the skin. The nose, gums, and gastrointestinal and urinary tract are common sites of bleeding. In fact, in acute DIC bleeding can occur from any site.

Traumatic Hemolytic Anemia. Problems are sometimes caused by the fibrin deposited in the small blood vessels. A traumatic anemia often occurs as circulating red cells are sliced apart by fibrin strands stretched across their path ("clotheslining").

Bilateral Necrosis of the Renal Cortex. A rare manifestation of DIC involves the deposition of fibrin in the glomeruli of the kidney. This cuts off the blood supply to the renal cortex, causing bilateral cortical necrosis and severe acute renal failure.

The clue to the diagnosis of acute DIC is the abrupt onset of bleeding in a sick patient who does not have a prior history of underlying clotting defect. In any such patient, acute DIC should be high on the list of possibilities.

CHRONIC DIC

Chronic DIC occurs when thromboplastic material is delivered into the bloodstream in a slow, steady trickle. It is less commonly diagnosed than acute DIC, but it is a subtle condition, and many cases perhaps go unrecognized.

Causes

Cancer. Malignant tumors are constantly discharging small amounts of thromboplastic material into the circulation. This material may be derived from cells that die within the tumor. It is responsible for the state of chronic DIC seen in many patients with cancer. Occasionally, it contributes to episodes of acute DIC in these patients. Acute DIC is a particular problem in patients with acute promyelocytic leukemia of the hypergranular variety (Ch. 23).

Missed Abortion. In some patients with missed abortion, thromboplastic substances leak only slowly from the dead fetus into the circulation. Such patients will develop a chronic rather than an acute form of DIC.

Giant Hemangioma (Kasabach-Merritt Syndrome). Giant hemangiomas can cause a state of chronic DIC. The mechanism is unclear, but it is thought that stasis of blood in the hemangioma may somehow contribute to the condition.

Antigen–Antibody Complexes. Chronic DIC can occur in diseases in which antigen-antibody complexes circulate on a long-term basis. Systemic lupus erythematosus is the best example of such a disease.

Symptoms

Thrombosis. The most frequent symptom of chronic DIC is thrombosis. The thrombi usually form in the veins (recurrent thrombophlebitis is the most typical manifestation of chronic DIC), but they sometimes form on the valves of the heart. The real hazard of thrombosis is the danger of pulmonary or arterial embolism, in which fragments of the thrombi are torn away and carried downstream by the circulation, plugging distant vessels.

Bleeding. Also common in chronic DIC, bleeding is less common than thrombosis. In contrast to acute DIC, the bleeding in chronic DIC is usually not widespread.

LABORATORY FINDINGS

DIC is associated with a characteristic pattern of abnormalities in the clotting function tests. These are listed in Table 15-1, together with their underlying mechanisms. The pattern given in the table is classic, but not invariable:

1. The fibrinogen level may be normal. This is because fibrinogen is an acute–phase reactant whose production increases during illness. Sometimes this increase in production is enough to offset the increase in consumption caused by the DIC, so fibrinogen remains within the normal range.

2. In chronic DIC, it often happens that the increases in platelet and clotting factor production that occur in response to the clotting disorder are enough to prevent the expected drop in their blood levels. For this

Table 15-1. Clotting Studies in DIC: Classic Pattern

Abnormality	Cause
Prolonged screening tests: PTT, PT, TT[a]	Decreased plasma clotting factor levels; elevated fibrin-split products
Low platelets	Consumption of platelets
Low fibrinogen	Consumption by the clotting cascade; destruction by plasmin
Elevated fibrin-split products	Destruction of fibrinogen by plasmin
Normal euglobulin lysis time	? Removal of plasminogen activator and plasmin from the circulation through binding to intravascular fibrin clots; action of α_2-antiplasmin

[a]Partial thromboplastin time, prothrombin time, thrombin time.

reason, many of the clotting tests may be normal in chronic DIC. Fibrin-split products, however, are usually elevated.

Measurements of clotting factors other than fibrinogen are of little help in diagnosing DIC. The levels of these clotting factors are supposed to behave in a predictable way when clotting takes place, but they actually vary widely in DIC and are only occasionally in agreement with what would be expected on theoretical grounds.

In addition to the clotting abnormalities, DIC shows the laboratory features of a traumatic hemolytic anemia. The hematocrit may be low, broken cells (schistocytes) are seen on the blood smear, and haptoglobin is reduced or absent. These and other manifestations of this type of anemia are discussed more fully in Chapter 9.

TREATMENT

There are three aspects to the management of DIC: the treatment of the underlying condition, the replacement of deficient clotting components, and the administration of heparin.
Treatment of the Underlying Condition. Treating the underlying condition is by far the most important aspect of management. DIC can sometimes be held in check by replacement therapy and heparin, but it can only be cured by eliminating the underlying disease.
Replacement of Deficient Clotting Components. If bleeding in DIC is accompanied by low blood fibrinogen or platelets, these

should be restored by transfusion: cryoprecipitate for fibrinogen deficiency, fresh frozen plasma to correct for possible deficiencies of other clotting factors, and platelets for thrombocytopenia. It may seem that this treatment is adding fuel to the fire by supplying more clotting components to a patient whose clotting system is already too active, but in fact bleeding patients do better, not worse, when their clotting deficiencies are corrected in this way.
Heparin Therapy. The treatment of DIC with heparin is a controversial matter. Theoretically, it should be possible to cure acute DIC by blocking ongoing coagulation with heparin, but in practice this mode of treatment has been far from an overwhelming success. The problems with use of heparin in acute DIC have been that bleeding can be aggravated by heparinizing patients who already have severe bleeding problems, and that the death rate in large groups of patients with acute DIC has not been improved by heparin. On the other hand, there have been numerous instances in which heparin appears to have saved the lives of individual patients with acute, severe DIC.

What is the current consensus among the experts with regard to the use of heparin in acute DIC? There is none. Some experts believe that heparin should be used in all patients with DIC. Others advise against its use under any circumstances. The middle view, perhaps the most widespread, holds that heparin need not be used routinely in DIC, but should be given as a life-saving measure to patients with truly severe DIC, to tide them over until other forms of treatment have had a chance to take effect. Patients with DIC who are given heparin must be monitored very carefully; bleeding must be watched for, and the status of the DIC should be followed by the fibrinogen level and the platelet count.

The use of anticoagulants may be of help in chronic DIC, when the problem is thrombosis rather than bleeding. Vitamin K antagonists are generally tried first, but they tend not to work in these patients. Low-dose heparin has proved effective in some patients. A full discussion of anticoagulants is given in Chapter 16.

PRIMARY FIBRINOGENOLYSIS

Primary fibrinogenolysis occurs when active plasmin is generated in the circulation at a time when the clotting cascade is not in operation. It is an occasional feature of certain diseases—most commonly severe liver disease—but once in a great while it is seen in cancer of the lung or prostate or in heat stroke. It is very rare.

The symptom of this disease is bleeding, which can be very severe. Bleeding occurs for two reasons: (1) because of depleted fibrinogen as it is split by the plasmin, and (2) because of the accumulation of "fibrin" (actually, fibrinogen)-split products, with their anticoagulant properties.

The condition that must be ruled out in order to make the diagnosis of primary fibrinogenolysis is DIC. At first glance this may appear difficult, because the laboratory findings in these two disorders have a number of similarities. The clotting factor screening tests—partial thromboplastin time (PTT), prothrombin time (PT), and thrombin time (TT)—

are prolonged in both disorders, fibrinogen levels are reduced, and fibrin-split products are found in the plasma. A traumatic anemia may also be present. There are, however, some distinct differences between the two (Table 15-2):

1. The platelet count is normal, not low, in primary fibrinogenolysis.

2. The euglobulin lysis time, a crude but useful measure of circulating plasmin, is shortened in primary fibrinogenolysis, but is often normal in DIC. The normality of the euglobulin lysis time in DIC is somewhat unexpected, because a great deal of active plasmin is generated in that condition. It may be that in DIC, most of the components of the plasmin system are associated with intravascular fibrin clots (both plasminogen activator and plasmin itself are known to bind avidly to polymerized fibrin), and are therefore left behind when blood is drawn for laboratory analysis.

3. The results of tests for fibrin-split products are different in the two conditions. Tests that detect split products by their structure (immunological or staphylococcal slumping assays) are positive in both conditions, whereas tests that depend on paracoagulation (ethanol or protamine gelation) are positive in DIC but negative in primary fibrinogenolysis. The reason is as follows. In DIC, the plasma contains fibrin monomers that are unable to form a fibrin gel because they are complexed to split products. When ethanol or protamine is added to this plasma, these complexes fall apart, and the liberated fibrin monomers polymerize to form the

Table 15-2. Differences between Primary Fibrinogenolysis and DIC

Parameters	Primary Fibrinogenolysis	DIC
Laboratory findings		
Platelet count	Normal	Low
Euglobulin lysis	Shortened	Normal
Fibrin-split products		
By structural assays	+	+
By paracoagulation tests	0	+
Treatment with ε-aminocaproic acid	Useful	Dangerous

telltale gel. In fibrinogenolysis, the split products are there, but the fibrin monomers are not, so a gel does not form upon the addition of ethanol or protamine.

Making the distinction between DIC and fibrinogenolysis is important for therapeutic reasons. Bleeding from fibrinogenolysis can be treated with ε-aminocaproic acid (or its structural cousin, tranexamic acid), which corrects the condition by inhibiting both plasmin and plasminogen activator. In DIC, however, these drugs are extremely dangerous, because that condition requires active plasmin to keep the blood vessels from filling with fibrin clot, and the administration of a plasmin inhibitor can cause a diffuse thrombotic disorder that leads rapidly to death.

THROMBOTIC THROMBOCYTOPENIA PURPURA

TTP is a mysterious and deadly disease in which plugs of fibrin and platelets appear in small blood vessels throughout the body, with little apparent activation of the clotting cascade or the fibrinolytic system. It is frequently preceded by a minor viral illness, but the connection between this minor illness and the catastrophe that follows is completely obscure. It also occurs in acquired immunodeficiency syndrome (AIDS), and as a complication of gastrointestinal infections caused by verotoxin-

---

TTP MAY BE ASSOCIATED WITH:

Infections
    Nonspecific viral infection
    AIDS
    Verotoxin-secreting *E. coli*

Drug treatment
    Mitomycin C
    Cyclosporin

MANIFESTATIONS OF TTP

Fever
Thrombocytopenia with bleeding
Traumatic hemolytic anemia
Acute renal failure
Severe CNS disturbances: fluctuating focal
    signs, seizures, coma

---

secreting strains of *Escherichia. coli*. A few cases have been associated with certain drugs: cyclosporin A, a powerful immunosuppressive, and the antitumor agent mitomycin C.

The disease has a rapid onset, with widespread manifestations appearing over the course of a day or two. In the classical case, these manifestations form what is referred to cabalistically as "the pentad" (Fig. 15-2).

1. Fever
2. Thrombocytopenia with bleeding
3. Traumatic hemolytic anemia
4. Acute renal failure
5. Severe central nervous system (CNS) disturbances: fluctuating focal signs, seizures, coma.

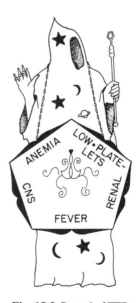

Fig. 15-2. Pentad of TTP.

The anemia, kidney failure, and CNS disturbances are probably attributable to the presence of fibrin in the blood vessels. The thrombocytopenia is presently unexplained, although some believe it is due to the appearance of an abnormal circulating protein, perhaps larger-than-normal multimers of von Willebrand factor, that precipitates the disease by causing platelets to aggregate within the blood vessels.

A milder form of what may be the same disease is typically seen in the young—especially infants and young children—and in pregnant women. It is frequently, but not invariably, heralded by an infection. This disorder features all the manifestations of TTP except for the CNS disturbances—a "tetrad" of symptoms—and is known by the descriptive name *hemolytic-uremic syndrome*. Elevated levels of plasminogen activator inhibitor (PAI-1) raise the possibility that the disease could be caused by a failure of fibrinolysis. Mortality in the hemolytic-uremic syndrome is significant, especially in adults, but is much lower than in TTP.

Laboratory findings are very helpful in making the diagnosis, and especially in making the

---

LABORATORY EVIDENCE OF TTP

Clotting abnormalities
    Low platelets
    Increased megakaryocytes
    Clotting tests otherwise normal
Traumatic hemolytic anemia
    Low hematocrit and hemoglobin
    Red cell fragments on smear
    Bilirubinemia
    Sometimes hemoglobinuria

---

sometimes difficult distinction between TTP and DIC (see box). The changes of traumatic hemolytic anemia are present, including a low hematocrit, fragmented red cells on the blood smear, and the other findings described in Chapter 9. The platelet count is low, but there are many megakaryocytes in the marrow, indicating that the reduction in platelets is attributable to increased consumption, rather than to decreased production. Other clotting studies are usually normal, an important distinction

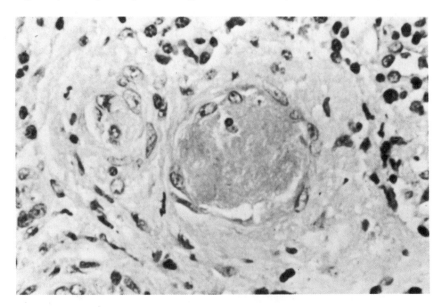

Fig. 15-3. Fibrin-plugged arteriole in gum biopsy from a patient with TTP. Note the absence of an inflammatory response around the arteriole. (From Pisciotta AV, Gottschall J [1980] Clinical features of thrombotic thrombocytic purpura. Semin Thromb Hemost 6:330, with permission.)

from DIC; screening tests are normal, fibrinogen levels are normal or increased, and split products are absent.

The diagnosis often has to be made on clinical grounds, but it can sometimes be made by biopsy, usually of the gum. The diagnostic finding is an arteriole that contains a mass of fibrin and platelets (Fig. 15-3). There is no evidence of inflammation (i.e., no cellular infiltrate surrounds the plugged arteriole), and there is no immunoglobulin or complement to be found. The finding of an arteriole filled with a bland plug is pathognomonic of TTP in this clinical setting.

TTP is usually treated by large-volume plasma exchanges, usually in combination with steroids. This form of therapy has decreased the mortality rate of TTP from 90 percent to something under 30 percent; no one knows why. In patients with TTP who have failed plasma exchange, a combination of steroids, antiplatelet agents, and emergency splenectomy has been used with some success. Platelet transfusions in these patients may cause acute arterial thrombosis and are strictly contraindicated.

SUGGESTED READINGS

Bick RL (1992) Disseminated intravascular coagulation. Hematol Oncol Clin North Am 6:1259

Colman RW, Robboy SJ, Minna JD (1979) Disseminated intravascular coagulation: a reappraisal. Annu Rev Med 30:319

McCrae KR, Samuels P, Schreiber AD (1992) Pregnancy-associated thrombocytopenia: pathogenesis and management. Blood 80:2697

Moake JL (1990) Recent observations on the pathophysiology of thrombotic thrombocytopenic purpura and the hemolytic-uremic syndrome. Hematol Pathol 4:197

Murgo AJ (1987) Thrombotic microangiopathy in the cancer patient including those induced by chemotherapeutic agents. Semin Hematol 24:161

Murphy WG, Moore JC, Warkentin TE et al (1992) Thrombotic thrombocytopenic purpura. McMaster University Medical Centre, Hamilton, Ontario, Canada. Blood Coagul Fibrinolysis 3:655

Ridolfi RL, Bell WR (1981) Thrombotic thrombocytopenic purpura. Medicine 60:413

Rosensweig JN, Gourley GR (1991) Verotoxic *Escherichia coli* in human disease. J Pediatr Gastroenterol Nutr 12:295

Rubin RN, Colman RW (1992) Disseminated intravascular coagulation. Approach to treatment. Drugs 44:963

Ruggenenti P, Remuzzi G (1990) Thrombotic thrombocytopenic purpura and related disorders. Hematol Oncol Clin North Am 4:219

Semeraro N, Colucci M (1992) Changes in the coagulation-figrinolysis balance of endothelial cells and mononuclear phagocytes: role in disseminated intravascular coagulation associated with infectious diseases. Int J Clin Lab Res 21:214

Thompson CE, Damon LE, Ries CA, Linker CA (1992) Thrombotic micrangiopathies in the 1980s: clinical features, response to treatment, and the impact of the human immunodeficiency virus epidemic. Blood 80:1890

16

Antithrombotic Therapy: Anticoagulants, Antiplatelet Drugs, and Fibrinolytic Agents

Diseases associated with thrombosis—heart attacks, strokes, pulmonary emboli, and so forth—are the most common causes of death in the developed countries. Current treatment of many of these diseases involves the use of drugs that counteract intravascular coagulation. These drugs fall into three categories: anticoagulants, which impede clotting through effects on the soluble clotting factors; fibrinolytic agents, which dissolve clots that have already formed; and the antiplatelet agents.

ANTICOAGULANTS

Anticoagulants are used for the treatment of conditions in which clotting occurs in the heart or blood vessels. They do not work equally well in all such conditions, however, and even when they do work, anticoagulants are hazardous to use because they can increase the risk of bleeding. The decision to use anticoagulants is therefore a serious matter, and the management of anticoagulated patients requires the utmost care and vigilance.

The two major types of anticoagulants are heparin and the vitamin K antagonists. Heparin is used to treat acute thrombosis; vitamin K antagonists are used for long-term anticoagulation.

Heparin

Heparin is a complex polymer of sugars and amino sugars containing a large number of acidic groups (carboxyl [—COO^-] and sulfate) that give it very high negative charge at biological pH (Fig. 16-1). Heparin is a member of a general class of acidic sugar polymers known as mucopolysaccharides. These mucopolysaccharides are abundant on cell surfaces and in the ground substance of connective tissues. Mucopolysaccharides similar to heparin are thought to be partly responsible for the anticoagulant properties of the endothelial surface (Ch. 13).

Heparin interferes with clot formation by causing the inactivation of all the clotting factors that work through proteolysis, with the exception of factor VIIa. It accomplishes this by a mechanism involving the plasma protein antithrombin III (AT III; Fig. 16-2). AT III has the ability to bind to proteolytic clotting factors in such a way as to block their active sites irreversibly. This reaction is slow, so that activated clotting factors may be able to do their job before AT III has a chance to interfere with their effects. What heparin does is to combine with AT III to form a complex of greatly

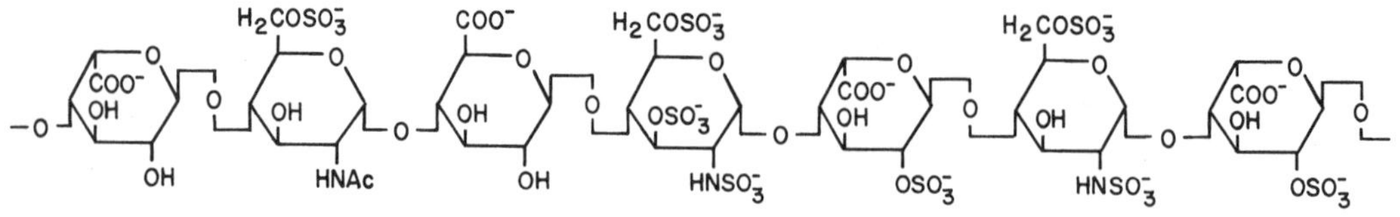

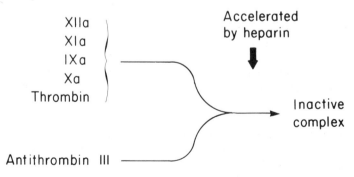

Fig. 16-1. Portion of the heparin molecule.

enhanced reactivity. In contrast to the slow action of free AT III, this complex is able to combine with clotting factors and block their effects almost as fast as the factors appear in the circulation.

The coagulation screening tests in heparinized patients are as expected from the action of the heparin–AT III complex. The partial thromboplastin time (PTT) and thrombin time (TT) are sharply altered. The prothrombin time (PT) is much less affected, because factor VIIa is resistant to the heparin–AT III complex. The bleeding time is not affected at all, as long as the platelet count is normal.

EFFECT OF HEPARIN ON COAGULATION SCREENING TESTS

Substantially prolonged: Partial thromboplastin time and thrombin time

Slightly prolonged: Prothrombin time

Unchanged: Bleeding time

CLINICAL USE

Because of its chemical nature, heparin cannot be absorbed from the intestine, so it must be given parenterally. The best way to administer heparin is continuously by vein. It is sometimes given by intermittent injections (intravenous or subcutaneous), but the risk of bleeding with intermittent therapy is higher than with continuous therapy, because adequate round-the-clock anticoagulation with intermittent therapy requires a dose of heparin large enough to cause a dangerous paralysis of clotting function for the first hour or two after administration. Heparin is cleared rapidly by the liver, having a half-life in the blood of about 1 hour, so intermittent therapy has to be given fairly often (every 4 to 6 hours is the rule).

It is generally necessary to give large doses of heparin at the start of treatment, because extensive clotting is going on, and large amounts of activated clotting factors have to be neutralized in the circulation. Once clotting is under control and the production of active clotting factors has fallen back toward normal, the

XIIa
XIa
IXa
Xa
Thrombin

Accelerated by heparin

Inactive complex

Antithrombin III

Fig. 16-2. How heparin works.

heparin dose must be cut back to avoid overanticoagulation and bleeding.

The degree of anticoagulation is usually determined by the PTT. The heparin dose is adjusted to give a PTT of 1.5 to 2 times control an hour before the next dose (intermittent therapy) or any time at all (continuous therapy). At these levels, heparin has little effect on the PT.

Heparin in very low doses can be used to prevent venous thrombosis in certain high-risk patients (e.g., patients about to undergo abdominal or chest surgery, or patients restricted to bed rest for congestive heart failure). Because the release of only a tiny amount of activated clotting factor in a vein is enough to trigger thrombophlebitis, a low dose of heparin is all that is needed to neutralize that tiny pulse of activated clotting factor and prevent formation of a clot. Once a clot does begin to form, however, major amounts of clotting factors are activated, and large doses of heparin are required to bring the ongoing clotting process under control. Low-dose heparin is given subcutaneously every 8 to 12 hours. It is not necessary to follow treatment with the PTT, since the doses given are too low to affect this test.

COMPLICATIONS

Bleeding

As with all anticoagulants, the major side effect of heparin is bleeding. This problem generally occurs when the patient is overanticoagulated, but it can also take place when the level of anticoagulation is in the therapeutic range as indicated by the PTT. Platelets are particularly important for clot formation in a patient whose soluble clotting system is partly paralyzed by heparin; to reduce the likelihood of bleeding in such a patient, antiplatelet agents are generally avoided.

Diagnosis of heparin toxicity is generally simple: Bleeding in a patient on heparin therapy who is found to have a long PTT can be considered a side effect of heparin, unless proved otherwise. Occasionally the diagnosis presents a problem, generally in patients in whom postoperative bleeding develops after cardiopulmonary bypass surgery. Patients on bypass are always given heparin during surgery to keep their blood from clotting in the pump. At the end of the operation, the heparin is neutralized with protamine, a group of positively charged proteins that form tight complexes with the negatively charged heparin molecules, preventing them from interacting with AT III. These patients sometimes bleed after surgery has been completed and the protamine has been given. Although there are a number of reasons why such bleeding may occur, the situation often boils down to the question: Does the patient have DIC, or has the heparin been incompletely neutralized? Routine testing may not answer this question: levels of fibrin-split products may be ambiguous, the split products themselves can mimic the anticoagulant activity of heparin, and the platelet count will be low in any postoperative patient who has received many units of blood. Fortunately, there is a test that can distinguish between these two possibilities (Fig. 16-3). This test, known as the *reptilase time*, is carried out by measuring how long it takes for plasma to clot after adding reptilase, the venom from the South American pit viper (*Bothrops jararaca*). Reptilase causes clot formation by splitting off fibrinopeptide A from fibrinogen, acting much like thrombin; in fact, the reptilase time is very similar in principle to the TT. Reptilase, however, is not affected by the heparin–AT III complex. Consequently, the reptilase time will be perfectly normal in heparin toxicity even though the TT may be infinite. Both times will be prolonged in DIC, however, because fibrin-split products will retard the assembly of fibrin monomers into a clot regardless of whether the monomers are produced by thrombin or reptilase.

As to treatment, mild bleeding caused by heparin toxicity can be managed by watchful waiting, since heparin is rapidly cleared from the bloodstream. For serious bleeding, heparin should be neutralized by protamine. Overneutralization should be avoided, however, since excess protamine itself may interfere with clotting. Transfusions should be used for blood replacement as necessary, but it should be borne in mind that *transfusions will not correct the clotting defect caused by heparin* and should therefore not be administered for that purpose.

Thrombocytopenia and Arterial Thrombosis; Osteoporosis

About 5 to 10 percent of patients on heparin will develop a low platelet count because of the appearance of a heparin-dependent anti-platelet antibody (see Ch. 30). *This is a very dangerous situation.* The reduction in the platelet count is usually mild, but it should raise an immediate alarm because patients with heparin-induced thrombocytopenia are paradoxically subject to arterial and venous thrombosis, with potentially catastrophic consequences that can include pulmonary emboli, strokes, heart attacks, and loss of limbs. If unexplained thrombocytopenia should develop in a patient on heparin, the heparin must be stopped immediately and the patient switched to oral anticoagulants. If necessary, the heparin can be replaced by a short course of *ancrod* (see p. 251), an experimental anticoagulant that is available for compassionate use. Because of the risk of thrombosis, platelet transfusions are absolutely contraindicated.

Patients on long-term heparin may develop osteoporosis (i.e., washed-out bones). This very rare complication has only been seen in patients who have been on high-dose heparin for 6 months or longer.

LOW MOLECULAR WEIGHT HEPARIN

Low molecular weight heparin is prepared by cleaving heparin into fragments about one-

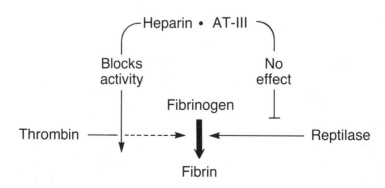

Fig. 16-3. Reptilase time versus thrombin time. AT-III, antithrombin III.

quarter the size of the original molecule. It differs slightly from native heparin in its spectrum of activities, and is not inhibited by platelet factor 4. Low molecular weight heparin has proved to be an effective anticoagulant, causing less bleeding than native heparin. It can be given as a daily subcutaneous dose without monitoring by PTT, making full-dose heparinization feasible in outpatients.

Vitamin K Antagonists

Vitamin K is necessary for the conversion of certain glutamate (glu) residues to γ-carboxyglutamate (gla) residues in factors II (prothrombin), VII, IX, and X. In the course of the glu $\rightarrow$ gla reaction, the vitamin undergoes oxidation, and has to be converted back to the reduced form before it can take part in the formation of another gla residue (Fig. 16-4). Vitamin K antagonists act by blocking the reduction of the oxidized vitamin, leading to a deficiency of reduced vitamin K. As a result, the glu $\rightarrow$ gla reaction is retarded, so the vita-

min K-dependent clotting factors are unable to acquire their γ-carboxyglutamate residues. Without these γ-carboxyglutamates, the clotting factors cannot bind Ca^{2+}, making them unable to function. The result is a state of impaired coagulation caused by an acquired deficiency of these four clotting factors. The clotting factors do not fall simultaneously, but are lost sequentially: factor VII first, because it turns over in the blood faster than any other clotting factor (its half-life in the blood is only 6 hours, as compared with the next shortest half-life, that of factor VIII, which is twice as long); factors IX and X next; and finally prothrombin, which requires 3 to 4 days to fall. The anticoagulated state is achieved only when all four clotting factors have reached their final levels.

As the active clotting factors decline, their gla-free precursors accumulate (1) in the liver, where they are manufactured; and (2) in the blood, where they are released from the liver and act as weak anticoagulants.

Vitamin K-dependent carboxylation is also needed to confer anticoagulant activity on pro-

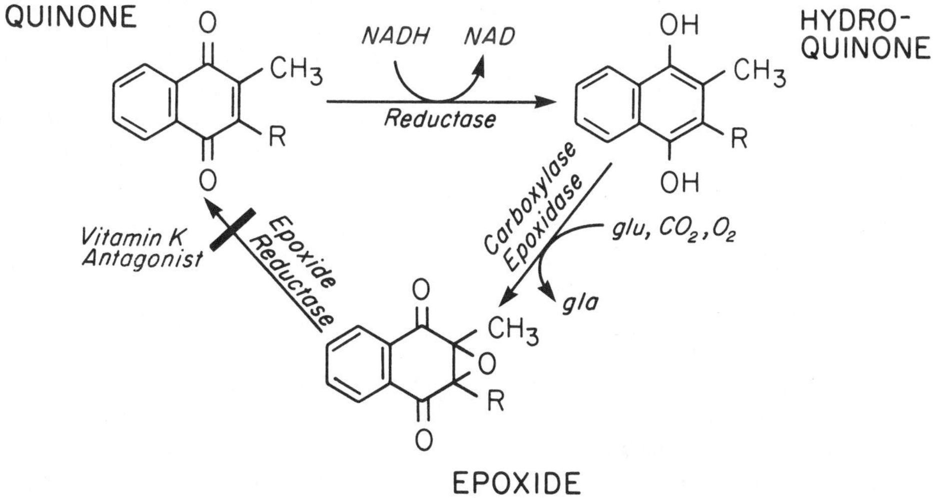

Fig. 16-4. The vitamin K cycle and the mechanism of action of vitamin K antagonists. Vitamin K in its reduced (hydroquinone) form is an essential cofactor for the carboxylation of glutamate (glu) to γ-carboxyglutamate (gla). During the course of this reaction, the vitamin is oxidized to the quinone epoxide and must be reconverted to the hydroquinone before it can participate again in the glu $\rightarrow$ gla reaction. Reconversion involves two sequential reductions: quinone epoxide $\rightarrow$ quinone, and quinone $\rightarrow$ hydroquinone. Vitamin K antagonists block the first of these reductions, thereby retarding the glu $\rightarrow$ gla conversion by depriving the reaction of its cofactor.

tein C and protein S. As with the vitamin K-dependent clotting factors, the activities of these anticoagulants decline in patients on vitamin K antagonists. The effect of this decline is to increase the tendency for blood to clot, but the procoagulant effect of the vitamin K antagonist is usually (though not always) overwhelmed by its anticoagulant effect.

All the effects of the vitamin K antagonists are reversed by a single dose of vitamin K, provided it is large enough. Carboxylation of glutamates begins as soon as the vitamin reaches the liver, and the clotting factor deficiency is completely corrected within 1 or 2 days. There is some evidence, in fact, for a transient overshoot as the accumulated precursors are rapidly carboxylated and released into the plasma as active clotting factors.

All the vitamin K antagonists in current use are derived from hydroxycoumarin (Fig. 16-5). They differ principally in their durations of action. At present, warfarin (Fig. 16-5) appears to be the vitamin K antagonist enjoying the widest use. The popularity of warfarin stems from the fact that its duration of action (5 to 7 days) offers the best compromise between the need for a stable level of anticoagulation and the conflicting need for a rapid response when the dose of the drug is changed.

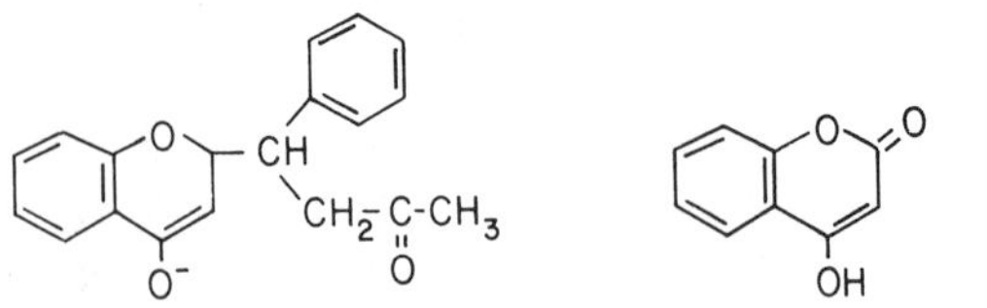

CLINICAL USE

Vitamin K antagonists have a very different role in anticoagulant therapy from that of heparin (Table 16-1). The latter is generally used to treat acute episodes of intravascular clotting, and the course of treatment is generally short (4 to 6 days or so). It is always given parenterally. In contrast, the vitamin K antagonists are used more to prevent future clotting than to treat immediate episodes of thrombosis.

Fig. 16-5. Warfarin and hydroxycoumarin.

The course of treatment is long, lasting months to years. The vitamin K antagonists are always given by mouth.

Patients are started on vitamin K antagonists at the dose considered necessary to maintain them at an adequate level of anticoagulation. A loading dose is not needed. The level of anticoagulation is evaluated by following the PT, which measures all the vitamin K-dependent clotting factors except factor IX. The prothrombin time is expressed as a ratio of the patient's PT to that of a normal control, correcting for the lot-to-lot variation in the potencies of the various thromboplastins used for measuring the PT by normalization against a World Health Organization standard. The normalized value, known as the *International Normalized Ratio (INR)*, is the figure used for the management of anticoagulant therapy. The anticoagulant dose is adjusted to achieve an INR appropriate for the condition being treated.

CAUSE OF POOR CONTROL

Even under the best of circumstances, anticoagulation therapy is a haphazard affair. The range of therapeutic anticoagulation is narrow, and patients will frequently move in and out of this range even on a constant dose of anticoagulant. In many cases, no reason can be found for these fluctuations in control. Nevertheless,

Table 16-1. Heparin and the Fibrinolytic Agents versus the Vitamin K Antagonists

	Heparin and the Fibrinolytic Agents	Vitamin K Antagonists
Purpose	Treatment of intravascular clotting	Prevention of future thrombosis
Route of administration	Parenteral	Oral
Duration of treatment	Days	Months to years

> **CLINICAL USE OF VITAMIN K ANTAGONISTS**
>
> Start at the estimated maintenance dose
> Follow prothrombin time daily. Adjust dose to achieve an International Normalized Ratio (INR) of 1.2 to 2.0 times normal
> Continue heparin until the anticoagulant effect of the vitamin K antagonist is established (generally 5 days)
> Once maintenance dose is determined, prothrombin time may be followed less frequently (eventually, every 2 to 3 weeks)

certain possibilities should be considered whenever control lapses in a patient on vitamin K antagonists. These include drug interactions, liver disease, change in diet, and noncompliance.

Drug Interactions

More than any other type of drug, the vitamin K antagonists are affected by other drugs that the patient may be taking. The four mechanisms by which these drug interactions take place are described below.

Accelerated Destruction of the Vitamin K Antagonist. Vitamin K antagonists are inactivated largely by the cytochrome P-450 system in the liver. The cytochrome P-450 system is an enzyme system (more accurately, a group of closely related enzyme systems) whose function is to oxidize drugs and other foreign chemicals so as to speed their elimination from the body. A property of this enzyme system is that it is induced by certain of the drugs it oxidizes, increasing in quantity whenever these drugs are present. This increase in the quantity of the cytochrome P-450 system naturally leads to an increase in the rate at which its substrates are metabolized. Specifically, it leads to accelerated destruction of the vitamin K antagonists. The result is an abrupt increase in the dose of anticoagulant required to maintain a given level of anticoagulation. Consequently, whenever a patient on anticoagulants takes a P-450-inducing drug, he escapes anticoagulation unless the dose is increased. Conversely, if an anticoagulated patient stops taking such a drug without adjusting the anticoagulant dose downward, he will become overanticoagulated as the P-450 level falls to its uninduced value, and is at increased risk of bleeding.

Decreased Destruction of the Vitamin K Antagonist. Certain drugs act, not as inducers of the cytochrome P-450 system, but as inhibitors of that system. Such drugs will slow the rate at which vitamin K antagonists are destroyed in the liver. The result is that a lower dose of anticoagulant is required to achieve a therapeutic effect. Patients on vitamin K antagonists who begin to take such drugs will require downward adjustment of their anticoagulant dose to avoid becoming overanticoagulated.

Displacement of the Anticoagulant from Plasma Albumin. In the circulation, anticoagulants are present in two freely exchangeable pools: a pool of unbound drug, and a pool of drug bound to plasma albumin. Although most of the drug by far is in the albumin-bound pool, it is the size of the tiny unbound pool that determines the degree of anticoagulation, because it is from this pool that the drug is taken up by the liver to exert its effect. When a patient on anticoagulants is given another drug that binds to albumin, the pool of anticoagulant increases as the new drug displaces some of the albumin-bound anticoagulant from the protein into free solution. Such a drug has the effect of increasing the potency of the anticoagulant and will throw the patient into an overanticoagulated state unless the dose of anticoagulant is cut.

Alterations of Intestinal Bacteria by Oral Antibiotics. A small amount of vitamin K is manufactured by the bacteria in the gastrointestinal tract. This makes no difference in patients on a normal diet, but in malnourished patients the intestinal bacteria can represent a significant source of the vitamin. Vitamin K deficiency can develop in these patients if their

Table 16-2. Interactions between Vitamin K Antagonists and Other Drugs

	Promotes Anticoagulant Effect		Opposes Anticoagulant Effect
Inhibition of Cytochrome P-450	Displacement of Anticoagulant from Albumin	Alteration of Intestinal Bacteria	Induction of Cytochrome P-450
Chloramphenicol	Long-acting sulfonamides	Neomycin	Barbiturates
Allopurinol	Phenylbutazone		Glutethimide
Cimetidine	Phenytoin		Rifampin
Fluoroquinolones	Aspirin (3 g/day)		
Metronidazole			

intestinal flora are suppressed by oral antibiotics. If these patients are placed on vitamin K antagonists, they will become overanticoagulated as the developing deficiency shifts the balance between the vitamin and the anticoagulant drug.

In Table 16-2, some of the more commonly used drugs that take part in these interactions are classified according to mechanism.

Liver Disease

Patients on anticoagulants are extraordinarily sensitive to the effects of liver disease on clotting factor production. Accordingly, the development of liver disease (e.g., drug-induced or viral hepatitis) is an occasional cause of sudden overanticoagulation in patients on vitamin K antagonists.

Change in Diet

In a patient on vitamin K antagonists, the level of anticoagulation depends on the balance between the dose of anticoagulant and the amount of vitamin K in the diet. A change in the diet may therefore throw an anticoagulated patient out of control and should be considered as a possibility whenever a patient on vitamin K antagonists lapses from control in either direction.

Noncompliance

The commonest cause of poor control in an anticoagulated patient is noncompliance: the patient fails to take the drug. The best way to diagnose noncompliance is to measure the level of anticoagulant in the blood. It takes several days for most of the commonly used vitamin K antagonists to be eliminated from the body, so a very low blood level suggests that the patient has not taken the anticoagulant for a number of days.

COMPLICATIONS

Bleeding

Bleeding is a common complication in patients on oral anticoagulants. It is particularly common in the overanticoagulated patient, but it may take place when the level of anticoagulation is in the therapeutic range. In the latter case, bleeding generally occurs from a preexisting lesion such as a healed duodenal ulcer or an intestinal polyp. Bleeding in overanticoagulated patients, however, can occur even in the absence of an underlying lesion. Minor bleeding can sometimes be managed by withholding the anticoagulant for a while and restoring the depleted clotting factors with fresh frozen plasma. It is often necessary, however, to neutralize the anticoagulant by giving vitamin K. A single dose of vitamin K is all that is needed to correct the clotting defect. Since correction requires the synthesis of new clotting factor, it takes 24 to 48 hours to reach completion. During this interval it may be necessary to give fresh frozen plasma (or factor IX concentrate)

> **MANAGEMENT OF BLEEDING CAUSED BY VITAMIN K ANTAGONISTS**
>
> Stop the anticoagulant
> Replace depleted clotting factors with fresh frozen plasma or, less desirably, with factor IX concentrate
> Give vitamin K if necessary
> Give transfusions as indicated

as a stopgap measure. Blood transfusions should be given as needed.

Decisions as to how to treat bleeding in chronically anticoagulated patients can be very difficult. Whereas stopping the bleeding is obviously essential, anticoagulation may be indispensable to prevent intravascular clotting in a high-risk patient (e.g., one with an artificial heart valve). The words of Hippocrates apply: "Art is long and life is short; the occasion instant, decision difficult and experiment perilous." Choosing among the therapeutic alternatives, with their uncertain benefits and imponderable risks, can tax the skills of the most able and experienced physicians.

Anticoagulation during Pregnancy

There are unusual hazards to the use of vitamin K antagonists during pregnancy. Vitamin K antagonists cross the placenta and enter the fetal bloodstream, leading to congenital anomalies if they are used during the first trimester. Maternal bleeding during delivery is also a problem. For these reasons, vitamin K antagonists should not be used during pregnancy, especially in the first and last trimesters. Long-term anticoagulation in pregnant women is generally carried out with heparin, which does not cross the placenta.

Other Anticoagulants

Two other agents are occasionally used as anticoagulants, one obtained from snake venom, and the other from bacteria. A third anticoagulant, presently experimental, is derived from a leech.

ANCROD

Ancrod is a highly specific protease isolated from the venom of the Malayan pit viper, *Agkistrodon rhodostoma*. It acts like reptilase, splitting fibrinopeptide A from the fibrinogen molecule. Fibrinogen altered in this way can no longer be acted on by thrombin. The blood is thus effectively stripped of fibrinogen (this process is called defibrination) and in this way is rendered unclottable.

The fibrinlike molecule produced by the action on fibrinogen is able to form a sort of clot, but the clot is weak and cannot be cross-linked by factor XIII. Its formation can be detected in clotting assays, but it is too weak to survive the powerful shearing forces in the circulation, so it breaks up in the blood vessels.

DEXTRAN

Dextrans are mixtures of high molecular weight glucose polymers secreted by certain bacteria. Dextran for clinical use is isolated from the medium in which these bacteria are grown. It exerts its anticoagulant effect mainly by coating the red cells, thereby reducing blood viscosity and decreasing stasis in the circulation. It also has an antiplatelet action. It is occasionally used to prevent venous thrombosis, especially postoperatively.

HIRUDIN

Hirudin is the anticoagulant produced by the medicinal leech, *Hirudo medicinalis*. It is a powerful and specific inhibitor of thrombin. Animal studies with recombinant hirudin suggest that bleeding is not likely to be a serious problem with this agent. Clinical trials on hirudin are currently under way.

FIBRINOLYTIC AGENTS

Like heparin, the fibrinolytic agents are used to treat acute thrombosis and embolism. They work by activating plasmin, the fibrin-dissolving enzyme of plasma. The plasmin opens clogged vessels by digesting any clot that has already formed, in addition to slowing further clotting by digesting factors V and VIII and by releasing fibrin-split products.

Agents in Current Use

Three fibrinolytic agents are currently in use: streptokinase, urokinase, and tissue plasminogen activator (t-PA). Each has advantages and disadvantages (Table 16-3).

Table 16-3. Fibrinolytic Agents

Agent	Source	Antigenicity	Cost
Streptokinase	Streptococci	High	Moderate
Urokinase	Cloned human	None	High
Tissue plasminogen activator	Cloned human	None	Very high

STREPTOKINASE

Streptokinase is a protein is made by group C streptococci, from which it is purified for clinical use. In the bloodstream, it combines with plasminogen (the precursor of plasmin) to form a complex with new and cannibalistic properties: The plasminogen in the complex is converted by the streptokinase into a highly specific protease that is able to convert free (i.e., not complexed to streptokinase) plasminogen into plasmin (Fig. 16-6). In practical terms, streptokinase has the disadvantage of being a foreign protein against which patients may have developed antibodies during a previous streptococcal infection. On the other hand, it is much less expensive than urokinase.

UROKINASE

A protein made by the kidney, urokinase is isolated from human urine. It is a protease that acts directly on plasminogen, converting it to plasmin (Fig. 16-6). As a human protein, urokinase is not antigenic, so patients do not make antibodies against it. However, it is about 10 times as expensive as streptokinase, so expensive that streptokinase is preferred over urokinase unless the patient to be treated has an allergy that prevents its use.

TISSUE PLASMINOGEN ACTIVATOR

t-PA, a major initiator of fibrinolysis in the normal circulation (Ch. 13), has recently become available in large quantities through gene cloning. It has attracted a great deal of attention as a fibrinolytic drug because, unlike streptokinase and urokinase, t-PA binds specifically to the fibrin in a blood clot, a process that both restricts its mobility and results in a sharp increase in its activity. As a result, t-PA will generate plasmin mainly at the site of a clot undergoing dissolution, while in contrast, streptokinase and urokinase will generate plasmin throughout the general circulation. Because the action of t-PA is localized while that of streptokinase and urokinase is generalized, the latter two have to activate much more plasmin than the former in order to dissolve the same amount of clot. This means that t-PA should theoretically generate the same clot-lysing power as streptokinase or urokinase with much less risk of bleeding. Clinical trials have shown, however, that the risk of bleeding is just as high in patients treated with t-PA as in those treated with other fibrinolytic agents. These findings, together with its very high cost, suggest that t-PA is probably not the fibrinolytic agent of choice, at least at the present time.

Clinical Use

Acute myocardial infarction is one of the major indications for fibrinolytic therapy. Patients with fresh myocardial infarctions benefit from a single intravenous dose of a fibrinolytic agent given within 6 hours of the onset of the illness: clots in the coronary arteries dissolve, myocardial damage is decreased, and survival improves. The chief complication of this therapy is bleeding, which occurs in a minority of patients and is occasionally severe.

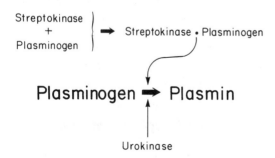

Fig. 16-6. How streptokinase and urokinase activate plasmin.

Fibrinolytic agents are also used in the treatment of severe thrombophlebitis. For this condition, the agent is usually given intravenously in fixed doses for 24 to 48 hours, after which the patient is switched over to heparin. In contrast to practice with other anticoagulants, treatment is generally not followed in the laboratory, because the dose is fixed. The existence of a fibrinolytic state, however, should be established early in treatment by some laboratory measure of fibrinolysis: a shortened euglobulin lysis time, a prolonged TT, elevated levels of fibrin-split products, or any other convenient test.

For treating thrombophlebitis, fibrinolytic agents appear to be the most effective of all the anticoagulants, but they are also the most dangerous with respect to bleeding. Even arterial lines can begin to leak blood in patients being given fibrinolytic agents. Consequently, these agents are rarely used for thrombophlebitis, and then only in its most serious forms, as in massive pulmonary embolism, or very extensive thrombophlebitis in young patients, for example. Fibrinolytic agents should be avoided in any patient with an increased risk of bleeding (e.g., postoperative patients, who can be anticoagulated with heparin or vitamin K antagonists under some circumstances but who should not as a general rule receive fibrinolytic agents).

Bleeding from Fibrinolytic Agents

When a patient on fibrinolytic therapy begins to bleed, the chances are overwhelming that the fibrinolytic agent is primarily responsible, and treatment should be directed accordingly. If bleeding is minor (e.g., a leak around an arterial line), it can sometimes be handled by local compression. If it is severe, or if it does not respond to local measures, fibrinolytic therapy should be stopped. This will restore fibrinolysis to normal levels within an hour or two, but a bleeding problem may still exist because of the secondary effects of fibrinolysis (i.e., low plasma fibrinogen, factors V and VIII, and circulating fibrin-split products). Fresh frozen plasma or cryoprecipitate can be used if necessary to treat these secondary problems. Blood transfusions should be given as required.

Occasionally bleeding caused by fibrinolytic therapy is massive or occurs in a critical location (e.g., inside the skull). This sort of bleeding problem constitutes a major emergency and requires the most rapid possible reversal of fibrinolysis, which is accomplished by giving ε-aminocaproic acid or tranexamic acid, inhibitors of plasminogen activation. The treatment carries with it the hazard of thrombosis and should only be used for the most serious forms of fibrinolysis-associated bleeding.

ANTIPLATELET DRUGS

In addition to the anticoagulants, which interfere with the formation and maintenance of the fibrin clot, a number of agents in clinical use work by interfering with platelet function. These anti-platelet agents are used mainly to prevent thrombosis on the arterial side of the circulation, where clots are generally thought to originate as intravascular platelet aggregates. They are less useful against thrombosis on the venous side, because venous thrombosis appears to result mainly from inappropriate activation of the clotting cascade, with platelets playing only a secondary role.

The anti-platelet agents in current use include aspirin, dipyridamole, and ticlopidine (Table 16-4). They are all much less potent than the anticoagulants, but they are also much less hazardous. Bleeding caused by impaired platelets is only a minor problem with aspirin and ticlopidine (although the ability of aspirin to cause serious GI bleeding through local irritation is well known) and is never seen with dipyridamole.

Aspirin

Aspirin blocks thromboxane production by irreversibly inactivating platelet cyclo-oxygenase. Through its effect on thromboxane production, aspirin prevents the secondary wave of aggregation undergone by platelets responding to primary stimuli. Its use as an antiplatelet agent is based on this effect.

In very high doses, aspirin blocks the production of prostacyclin, a natural inhibitor of platelet aggregation, by inactivating the cyclo-oxygenase of the vascular endothelium. In the absence of prostacyclin, platelet aggregation is extremely efficient—enough to more than off-set the direct effect of aspirin on the platelets. Theoretically, then, high doses of aspirin would have an effect diametrically opposed to that desired—that is, the drug would act to promote platelet aggregation, not inhibit it. However, doses of aspirin sufficient to achieve this reversed effect are not used in practice.

Other Agents

DIPYRIDAMOLE

The function of platelets is controlled in part by the internal concentration of cyclic adenosine monophosphate (cAMP), which acts as a general suppressant of platelet function, inhibiting aggregation and release. AMP, made from adenosine triphosphate (ATP) by adenyl cyclase, is destroyed by phosphodiesterase in a ring-opening reaction that converts the cyclic nucleotide to AMP (Fig. 16-7). Dipyridamole interferes with platelet function by inhibiting phosphodiesterase, causing cAMP to build up in the platelet.

TICLOPIDINE

Ticlopidine blocks the response of platelets to adenosine diphosphate (ADP) and collagen. Like aspirin, it acts irreversibly. Its mechanism of action is unknown. It is a clinically useful antiplatelet agent, but it causes severe neutropenia in a small number of patients. Fortunately, the neutropenia corrects itself when the drug is discontinued.

INDICATIONS FOR TREATMENT

Venous thrombosis and pulmonary embolism are the most frequent indications for

Table 16-4. Antiplatelet Agents

Agent	Effect	Mechanism of Action
Aspirin	Decreased thromboxane production	Inactivation of cyclo-oxygenase (*ir*reversible)
Dipyridamole	Increased cAMP	Inhibition of phosphodiesterase
Ticlopidine	Increased cAMP	Blocks ADP receptor-dependent signal
	Decreased fibrinogen binding	transduction

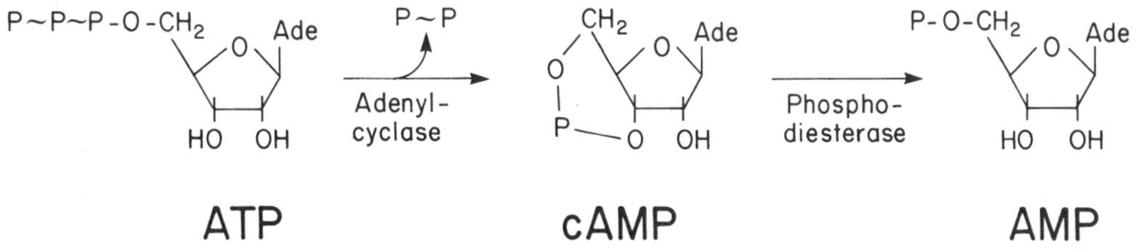

Fig. 16-7. Cyclic AMP metabolism. For the sake of clarity, some phosphate-bound oxygen atoms have been omitted.

anticoagulant treatment (Table 16-5). Because they are so subtle, so often difficult to diagnose, and especially because they are so common, they will be discussed more fully than the other indications for anticoagulation.

Thrombosis and Embolism

VENOUS THROMBOSIS

Venous thrombosis usually involves the veins of the legs and pelvis. It occurs most often when there is stasis of blood in the veins—notably, in pregnant women and in patients placed at bed rest. The likelihood of this event is increased if the patient has had a recent operation or suffers from congestive heart failure or any of the conditions associated with chronic disseminated intravascular coagulation (DIC). In addition, there are certain uncommon diseases, almost all hematologic, in which venous thrombosis may be a major problem. All these conditions that predispose to venous thrombosis are said to induce a "hypercoagulable state."

The diagnosis of venous thrombosis is difficult to make on clinical grounds. The leg on the affected side may ache and swell, and there may be tenderness over the course of the vein, but these symptoms are seen in other conditions as well. Moreover, venous thrombosis often occurs without any clinical manifestations whatsoever. It is therefore important to be able to make the diagnosis by more accurate techniques.

A screening test that may help select patients for further diagnostic studies is the *plasma D-D dimer* level. In a patient with venous thrombosis, the clot is under constant attack by plasmin, which releases D-D dimers continuously into the plasma as it attempts to dissolve the clot. A high plasma D-D dimer level does not necessarily mean venous thrombosis, however, because D-D dimers also arise from other sources. On the other hand, a low D-D dimer level is strong evidence against

---

UNCOMMON CAUSES OF A HYPERCOAGULABLE STATE

Coagulation disorders
    Antithrombin III deficiency
    Protein C deficiency
    Protein S deficiency
    Abnormal plasminogen
    Defective release of plasminogen activator
    Dysfibrinogenemia

Stem cell diseases
    Polycythemia vera
    Essential thrombocythemia
    Thrombocythemia secondary to myelofibrosis or chronic myelogenous leukemia
    Paroxysmal nocturnal hemoglobinuria

Vessel wall disease
    Homocystinuria

Table 16-5. Indications for Anticoagulants and Antiplatelet Drugs

	Full-Dose Anticoagulation	Low-Dose Warfarin	Antiplatelet agents	Low-Dose Heparin	Fibrinolytic Agents
Prophylactic					
Against arterial thrombosis					
Postmyocardial infarction			+		
Postcerebrovascular thrombosis			+		
Saphenous vein bypass grafts			+		
Against arterial embolism			+		
Valves and grafts	+		+ (mechanical)		
Against venous thrombosis					
Patients put to bed				+	
Before chest or abdominal surgery				+	
Broken hip or before hip surgery	+				
Therapeutic					
Venous thrombosis and pulmonary embolism	+				
Arterial embolism	+ (old)				+ (fresh)
Atherosclerosis					
Myocardial infarction	+ (new)		+ (old)		+ (new)
Unstable angina			+		
Stroke-in-evolution	+				
Transient ischemic attacks			+ (aspirin)		
Thrombocytosis			+ (?)		
Atrial fibrillation		+			

venous thrombosis, and suggests that the patient may not require further investigation.

A number of methods (described below) are available to establish the diagnosis of venous thrombosis (Fig. 16-8).

Venography

In venography, radiography is used to visualize obstructed vessels after the injection of a radiopaque dye into the veins of the legs. This procedure is the surest way to diagnose venous thrombosis, but it is an invasive technique, and may sometimes be complicated by thrombosis of a previously normal vein.

^{125}I-Fibrinogen Scanning

When given intravenously to a patient with ongoing venous thrombosis, ^{125}I-fibrinogen will be incorporated into the clot, where it can be detected by external radiation monitoring. This is a less invasive procedure than venography and is commonly used in some areas of the world to diagnose venous thrombosis. Its disadvantages are that (1) it takes about 3 days for enough radioactivity to be incorporated so the clot can be seen by external monitoring and (2)

it is unreliable in picking up clots in the deep veins of the pelvis and thigh, although it is quite accurate for calf vein thrombosis.

Impedance Plethysmography

In impedance plethysmography, the leg is made to fill with excess blood by occluding the veins of the upper thigh through the use of an inflatable cuff. The cuff is then abruptly deflated, and the rate at which the excess blood drains from the leg is determined by measuring the rate of fall in the volume of the engorged leg as it returns to its original size, using the electrical resistance across the leg (i.e., the impedance) as the volume indicator. This method is best for detecting obstructing thrombi in the large veins of the thigh and pelvis; it is not reliable for calf vein thrombosis.

Doppler Ultrasound

High-frequency sound (ultrasound) may be used to determine whether blood is flowing in a vein. A beam of ultrasound is aimed at the vein, causing some of the sound to be reflected from the red cells in the vein as an echo. If the red cells are moving, the pitch of the echo will

Venography

^{125}I - fibrinogen
scanning

Impedance
plethysmography

Doppler
ultrasound

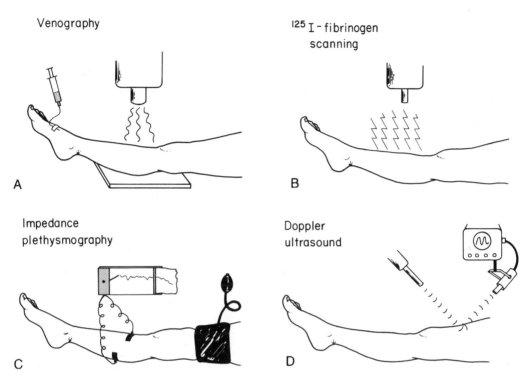

Fig. 16-8. Methods of diagnosing venous thrombosis. (**A**) Venography. Veins are visualized by radiography after the intravenous injection of a radiopaque dye. (**B**) ^{125}I-fibrinogen scanning. ^{125}I-fibrinogen taken up into a clot is detected by external radiation monitoring. (**C**) Impedence plethysmography. When the cuff is inflated, venous drainage from the leg is blocked, causing the leg to swell as it fills with excess blood. Deflation of the cuff permits excess blood to drain off, restoring the leg to its original size. The rate at which the leg returns to its original size is measured electrically. (**D**) Doppler ultrasound. A beam of ultrasound is directed at the vein in the leg. The pitch of the echo from the beam indicates whether blood is flowing through the vein.

be different from that of the original beam because of the Doppler effect (the same effect that causes the pitch of a locomotive whistle to drop as the train passes). If, however, the red cells are at rest because of a clot in the vein, the beam and the echo will have the same pitch. Like impedance plethysmography, the ultrasound test is sensitive to thrombi in the large veins of the thigh and pelvis, but cannot pick up calf vein thrombi.

PULMONARY EMBOLISM

The real danger posed by a clot in the veins of the leg or pelvis is that a piece of the clot can break away from its original mooring, travel to the lungs, and lodge there as a plug in the pulmonary circulation. A piece of clot that breaks loose in this way is known as an *embolus*, and the occlusion of a pulmonary vessel by such a piece of clot is called *pulmonary embolism*.

The symptoms of pulmonary embolism usually begin abruptly, and include various combinations of cough, chest pain, and breathlessness. A large embolus blocking both main branches of the pulmonary artery (a so-called saddle embolus) will cause acute, crushing chest pain like that of a heart attack and can prove fatal within minutes unless treated immediately. A smaller embolus can present with cough, shortness of breath, or both; if small enough, it may cause no symptoms at all. If an embolus affects a region of the lung whose blood supply is already impaired, it can cause the death of a segment of lung tissue (pulmonary infarction). Symptoms in this case are hemoptysis and "pleuritic" chest pain (i.e., pain aggravated by respiration, attributable to inflammation of the pleura overlying the dead lung). Chronic recurrent pulmonary emboli can lead to pulmonary hypertension and ultimately right heart failure.

Like the diagnosis of venous thrombosis, the diagnosis of pulmonary embolism must be established by special tests.

Ventilation/Perfusion Lung Scan

The lung scan shows the distribution of blood and air in the lungs. Both are determined by giving the patient a suitable radioactive tracer and then measuring the distribution of the radioactivity in the lungs with a scanning device. To look at the distribution of blood, ^{125}I-labeled aggregated albumin given by vein is often used as a tracer; the distribution of air is determined with ^{133}Xe given by inhalation. Certain abnormalities in the distribution patterns will indicate a high likelihood of pulmonary embolism.

Pulmonary Angiography

In pulmonary angiography, the pulmonary blood supply is directly visualized by radiography after the injection of a radiopaque dye into the pulmonary artery through a right heart catheter. The presence of cut-off vessels (Fig. 16-9) is virtually diagnostic of pulmonary embolism. Pulmonary angiography is much less dangerous than it sounds and is frequently used to establish the diagnosis of pulmonary embolism with certainty before committing a patient to a hazardous course of anticoagulant therapy.

TREATMENT

Once the diagnosis of venous thrombosis or pulmonary embolism is made, anticoagulant treatment is started. As a general rule, patients are begun on heparin (or, less frequently, fibri-

nolytic drugs followed by heparin), and then switched to a vitamin K antagonist after 7 to 10 days. Treatment with a vitamin K antagonist is continued for 3 months or so, and then stopped, unless the patient is particularly at risk for recurrent venous thrombosis. In that case, anticoagulation should be continued indefinitely.

Other Indications

ARTERIAL EMBOLISM

Arterial embolism (i.e., obstruction of an artery by a clot that has traveled there from somewhere else) is always an indication for anticoagulation. If the embolus is fresh, fibrinolytic agents should be used. Otherwise, treatment is similar to that used for pulmonary embolism. If the patient has an underlying condition that is regularly associated with arterial embolism—for example, a mechanical heart valve, or chronic atrial fibrillation from any cause—prophylactic anticoagulation should be

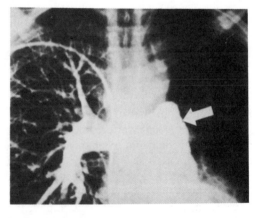

Fig. 16-9. Pulmonary angiogram showing cut-off left pulmonary artery (*arrow*). A column of dye that should normally fill that artery and its branches is abruptly blocked by an embolic plug located at the point of the cut-off. This x-ray finding is virtually diagnostic of pulmonary embolism. (From Shuck JW, Walder JS, Kam TH, Thomas HM [1980] Chronic persistent pulmonary embolism: Report of three cases. Am J Med 69:790, with permission.)

started with a vitamin K antagonist for an indefinite period to prevent the first episode of embolism from occurring. For bioprosthetic heart valves, 3 months of anticoagulation with moderate-dose warfarin is enough.

FRACTURED HIP AND HIP SURGERY

Venous thrombosis and pulmonary embolism are especially common in patients who have fractured their hips or who require hip surgery. These patients should be anticoagulated with moderate-dose warfarin (INR 2 to 3 times normal) or heparin during their convalescence.

LOW-DOSE HEPARIN

Low-dose heparin is an unusually benign method for preventing venous thrombosis that should be considered in all patients at risk of developing this condition. Examples are patients about to undergo chest or abdominal surgery and patients on bed rest because of chronic heart failure or malignancy.

ATHEROSCLEROTIC HEART DISEASE OR CEREBROVASCULAR DISEASE

Whether to anticoagulate patients for angina, heart attacks, or strokes has been a vexed question since anticoagulants were first introduced into medical practice. Opinion has cycled over the years, depending on the results of the most current studies. Very large scale clinical trials, however, are just now beginning to provide some reasonably firm answers to these difficult questions. Currently there appears to be no indication for heparin or vitamin K antagonists in any form of atherosclerotic disease affecting the brain, except perhaps in stroke-in-evolution. In myocardial infarction, treatment with low-dose heparin is now recommended unless the risk of embolism is high (e.g., in a patient with atrial fibrillation); in these patients, moderate-dose warfarin anticoagulation is used. Further recommendations will depend on the results of future clinical trials.

Antiplatelet Drugs

THROMBOCYTOSIS

Intravascular clotting is a problem when there are too many platelets in the circulation, particularly if the platelets are functionally abnormal. Antiplatelet agents are often given to control clotting in thrombocytosis. Evidence as to their effectiveness is scanty, but their use under these conditions constitutes a valid approach to therapy.

BLOOD VESSEL GRAFTS

Clots will always form on blood vessel grafts, with arterial embolism as the inevitable sequel, unless patients with such grafts are anticoagulated prophylactically. Arterial grafts are kept open with aspirin or coumadin, depending on the size of the artery. Saphenous vein bypass grafts are kept open with aspirin plus dipyridamole, and atrioventricular shunts with aspirin alone.

ATHEROSCLEROTIC HEART DISEASE OR CEREBROVASCULAR DISEASE

Antiplatelet agents have been studied as intensively as anticoagulants to find a role for them in the treatment of heart attacks and strokes. These studies show that aspirin is useful in cerebrovascular disease to reduce the frequency of attacks and prevent full-blown strokes in patients who suffer from so-called transient ischemic attacks (i.e., brief episodes of neurologic symptoms caused by atherosclerosis of the blood vessels that supply the brain) and that ticlopidine reduces the likelihood of second strokes in patients with prior cerebral thrombosis. In coronary artery disease, antiplatelet agents (1) are useful in unstable angina and (2) will reduce the mortality rate after a heart attack. Beyond these limited indications, no other use has yet been found for antiplatelet agents in managing the complications of atherosclerosis.

PREVENTION OF ATHEROSCLEROSIS

The role postulated for platelets in the development of atherosclerosis has raised considerable interest in the possibility that antiplatelet drugs might be useful in preventing this disease. Despite the claims of certain widely publicized studies, however, the answer to this question is not clear. While aspirin may well turn out to be an effective prophylaxis against heart attacks, it remains to be seen whether this benefit will result in an increased life expectancy, or offset the dangers of acute GI bleeding in patients on chronic aspirin therapy.

SUGGESTED READINGS

ACCP-Third Consensus Conference on Antithrombotic Therapy (1986) Chest 102:303

Bauer KA, Rosenberg RD (1987) The pathophysiology of the prethrombotic state in humans: insights gained from studies using markers of hemostatic system activation. Blood 70:343

Bell WR, Meek AG (1979) Guidelines for the use of thrombolytic agents. N Engl J Med 301:1266

Bern MM (1992) Considerations for using lower doses of warfarin. Hematol Oncol Clin North Am 6:1105

Boisclair MD, Ireland H, Lane DA (1990) Assessment of hypercoagulable states by measurement of activation fragments and peptides. Blood Rev 4:25

Brozovic M (1976) Oral anticoagulants, vitamin K and prothrombin complex factors. Br J Haematol 32:9

Brozovic M (1978) Oral anticoagulants in clinical practice. Semin Haematol 15:27

Clin Hematol (1981) v 10 (2) Thrombosis

Collen D, Lijnen HR (1991) Basic and clinical aspects of fibrinolysis and thrombolysis. Blood 78:3114

Coller BS (1990) Platelets and thrombolytic therapy [see comments] N Engl J Med 322:33

Graham DY, Smith JL (1986) Aspirin and the stomach. Annu Rev Med 104:390

Greaves M, Preston FE (1991) The hypercoagulable state in clinical practice. Br J Haematol 79:148

Hirsh J (1981) Blood tests for the diagnosis of venous and arterial thrombosis. Blood 57:1

Hirsh J (1991) Heparin. N Engl J Med 324:1565

Hirsh J (1991) Oral anticoagulant drugs. N Engl J Med 324:1865

Hirsh J, Levine MN (1992) Low molecular weight heparin. Blood 79:1

Hirsh J, Dalen JE, Fuster V et al (1992) Aspirin and other platelet-active drugs. The relationship between dose, effectiveness, and side effects. Chest 102(suppl.4): 327S

Hull R, Hirsh J (1981) Advances and controversies in the diagnosis, prevention and treatment of venous thromboembolism. Progr Hematol 12:73

Kelton JG, Hirsh J (1980) Bleeding associated with antithrombotic therapy. Semin Hematol 17:259

Koller RL (1991) Prevention of recurrent ischemic stroke. Postgrad Med 90:81, 89, 93

Lewis SM (1987) Thromboplastin and oral anticoagulant control. Br J Haematol 66:1

Marder V (1979) The use of thrombolytic agents: choice of patient, drug administration, laboratory monitoring. Ann Intern Med 90:802

Oates JA, Wood AJJ, FitzGerald GA (1987) Drug therapy. Dipyridamole. N Engl J Med 316:1247

Preston FE (1985) Platelet suppressive therapy in clinical medicine. Br J Haematol 60:589

Prog Cardiovasc Dis (1972) 21(4 and 5). Fibrinolysis

Rosenberg RD (1977) Biologic actions of heparin. Semin Hematol 14:427

Sasahara AA, St Martin CC, Henkin J, Barker WM (1992) Approach to the patient with venous thromboembolism. Treatment with thrombolytic agents. Hematol Oncol Clin North Am 6:1141

Schaefer AI, Handin RI (1980) The role of platelets in thrombotic and vascular disease. Progr Cardiovasc Dis 22:31

Schafer AI (1985) The hypercoagulable states. Ann Intern Med 102:814

Sharma GVRK, Cella G, Parisi A et al (1982) Drug therapy: thrombolytic therapy. N Engl J Med 306:1268

Ticlopidine [editorial] (1991) Lancet 337:459

Verstraete M, Collen D (1986) Thrombolytic therapy in the eighties. Blood 67:1529

Verstraete M (1978) Biochemical and clinical aspects of thrombolysis. Semin Hematol 15:35

Warkentin TE, Kelton JG (1990) Heparin and platelets. Hematol Oncol Clin North Am 4:243

Webster MW, Chesebro JH, Fuster V (1990) Platelet inhibitor therapy. Agents and clinical implications. Hematol Oncol Clin North Am 4:265

Wessler S, Gitel SN (1979) Heparin: new concepts relevant to clinical use. Blood 53:525

Willard JE, Lange RA, Hillis LD (1992) The use of aspirin in ischemic heart disease. N Engl J Med 327:175

Section III

White Blood Cells and Their Diseases

Although white blood cells are no whiter than any other unpigmented tissue cells, the term *white cell* was concocted by nineteenth century microscopists to distinguish these actually colorless cells from the red-tinted erythrocytes. The blood contains three principal types of white blood cells: the polymorphonuclear leukocytes, the monocytes, and the lymphocytes. These white cells or leukocytes arise from pluripotent stem cells in the bone marrow (Ch. 1) and differentiate into those forms that are easily distinguished and different numbers of which circulate in the blood (Table III-1). Each type has a very different life history, function, and fate. The enumeration of leukocytes, usually called the *white blood cell count*, is one of the most frequently obtained laboratory values in medicine, because it is extremely informative as to the state of health of the host. The total white blood cell count is determined automatically by means of an electronic counter in most laboratories in the United States. The differential count, which identifies the different blood cell types, is usually done by an examination of Wright's stained smears, although automated counters for this purpose are now available. The physician obtaining a white blood cell count and differential count receives a report of (1) the white blood cell count in cells per microliter (µl) or, as sometimes stated, per cubic millimeter (mm^3) and (2) the percentage differential of the total of each white blood cell type. A convention being promoted for expressing loboratory values in medicine, known as the *SI system* (International System of Units; le Systéme International d'Unites), recommends that the number of white blood cells be expressed as cells per liter and that the *fraction* rather than the *percentage* of blood cells be enumerated. In other words, 5,000 white blood cells per microliter becomes 5×10^9 cells/L, 50 percent neutrophils becomes 0.5 neutrophils, or 3 percent eosinophils becomes 0.03 eosinophils.

Table III-1. Numbers of White Blood Cells in Normal Blood

Total white blood cells	4,500–11,000/μl
Band-form (immature) neutrophilic polymorphonuclear leukocytes	3%
Segmented (mature) neutrophilic polymorphonuclear leukocytes	40–70%
Lymphocytes	25–45%
Eosinophilic polymorphonuclear leukocytes	3%
Basophilic polymorphonuclear leukocytes	0.5%
Monocytes	4%

The principal known function of white blood cells is in defending the organism against microbes. In this activity, the white blood cells are deployed in two major categories: the phagocytes and the lymphocytes. To defend against infection, there is considerable cooperation between these classes of white blood cells.

DEFINITIONS

Some of the terms used to describe white blood cell abnormalities over the years arose when white blood cell physiology and pathophysiology were not as well understood as today, so that some of the names are now not accurately descriptive, creating the potential for confusion. Some of the terms are highlighted here to help alleviate the confusion.

Leukocytosis: increased number of circulating white blood cells. *Neutrophilic leukocytosis* refers to a specific elevation in the number of neutrophils; *monocytosis, lymphocytosis, eosinophilia*, and *basophilia* refer to increases in the numbers of monocytes, lymphocytes, eosinophils, and basophils, respectively.

Leukopenia: decreased number of circulating white blood cells. *Neutropenia, monocytopenia, lymphopenia*, and *eosinopenia* indicate reductions in neutrophils, monocytes, lymphocytes, or eosinophils, respectively. Severe neutropenia is also designated *agranulocytosis*.

Mononucleosis: a group of usually self-limited diseases caused by viruses in which morphologically abnormal white blood cells appear in the circulation (Ch. 19). These cells are actually *atypical lymphocytes*, and the term "mononucleosis" is meaningless.

17

Immunoproteins and Immunoprotein Disorders

IMMUNOPROTEINS: PLASMA PROTEINS IMPORTANT TO THE PHAGOCYTIC AND LYMPHOID SYSTEMS

A chapter describing the plasma immunoproteins is interpolated at this point in the section on white blood cells for two reasons. First, the major class of circulating immunoproteins, the immunoglobulins, is produced by a set of lymphoid cells, the plasma cells. Other lymphocytes produce but do not secrete immunoglobulins, and the production and disposition of immunoglobulins by lymphocytes is intimately linked to their state of differentiation. Therefore, a comprehension of the stucture and function of immunoglobulins aids considerably in understanding lymphoid cell development. Second, the cells of the phagocytic and lymphoid systems depend to a large extent on recognition mechanisms that help them identify and respond to foreign invasion. In large measure, this surveillance is mediated by circulating immunoproteins. These proteins are remarkably versatile in that they can be involved simultaneously with white blood cells and pathogens.

Normal Structure and Function of the Immunoproteins

IMMUNOGLOBULINS

Immunoglobulins, or antibodies, are a class of proteins of very similar structure that are secreted by plasma cells. The composition of all normal immunoglobulins is an assembly of two pairs of polypeptides; two larger ones are called *heavy chains*, and two smaller ones are designated *light chains* (Fig. 17-1). Disulfide bonds connect the heavy chains to each other, and each heavy chain to one light chain. Despite the general similarity in the structure of immunoglobulins (Igs), small differences in the amino acid sequences of the heavy chains create important variations in the function of the immunoglobulins in their specific interactions with the immune system. These variations determine five classes of heavy chains, designated μ, γ, α, δ, and ε, which comprise immunoglobulins classified as IgM, IgG, IgA, IgD, and IgE, respectively (Fig. 17-2). Similar small differences in the amino acid sequences of the light chains define two classes called κ and λ. The importance of κ and λ light chains in immune functions is unknown, but as amplified in Chapter 19, they are highly relevant for defining an origin of immunoglobulins from a single clone of lymphoid cells and for diagnosing certain neoplasms of lymphoid cells.

Alterations in the primary structure of the heavy chains and light chains near the region of the immunoglobulin where the heavy chains and light chains overlap confer the most remarkable feature on the immunoglobulins—their incredibly specific binding to all sorts and conditions of substances, which become defined as antigens. The domains in which the binding to antigen takes place is known as the *Fab region*. Bound to antigens by their Fab sites, the class of heavy chain and the opposite end of the immunoglobulins called the *Fc region* determine what will happen to the antigen–antibody complex (Fig. 17-1). The very similar amino acid sequences of about one-half the light chains and heavy chains in the Fab region and all the Fc region define what is called the *constant domains* of immunoglobulin molecules (shaded area, Fig. 17-1). The specificity for antigens arises from very different amino acid sequences in the other half of the Fab regions of the light chains and heavy chains, denoted as the variable domains. Most of the differences are clustered into four sequences of the variable regions, called the *hypervariable domains*. These combinations and permutations of amino acid sequences modify the final folding of the Fab region of the immunoglobulin molecule sufficiently to confer the exquisite specificity for antigen-binding characteristic of antibody molecules. How immunoglobulins are synthesized and how their antigen binding specificity is achieved are explained in Chapter 19.

Immunoglobulins are found in all protein-containing internal body fluids. External secretions, such as tears, saliva, and gut fluids, contain principally immunoglobulin A (IgA) because of a unique carbohydrate-containing sequence called *secretory piece* that enables the immunoglobulin to be secreted. The function of secretory IgA is not known with certainty. IgG and IgA, but not IgM, cross the placenta. Therefore, newborns have maternal IgG and IgA in their plasma, but not IgM. On the other hand, IgM is made by newborns before they have the capacity to produce IgA or IgG.

The catabolism of immunoglobulins is proportional to their concentration in the plasma. Therefore, persons with high concentrations of immunoglobulins in their plasma degrade these

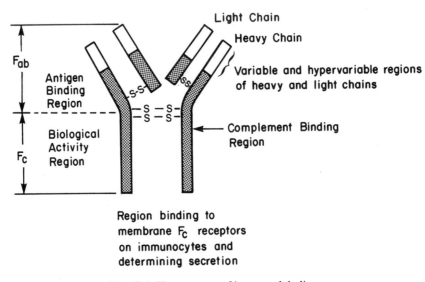

Fab

Antigen
Binding
Region

Biological
Activity
Region

Fc

Light Chain

Heavy Chain

Variable and hypervariable regions
of heavy and light chains

Complement Binding
Region

Region binding to
membrane F$_c$ receptors
on immunocytes and
determining secretion

Fig. 17-1. The structure of immunoglobulin.

Class	Heavy Chain Class	Serum Concentration mg/ml	Structure		Major Functions
IgG	γ	12	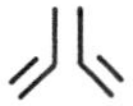	Monomer	Antitoxin Virus neutralization Opsonization
IgA	α	3	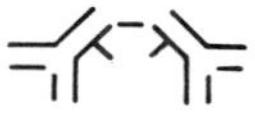	Dimer, joined by "J-chain"	Immune functions in Secretions ? Prevent attachment of pathogens to mucosal surface
IgM	μ	1	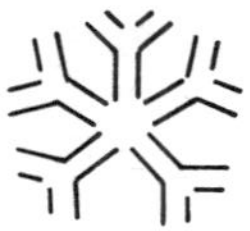	Pentamer	Complement activation Agglutination reactions
IgD	δ	0.03	B-cell membrane	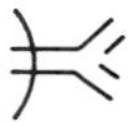 Monomer	Unknown
IgE	ϵ	0.0001	Mast cell & Basophil membrane	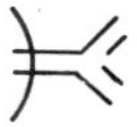 Cell bound "Cytophilic"	Mediator release

Divided into subclasses IgG$_1$ - IgG$_4$ with different participation in these functions

Fig. 17-2. Classes of immunoglobulin.

molecules more rapidly than do those with low concentrations of the proteins.

COMPLEMENT

At least 20 proteins make up the *complement system* (Fig. 17-3); most of the proteins are designated by a number preceded by the capital letter C. Complement resembles the coagulation system (Ch. 13) in that it operates as a cascade, wherein proteins become sequentially activated. The consequences of activation of parts of the cascade are directed, like antibody, toward conferring recognition on foreign objects so they can be dealt with by white blood cells or, in some cases, even to cause the lysis of the foreign cells. In certain circumstances, immunoglobulin antibodies cause the initial activation of the complement system (Fig. 17-3A). In such instances, antibody provides recognition, whereas complement generates or amplifies the effector response initiated by the recognition with antibody.

The Fc region of certain immunoglobulins bound to an antigen that usually is on a cell surface binds C1, which is actually a complex of protein subunits. The assembly of the C1 complex on the cell surface activates an enzymatic activity in the C1 complex called *esterase* of the C1 protein. This enzyme catalyzes the splitting of the C2 and C4 complement components into fragments. Pieces of C2 and C4 called C2b and C4b bind to the cell surface. C3 is the complement protein found in highest concentration in the blood. The C4b–C2b complex, known as the *classic pathway C3 convertase*, binds and splits C3 into fragments called C3a and C3b. C3a leaves the site at which it was cleaved, but it has the capacity to cause contraction of smooth muscle and to increase permeability, rendering it a mediator of inflammation. C3b bound to the cell surface is recognized by phagocytes and can cause phagocytosis or destruction of the cell to which it is bound by phagocytic cells. Of chemical interest in the binding of C3 to target objects is the fact that C3 cleavage results in the exposure of a previously buried cysteinyl

sulfydryl group esterified to a nearby glutamate residue and the scission of this internal thioester linkage. The exposed glutamate then becomes covalently linked by a transacylation reaction to a hydroxyl or amino group on the target surface.

C3b is also an initiator of a more primitive limb of the complement pathway, the *alternative pathway* (historically known as the properdin system; Fig. 17-3B). In this system, proteins called *factor B* and *factor D*, which are similar to C2 and C4, enter the complement sequence without a requirement for antibodies. These and other alternative pathway proteins complete a loop by eventually binding and cleaving C3. The surfaces of microorganisms such as the lipopolysaccharide that is the endotoxin of gram-negative bacteria, yeast cell walls, and membranes of certain mammalian cells, especially after damage or alteration in various diseases, bind the components of the alternative pathway that cause the fixation of C3, the alternative pathway C3 convertase. C3b binds and cleaves C5 to C5a and C5b. The former is a potent chemotactic factor for attracting phagocytic cells. The latter reacts with the rest of the complement components, C6–C9. The C6–C9 aggregate can punch holes in membranes of susceptible cells; it is called the *lytic* or *membrane attack complex*. The actual lytic agent is a circular polymer of C9 molecules the assembly of which forms a pore, 10 nm in diameter, in the target cell plasma membrane.

Complement components are found in most protein-containing body fluids. The major source of plasma C3 is synthesis by hepatocytes. The origin of other circulating complement proteins is not entirely certain, but macrophages are capable of synthesizing many of them.

To counteract the possibility of uncontrolled complement activation, the plasma contains inhibitor proteins that block the complement sequence at various control points. Acting as dampers, these inhibitors prevent low levels of complement activation when the inciting stimulus is small, but do not stop activation by strong stimuli.

An inhibitor of C1 esterase prevents the cleavage of C1. Persons who are genetically deficient in C1 esterase suffer from recurrent attacks of edema (hereditary angioneurotic edema). Two other proteins, factors H and 1, respectively, act to dissociate activated factor B from C3b, thereby inhibiting the autocatalytic feedback loop that initiates the alternative pathway of complement activation. The decay of the alternative pathway C3-converting complex is also enhanced by a molecule on the surface of target cells called *decay-accelerating factor* or *DAF*. DAF is interesting because it is one of a class of surface membrane proteins anchored

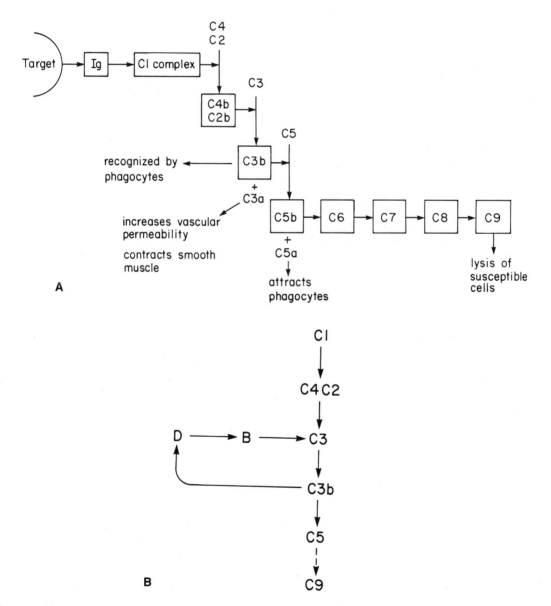

Fig. 17-3. (A) Classic complement sequence. Components within boxes remain entirely or partly attached to the target cell surface. **(B)** Alternative complement pathway and its relationship to the classic sequence.

to the lipid bilayer through a sugar–inositol linkage and because its deficiency contributes to the pathogenesis of a blood disease called paroxysmal nocturnal hemoglobinuria (Ch. 22). In addition to dissociating the C3 convertase, H and I promote the sequential degradation of C3b to a number of fragments called iC3b, C3c, and C3d. Phagocytes and lymphocytes, respectively, have surface receptors that bind objects to which iC3b and C3d are affixed. Deficient expression of a receptor for iC3b is the cause of a genetic disorder (Ch. 18). C3c is released from the surface of the target cell and has no known functional significance. The plasma antiproteases and a plasma carboxypeptidase inhibit the action of the complement chemotactic factor, C5a. Another inhibitor, known as *protein S* (a different protein S than the vitamin-K-dependent protein S that is a component of the coagulation system!), binds to C6, preventing binding of C7, and therefore the completion of the formation of a lytic complex. In addition, there is a C8-binding protein that inhibits the contribution of this C component to lytic activity.

Measurement of Plasma Immunoproteins

COMPLEMENT

In the clinical setting, blood complement components are commonly assayed by two techniques. The first is a functional test for the entire sequence of components C1–C9 that measures the capacity of the system to lyse susceptible cells. Sheep red cells are coated with IgM antibody and reacted with a test serum; the quantity of hemoglobin released from the red cells after a suitable incubation period is then determined. This release of hemoglobin depends on the entire complement sequence being activated and producing lysis of the cell; this assay can be standardized in various ways. Usually the quantity of serum required to lyse 50 percent of the erythrocytes is measured, and the result is reported as CH_{50} units. This test serves as a screening assay for reductions in the levels of one or more compo-

nents of the complement sequence. It is also possible to measure levels of certain complement components immunochemically as described for immunoglobulins.

IMMUNOGLOBULINS

The concentration of immunoglobulins can be measured immunochemically by using specific antibodies directed against them. The immunochemical measurement of the immunoglobulin concentration is determined by the density of precipitate formed in mixtures of test serum and specific antibody.

The concentration of plasma immunoglobulin, and of certain other plasma proteins, can also be assayed by the electrophoretic technique, *protein electrophoresis*. For convenience, blood is permitted to clot, and the serum rather than plasma is analyzed. Serum is placed in a narrow strip on a porous matrix, such as paper or an agar gel, and then subjected to an electrical field. The proteins migrate in the electrical field according to their net charge. After an appropriate time, the matrix is fixed and stained, enabling the position of the separated proteins to be visualized (Fig. 17-4A). Albumin is well separated from the more cationic serum proteins collectively called *globulins*. The globulin fraction of plasma is further classified into α, β, and γ regions on the basis of distance migrated (Fig. 17-4A). Immunoglobulins migrate in the γ range and are referred to as γ-globulins, although not all γ-globulins are immunoglobulins.

From the information gained by electrophoresis of purified proteins, the position of normal serum protein components is known. The relative concentrations of the components can be quantified by shining a light through the matrix as it moves across a photometer. The stained regions absorb light in proportion to the amount of protein present, and the changes in absorbance of light by the stain are charted on a strip recorder (Fig. 17-4A). The total protein in the serum can be measured chemically, allowing its absolute quantity to be determined. For example, if the total protein is 6 g/dl and the albumin is 60 percent of the density of the

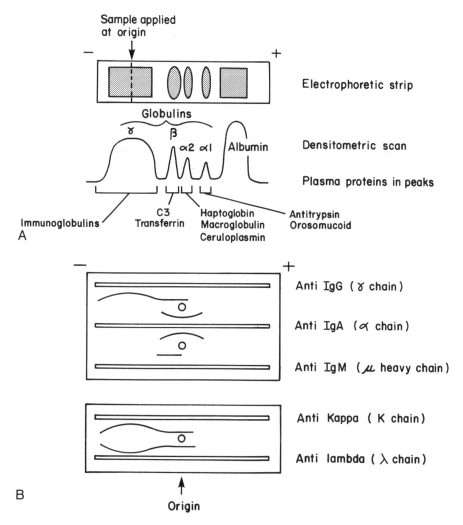

Fig. 17-4. (**A**) Serum protein electrophoresis. (**B**) Immunoelectrophoresis. Serum samples are put in wells at the origin, subjected to electrophoresis, and then allowed to diffuse toward specific antibodies added to the troughs. The arcs indicate the position of precipitin reactions.

scan, the albumin concentration in the sample is 3.6 g/dl.

Immunoglobulins in an electrophoretic field remain as a diffuse band near the negative electrode and even move in the opposite direction, as demonstrated schematically in Figure 17-4A. This finding indicates that immunoglobulins tend to have a relative net positive charge. Figure 17-4A also shows that the immunoglobulins form a broad band in comparison with other components of the serum. This indicates that normal plasma contains a wide range of

antibodies with various specificities. The reason for this lack of homogeneity is the wide repertoire of primary structures of serum immunoglobulins programmed in the variable sequences of the normal immunoglobulin molecules.

This electrophoretic technique is only sensitive enough to detect the major serum protein classes; it does not discriminate among the different classes, subclasses, or subunits of immunoglobulins. To detect these entities, an immunological method, *immunoelectrophore-*

sis, is used. This technique combines the separate powers of electrophoresis with the specificity of antigen–antibody reactions. A serum sample is subjected to electrophoresis in an agar matrix and then reacted in a different direction against antibodies specific for components being sought, for example, an antibody class or a light chain type. The presence of a precipitin arc demonstrates the existence and electrophoretic mobility of the serum protein in question (Fig. 17-4B). Immunoelectrophoresis is sufficiently sensitive to distinguish the different antibody classes when whole serum is reacted against antibodies acting with whole serum. To achieve a better resolution, monospecific antibodies, raised in animals injected with purified proteins, are used. The resulting immunoelectrophoretic pattern is much simpler and easier to interpret quantitatively (Fig. 17-4B)

DISORDERS OF PLASMA PROTEINS

Reactive Changes in Plasma Proteins and Immunoproteins

In response to infection or inflammation, changes occur in the concentration of certain serum proteins. The magnitude of the variation is a function of the nature, intensity, and duration of the provocation. Proteins that alter their concentrations in this way have been named *acute-phase reactants.* Of the proteins mentioned in Chapter 1, haptoglobin, macroglobulin, ceruloplasmin, complement proteins, and immunoglobulins increase during inflammatory diseases. The concentration of the coagulation protein, fibrinogen, also rises. This protein is elongated in structure and has a tendency to coat red blood cells, causing them to clump. The clumped red cells settle rapidly when anticoagulated blood is left standing. This phenomenon is the basis of the long-known fact that the red cell sedimentation rate rises in inflammatory diseases.

The increased immunoglobulin levels may reach extremely high values, as much as four to five times the baseline normal concentrations. Examples of chronic infections or inflammatory diseases associated with hypergammaglobulinemia are listed in the box below. Occasionally the stress of these processes on the immunological system can lead to the expression of abnormal immunoproteins called *paraproteins,* as will be seen later in this chapter.

The changes in complement proteins vary, depending on the disease process. Chronic infections usually promote a moderate rise in the complement components. However, in disorders characterized by immune complex formation, for example, systemic lupus erythematosus (SLE), complement components can be consumed and their levels may actually fall if production does not keep up. In contrast to other acute-phase proteins, the concentration of transferrin falls during infection and inflammation (see also Ch. 4).

Paraproteins

A given immunoglobulin molecule is the product of a single clone of lymphocytes (Ch. 19). The many immunoglobulins in normal plasma and other body fluids reflect the production of numerous lymphoid clones.

SOME MANIFESTATIONS OF SYSTEMIC AMYLOIDOSIS

Peripheral neuropathy

Cardiomyopathy

Nephrotic syndrome

Purpura

Macroglossia

Polyarthropathy

Coagulation factor X deficiency

Therefore, normal serum immunoglobulins and hypergammaglobulinemia are said to be *polyclonal*. Under certain conditions, a single clone of immunoglobulin-producing cells can proliferate sufficiently to result in the accumulation of significant amounts of immunoglobulins with the identical primary sequence, constituting a paraprotein.

TYPES OF PARAPROTEINS

The monoclonal immunoglobulin detected by electrophoresis of the serum is a single band of protein in the diffuse γ-globulin region (Fig. 17-5); the paraprotein is called an *M component*, and when the M component is associated with disease, its presence defines a monoclonal gammopathy.

Further analysis of the M component by immunoelectrophoresis characterizes it as to its class of heavy chains and light chains (Fig. 17-5). The heavy chains may be of any class (i.e., μ, α, γ, δ, or ε), but the light chains of a given M component will be only either κ or λ. In some cases, the abnormal clone will produce only heavy chains, heavy chain fragments, or only light chains. The light chains, being of relatively low molecular weight, are filtered readily by the glomerulus, and enter the urine. The presence of immunoglobulin light chains in the urine has historically been called *Bence Jones proteinuria*. It is worth noting that Bence Jones protein in the urine is not detectable by commercial "dip-stix" used to screen the urine for albumin, but can be detected by heat coagulation or sulfosalicylic acid tests for urine protein. Sometimes the paraprotein will be present in small amounts, and it is necessary to concentrate the serum or urine in order to detect it.

M components made up of isolated heavy chains of the μ, γ, or α class or fragments thereof may migrate in an electrophoretic field to a region other than that characteristic of immunoglobulins. By the process of immunoelectrophoresis, the M component can be identified as being immunoglobulin by its immunological reaction in forming a precipitin line with anti-immunoglobulin of the appropriate class. However, the protein will not form a precipitin arc against anti-λ or anti-κ antibodies, indicating that only heavy-chain determinants and not light-chain sequences are present.

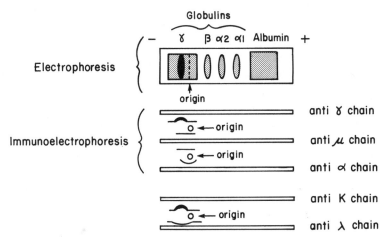

Fig. 17-5. Protein electrophoresis and immunoelectrophoresis of a paraprotein-containing serum. Protein electrophoresis shows M component in the γ region. Immunoelectrophoresis defines M component as having γ heavy chains and κ light chains. Paraprotein is therefore an IgG–K.

CAUSES OF PARAPROTEINS

An M component is often the product of a malignant neoplasm of the antibody-secreting cells. The lymphoid cell neoplasm most often associated with paraproteins is *multiple myeloma,* which is described in Chapter 29. Under these circumstances, the M component is present in fairly high concentrations, greater than 2 g/dl (or greater than 6 g/dl of Bence Jones protein in the urine). Its concentration increases with time, and there is other evidence of the underlying malignancy. In the setting of lymphoid neoplasms producing M components, the normal polyclonal immunoglobulin levels are often reduced.

M components can also appear in various inflammatory and degenerative immunologic disorders. In these situations, the balance of regulatory factors that ordinarily prevent any one clone of immune cells from expressing itself above the background of its fellows becomes deranged, and for some reason, a clone of antibody-forming cells becomes unusually active. M components are also found in a few apparently healthy persons. In this setting, the concentration of the M component is usually less than 1 g/dl (or less than 6 g/dl of Bence Jones protein in the urine), and the level remains constant with time. The incidence of this benign monoclonal gammopathy rises with age, reaching nearly 6 percent of the population of octogenarians and their older brethren. Most persons with such incidentally detected M components do not proceed to develop lymphoid neoplasms, but in slightly more than 10 percent of cases a malignant lymphoid disease does appear with time.

EFFECTS OF M COMPONENTS

Kidney Damage

Bence Jones proteins can accumulate in renal tubular cells. This accumulation may result in obstruction of the tubular lumen and can lead to necrosis of the tubular cells. In some cases, there is a selective preference for damage to proximal convoluted tubules, giving rise to amino aciduria, glucosuria, uricosuria, and phosphaturia. Light-chain deposition can also damage distal convoluted tubules, leading to acidosis and inability to concentrate the urine. Progressive necrosis of renal tissue can result in chronic renal failure. Kidney failure is a common complication of multiple myeloma (Ch. 29).

It is not clear why the toxicity of immunoglobulin light chains for the kidney varies so in its incidence and distribution of effect within the organ. Presumably, the differences in the primary structure of the different light chains account for this variability. Recently it was shown that infusion of human Bence Jones protein into rats led to renal lesions resembling the human nephropathy, raising the possibility that some insight into pathogenesis may be possible.

In addition to the direct toxicity of light chains for the kidneys, amyloidosis, a complication of paraprotein production, described in detail below, can produce renal damage.

Hyperviscosity Syndrome

The viscosity of the blood is determined by the concentrations of formed elements and of the plasma proteins. The molecular dimensions of normal immunoglobulin molecules are sufficiently small that they do not appreciably affect the flow properties of the blood. However, if the immunoglobulins aggregate, they can significantly impede blood flow. IgM, because it exists as a pentamer and therefore has the highest molecular weight, is the paraprotein most frequently associated with hyperviscosity syndrome (see Fig. 17-2). IgA molecules also have some tendency to aggregate, and therefore IgA paraproteins are sometimes also associated with hyperviscosity syndrome. IgM aggregates increase the viscosity of the blood to a marked degree, over five times that of normal plasma, when their concentration rises to levels of 5 to 8 g/dl. Once these levels are achieved, symptoms begin to appear.

The clinical effects of hyperviscosity are usually manifested by impaired blood flow to the brain. A patient with the hyperviscosity syndrome will complain of dizziness, loss of consciousness, and visual disturbances.

Ophthalmoscopic examination of the microcirculation in the retina can detect engorged vessels, dilated to form what are termed "sausages." A patient with a hyperviscosity syndrome may also have impaired circulation to the fingers and toes and may complain of numbness and coldness at the periphery of the extremities. The association of serum hyperviscosity with high serum IgM concentrations in the setting of a lymphoid neoplasm was first described by the Swedish hematologist Jan Waldenström; this entity continues to bear the designation macroglobulinemia of Waldenström. In nonneoplastic inflammatory or immunological disorders such as SLE, the increased concentration of polyclonal immunoglobulins can occasionally aggregate to produce a hyperviscosity syndrome.

Impaired Hemostasis

Paraproteins, especially IgM, can have deleterious effects on platelet function and on the actions of coagulation proteins, leading to hemorrhages of the skin and mucous membranes. The clinician may be able to see these hemorrhages as well as the dilated vessels on ophthalmoscopic examination of the retina.

Impaired Phagocyte Function

Paraproteins, especially IgA aggregates, interfere with the movement of wandering phagocytes. Immunoglobulin paraproteins have also been shown to bind to complement components, thereby impeding the activation of complement required for optimal phagocytic function.

Inflammation

The normal function of immunoglobulins and complement proteins is to confer the ability to recognize foreign substances as nonself, when appropriate, and to attract cells of the immune system to the foreign matter so these cells can kill, degrade, and eliminate pathogens. It is extremely unusual for paraproteins associated with lymphoid neoplasms to have true specificity for any particular sub-

stance. Insofar as paraproteins are products of disordered cellular machinery, that is, of malignant lymphoid cells, sometimes these immunoglobulins begin to react with normal proteins, as well as with each other. The abnormal immunoglobulins of the IgM class occasionally form complexes with IgG, a phenomenon seen in rheumatoid arthritis, in which case the IgM is designated a *rheumatoid factor*.

Paraproteins or aggregates of paraproteins and other proteins can react with complement components to initiate inappropriate inflammatory responses in the skin, kidney, blood vessels, or for that matter, anywhere. Occasionally, lowering of the temperature of the blood below the core body temperature of 37°C causes these reactions to occur. If the cooling produces a frank precipitate of plasma protein, a *cryoprecipitate* is said to be present, and the proteins in the precipitate are *cryoproteins*.

The structure of a paraprotein will determine its reactions with other components of the immune system. Because the possible permutations of structure of these proteins are so vast, the manifestations of cryoprotein states, such as immune complex disease, can be truly protean, ranging from none to a fulminant vasculitis. The paraproteins are not necessarily directed against known specific antigens, so these cryoprotein complexes need not be, strictly speaking, immune complexes, although they may be antibodies against the antigen-combining site of other immunoglobulins, so-called *anti-idiotype antibodies*. The M component can be detected by immunoelectrophoresis in such complexes, provided the various components in the complex can be appropriately dissolved. These autoaggressive inflammatory expressions of paraproteins arise most often in non-Hodgkin's lymphomas.

Paraproteins have been rarely the causes of unusual pathological effects. One patient with a lymphoid neoplasm developed yellow coloring of the skin and mucous membranes, because the IgG M component present in high concentrations bound the yellow vitamin riboflavin with high affinity. The riboflavin–protein complex deposited in the skin was responsible for the peculiar pigmentation of the patient. In another case, an IgG paraprotein was believed to have had some specificity for peripheral nerve myelin and was thought to be responsible for a peripheral neuropathy in that patient. Hypoglycemia caused by an insulin-binding paraprotein immunoglobulin has also been documented in one case and muscle hypertrophy in another. Pemphigus and other cutaneous abnormalities have also been described in patients with paraproteins.

The reactive biological effects of paraprotein complexes cited here are encountered in nonneoplastic conditions associated with abnormal concentrations or structures of immunoglobulins, as well as in diseases primarily affecting antibody-forming cells. For example, cryoprecipitates can be demonstrated in patients with circulating hepatitis B virus antigen; the antigen appears in the cryoprecipitates along with IgG. This finding suggests that the chronic presence of certain infectious antigens can modify the behavior of immunoglobulins so as to promote these abnormal reactions.

Amyloidosis

Amyloidosis is a rather nonspecific pathological entity in which tissues become infiltrated with a waxy substance having a fibrillar ultrastructure and that stains green after reacting with Congo red dye. This infiltration can impair the function of organs and, depending on the extent of the process and the organs involved, amyloidosis can be a serious and fatal condition. The disorder can arise in a number of unrelated settings. This fact and the finding that the infiltrative material has a variable chemical composition shows that amyloidosis is really more than one disease. In one instance in which the amyloidosis is a genetic disorder, for example, and in which the patients suffer a progressive neuropathy, the amyloid is a polymer of a mutant plasma protein called *transthyretin* (or *prealbumin),* a thyroid hormone-binding protein. In another, characterized by corneal lattice dystrophy and cranial neuropathies, the amyloid contains a mutant extracellular actin-binding protein called *plasma gelsolin.*

Nevertheless, it is clear that (1) most amyloid deposits of importance in hematology contain pieces of immunoglobulin molecules and (2) amyloid appears in patients with high circulating levels of immunoglobulins, including patients with paraprotein M components. The pattern of tissue deposition in such patients is variable. Any tissue or organ can be affected, but certain characteristic syndromes are relatively common. In patients with Bence Jones protein in the urine, amyloid deposits are found in the kidney parenchyma and can impair renal function. The damage primarily affects the renal glomerulus such that proteinuria sufficient to cause the nephrotic syndrome is common. Amyloid deposition in the peripheral nerves causes a neuropathy with a stocking-glove distribution. Cardiac involvement may lead to congestive cardiac arrhythmias. Infiltration of the skin can cause it to lose its elasticity and render it susceptible to hemorrhage, especially in intertriginous regions. In some cases the joints are affected and are even seen to become enlarged and limited in range of motion. A classic finding is enlargement of the tongue, known as macroglossia, a complication that can impair the ability to swallow. A

DISEASES ASSOCIATED WITH SERUM M COMPONENTS

Plasma cell neoplasms: multiple myeloma, plasmacytoma

Non-Hodgkin's lymphoma: macroglobulinemia of Waldenström, heavy-chain disease

Chronic lymphocytic leukemia

Other neoplasms

Cirrhosis of the liver

Chronic infections

Autoimmune disorders

Immunodeficiency disorders

complication of special interest to the hematologist is the development of coagulation factor X deficiency. For some reason, amyloid deposits absorb this coagulation factor.

Our understanding of the mechanism of immunoglobulin-derived amyloid formation is far from complete. It appears that the final common pathway of amyloid formation is the assembly of protein fragments into a linear array called a β-pleated sheet structure. Something about the primary and secondary characteristics of amyloidogenic proteins causes them to aggregate in this fashion. In patients with circulating Bence Jones protein, these immunoglobulin fragments form the bulk of the amyloid structure. The amyloid in such cases is designated AL type. In other patients, the source of the precursor subunits, called SAA protein, is a mixture of serum proteins of undetermined origin and intact immunoglobulin molecules. The amyloid in these patients is said to be of the AA type. It is now believed that abnormalities in the degradation of immunoglobulins and other proteins by mononuclear phagocytes plays an intermediate role in the pathogenesis of secondary amyloidosis (Fig. 17-6). These cells normally are responsible for the degradation of serum proteins (Ch. 18). The presence of abnormal immunoglobulin fragments secreted by neoplastic plasma cells presents the macrophages with proteins that they cannot degrade appropriately. This situation leads to the accumulation of protein breakdown products that have the chemical propensity to form the amyloid deposits.

POEMS Syndome

A rare clinical complex of multiple endocrine organ failure and peripheral neuropathy in association with plasma cell disorders leading to M components has been designated *POEMS syndrome*, an acronym for *p*olyneuropathy, *o*rganomegaly, *e*ndocrinopathy, *M* proteins, and *s*kin changes. The neuropathy begins with distal sensorimotor loss of function that spreads centrally. The enlarged organs are the liver, spleen, and lymph nodes. Gonadal, thyroid, and pancreatic endocrine deficiencies are most frequently encountered. Skin abnormalities include alopecia, hyperpigmentation, and thickening.

TREATMENT OF DISEASE CAUSED BY PARAPROTEINS

When the presence of a paraprotein is the result of an underlying infectious, inflammatory, or neoplastic disorder, the ideal treatment is to eradicate the underlying disease. In such

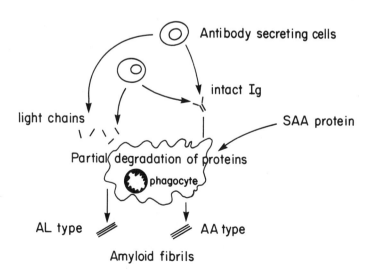

Fig. 17-6. Pathogenesis of amyloidosis.

cases, treatment may reverse amyloid deposition in tissues, when it is present. However, such definitive treatment is not always possible and, in the case of lymphoid neoplasms, may only be of temporary benefit. In these circumstances, it may be possible literally to wash the paraprotein out of the patient by means of a procedure called *plasmapheresis*. With this technique, whole blood is removed from the patient in amounts that are tolerable, the formed elements and plasma are separated, and the formed elements are returned to the patient. The fluid volume removed with the paraprotein-containing plasma is repleted by infusion of normal plasma, albumin, or electrolyte solutions. Depending on the cardiovascular status of the patient, the distribution of the paraprotein, and the intensity of symptoms, this type of treatment can be repeated for long periods of time. With plasmapheresis, it is possible to alleviate the symptoms of the hyperviscosity syndrome or to reduce the manifestations of cryoproteinemia. IgG antibodies are distributed throughout the extracellular fluid, whereas IgM is localized to the vascular system. Therefore, it is clearly easier to remove IgM by plasmapheresis than it is to remove IgG or IgA.

SUGGESTED READINGS

Alper CA (1974) Plasma protein measurements as a diagnostic aid. N Engl J Med 291:287

Burton DR, Woof JM (1992) Human antibody effector function. Adv Immunol 51:1

Buxbaum JN, Chuba JV, Hellman GC, Solomon A, Gallo GR (1990). Monoclonal immunoglobulin deposition disease: light chain and heavy chain deposition diseases and their relation to light chain amyloidosis: clinical features, immunopathology, and molecular analysis. Ann Intern Med 112:455

Case 39-1992 (1992) Case records of the Massachusetts General Hospital. N Engl J Med 327:1014

Kyle RA, Lust JA (1989) Monoclonal gammopathies of undetermined significance. Semin Hematol 26:176

Müller-Eberhard HJ (1988) Molecular organization and function of the complement system. Ann Rev Biochem 57:321

Sipe JD (1992) Amyloidosis. Ann Rev Biochem 61:947

Solomon A, Weiss DT, Kattine AA (1991) Nephrotoxic potential of Bence Jones proteins. N Engl J Med 324:1845

18

Phagocytes and Nonneoplastic Phagocyte Diseases

Phagocytosis, the capacity to engulf particulate matter, is a property possessed by many types of cells. Certain cells are uniquely adept at this function—the polymorphonuclear leukocytes and the mononuclear phagocytes—and therefore have been called "professional" phagocytes. Phagocytes develop from a common committed stem cell called the *granulocyte–macrophage stem cell*. This stem cell differentiates into branches that lead to the formation of three classes of polymorphonuclear leukocytes and to mononuclear phagocytes (Fig. 18-1).

POLYMORPHONUCLEAR LEUKOCYTES

The class of phagocytes called *polymorphonuclear leukocytes* are called such because the nuclei of the cells in the circulation are segmented to form two or more lobes. The polymorphonuclear leukocytes are also called granulocytes for the numerous granules in their cytoplasm. The coloration of these granules after reaction with Wright's stain determines the further subdivision of polymorphonuclear leukocytes into three classes: *neutrophilic* polymorphonuclear leukocytes, in which the granules are essentially colorless; *eosinophilic* polymorphonuclear leukocytes, in which the granules stain red; and *basophilic* polymorphonuclear leukocytes, in which the granules are blue-black after staining. These cells may also be called neutrophils, eosinophils, and basophils, respectively. The hematological importance of these three classes of polymorphonuclear leukocytes is quite different, as are their numbers in the peripheral blood.

Neutrophils

The neutrophilic polymorphonuclear leukocytes, often called "polys" by physicians, are the most numerous polymorphonuclear leukocytes, normally making up 50 to 80 percent of the leukocytes. Their function is to enter the tissues and to kill invading microorganisms. The mature polymorphonuclear leukocyte in the circulation is a cell capable of sticking to the capillary wall adjacent to such sites of invasion, passing through the capillary into the tissues by active ameboid motion, and finding and killing pathogens in these tissues. The life cycle of the neutrophilic polymorphonuclear leukocyte is geared toward the development and execution of these functions.

279

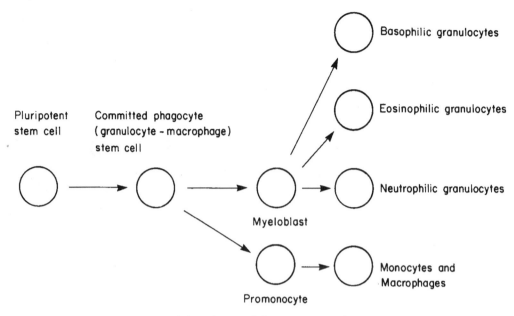

Pluripotent stem cell

Committed phagocyte (granulocyte - macrophage) stem cell

Myeloblast

Promonocyte

Basophilic granulocytes

Eosinophilic granulocytes

Neutrophilic granulocytes

Monocytes and Macrophages

Fig. 18-1. Pathways of phagocyte maturation.

DEVELOPMENT OF NEUTROPHILIC POLYMORPHONUCLEAR LEUKOCYTES

The neutrophilic polymorphonuclear leukocyte matures from the bone marrow committed phagocyte stem cell. During this time, ordinarily requiring 10 days, the cells undergo characteristic changes in appearance that have arbitrarily led to the classification of stages of maturation (Fig. 18-2). The major characteristics permitting the identification of the developmental stages are nuclear shape and the presence or absence of granules.

The first stage of maturation recognizable by the appearance of the cells in stained bone marrow smears is the *myeloblast*. The myeloblast is a large cell having a large nucleus and multiple distinct nucleoli. The normal marrow contains few myeloblasts, and the myeloblast is not highly distinctive in appearance in comparison with other very immature cells. Therefore, it is not always easy to identify myeloblasts with certainty. After a time, the myeloblast begins to synthesize granules. This granulated myeloblast is designated the *promyelocyte*. The granules in the promyelocyte arise from the Golgi apparatus by the

same mechanism described for various secretory cells, such as the pancreas or the salivary gland, in which secretory products are packaged in granules. Being the first granules to appear, they are called *primary granules.* Because the promyelocyte granules stain with an azure hue, they are also called azurophilic, as well as primary granules. These granules contain enzymes that can degrade protein (proteases), fats (lipases), and carbohydrates (glucosidases and mannosidases), as well as a heme-containing peroxidase, often called *myeloperoxidase,* important in killing microorganisms. This enzyme has a green color, which is responsible for the greenish hue of pus.

In the next developmental stage, the nucleus becomes rounder and the nucleoli less distinct. Azurophilic granule synthesis ceases. The cells of this stage, *myelocytes,* continue to divide as they synthesize another set of granules that will have the distinct staining characteristics of mature neutrophilic, eosinophilic, or basophilic polymorphonuclear leukocytes. Therefore, these granules are called *specific* or *secondary granules.* The myelocytes continue to undergo cell division after ceasing to make azurophilic granules. This process dilutes the concentration

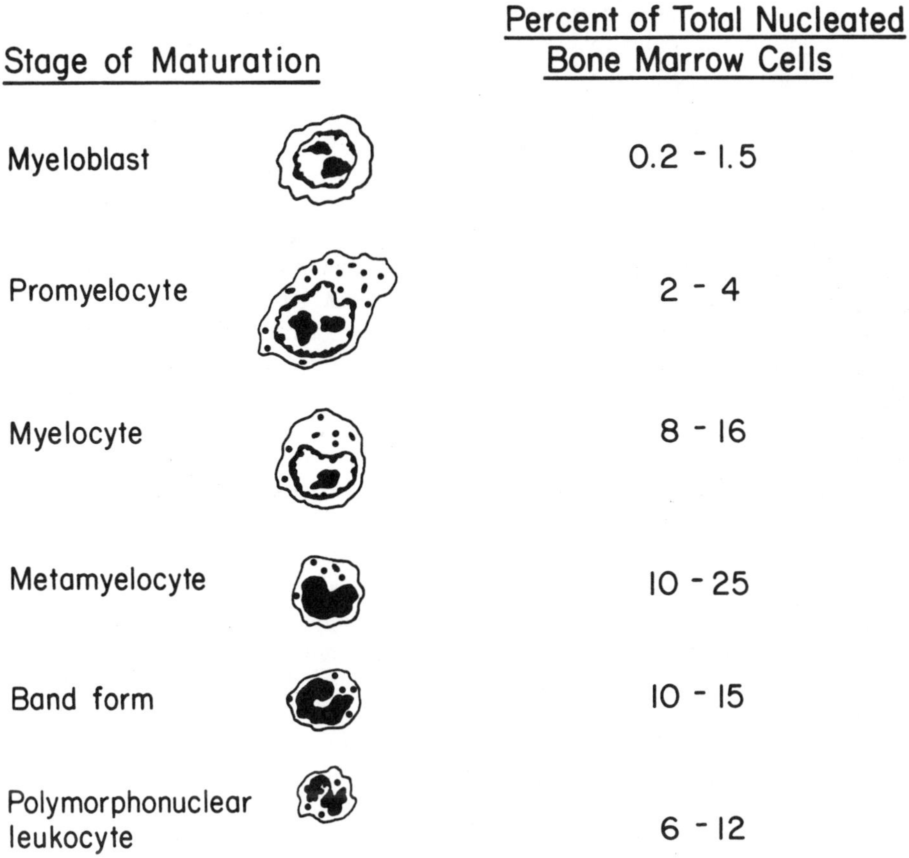

Stage of Maturation		Percent of Total Nucleated Bone Marrow Cells
Myeloblast		0.2 - 1.5
Promyelocyte		2 - 4
Myelocyte		8 - 16
Metamyelocyte		10 - 25
Band form		10 - 15
Polymorphonuclear leukocyte		6 - 12

Fig. 18-2. Maturation of neutrophils.

of azurophilic granules relative to that of specific granules. Therefore, azurophilic granules are not visible in stained smears of mature polymorphonuclear leukocytes. As can be expected from their variable staining properties, the content of the specific granules differs among the different classes of polymorphonuclear leukocytes. Depending on the appearance of the specific granules, myelocytes can be designated neutrophilic, eosinophilic, or basophilic. In the neutrophilic polymorphonuclear leukocyte, the secondary granules are smaller than the azurophilic granules. They contain lysozyme, an enzyme that degrades cell wall mucopeptides of certain gram-positive bacteria, a vitamin B_{12}-binding protein, and an iron-binding protein called *lactoferrin*.

Myeloblasts, promyelocytes, and myelocytes can divide. They make up the mitotic compartment of granulocyte development. Beyond the myelocyte stage, the granulocytes are incapable of cell division and therefore constitute the postmitotic compartment. The major changes from this point on in the development of neutrophilic polymorphonuclear leukocytes involve progressive segmentation and condensation of the nucleus. An indentation of the round nucleus of the myelocyte defines the neutrophilic *metamyelocyte*. Further nuclear condensation and development of the indentation make the nucleus bilobed, indicating the *band form* or *stab form*. The final polymorphous form of the nucleus heralds the complete development of the neutrophilic, polymorphonuclear leukocyte. It is possible that the segmented nucleus permits the neutrophils to fit through small spaces as they crawl in the tissues.

Occasionally, the majority of peripheral blood neutrophils are found to have a peculiarity of nuclear shape. Instead of being organized into several lobes, the segmentation is limited to two lobes that appear quite round (Fig. 18-3). These two lobes may overlap to give the appearance of a single round nucleus with the dense staining of the usual mature neutrophil nuclei. This nuclear configuration, called *the Pelger-Hüet anomaly*, appears in two circumstances. One is inherited. It is passed as an autosomal recessive trait and is not associated with any significant abnormalities in the functioning of the mature neutrophils. The second setting in which these so-called Pelger-Hüet cells appear is in the blood of some patients who have acute granulocytic leukemias (Ch. 23) or who have myelodysplastic syndromes (Ch. 22). In this context, the anomaly appears to be the result of an acquired derangement in the genetic material of the phagocytic stem cell.

FATE AND FUNCTION OF NEUTROPHILIC POLYMORPHONUCLEAR LEUKOCYTES

The maturation of the neutrophil from myeloblast to a segmented form in the bone marrow takes about 1 week. After release from the bone marrow into the circulation, some polymorphonuclear leukocytes traverse the axial stream, the main column of formed elements coursing in the middle of blood vessels. These cells are readily removed during venipuncture and measured as the peripheral blood neutrophil count. Such cells are said to constitute part of the *circulating neutrophil pool*. In a person of average size, this pool contains 25 billion cells. Other neutrophils roll along the sides of the vessels, peripheral to the main column of streaming cells in the center of the lumen. At any given time, about one-half the given neutrophils in the vascular compartment are not found in samples of peripheral blood. This hidden population of neutrophils has been called *the marginal pool,* with the idea that it is the cells that roll along the vessel walls. It is now believed that most of these "marginated" neutrophils are actually sequestered in the lungs, spleen, and elsewhere. These cells mix freely with the circulating cells. Rolling along the endothelium, in fact, is not the result of passive hemodynamic properties of blood flow but rather is the first step in a concerted series of active sensory, motor, and secretory events that permit phagocytes (and lymphocytes too) to leave the circulation in precise locations where they are called.

The total number of polymorphonuclear leukocytes going through this emigration process out of the circulation into the tissues, called *diapedesis* (Fig. 18-4), is on the order of 100 billion cells/day in a 70-kg person. It follows that to maintain the normal level of circulating polymorphonuclear leukocytes, an equivalent number of cells must leave the bone marrow. The life cycle of the polymorphonuclear leukocyte therefore depends on a high turnover. The average polymorphonuclear leukocyte circulates in the blood for less than 12 hours. Compare this short circulation time of the neutrophil with those of red blood cells (120 days) and of platelets (7 days).

Sensory Aspects of Phagocyte Function

Rolling of leukocytes along the walls of blood vessels takes place when *L-selectins,* membrane receptors constitutively present on the surface of neutrophils, bind to fucosyl and sulfatidyl groups on molecules externally disposed on the endothelial cells of postcapillary

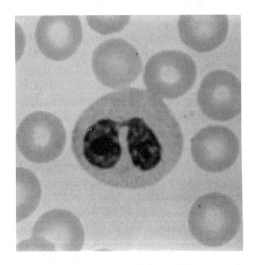

Fig. 18-3. Pelger-Hüet cell.

venules (Figure 18-4). At the same time, similar molecules, called *P-* and *E-selectins*, become expressed when the blood vessels encounter cytokines, such as interleukin-1 or tumor necrosis factor, released by mononuclear phagocytes in the connective tissue that interact with microorganisms or other inflammatory stimuli, and the E-selectins bind to sugars, specifically fucose-containing oligosaccharides, and to sulfatide-bearing glycolipids on the leukocyte surface. The selectins are named after the fact that they have structures characteristic of calcium-dependent carbohydrate-binding proteins, known as *C-type lectins.*

The activated endothelial cells, and tissue macrophages as well, also release other cytokines, such as *interleukin-8* and the arachidonic acid metabolite *platelet-activating factor,* which cause the rolling neutrophils to spread, acquire motility, and release their own bioactive reactants that induce separation of endothelial cell junctions, permitting the neutrophilic polymorphonuclear leukocytes to crawl into the surrounding connective tissues in a directed manner toward the source of inflammation. This sensing and response by polymorphonuclear leukocytes to the gradient of factors elaborated by microbial invasion or

injury is called *chemotaxis,* and the molecules in the gradient are termed *chemotactic factors* (Fig. 18-4).

The chemotactic factors that attract polymorphonuclear leukocytes are many and varied (Fig 18-4). This abundance is reasonable in light of the importance of polymorphonuclear leukocyte chemotaxis for survival against infection. These factors include, in addition to interleukin 8 and related cell-derived molecules, *N-formyl-oligopeptides*, released by microorganisms or by damaged mitochondria. In addition, the systems of inflammatory mediators elaborate compounds that attract polymorphonuclear leukocytes. These systems include C5a, a fragment of C5 in the complement system (Ch. 17), *fibrinopeptides* derived from the coagulation and fibrinolytic system, leukotriene B4, an icosanoid product of arachidonic acid oxidation reactions that occur in the membranes of many cells, including phagocytes and platelets (Ch. 14, Fig. 18-10, and below).

Chemotactic factors act by binding to *chemotactic factor receptors* on the outer surfaces of the membranes of the polymorphonuclear leukocytes. These receptors are similar in structure to the seven-spanning thrombin

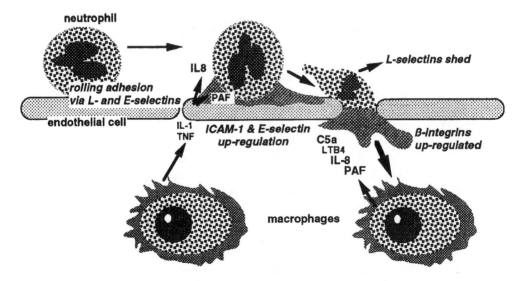

post-capillary venule lumen

Fig. 18-4. Diapedesis and chemotaxis.

receptor of platelets. The binding of chemotactic factors to their receptors on leukocytes activates *signaling* or *stimulus–response coupling*. This signaling process has been extensively analyzed in phagocytes because of the many rapid and easily measurable responses elicited by agonists, and the findings are in large part also applicable to the way in which agonists stimulate platelets to undergo shape changes and secretion (Ch. 14) and in which a large variety of cells are induced to undertake mitosis in response to growth factors (Ch. 21).

Two major and interrelated classes of signals are generated when agonists such as chemotactic factors engage receptors (Fig. 18-5). One of these signal systems is the breakdown and resynthesis of a class of membrane phospholipids, the *polyphosphoinositides*. Another is a change in the cytosolic concentration of ions, especially *calcium*. The initial event in phosphoinositide metabolism following receptor perturbation involves the hydrolysis of the polyphosphoinositide, *phosphatidylinositol*-bis-*phosphate* (PIP_2), by an enzyme called phospholipase C. Phospholipase C attacks the phosphodiester bond between the phosphorylated inositol ring in PIP_2 and its diacylglycerol backbone, generating *diacylglycerol* (*DAG*) and *inositol triphosphate* (*IP$_3$*). Phospholipase C ordinarily requires higher concentrations of calcium than are found in the unstimulated (resting) phagocyte for significant activity, but following stimulation of the receptor, a cytosolic gaunosine nucleotide-binding protein, known as a *G-protein*, exchanges guanosine diphosphate (GDP) for guanosine triphosphate (GTP) and then binds phospholipase C and other cellular molecules (designated E in Fig 18-6), permitting these effectors to be active (E*). The G-protein then hydrolyzes GTP to GDP and orthophosphate (Pi) and loses effector-activating ability. Cellular factors can accelerate this hydrolysis and are called GTPase-activating proteins, or GAPs.

There are two classes of G-proteins. One is called hetertrimeric because the proteins contain three subunits, designated α, β, and γ, which associate reversibly depending on the activation state of the complex (Fig 18-6A). The second class, called small G-proteins or *ras*-related proteins, was originally discovered as transforming oncogenes (Fig 18-6B) (Ch. 21). Some cellular proteins (GDIs) accelerate, whereas other (GDSs) inhibit the cyclic activation of these G-proteins. Both types of G-proteins serve as amplifiers to permit ligation of a single receptor to activate many intracellular effectors.

A second mechanism for activating phospholipase C and other cellular effectors is when receptor ligation induces the phosphorylation of intracellular proteins. A common theme is for the receptor itself to have protein kinase activity in its cytoplasmic domain that phosphorylates tyrosine residues on the receptor (autophosphorylation). The phosphotyrosines serve as ligands for intracellular effectors such as phospholipase C, which in turn become activated by phosphorylation.

The IP_3 released by the breakdown of PIP_2 diffuses to cytoplasmic vesicles that contain abundant calcium *(calciosomes)* and causes these structures to release the stored calcium into the cytoplasm. This rise in cytosolic calcium, in addition to potentiating the activity of phospholipase C, activates a number of intracellular reactions involved in phagocyte responses, such as the contractile activity of myosin. The other product of PIP_2 hydrolysis, DAG, activates an enzyme called *protein kinase C,* and this enzyme presumably stimulates other reactions by phosphorylating key intracellular proteins. DAG is also the substrate for the enzyme phospholipase A_2, which generates arachidonic acid for disposal into the leukotriene and prostaglandin pathways.

A different set of reactions terminates or reverses the processes set in motion by the breakdown of PIP_2. A series of kinases catalyze the phosphorylation of phosphatidylinositol (PI) and phosphatidylinositol monophosphate (PIP), resulting in the resynthesis of PIP_2. Adenosine triphosphate (ATP)-dependent pumps in the plasma membrane and in the intracellular calcium storage vesicles efficiently restore the increased cytosolic calcium levels to baseline values.

Motor Aspects of Phagocyte Function

These intracellular signalling events cause the phagocytes to shed their selectins and concomitantly express more copies of a class of two-chain receptors that are members of a widely distributed family of cell–cell and cell–surface adhesion molecules (CAMs) called *integrins* (Figure 18-4). The activated integrins of phagocytes are designated β2-integrins, and one of the most important is named *CD11b/CD18*. CD11b/CD18 on phagocytes binds to specific receptors, *ICAM-1* and *ICAM-2* on endothelial cells and to a variety of connective tissue components. Another integrin (*VLA*) binds to a molecule named *VCAM-1* on endothelial cells. The adhesion of leukocytes to endothelial cells and to fibers of the interstitial spaces provides the frictional force by which leukocytes can move toward the source of the chemotactic factor gradient. Leukocytes, therefore, *crawl* rather than swim.

The cells employ a tank-tread mechanism to move the sites on their membranes that are adherent to extracellular fibers toward the rear of the cell, whereupon the adhesive sites become detached. The formation and destruction of a system of actin fibers beneath the cell membrane at the leading edge of the cell provide the motor forces for this translational movement, and the system serves as an anchor for the internal fixation of cell–surface adhesion molecules described above.

Should the cells leaving the circulation encounter microorganisms, they ingest them if they recognize the microbes appropriately as foreign. An important mechanism for rendering microbes recognizable is a process whereby serum components coat the microbes. The molecules that coat organisms are called *opsonins* (from the Greek, meaning "to prepare for dining"). These molecules are normal constituents of plasma. The major plasma opsonins are IgG and the C3 fragments C3b and iC3b, which become deposited in the microorganisms by the action of the classic or alternative pathways of complement activation, as described in Chapter 17. The opsonins bound to microorganisms engage membrane receptors on the surfaces of the phagocytes. IgG binds to three classes of receptors for the Fc portion of the immunoglobulins *(Fc receptors)*; Fc-receptor type I (FcR1, CD64) is only on certain mononuclear phagocytes following or on neutrophils exposed to interferon-γ; it binds monomeric IgG with high affinity, whereas FcRII and FcRIII (CD16) are expressed constitutively on neutrophils and mononuclear phagocytes and bind IgG aggregates. C3b binds to a specific receptor designated *CR1* (CD), and iC3b binds the integrin CD11b/CD18. These binding interactions cause the membrane to extend pseudopodia that envelop the opsonized objects within a *phagocytic vacuole* or *phagosome*. As in locomotion, these movements are driven by actin assembly beneath the cell membrane. Concomitantly, the granules are secreted into the forming vacuole or *phagolysosome*.

Effector Aspects of Phagocyte Function

One metabolic reaction of great importance for antimicrobial function arises from an enzyme system, *the NADPH oxidase*, that takes electrons from the reduced pyridine nucleotide (NADPH) and adds them to oxygen sequentially to form reactive metabolites. The first product of oxygen metabolism is *the superoxide anion* (O_2^-), a one-electron reduction product of oxygen; the second product is *hydrogen peroxide* (H_2O_2).

The NADPH oxidase assembles from several components that ultimately come to reside in the plasma membrane of the phagolysosome. These components include a flavin- and heme-binding cytochrome b_{558}, which comprises two subunits, p22 and gp91, two phosphoproteins, $p47_{phox}$ and $p67_{phox}$, and low molecular weight G-proteins (Fig. 18-7A). Secretion of granule contents, superoxide, and hydrogen peroxide begins before the vacuole is closed, so that the environment of the phagocyte is also exposed to granule enzymes and to reactive oxygen metabolites. These neutrophil products damage normal tissues and therefore are important mediators of inflammation. In this region, the

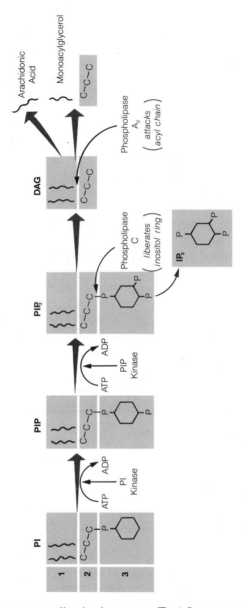

Fig. 18-5. Stimulus–response coupling in phagocytes. (**Top**) Structures and reactions of phospholipids involved in transmembrane signaling. Phosphatidylinositol (PI), the source of signal phospholipids, has two fatty acids (*1*) linked to a glycerol backbone (*2*) and an inositol ring (*3*) bound to the third carbon by a phosphodiester bond. Successive phosphorylation of the inositol ring in the 4 and 5 positions by ATP-requiring kinases generates phosphatidylinositol phosphate (PIP) and phosphatidylinositol *bis*-phosphate (PIP$_2$) respectively. PIP$_2$ is the target of a phosphodiesterase enzyme, phospholipase C, which liberates the inositol ring containing three phosphates, inositol triphosphate (IP$_3$) into the cytoplasm, leaving diacylglycerol (DAG) at the plasma membrane. The phospholipids are all potential substrates of phospholipase A$_2$ enzymes, which attack the second acyl chain, usually an arachidonic acid, producing free arachidonic acid and, depending on the species hydrolyzed, monoacylglycerol or else a phospholipid missing one fatty acid (called a lysophospholipid). For

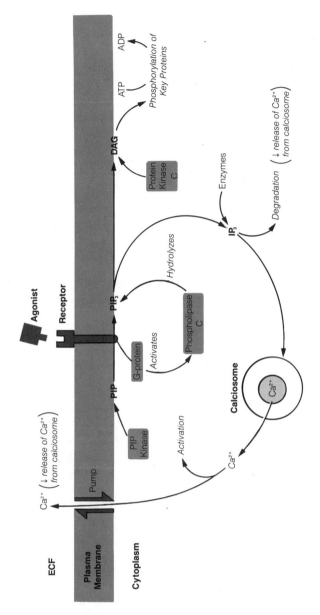

simplicity, only the hydrolysis of DAG is shown in the diagram. (**Bottom**) Signaling reaction cycles. Agonist binding to the external portion of a receptor causes a conformational change in the transmembrane portion of the receptor such that the cytoplasmic region interacts with a G-protein, which in turn activates phospholipase C. Phospholipase C hydrolyzes PIP_2 to produce IP_3 and DAG. IP_3 interacts with calciosomes to release ionized calcium into the cytoplasm where it activates a variety of enzymes and structural proteins involved in phagocyte responses. A cytoplasmic enzyme, protein kinase C, binds DAG at the plasma membrane and phosphorylates other enzymes or structural proteins important in phagocyte responses. Dissipation of the activation signals is brought about by membrane pumps that extrude calcium, by enzymes that degrade IP_3, thereby stopping the release of calcium from calciosomes, and by the enzymatic breakdown of DAG. Activation of PI kinases regenerate PIP_2 for further signaling. PIP_2 also interacts with cytoplasmic actin-regulating proteins.

287

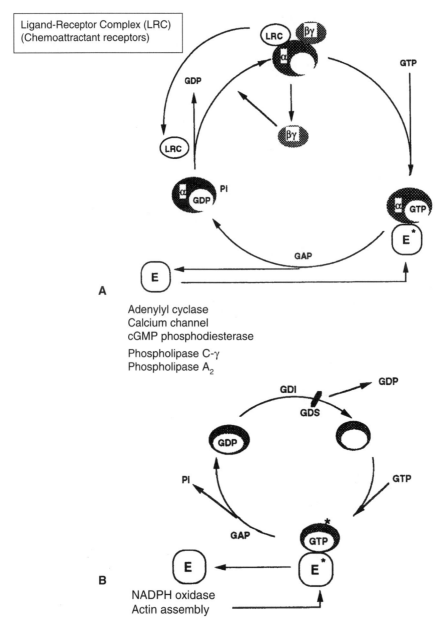

Ligand-Receptor Complex (LRC)
(Chemoattractant receptors)

A

Adenylyl cyclase
Calcium channel
cGMP phosphodiesterase

Phospholipase C-γ
Phospholipase A₂

B

NADPH oxidase
Actin assembly

Fig. 18-6. Heterotrimeric (**A**) and *ras*-related (**B**) G-proteins.

toxic properties of the lytic granule enzymes, the oxygen metabolites, and a potent microbicidal system composed of the azurophil granule enzyme myeloperoxidase and hydrogen peroxide work to kill the microorganism (Fig. 18-8).

The segregation of degradative enzymes and oxygen metabolites away from the cytoplasm of the polymorphonuclear leukocyte helps pre-

vent damage to the phagocyte as it attacks microbes. However, superoxide anions and hydrogen peroxide diffuse easily across membranes. The cytoplasm of the neutrophil contains the enzymes *superoxide dismutase* and *catalase* and the metabolite *reduced glutathione (GSH)*, which detoxify these compounds should they enter the cell. Superoxide

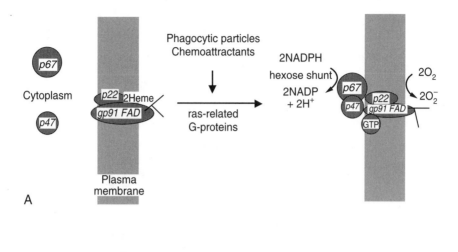

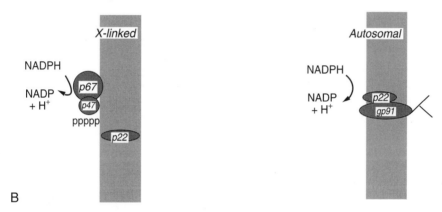

Fig. 18-7. (**A**) Activation of the superoxide-forming oxidase. (**B**) Pathogenesis of different focus of chronic granulomatous disease.

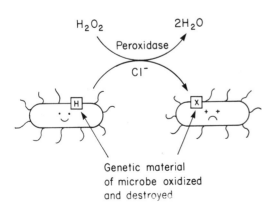

Fig. 18-8. Hydrogen peroxide–halide–peroxidase microbicidal system.

dismutase converts superoxide to hydrogen peroxide; catalase and reduced glutathione destroy hydrogen peroxide. Recall that these are the same protective systems that operate in erythrocytes for destroying oxidants. Reduced glutathione is regenerated, as in the erythrocyte, by reactions coupled to the hexose-monophosphate shunt of the glycolytic pathway (Fig. 18-9).

Another important effector system activated by phagocytic recognition is the elaboration of bioactive arachidonic acid metabolites known as *icosanoids*. The initial steps in this process are identical to those described for platelet icosanoid metabolism in Chapter 14 and involve the release of arachidonic acid from membrane phospholipids. Instead of the dominance of cyclo-oxygenation that converts

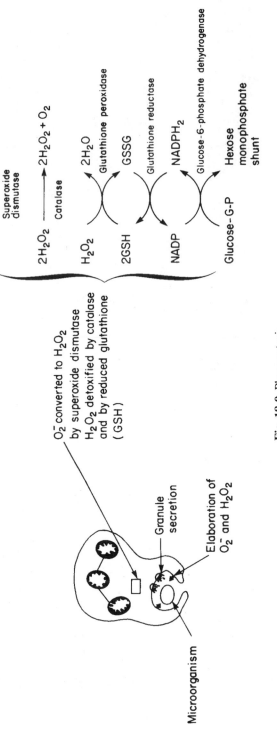

Fig. 18-9. Phagocytosis.

arachidonate to prostaglandins and thromboxanes in platelets, a different set of enzymes converts arachidonic acid to compounds known as *leukotrienes*, although phagocytes can also produce the prostaglandins and platelet-activating factor (Fig.18-10). A large number of leukotriene intermediates have been identified. A few of these are of particular interest; leukotrienes B$_4$, C$_4$, and D$_4$ (LTB$_4$, LTC$_4$, and LTD$_4$). LTB$_4$, as mentioned above, is a potent chemotactic factor for neutrophils and monocytes. LTC$_4$ and LTD$_4$, historically known as "slow-reacting substances of anaphylaxis," have strong smooth muscle constricting effects. Therefore, these agents contribute importantly to the inflammatory effects of phagocytic infiltration of tissues during infection and injury.

Eosinophilic Polymorphonuclear Leukocytes

The eosinophilic polymorphonuclear leukocytes develop in the bone marrow through the same maturation steps as the neutrophilic polymorphonuclear leukocyte. Eosinophil maturation is promoted by interleukins 4 and 5. The specific granules of the eosinophilic polymorphonuclear leukocyte are very large. The red staining of the eosinophil granule arises from its abundant quantities of a basic protein, that is, one having many positively charged amino acids. The segmentation of the nucleus of the mature eosinophil tends to be less marked than that of the other granulocytes, so that the mature eosinophil has a bilobed nucleus with a

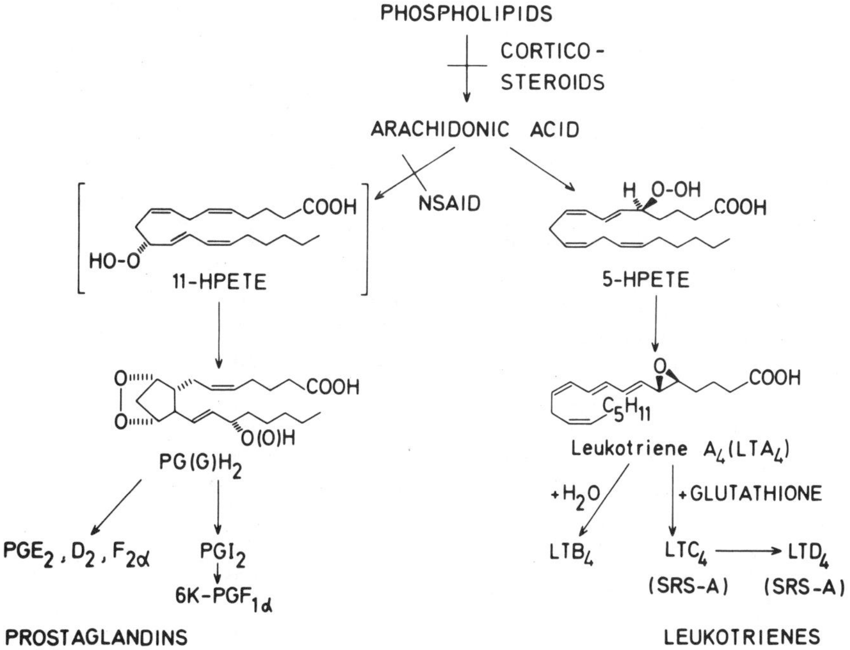

Fig. 18-10. Pathways for the production of prostaglandins and leukotrienes in phagocytes. An enzyme called *phospholipase A$_2$* releases arachidonic acid from the second carbon in the glycerol backbone of membrane phospholipids. Corticosteroids are believed to inhibit this reaction. A cyclo-oxygenase enzyme sensitive to inhibition by nonsteroidal anti-inflammatory chemicals such as ibuprofen converts arachidonate to prostaglandin H$_2$ (PGH$_2$) via an intermediate, 11-hydroxy pentaeonic acid (11-HPETE). PGH$_2$ is then further metabolized to other prostaglandins. A different pathway involves an enzyme called 5C lipoxygenase, which oxidizes arachidonate into 5C hydroxypentaeonic acid, the precursor of the leukotrienes. LTC$_4$ and LTD$_4$ are sulfur-containing lipids, and the source of the sulfur is glutathione.

thinner stalk between the lobes than that observed for the band form of the neutrophil.

The eosinophilic polymorphonuclear leukocyte has capabilities similar to those of the neutrophilic polymorphonuclear leukocyte for chemotaxis, phagocytosis, and microbicidal activity. Nevertheless, representing ordinarily a small proportion of the total polymorphonuclear leukocyte population, its role in defense against bacterial infection is uncertain. Because the eosinophil count rises in certain parasitic infestations and allergic states, it is widely believed that the eosinophil has a special role in combating parasites or in controlling allergic insults.

Basophilic Polymorphonuclear Leukocytes

The specific granules of the basophil are also very large. The blue staining of the basophilic specific granules derives from large amounts of acidic (negatively charged) polysaccharides with many sulfate and carboxyl groups, such as heparin.

The basophil contains the bulk of the histamine found in the blood. When appropriately stimulated, the basophil releases histamine. The circulating basophil has receptors for IgE on its surface. Antigens reacting with IgE on the basophil surface are potent inducers of histamine release. It may be that the tissue mast cell, which also releases histamine and other vasoactive substances after exposure to IgE and antigens reactive with it, is related to the circulating basophil. The consequences of release of these mediators are manifestations of allergy, such as rhinitis, bronchospasm, urticaria, angioedema, and anaphylaxis.

MONONUCLEAR PHAGOCYTES

In many ways the mononuclear phagocytes behave like the polymorphonuclear leukocytes. Both arise from the bone marrow, circulate, enter the tissues in response to chemotactic factors, are actively phagocytic, and kill microbes by means of an oxygen-dependent mechanism. The major difference between these phagocytes is the longevity of the mononuclear phagocytes, in contrast with the brief, hectic life span of the polymorphonuclear leukocytes.

Development

The mononuclear phagocyte does not develop through a series of morphologically discrete stages as does the polymorphonuclear leukocyte, but rather appears to mature continuously under stimulation by granulocyte–macrophage colony-stimulating factor (GM-CSF) and especially M-CSF. The marrow phase of mononuclear phagocyte development is ordinarily much less distinctive than that of polymorphonuclear leukocytes. The promonocyte, the monocyte precursor, is very difficult to find or identify in the bone marrow. It is believed that this cell remains in the marrow only a few days and then enters the circulation as a monocyte.

The blood monocyte is recognizable in Wright's stain smears on the basis of certain characteristic features. The nucleus seems to wrap around itself. The cytoplasm is gray and occasionally contains vacuoles and granules. The cell shape is oval or irregular. In the transition to the tissue macrophage, the mononuclear phagocyte becomes progressively larger than the monocyte. The nucleus becomes round, and distinct nucleoli appear. The cytoplasm becomes blue and may contain azurophilic granules (Fig. 18-11).

Function and Fate

The mononuclear phagocytes have much in common with neutrophilic polymorphonuclear leukocytes. They have the same receptors for, and response to, chemotactic factors and opsonins as polymorphonuclear leukocytes. They kill microorganisms by immolating them with degradative enzymes, derived from cytoplasmic granules, superoxide, and hydrogen peroxide. Monocytes, like polymorphonuclear

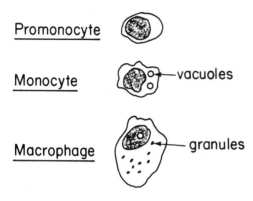

Promonocyte

Monocyte — vacuoles

Macrophage — granules

Fig. 18-11. Development of the mononuclear phagocyte.

leukocytes, crawl to sites of infection and injury.

After 24 to 36 hours, the monocyte leaves the capillary system, entering either the tissues, as does the polymorphonuclear leukocyte, or certain organs important for filtering and immunologic function, such as the liver, spleen, lymph nodes, and lungs. The macrophages in the liver, spleen, and lymph nodes are organized so as to be in intimate contact with matter percolating through the blood and lymphatic circulation of these organs. Constituting a sentry network to engulf microbes that gain access to the gates and alleyways of the body, they also trap and destroy aged or prematurely damaged blood cells. This filtering function of mononuclear phagocytes was called the reticuloendothelial system for many years, although this term is now relatively meaningless, as it is now known that macrophages, not endothelial cells, are responsible for this filtering function.

The large mass of macrophages in contact with the circulation is also strategically located to interact with normal and abnormal plasma proteins. In the former case, the macrophages have the capacity to internalize large quantities of soluble proteins by the process called *pinocytosis*. The cells pinch off tiny vesicles of membrane containing the plasma and carry it to the cell interior, from which granules containing proteolytic enzymes fuse with the vesicles.

The ingested proteins are then rapidly degraded. In this way, the mononuclear phagocyte system is responsible for catabolizing plasma proteins. The internalization of soluble material is called *fluid-phase pinocytosis*. Macrophages also take up other proteins that bind to their membranes. This process is called *adsorptive pinocytosis*, or more commonly, *receptor-mediated endocytosis*. Proteins that bind to specific membrane receptors, such as mannose-containing glycoproteins, oxidized lipoproteins (which cause macrophages to turn into foam cells causing atherosclerosis), aggregated proteins, immune complexes, and complexes of activated clotting factors, are cleared from the circulation in this way. Macrophages also cooperate with lymphoid cells to assist them in performing complex immunological functions, such as the generation of specific antibodies and the mounting of cell-mediated immune reactions (Ch. 20). The macrophages also have a role in containing and inactivating certain parasites, such as mycobacteria, viruses, and trypanosomes. In such cases, the lymphoid system arms the macrophages by enabling them to secrete large quantities of hydrogen peroxide after phagocytosing these parasites. Macrophages also secrete nitric oxide, which has antimicrobial as well as numerous vasoactive effects. Additionally, macrophages produce a wide variety of cytokines, including hematopoietic growth factors (see Table 1-1). Tumor necrosis factor and interleukin-1 released by macrophages in states of infection and inflammation probably account for many of the systemic signs and symptoms of septic shock.

REGULATION OF THE PHAGOCYTE LIFE CYCLE

The principal purpose of phagocytosis is to defend against microorganisms and to clean cellular debris after injury. It is therefore reasonable that a major stimulus for phagocytic maturation, release, and disposition to the tissues is the presence of chemotactic factors or substances released from microorganisms, such as cell-wall endotoxins. In addition, infection induces the synthesis and release of phagocyte growth factors, G-CSF, GM-CSF, and others (Ch. 1). These substances can be found in both serum and urine. The presence of infection, tissue damage, or other inflammatory states markedly increases—by as much as tenfold—the maturation rate, the size of the marrow precursor pool, and the daily turnover rate of phagocytic cells.

REACTIVE CHANGES IN PHAGOCYTES

The number of peripheral blood phagocytes, principally the neutrophils, changes rapidly in response to stress. Depending on the magnitude and type of stress, the counts rise or fall variably within a matter of hours. An increase in the neutrophil count above 10,000/µl defines a neutrophilic leukocytosis or *neutrophilia;* a drop below 1,500/µl is designated *neutropenia,* although this definition is somewhat arbitrary. *Monocytosis* describes an elevation of the monocyte count above normal, and *monocytopenia* is a decrease below normal. The set at which the peripheral blood neutrophil count is maintained in the "normal" state depends on the population studied. The normal values given in Table III-I are based on samples of blood taken from white persons of European origin. Although the range of normal thus established is applicable to many populations, many blacks and certain Mideastern populations have average neutrophil counts considerably lower than the normal levels listed here. This fact must be kept in mind when evaluating neutrophil counts. A healthy black person displaying no evidence of blood disease but having a neutrophil count below the normal range is actually normal. Some of the usual stresses that affect phagocytes encountered in medical practice are described below.

Adrenergic Stimulation

Adrenergic agents such as epinephrine raise the peripheral white blood cell count as much

as twofold within minutes. Both neutrophilic polymorphonuclear leukocyte and lymphocyte counts increase. The rise in neutrophils is the result of a mobilization of the cells from the marginal pool. This shift in distribution occurs because the stimulation of adrenergic receptors on the leukocytes reduces their intrinsic stickiness. The elevation in neutrophil and lymphocyte counts may persist for hours. On the other hand, the eosinophil count falls, rather than rises, in response to adrenergic stimulation.

Infection, Inflammation, and Necrosis

The presence of microbes or damaged tissues releases certain chemotactic factors, eliciting polymorphonuclear leukocytes from the bone marrow as well as the marginal pool. If the stimulus is persistent, bone marrow production of phagocytes increases and contributes to the elevated circulating level of neutrophilic polymorphonuclear leukocytes and monocytes, that is, neutrophilia and monocytosis. An example of this phenomenon may be the fact that cigarette smokers can have on average somewhat higher neutrophil counts in the blood than nonsmokers. Presumably chronic pulmonary inflammation in response to components of the smoke account for this finding.

If the inflammatory stimulus is strong, the level of circulating neutrophils may rise as much as tenfold, and immature forms may appear in the blood. Such extreme elevations in the blood neutrophil count, especially if associated with the appearance of immature forms, are sometimes called a *leukemoid reaction.* When nucleated red cell precursors are present together with the immature neutrophils, the picture is defined as a *leukoerythroblastic reaction.* Leukoerythroblastic reactions occur in states of acute hypoxia and in some disorders involving invasion of the bone marrow. Processes of this kind that characteristically cause leukoerythroblastic reaction are cancers that invade the bone marrow and fibrosis of the bone marrow.

The emergence of immature neutrophils usually occurs in reverse order of maturation, bands being most frequently encountered, but metamyelocytes, myelocytes, and even promyelocytes and myeloblasts can appear in extreme states of stress. This peripheral blood neutrophilic polymorphonuclear leukocyte immaturity is commonly called a *shift to the left*. Presumably this terminology arose from a convention wherein developing forms have been diagrammed in textbooks from left to right in order of increasing maturity.

Sometimes infections and related stresses cause a drop rather than a rise in the neutrophil count. This fall occurs most often in cases of viral infections. The decrease in counts is presumably the result of a direct toxic effect of the virus infection on the production of phagocytes in the bone marrow. A drop in the neutrophil count may occasionally take place in bacterial infections, especially of an overwhelming nature. A bacterial infection characteristically displaying this effect is septicemia caused by gram-negative organisms, especially typhoid fever. The mechanism of the fall in the neutrophil count is an increase in the fraction of cells that become too sticky for proper function and that enter the marginal pool. Toxins produced by the infection may also inhibit the production of neutrophils in the bone marrow.

The eosinophil counts may or may not parallel changes of neutrophil counts during bacterial infection. In parasitic infections caused by worms, such as trichinosis (but not protozoa), the eosinophils may increase and may become the major blood white cells. This state is called *eosinophilia*. The eosinophil count can also rise in allergic states such as asthma.

The monocyte count usually rises somewhat in parallel with the neutrophil counts in acute infection and inflammation. However, a marked monocytosis, elevation of the monocyte concentration, does not ordinarily occur. Persistent increases in the monocyte count are encountered in chronic inflammatory diseases, such as tuberculosis, sarcoidosis, and subacute bacterial endocarditis.

In addition to changes in neutrophil numbers and in the appearance of immature forms in the blood during infection, inflammation, and necrosis, some alterations in the appearance of neutrophilic polymorphonuclear leukocytes can also take place. Greenish blotches can be seen in the cytoplasm of some neutrophilic polymorphonuclear leukocytes. These are aggregates of rough endoplasmic reticulum called *Döhle bodies* in deference to their first observer. Ordinary granules are barely visible in neutrophilic polymorphonuclear leukocytes because of their neutral staining characteristics. However, in these states of stress, blue-black granules become visible in the neutrophil cytoplasm. These so-called *toxic granules* are much smaller than the specific granules of basophils and are therefore not easily confused with the latter. The toxic granules may be remnants of circulating matter that were ingested and partially degraded by the neutrophil.

Alkaline phosphatase is an enzyme of unknown physiological function that splits phosphate off from a variety of synthetic esters at a very alkaline pH. The hydrolysis of phosphate esters can be measured chemically in extracts of polymorphonuclear leukocytes or, more conveniently, can be semiquantitatively estimated on fixed blood smears by means of a histochemical staining reaction. The phosphate liberated is colored by suitable reagents, and the number of cells so stained and the intensity of the staining are noted to establish a *leukocyte alkaline phosphatase* (LAP) score. This alkaline phosphatase activity of neutrophilic polymorphonuclear leukocytes in reactive states, polycythemia vera, and idiopathic myelofibrosis is usually elevated above normal, but is low or absent in chronic granulocytic leukemia (Ch. 22).

MEDICATIONS AND PHAGOCYTE DISEASES

The first or major side effect of many medications is often a change in the leukocyte count. Often, the toxic effect of medications is to lower the leukocyte count either by a direct toxic effect on the production of neutrophils in the bone marrow (Ch. 21) or by generating antibodies that can react with phagocytic white blood cells (Ch. 30).

A few drugs raise the phagocyte count. Corticosteroids increase the neutrophil count by releasing neutrophils from the bone marrow and stimulating the bone marrow production of neutrophils. The mechanism for this effect is in part the action of corticosteroids to inhibit neutrophils from sticking to endothelium and crawling into the tissues. The reduction in tissue neutrophils secondarily causes an increase in the release of tissue chemotactic factors.

The effect of corticosteroids on eosinophils is the opposite of the effect on neutrophils. Corticosteroids lower the eosinophil count, whereas corticosteroid deficiency, as observed in Addison's disease (adrenal cortical insufficiency), causes a rise in the eosinophil count.

Lithium carbonate, a drug used by psychiatrists to treat manic-depressive disease, raises the blood neutrophil count without impairing neutrophil delivery to the tissues.

ALTERATIONS IN PHAGOCYTE ACTIVITY

The concept of phagocyte activity refers to the process whereby microorganisms and phagocytes come into contact with one another, killing or containing the microbes. Normal phagocyte activity requires both adequate numbers and proper functioning of phagocytic cells. The activities of phagocytes in the defense against microorganisms can be summarized by two generalizations.

The first rule is that the defense against high-grade encapsulated pathogens, such as *Streptococcus*, *Pneumococcus*, *Meningococcus*, and *Haemophilus*, primarily involves macrophages of the filter organs, the spleen, liver, and lung, and the opsonins of serum, lgG, and opsonic fragments of C3.

The second generalization about phagocytes in host defense against infection is that the protection against low-grade resident microorganisms, microbes that infest the skin and mucosal surfaces, for example, *Staphylococcus aureus* and gram-negative enteric flora, requires a constant flow of wandering phagocytes, the mono-

cytes and especially the polymorphonuclear leukocytes into the tissues. Patients with congenital or acquired abnormalities of opsonins of macrophages acquire unusually frequent and severe infections, specifically septicemias, pneumonias, and meningitis, caused by the encapsulated organisms.

Disorders of Opsonins

Immunoglobulin deficiency is encountered as a physiological concomitant of infancy. Maternal IgG crosses the placenta but is depleted before the infant is able to mount an antibody response with IgG. The low point of infant IgG occurs at about 6 weeks of age. Therefore, the 6-week-old infant is at high risk of infection with the encapsulated pathogens cited. Furthermore, even older infants and children lack a well-developed repertoire of anticapsular antibodies, as compared with adults, and are therefore more susceptible to such infections than are adults. A pathological diminution or absence of immunoglobulins occurs in the congenital antibody deficiency syndromes and acquired disorders of antibody formation associated with diseases of the lymphoid system. Some diseases of complement predispose to recurrent infections with encapsulated pathogens. For example, patients having the rare genetic diseases in which the major opsonin of complement C3 is not synthesized or is destroyed with abnormal rapidity suffer from recurrent infections caused by high-grade microorganisms. Infection is occasionally the presenting problem in an immune complex disorder such as systemic lupus erythematosus, in which the C3 protein gets consumed abnormally.

Disorders of Clearance by Macrophages

SPLENECTOMY

Because of its abundant blood flow and its unique circulation, which puts blood in contact with many macrophages, the spleen is an efficient organ of clearance. Other clearance organs such as the liver can match the efficiency of the spleen only if the material to be cleared is very recognizable to the hepatic macrophages. Such recognition is possible only with heavily opsonized cells or microorganisms, that is, those that have been massively coated with IgG, C3b, or both. Removal of the spleen creates a small but definite risk of serious bloodstream infection by encapsulated pathogens. These infections may be fulminant and rapidly fatal. The danger of such infections is greater in splenectomized infants and young children than in adults, because the former have lower quantities of specific anticapsular antibodies, which permit the liver and other macrophage-rich organs to compensate for the absence of the more efficient spleen. Splenectomy is an example of macrophage ablation.

CIRRHOSIS OF THE LIVER

Although a less efficient clearance organ than the spleen, the liver contains a large number of macrophages that can clear microorganisms from the portal blood. In severe liver failure, a sizeable fraction of the portal circulation circumvents the liver parenchyma and its macrophages, reducing the total clearance function of this macrophage system. Hepatic cirrhosis is therefore an example of macrophage bypass. Patients with certain forms of severe liver disease may have low levels of C3 in their serum as well, because the hepatocyte is the source of C3 and many other proteins that circulate in the blood. It is not surprising, therefore, that patients with advanced cirrhosis of the liver are highly susceptible to bacterial infections.

HEMOLYTIC DISORDERS

In diseases characterized by large numbers of chronically damaged red blood cells, such as sickle cell anemia or the thalassemia syndromes, the macrophage system is diverted from its task of clearing microorganisms. The macrophages have to ingest the abnormal red blood cells, eventually depleting membrane from their surfaces and saturating their capaci-

> ### DISORDERS OFTEN LEADING TO SERIOUS RECURRENT OR SEVERE INFECTIONS WITH VIRULENT ENCAPSULATED PATHOGENS
>
> Antibody deficiency syndromes
>   Transient infantile antibody deficiency
>   Congenital antibody deficiency
>   Acquired antibody deficiency
>   Associated with lymphoid neoplasms
>   Protein-losing syndromes
> Complement disorders
>   Congenital deficiency of C3 or other components
>   Acquired deficiency of C3 or other components caused by immune complex diseases (systemic lupus erythematosus, acute glomerulonephritis)
> Mononuclear phagocyte disorders
>   Macrophage ablation: splenectomy
>   Macrophage bypass: hepatic cirrhosis
>   Macrophage diversion: sickle cell anemia; other hemoglobinopathies with unstable erythrocytes
> Combined disorders
>   Hepatic cirrhosis: macrophage bypass and impairment of C3 synthesis

ty to ingest anything else. The association between infection and hemolysis is most frequently seen in sickle cell anemia, in which the hemolytic state is constant and lifelong. The diversion of the macrophage system is further exacerbated by infarction of the spleen, which follows frequent occlusions in the splenic circulation. As in the case of splenectomy alone, the susceptibility to infection in severe hemolytic anemia is most marked in infancy and early childhood.

Disorders of Neutrophil and Monocyte Activity

The flow of neutrophils and monocytes into the tissues on which normal neutrophil and monocyte phagocytic activity depends is equivalent to the large turnover of polymorphonuclear leukocytes and monocytes. A sufficient diminution in the number of available wandering phagocytes or in the ability of these cells to function properly predisposes the patient to unusually recurrent or severe infections with low-grade pathogens.

REDUCTIONS IN NEUTROPHIL TURNOVER

It cannot be overemphasized that the neutrophil count of the peripheral blood may not be a reliable indication of the neutrophil turnover from blood to tissues. For example, a low neutrophil count in the blood could result from a redistribution into the marginal pool, in which case the delivery of neutrophils into the tissues might be normal. One way to test for tissue penetration of neutrophils into peripheral tissues is to make an abrasion on the forearm that scrapes off the superficial epidermis without causing bleeding and to place a glass coverslip over the abrasion. The tissue damage produced by this technique releases chemotactic factors that attract neutrophils. The neutrophils stick to the glass coverslip. By 5 hours, the coverslip should be covered with neutrophils. If this coverslip is replaced with another, monocytes as well as neutrophils will be on it by 12 to 24 hours. This dermal abrasion technique is called the *Rebuck skin window*.

Decreased neutrophil turnover can be caused by impaired neutrophil production, destruction of mature neutrophils, or a combination of these mechanisms. Destruction of mature neutrophils sufficient to predispose to recurrent infections occurs infrequently, because of the immense productivity of the bone marrow for neutrophils. However, a reduction of neutrophil formation frequently results from many causes of bone marrow failure. In these disorders of neutrophil synthesis, the neutrophil blood count can reflect the turnover directly, and the risk of infection begins to mount when the neutrophil count falls below 500 cells/μl. The infections occur most frequently in those areas where microorganisms are in contact with the tissues: the skin, the anus, the mouth, and the respiratory passages.

DISORDERS OFTEN LEADING TO RECURRENT OR SEVERE INFECTIONS WITH RESIDENT PATHOGENS

Deficiency of neutrophils and monocytes
  Congenital neutropenia
  Autoimmune neutropenia
  Medication-induced neutropenia
  Generalized bone marrow failure secondary to aplastic anemia, metastatic cancer, acute leukemia, marrow fibrosis, effects of toxins, and ionizing radiation
Disorders of phagocyte structure and function
  Various genetic diseases in which neutrophil adhesion, locomotion, and phagocytosis are impaired
  Chronic granulomatous disease
  Chédiak–Higashi syndrome

In the presence of a normal neutrophil production rate, the flow of neutrophils into the tissues can be reduced if the neutrophils are defective in their ability to leave the circulation and enter the tissues. Theoretically, failure to elaborate chemotactic factors could cause such an impairment in neutrophil turnover, but in fact the great number of chemotactic factors produced during infection prevent this possibility from being a real problem. On the other hand, congenital and acquired abnormalities of neutrophils can prevent these cells from responding properly to chemotactic factors. In that case, the blood neutrophil count increases, tissue neutrophils decrease, and skin and mucosal infections occur. Corticosteroids have this effect on neutrophils. In addition, a rare genetic disorder exists in which this situation arises because structural components of neutrophils are defective.

Leukocyte adhesion deficiency is an autosomal recessive disease in which affected patients suffer from recurrent infections caused by low-grade pathogens. The phagocytes of these patients are defective in adhesion to surfaces and in phagocytosis of iC3b-coated particles, because the cells express variably diminished amounts of the integrins that mediate phagocytosis of iC3b-coated bacteria and adhesion of phagocytes to many surfaces, especially to ICAM on endothelial cells. The degree of expression of these β2-integrins correlates inversely with the susceptibility to recurrent infections. The heterogeneity of this disorder and analysis of affected leukocytes at the molecular level indicate that leukocyte integrin deficiency results from a spectrum of specific genetic defects in which either the β-chain of phagocyte integrin is not synthesized or an abnormal chain is generated.

If the neutrophils that reach the tissues have a reduced capacity to kill microorganisms, susceptibility to infection is also increased. Such a reduction in killing capacity is found in the genetic disorder *chronic granulomatous disease,* usually inherited as an X-linked recessive trait. In this condition, the polymorphonuclear leukocytes and monocytes do not produce superoxide and hydrogen peroxide, the toxic products of oxygen required for efficient killing of bacteria and fungi. This failure is the result of a variety of possible molecular defects (Fig 18-7B). In most families with the disease, the X-linked deficiency b-cytochrome subunits that couple NADPH oxidation to oxygen reduction to superoxide are either missing or mutated. In other families in which the disease is transmitted as an autosomal recessive, the cytochrome is incapable of activation because of deficiency in expression of the phox 47 and phox 67 activating components in the affected cells. Alternatively, in rarer instances in which the leukocytes have nearly a complete deficiency of the enzyme glucose 6-phosphate dehydrogenase, the capacity of the cells to regenerate NADPH from NADP, thereby providing reducing equivalents for the superoxide-forming enzyme, may be sufficiently impaired to render the neutrophil unable to synthesize superoxide and hydrogen peroxide.

Patients with all these variants of chronic granulomatous disease may suffer from recurrent episodes of lymphadenitis, pneumonia, osteomyelitis, and abscesses affecting the skin, liver, and other organs. Histologically, the affected tissues frequently contain granulomas, hence the name of this disease. The microorganisms causing the infections in these patients are gram-positive and gram-negative bacteria and fungi, predominantly of low grade, that is, organisms that do not ordinarily cause infections in normal persons. Interestingly, phagocytes in these patients have the capacity to kill streptococci, pneumococci, and a variety of other organisms. This ability is explained by the role of oxygen metabolites in the pathogenesis of this disease.

Aerobic organisms such as *Streptococcus* and *Pneumococcus* elaborate hydrogen peroxide as part of their normal metabolism. In the free-living state this production of potentially toxic compounds does not appear to harm the microorganisms. However, in the narrow confines of phagocytic vacuoles of phagocytes from patients with chronic granulomatous disease, the hydrogen peroxide synthesized by the bacteria is sufficient to cause their own suicide. The granule enzyme myeloperoxidase enters the phagocytic vacuole by fusion in the normal fashion in phagocytes of patients with chronic granulomatous disease and works with hydrogen peroxide to kill the bacteria. However, many aerobic microbes, including *Staphylococcus aureus* and most gram-negative enteric organisms, produce the enzyme catalase. This enzyme destroys the hydrogen peroxide generated by the bacteria. Unlike catalase-negative microbes, these microbes therefore do not destroy themselves. Therefore, chronic granulomatous disease neutrophils and monocytes cannot kill catalase-producing organisms, and the patients afflicted with this disorder suffer from recurrent infections with such microorganisms (Fig 18-12).

The diagnosis of chronic granulomatous disease can easily be made by means of biochemical and histochemical techniques that detect the ability of blood neutrophils to metabolize oxygen. One such test, called the *NBT test,* mixes blood neutrophils with a dye called nitroblue tetrazolium (NBT) in the presence of microorganisms. If the phagocytes are normal, they reduce the yellow dye to a blue product called *forrmazan,* and precipitates of this material can be seen in the light microscope. Neutrophils of patients with chronic granulomatous disease fail to reduce the dye. Female carriers of the disease will show that approximately one-half their cells possess the chronic granulomatous disease gene, because only one-half their cells reduce the dye in this test.

Two other genetic diseases affecting phagocyte function are interesting and worthy of brief description. In *hereditary myeloperoxidase deficiency*, an autosomal recessive condition, the azurophilic granules lack the enzyme myeloperoxidase. The microbicidal power of myeloperoxidase in the presence of hydrogen peroxide is missing in the affected neutrophils, and they are somewhat impaired in their capacity to kill microbes. Unlike chronic granulomatous disease, however, this deficiency is not associated with serious susceptibility to bacterial infection, but may predispose to infection by the fungus *Candida albicans*. It may be inferred that the main role of the peroxidase system is in the killing of this ubiquitous fungal organism.

The *Chédiak-Higashi syndrome* is an autosomal recessive disorder of unknown cause. The most distinctive feature of the Chédiak-Higashi syndrome is the fact that white blood cells and many other cells possess large abnormal granules that represent fusions of certain normal cytoplasmic granules. This granule aggregation in dermal melanocytes causes a partial albinism and a silvery gray hair color. The giant granules in mature neutrophils fuse abnormally slowly with phagocytic vacuoles after ingestion of microorganisms, causing a small delay in microbicidal activity by the cells. The major clinical consequences of the Chédiak-Higashi syndrome relate to cellular dysfunctions that cannot as yet be explained either anatomically or enzymatically. Patients with this disease have variable degrees of neutropenia and impairment of neutrophil locomotion, leading to decreased neutrophil activity in the tissues. The result is recurrent infections with low-grade pathogens. There are also minor abnormalities of platelet function, renal

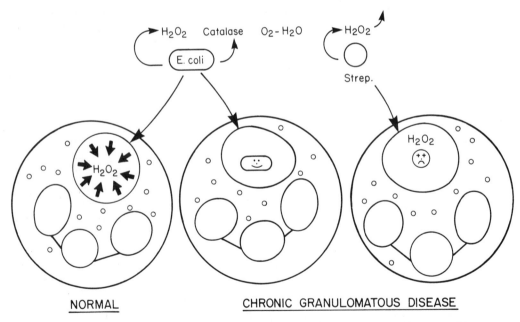

NORMAL   CHRONIC GRANULOMATOUS DISEASE

Fig. 18-12. Pathogenesis of chronic granulomatous disease. *Streptococcus* and other aerobic catalase-negative organisms accumulate hydrogen peroxide in phagocytic vacuole of chronic granulomatous disease (CGD) phagocyte and are killed by it. The catalase-positive organisms have no net accumulation of hydrogen peroxide and are not killed. A normal phagocyte makes enough hydrogen peroxide to overcome the protective effect of catalase produced by the microorganism.

tubular function, and variable changes in neuronal function, which can sometimes lead to neurological deficits. Many patients with the Chédiak-Higashi syndrome develop what has been called an accelerated phase of the syndrome, characterized by fever, pancytopenia, and organ enlargements caused by proliferations of macrophagelike cells. The accelerated phase leads inexorably to death by infection and wasting. Genetic diseases closely resembling the Chédiak-Higashi syndrome exist throughout the animal kingdom. Species known to carry the genes include mice, cattle, mink, and even killer whales.

STORAGE DISEASES

Storage diseases encompass a large family of genetic disorders caused by the absent or significantly reduced activity of enzymes that reside in cellular lysosomes. The consequence of this hypoactivity is the accumulation within cells of substances ordinarily degraded by these enzymes, usually complex lipids, glycolipids, or mucopolysaccharides. This accumulation is often toxic, and the susceptibility of a given cell type to this toxicity determines the clinical manifestation of the storage disorder. Nearly all lysosomal storage diseases are inherited in an autosomal recessive manner.

Many storage diseases cause neurological and skeletal dysfunction. Only one, a variant of Gaucher's disease, is frequently encountered by the hematologist, because this form of Gaucher's disease is characterized by splenomegaly and hypersplenism or bone marrow failure, or both. The blood, however, is often relevant in other types of storage diseases, because blood leukocytes may also lack the enzyme in question, permitting biochemical measurements of peripheral blood leukocytes to establish the diagnosis. In addition, products accumulating abnormally in leukocyte lysosomes can cause visibly distinct inclusions or cytoplasmic vacuoles to appear in blood cells. The inclusions appearing in leukocytes of patients with storage diseases carry the name Alder-Reilly bodies. In mucopolysaccharide

storage disorders the inclusions are metachromatic, that is, they appear bluish-purple after the cells are stained with toluidine blue dye.

The bone marrow contains foam cells in many storage diseases. Foam cells are macrophages laden with vacuoles containing undigested matter. Although not entirely specific for storage disorders, the appearance of foam cells in a bone marrow aspirate or biopsy specimen may help establish the diagnosis in the appropriate clinical setting.

Gaucher's Disease

The first storage disease was recognized by Philip C.E. Gaucher in 1882 as an epithelioma of the spleen. The variant of Gaucher's disease encountered by the hematologist is called type I; its clinical manifestations are caused by deficiency of glucocerebrosidase activity in cells of the mononuclear phagocyte system. The recessive gene for Gaucher's disease, which resides on chromosome 1, is most prevalent in Ashkenazi Jewish populations. Gaucher's disease types II and III are uncommon and involve the nervous as well as the mononuclear phagocyte systems.

Sphingolipids are components of normal plasma membranes. They consist of the alcoholic compound sphingosine linked to fatty acids. They may be linked to sugars, phosphate, or sulfate. This general compound is also designated a ceramide. The glycoprotein enzyme glucocerebroside β-glucosidase (glucocerebrosidase) creates a glucose residue from the one-carbon of sphingosine. This degradation is part of the general digestive process that occurs after senescent blood cells are internalized by macrophages of the spleen and other clearance organs and during the normal turnover of blood cells in the bone marrow comprising the effective hematopoiesis. The inability to degrade a variety of blood cell glycolipids by the enzyme-deficient macrophages results in an accumulation of the undigested glycolipid in the cytoplasm of the macrophages. The undigested matter takes on the appearance of a series of wrinkled tubules, 6 nm in diameter, which contain cholesterol, phospholipid, and protein as well as glucocerebroside. The wrinkled inclusions are distinctive, and macrophages laden with them are called *Gaucher cells* (Fig. 18-13). The diagnosis of Gaucher's disease is easily made without requiring a bone marrow examination by measuring the activity of glucocerebrosidase in peripheral white blood cells using fluorescing β-glucoside substrates.

Gaucher cells may also be visible in bone marrow specimens of patients with diseases associated with very high blood cell turnover, such as in the homozygous β-thalassemias or in chronic granulocytic leukemia. In this setting, it may be that the mass of blood cell membranes to be processed outstrips the digestive capacity of normal macrophages, and that glucocerebroside or other membrane constituents accumulate in these macrophages.

The clinical manifestations of type I Gaucher's disease vary in severity and are the result of an accumulation of Gaucher cells in the spleen, liver, and bone marrow. Splenic enlargement may cause either discomfort in the left upper quadrant or gastric compression, or both. Anemia, leukopenia, and/or thrombocytopenia can occur as a consequence of hypersplenism. The accumulation of Gaucher cells in the bone marrow may superimpose an element of bone marrow failure on the shortened survival of blood cells due to hypersplenism.

The nonhematological consequences of Gaucher's disease occur in the liver and the skeleton. Enlargement of the liver and impairment of liver excretory function are secondary to encroachment on the liver parenchyma by Gaucher cells. Erosion of long bones by Gaucher cells originating in the marrow can lead to pathological fractures and to deformities. A characteristic bone abnormality visible on x-ray films of the limbs is a widening on the epiphyses, called the *Erlenmeyer flask deformity*.

The variability of clinical manifestations of Gaucher's disease results from different defects in the glucocerebrosidase gene, although even siblings with the same gene defect can have different clinical courses. The mild forms of the disorder usually presenting in mid- to late childhood and early adulthood are often not progressive and may be compatible with a normal life span. The hematological complications of anemia or thrombocytopenia with attendant bleeding have responded to splenectomy. However, if bone lesions are a prominent feature of the disease, considerable morbidity can occur. Recently, recombinant glucocerebrosidase has become available for infusion into patients with Gaucher's disease. The enzyme is taken up by macrophages via mannose receptors and enters lysosomes, where it degrades the stored ceramide. The effectiveness of this treatment in reversing organomegaly and bone changes of Gaucher's disease proves that enzyme replacement can work in patients and sets the stage for gene replacement therapy in the future. An interesting event in this regard was the amelioration of Gaucher's disease in a patient receiving a liver transplant. Donor-derived macrophages survived in the recipient and evidently degraded glucocerebroside deposits.

SUGGESTED READINGS

Beutler E (1993) Gaucher disease as a paradigm of current issues regarding single gene mutations of humans. Proc Nat Acad Sci USA 90:5384

Gallin JL, Goldstein I, Snyderman R (1992) Inflammation. Basic Mechanisms and Clinical Correlates. 2nd Ed. Raven Press, New York

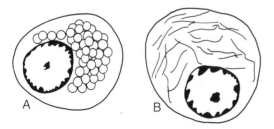

Fig. 18-13. Foam cell (**A**); Gaucher cell (**B**).

Gleich GJ, Adolphson CR (1986) The eosinophil leukocyte: structure and function. Adv Immunol 39:177

Horesçi V (1991) Surface antigens of human leukocytes. Adv Immunol 49:75

Lawrence MB, Springer TA (1991). Leukocyte rolling on a selectin at physiologic flow rates. Cell 65:869

Starzl TE et al (1993) Chimerism after liver transplantation for type IV glycogen storage disease and type I Gaucher's disease. N Engl J Med 328:745

Stossel TP (1993) On the crawling of animal cells. Science 260:1086

19

Lymphoid Cells and Immune Reactions Associated with Defense and Disease

Lymphoid cells are more uniform in appearance on Wright's-stained blood smears than are phagocytic leukocytes. However, these cells are exceedingly diverse and complex and are the "brains" of the immune system. They discriminate self from nonself, generate specificity in the attack on offending microorganisms, and are the repositories of memory, permitting a rapid response to invasion. Unlike the phagocytes, which have a life cycle that tends to be a one-way street from bone marrow to blood to tissues, many lymphoid cells circulate and recirculate among bone marrow, blood, lymphatics and lymphoid organs, the lymph nodes, and the spleen.

LYMPHOCYTES IN NORMAL BLOOD AND TISSUES

Most lymphocytes are found in the lymphatic system, or lymphon, a network of channels interspersed by aggregates of lymphocytes together with other cells. These aggregates are lymph nodes of lymph glands and the spleen. The lymphatic system communicates directly with the blood vasculature at the thoracic duct, where the lymph enters the subclavian vein. The blood and lymphatic systems are also in intimate contact in the spleen, where the blood percolates through rich lymphoid collections, called *white pulp*, of this organ. Figure 19-1 shows the locations of lymph nodes, the sizes of which can be ascertained by the clinician employing observation and palpation during the physical examination. These nodes include the tonsils and the cervical, axillary, epitrochlear, subclavian, and inguinal glands. Of the internal lymph nodes, the mediastinal nodes may be visualized, especially if enlarged, on x-ray films of the chest. Special procedures including lymphangiography and computed tomography are required to evaluate the size of abdominal lymph nodes.

The architecture of lymph nodes features a *capsule* surrounding glandular substance divided into outer *(cortical)* and inner *(medullary)* regions (Fig. 19-2A). Lymphatic channels bringing lymph into the gland (afferent vessels) enter the cortex, delivering the lymph to a subcortical space. The cortex contains clumps of cells, *the germinal follicles*, the site of anti-

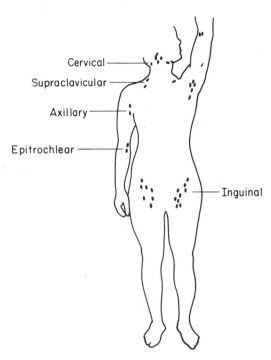

Fig. 19-1. Location of lymph nodes.

body-forming lymphoid cells. Lymph percolates into the medulla and leaves by efferent vessels at the hilum of the node. The different types of normal and abnormal lymphocytes prefer to reside in discrete areas of the lymph node (Fig. 19-2B).

In the healthy adult, the blood contains 1,500 to 3,500 lymphocytes/μl. Early in life, the number of lymphocytes may be much higher, up to 15,000/μl; the concentration of these cells falls progressively, reaching the adult level by adolescence. Similarly, the lymphoid organs, the lymph nodes and spleen, of young children tend to be relatively large and diminish in size until, by adulthood, they are impalpable or barely so. The typical blood lymphocyte observed on a Wright's-stained smear of the blood is a relatively small leukocyte, essentially characterized as a dense nucleus with clumped chromatin and an indistinct nucleolus with a bit of blue cytoplasm peeking around it (Fig. 19-3). If the nuclear chromatin is less dense, the nucleoli are more obvious, the quantity of cytoplasm is increased, and the lymphocyte is called *atypical* (Fig. 19-3). Up to 5 per-

cent of the lymphocytes of normal persons may be atypical. What appears simply as typical and atypical lymphocytes to the morphologist in reality represents a complex of many populations of cells having very different life histories and functions. The principal categories of lymphoid cells are thymus-derived lymphocytes (*T cells*) and bone marrow-derived lymphocytes (*B cells*).

Thymus-Derived Lymphocytes

During fetal development, a population of lymphocytes arises from the bone marrow and migrates to the thymus gland (Fig. 19-4). There, in response to interactions with the epithelial cells of this organ, the cells acquire the ability to perform their specific immunological functions. The cells leave the thymus and percolate in the blood and lymphatic circulation until they reach specific areas of the spleen and lymph nodes called the *paracortical region* (Fig. 19-2B). These T cells recirculate periodically out of the lymphoid organs into the circulation and have the capacity, like phagocytes, to enter the tissues, although their motility is slower than that of phagocytes. Eventually, the lymphocytes return to the lymph nodes and spleen. Of the blood lymphocytes, about two-thirds are T cells in the normal state. During the course of their meanderings, the cells may encounter an antigen, such as a microorganism, to which they are able to respond. The confrontation causes the lymphocyte to increase in size and undergo division, generating a clone of cells reactive to that antigen (see below). These changes in morphology of the lymphocytes, which correspond to those of the atypical lymphocytes seen in the peripheral blood, are accompanied by DNA synthesis and eventually by cell division. The phenomenon, called *blast transformation,* can be measured in the laboratory by observing the incorporation of radioactively labeled thymidine into cellular DNA.

T cells are particularly important in the destruction of foreign cells and are the principal agents for the rejection of grafts in the set-

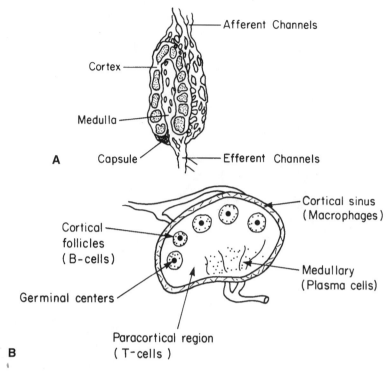

Fig. 19-2. Architecture of a lymph node. (**B**) Distribution of cell types in a lymph node.

ting of purposeful or accidental transplantation of cells and organs. The particular response of the activated T cell depends on its programming in the thymus. T cells as a whole are functionally very versatile. The many different functions they perform are done by different subsets of T lymphocytes. Certain T-effector cells may directly participate in the killing of facultative intracellular parasites by killing the cells in which the parasites reside, for example, virus-containing cells. Such cells are designated *cytotoxic* or *killer T cells.* Killer T cells may recognize their targets because of the specificity built into them during differentiation. Alternatively, the T cells can recognize and kill target cells that are coated with specific antibodies directed against the target cell. One of the mechanisms by which the killing occurs is the secretion by the cytotoxic or killer T cell of proteins called *perforins,* which punch holes in target cells. The perforins resemble the terminal component of the complement sequence C9 (Ch. 17). A second function of T cells is to elaborate substances, lymphokines, that act on other cells. One set of lymphokines, activates macrophages, enabling the latter to kill facultative intracellular parasites within them. One of the most important macrophage-activating lymphokines is interferon-γ. Cytoxic/suppressor cells also elaborate tumor-necrosis factor (TNF) as well as other cytokines.

Another cytokine, interleukin-2 (IL-2), acts as a B-cell growth factor; in this respect it is important in the setting of a third function of the T cell, in which another subclass of these cells, called *helper cells,* cooperates with B cells to stimulate their differentiation into plasma cells producing specific antibodies. There are at least two classes of helper T cells, designated TH1 and TH2. TH1 cells primarily promote the development of IgG-producing plasma cells and resemble T suppressor/cytotoxic cells in synthesizing macrophage-activating cytokines. TH2 cells induce plasma cells that make IgE, and they promote the growth of eosinophils and mast cells. Therefore TH2 cells

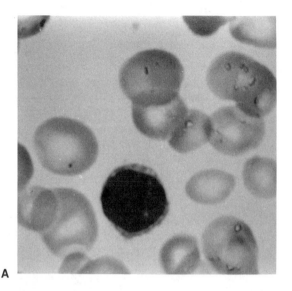

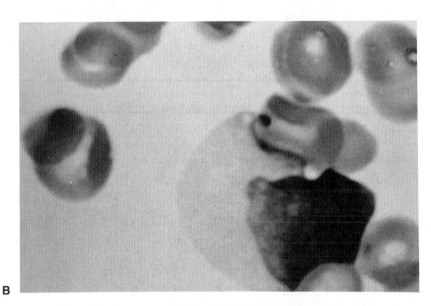

Fig. 19-3. Appearance of typical (**A**) and atypical (**B**) lymphocyte.

are important in the generation of immediate hypersensitivity responses.

IL-2 also induces cytotoxic activity of certain T cells. The attempt to activate such T cells by recombinant IL-2 into "killer (LAK) cells" against tumor cells has been used as a form of experimental cancer therapy. An additional lymphokine, TNF, has multiple toxic metabolic effects. A fourth function of certain T cells is to control or suppress the production of antibodies by B cells, preventing uncontrolled or inappropriate immune reactions. Such cells are designated *suppressor cells* (Fig. 19-4).

If the thymus is removed from or destroyed in an animal or human before or shortly after birth, the subject lacks T cells and lacks the ability to express cell-mediated immunity. The specificity programmed into B and T lymphocytes persists after an encounter with antigen in

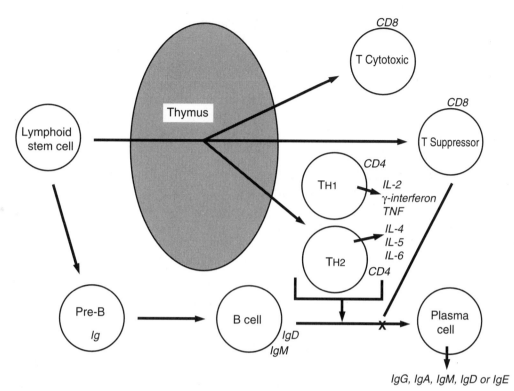

Fig. 19-4. Ontogeny of lymphoid cells.

the form of immunological memory. Progeny of the specific clones persist for many years in a dormant state. On subsequent encounter with the original antigen, clonal expansion occurs again, but with greater efficiency, and this secondary response in terms of cell-mediated immunity or antibody production is the basis of specific immunity and provides the rationale for vaccination.

Bursa or Bone-Marrow-Derived Lymphoid Cells

In birds, an organ associated with the gastrointestinal tract, the bursa of Fabricius, participates in the education of undifferentiated lymphoid cells into B cells, a function analogous to the activity of the thymus for the development of T cells. Lymphocytes arising from the bone marrow migrate to this organ and acquire the eventual capacity to differentiate into *plasma cells* that secrete specific antibod-

ies. These cells have been named B cells after the bursa of Fabricius. Birds from which the bursa is removed before hatching have no B cells and no antibodies.

Mammals do not have a bursa of Fabricius; presumably, the bone marrow itself assumes this function of conditioning certain lymphocytes for subsequent antibody formation.

One of the earliest identifiable cells of B-cell lineage is called a pre-B cell (Fig. 19-4). Mature B lymphocytes circulate in the blood and lymphatics but are found primarily in the germinal centers of the cortex of lymph nodes and in the white pulp of the spleen. Of blood lymphocytes, fewer than one-fifth are B cells. They are typical lymphocytes in their morphological appearance. Responding to antigens, B lymphocytes proliferate and differentiate into clones of plasma cells that secrete specific antibodies directed against the antigens. Plasma cells have a characteristic morphology (Fig. 19-5). They are ovoid to rhomboid in shape. Their nucleus is round, and in an off-center location; clumps of nuclear chromatin are visibly located around the edges of the nucleus in a spoke-wheel pattern in formalin-fixed and hematoxylin and eosin-stained specimens. The peripheral cytoplasm stains dark blue in Wright's-stained smears because of abundant ribosomes involved in the synthesis of immunoglobulins. A distinct light perinuclear halo is the location of a Golgi complex.

During the course of antibody production against a new antigen, the B-cell system makes IgM first, followed by other classes of immunoglobulin. A mature plasma cell secretes only one class of immunoglobulin, with specificity for only one antigen. This means that the cell makes one class of heavy chains—either μ, γ, α, δ, or ε—and one class of light chains ending up as IgM, IgG, IgA, IgD, or IgE antibodies. However, during development, B cells make various classes of immunoglobulin and express them in different ways. For example, pre-B cells have immunoglobulins in their cytoplasm but not on their membranes, and they do not secrete these immunoglobulins. During maturation, B cells express at varying times IgM and IgD on their surfaces. The surface immunoglobulin of a given B cell will have either λ or κ light chains, but the normal B-cell population, like the populations of immunoglobulins in the circulation, will express a mixture of κ and λ light chains in a ratio of 2:1. As the lymphocyte matures into a plasma cells it switches over to making a particular immunoglobulin class that it secretes; the conversion in type of antibody made by developing B lymphocytes is called *class* or *isotype switching*. This sequence of changes in the expression of immunoglobulins during B-cell development is diagrammed in Figure 19-4.

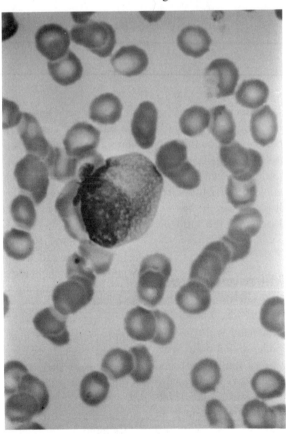

Fig. 19-5. Plasma cell.

Other Cells of the Lymphoid System

A population of lymphocytes that cannot be characterized as either T or B cells as defined by surface Ig expression or cosetting with sheep red cells are designated *null cells*. These cells are very immature lymphocytes, not committed yet to either B- or T-cell lineage. They may even be stem cells. Some of these cells contain terminal deoxyribonucleotide transferase, an enzyme that catalyzes the addition of deoxyribonucleoside triphosphate bases, such as deoxy-ATP, into the 3'-hydroxyl end of single-stranded polynucleotides. This DNA polymerase is unique in mammalian DNA synthesis in not requiring a template for its function. It is a very useful marker for immature cells and for the diagnosis of certain lymphoid neoplasms. Ten to 20 percent of blood lymphocytes are null cells.

A class of cells important in immune reactions are *natural killer (NK)* cells. These cells have the ability to kill abnormal cells, such as damaged cells, virus-infected cells, and possibly cancer cells without being primed by previous recognition of the antigen or without requiring a specific antibody for their action. Interferon-γ stimulates the cytotoxic action of natural killer cells.

Cells with long processes called *dendritic cells* are important for the complex communication described below that goes on between B cells, T cells, and macrophages during the generation of specific antibody responses.

IDENTIFICATION OF LYMPHOID CELLS

The different types of lymphocytes can be identified by receptors on their membranes, usually defined by the CD designation (see footnote on p. 11, Ch. 1). The receptors may bind particular antibodies or certain types of red blood cells. These surface markers define the various populations of lymphoid cells (Table 19-1).

The most straightforward method for identifying B cells is to detect immunoglobulin molecules in or on them. This can be done by reacting the cells with fluorescein-tagged anti-immunoglobulin antibody, washing off excess reagent, and looking for cell-associated fluorescence in a fluorescence microscope or with a flow cytometer. B cells also bind to erythrocytes coated with the third component of complement. The erythrocytes surround the lymphocyte. From the floral resemblance, this tableau is called *a rosette*. Phagocytes also form rosettes with complement-coated erythrocytes, but unlike B lymphocytes, they can phagocytize the complexes under appropriate conditions.

T cells form rosettes with sheep erythrocytes; the formation of these E rosettes, once the principal assay for T lymphocytes, has been supplanted by tests for specific T-cell antigens, for example, the specific receptor molecule on the T cells for sheep red blood cells. In addition, T cells specifically undergo blast transformation in response to concanavalin A, a lectin (protein that binds to sugars, specifically to

Table 19-1. Some Functional and Immunochemical Markers of Lymphoid Cells

Cell Type	Functional Marker	Immunochemical Definition
Immature T cell	Terminal deoxynucleotide transferase	CD3
T cell	Responds mitogenically to concanavalin A	CD2,CD3,CD5,CD6,CD7
Helper cell	Promotes synthesis of antibodies by B cells	CD4
Suppressor cell	Inhibits synthesis of antibodies	CD8
Pre-B cell	Rearranged Ig genes	Cytoplasmic Ig, CD10
Immature B cell	Expresses C3b receptors, IgM, IgD	CD19, CD20, CD22
Mature B cell	Expresses class II MCH receptors (Ia antigen)	CD19, CD20
Plasma cell	Secretes Igs	PCA1, PCA2

mannose residues). Antibodies can be raised in animals against antigens on the surface of lymphoid cells of unrelated species; these antibodies can be tagged with fluorescein and can be used to identify T cells, B cells, and subsets of T cells, the helper and suppressor cells (Table 19-1). When antibodies against antigens on cells of one species are generated in another species, these antibodies are said to be *heterologous*. The antibodies are generated by the lymphoid system of an organism exposed to the foreign cells. The process that goes into the production of these antibodies involves a selection and the development of multiple clones producing antibodies of varying avidity for the antigen. Furthermore, unless the antigen is perfectly pure, the organism will almost certainly generate antibodies reactive against multiple antigens in the preparation used to immunize the animal. In the case of cells containing multiple surface antigens, this is a serious problem. The development of antibodies for use in detection of certain types of cells by this technique therefore requires that the immunoglobulin preparation be absorbed with various cells until a desired specificity for a particular cell is achieved. With this complex methodology, the specificity of the antibodies is always in question and is hard to reproduce from one laboratory to another.

It is therefore preferable for diagnostic purposes to produce antibodies in tissue culture in large quantities that are specific for a single part of a single antigen. These antibodies are derived from a single clone of B cells. These *monoclonal antibodies* are made by fusing spleen cells from a mouse immunized with the antigen to a mouse lymphoid tumor cell. The tumor cell confers immortality on the fusion product, called a *hybridoma,* which permits it to undergo continuous replication and secrete large quantities of antibody derived from the B-cell genes operative in the hybridoma. In developing a hybridoma antibody, the fusion products must be separated and cultivated separately and analyzed for their antibody specificity. Once the desired antibody is found, its specificity is more definite. Monoclonal antibodies directed against components of the sur-

face of lymphoid cells are now the principal tools for identification of lymphoid cell subsets. Certain of these antibodies are specific for the various functional subsets of lymphoid cells, for example, for helper T cells, suppressor T cells, and other types of lymphocytes. These antibodies can assist the clinician in determining whether the lymphocyte subpopulations are altered in various disease states and whether an elevation in the blood lymphocyte count or an infiltrate of lymphocytes in the tissues represents the expansion of a particular type of lymphoid cells.

Some of the antibodies are relatively specific for particular stages of lymphoid maturation, whereas others have a broader specificity, for example, for all types of B or T cells. A somewhat confusing situation has arisen from the fact that several commercial sources market monoclonal antibodies and have given them different names. In addition, some of these antibodies may react with different regions of the same surface molecules. Table 19-1 lists some of the different designations as well as the CD nomenclature. In normal blood, about one-half the lymphocytes can be identified as T cells and about one-third as B cells. The remainder, bearing neither T- nor B-cell markers, are classified as null cells. It must be emphasized that the marker systems for identifying lymphoid cells are in constant evolution as new insights develop concerning the complexities of the lymphoid system. The catalog summary of lymphoid cell types and their markers (enumerated in Table 19-1) should therefore be viewed as an initial convenience for learning; the student must be prepared to revise and juggle these concepts. Nevertheless, the use of markers to classify lymphoid cell types is becoming increasingly useful in identifying aberrations in lymphoid cell populations, especially in lymphoid neoplasms.

THE ACQUISITION OF SPECIFIC ANTIGEN RECOGNITION BY LYMPHOID CELLS

How do a large but finite number of B cells have the capacity to regenerate clones of plasma cells, producing antibodies to the apparently infinite number of antigens in the environment, and how do stimulated T cells acquire the capacity to mount cell-mediated immune responses against specific antigens? Why do some individuals make immune responses to certain antigens more readily than others? The answers lie in a set of remarkable mechanisms in which some lymphoid cells shuffle parts of genes encoding recognition molecules, immunoglobulins on B cells and T-cell receptors on T cells, to generate combinations that bind to antigens with high avidity. Engrafted on this selection process is a recognition filter for antigens that varies subtly from one individual to another. Cells such as macrophages and dendritic cells *process* molecules and *present* them in their entirety or in fragments as the ultimate antigens to which the lymphocytes will acquire specific responsiveness. These collaborating cells are designated *antigen-presenting cells (APC)*. The cellular machinery controlling processing and presentation is highly complex, exerting another level of control.

Generation of Effector Specificity

The immunoglobulin molecules expressed on the surfaces of immature B cells serve as crude antigen receptors. When a threshold in the avidity of binding between some of these receptors and antigen is achieved, the selected B cell begins to differentiate and proliferate. Usually this process involves the cooperation of macrophages and a subset of T cells (see below). During differentiation and proliferation the specificity of the reaction between the cell and the antigen must increase. In the case of antibody formation (1) gene recombinations or mutations in the genes coding for variable and hypervariable regions of immunoglobulin molecules permit a testing of different immunoglobulins on the surface of the various B cells and (2) the greater avidity of binding between these molecules and the antibody somehow stimulates proliferation of the B-cell clone with the highest specificity.

The task by which lymphoid cells employ a limited number of genes to produce an enormous quantity of antibody protein molecules, each differing in primary structure, is accomplished by the separation of genes coding for regions of immunoglobulin molecules into different parts of cellular DNA and the subsequent recombination of these genes to yield products that code for different immunoglobulins. The recominbation of genes leading to synthesis of the variable region of heavy chains occurs first, followed by light chain gene recombination. Figure 19-6 shows a scheme for the synthesis of an immunoglobulin light chain. The light chain DNA, located on chromosome 2, contains a small number of base pair sequences that code for the constant region of the molecule, indicated by C, and a larger number of sequences coding for variable region, designated V. In addition, a number of sequences encode the region that joins the constant and variable domains and are shown by the letter J. The recombination of 150 V genes to 1 of 5 J genes can yield 750 different genes for the variable region of the light chain. This variability can be increased further by a factor of, say 10, by imprecise splicing at the J–V recombination locus. Following the transcription of the recombined DNA to RNA, intervening sequences, indicated by the broken lines, are spliced out to produce the final RNA product. This RNA can then be translated to synthesize the completed immunoglobulin molecule. The scheme for antibody diversity outlined in the figure for the case of a light chain is even more complex for the heavy chain. The heavy chain gene, located on chromosome 14, also contains sequences involved in recombination, called D for diversity.

Given the information that there may be as many as 80 embryonic heavy-chain V genes, 50 D genes, and 6 J genes, there are 24,000 possible combinations that can be multiplied by another factor of 100 to allow for recombinational variations. These 2.4 million possible different heavy chains combined with 7,500 possible light chains lead to the theoretical possibility of 18 million antibodies.

The way in which T cells develop the ability for specific recognition of targets is analogous

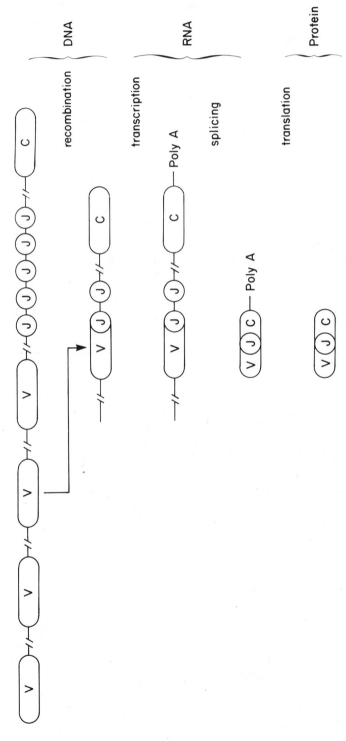

Fig. 19-6. Sequence of changes in the expression of immunoglobulins during B-cell development.

to the generation of antibody specificity by B cells. Instead of surface immunoglobulin serving as an antigen receptor that undergoes regulated mutation into a more specific receptor that eventually becomes secreted to act extracellularly, a family of molecules, known as the *T-cell receptor,* undergoes similar rearrangements but remains affixed to the T-cell membrane. The T-cell receptor resembles immunoglobulin in having two sets of polypeptide chains, each of which has constant and variable regions. The constant regions are anchored in the plasma membrane of the T cell, and, as with immunoglobulins, there are several types of constant domains: most T cells express a and b constant regions while a minority make pairs with somewhat different structure designated δ, γ. The variable domains of the T-cell receptor dimers extend into the extracellular space. As with immunoglobulin genes, a limited number of germline T-cell receptor genes rearrange to generate as many as 10^{15} variable sequences in the variable region of the T-cell receptor molecule. The production of antigen specificity involves the selective activation of T-cell clones with T-cell antigen receptors that react progressively more avidly with the antigen.

The recombination of gene fragments to yield antibodies or T-cell receptors with particular specificities has been shown to be catalyzed by enzymes called *recombinases*, and which are activated by genes named *RAG-1* and *RAG-2*. These genes were discovered by transfecting lymphoid DNA into fibroblasts expressing immunoglobulin gene sequences and isolating the specific genes that caused these sequences to recombine. Transgenic mice in which the *RAG-1* and *RAG-2* genes are inactivated are severely deficient in generating specific immune responses. Class switching of immunoglobulin genes occurs later than the development of antigen specificity. The genes encoding the constant regions determining the different heavy chains are strung out downstream, in the 3′-direction, of the recombined V–D–J genes. By splicing one of the constant genes to the V–D–J sequence, a B lymphocyte generates an antibody of a particular class with a specific recognition site.

Antigen Recognition

Antigen recognition takes place at both afferent (sensory) and efferent (effector) limbs of the immune response. In the afferent limb, lymphoid cells transform rudimentary recognition into highly targeted specific recognition. In the efferent limb, antibodies and T lymphocytes detect target antigens for clearance or destruction.

Some antigens are capable of inducing B-cell differentiation into specific antibody-producing plasma cells without help from other cells. For other antigens, T cells and macrophages interact with the antigens and the B cells to promote differentiation of the B cells in response to antigens. In both cases the membranes of the reacting cells sense antigens through externally disposed receptors mostly produced by genes residing within what is called the *major histocompatibility complex (MHC)* on the short arm of chromosome number 6. Considerable person-to-person variation in the primary amino acid sequences of the extracellular portions of these *major histocompatibility complex proteins* accounts for much of the selectivity in responses of lymphocytes to antigens. These proteins were first discovered as antigens on human lymphocytes reacting with antibodies in the serum of persons who had been exposed to foreign tissues: women who have had numerous pregnancies, persons who had had many blood transfusions, and others who had rejected tissue grafts. These *human lymphocyte antigens (HLA)* were recognized as important mediators of graft rejection following transplantation of tissues from one person to another (Ch. 32). Subsequently, it became clear that one's MCH genotype could predict immune responsiveness to certain antigens and susceptibility to selected autoimmune diseases. MHC proteins are important in both afferent and efferent aspects of the immune response.

MCH proteins divide into two classes. *Class I* MCH proteins are believed to mediate recognition of intracellular antigens that will lead to humoral and cellular immune responses, and they participate in the recognition process when killer T cells attack virus-infected target cells. They are expressed at constant levels on the surfaces of most cells. *Class II* MCH proteins are thought to be more important for antigens derived from outside of cells, and they are particularly important in cooperation between T-helper cells and B cells and for determining individual immune responses to specific antigens. They are normally detectable only on B cells and mononuclear phagocytes, although their expression on these cells can be increased and their appearance induced on other cells following exposure of the cells to interferon-γ and other cytokines. Both MCH proteins bind to the T-cell receptors. Like T-cell receptors and immunoglobulins, MHC proteins consist of two polypeptide chains and have constant and variable regions. The constant domains reside in the intracellular and membranous portion of the molecules, and the variable parts are external. The chains of class II are designated α and β; one of the chains of class I was originally discovered as a circulating protein and named β_2-microglogulin, because it is shed from cells. (See its use as a prognostic marker in multiple myeloma—Ch. 29).

Unlike immunoglobulins or T-cell receptors, however, the variable regions of MHC do not arise from gene rearrangements but derive from differences in inherited genes. The variable sequences account for subtle variations in the three-dimensional structure of a pocket in the extracellular domain where antigenic peptides bind. These variations, especially in class I MHC molecules, account for the fact that tissues transplanted into unrelated recipients elicit immune responses on the one hand and on the other for the fact that cytotoxic T cells recognize self but not nonself virus-infected target cells∇ in the former cases the immune system plays on differences between MHC molecules and in the latter case on identity of MHC molecules. Variations in class II MHC molecules explain differences in antigen presentation from person to person that lead to variability in immune responsiveness to vaccines and grafts and in susceptibility to autoimmune disease (Ch. 20).

Yet another level of regulation is conferred by genes first discovered as "class I modifiers," genes that caused experimental animals with identical class I genes to exercise different immune responses. These genes have now been shown to encode proteins that regulate the transport of intracellular peptides into the cell's endoplasmic reticulum or Golgi compartments where the MHC molecules are assembled. The presence of peptide is very important for stabilization of the MHC in these compartments and their eventual transit to the cell surface, since in the absence of peptide, MHC I may not leave the Golgi complex where they first reside following synthesis or may be degraded. Since the transport genes are highly polymorphic between individuals, there exist differences in the way peptides gain access to MHC, creating an additional control mechanism for generation of immune responsiveness. The breakdown of intracellular proteins into peptides that become transported is the function of a multi-subunit proteolytic enzyme complex called the *proteasome*. This remarkable structure evidently moves proteins around its surface, a process energized by hydrolysis of adenosine triphosphate (ATP), until suitable conformations occur that permit cutting of peptide bonds.

Before combination with antigens, a third subunit of the MHC II, the γ-chain, stabilizes the MHC II $\alpha\beta$ dimers. Extracellular antigens enter the cell by receptor-mediated endocytosis (Ch. 18), which results in intracellular digestive vesicles containing the internalized antigens and their degradation products. These vesicles fuse with various intracellular membrane compartments including Golgi-derived vesicles containing newly synthesized MHC II that then go to and fuse with the cell's surface membrane (Fig. 19-7). Cell-to-cell variations in the nature of intracellular membrane traffic may influence the efficiency of MHC II–antigen combination.

Not all antigens work in the same way to induce immune responses. For example, some antigens, known as *superantigens*, include some viruses and toxins produced by certain strains of bacteria. Superantigens induce high levels of antigen-specific T cells. In contrast to other antigens they interact primarily with the β-subunit of the T-cell receptor, and they do not have the usual requirements for MHC compatibility associated with other types of antigens.

In addition to MHC–T-cell receptor pairing, *accessory molecules* are required for efficient antigen presentation and for effector responses involving T cells (Fig. 19-8). These accessory molecules include a complex immunochemically defined as *CD3* and known to consist of four different polypeptides, designated δ, γ, ε, and ζ. In cytotoxic/suppressor T cells, another adhesion molecule, *CD8*, also binds to MHC class I, whereas in helper T cells a molecule named *CD4* binds MHC class II molecules. CD4 is also important as the receptor that

mediates the internalization of the human immunodeficiency virus (HIV)-1 (acquired immunodeficiency syndrome [AIDS]-causing) virus (Ch. 21). A receptor of the integrin class (Ch. 18), *CD11a/CD18* (also called *LFA-1*) on lymphocytes binds receptors of the immunoglobulin superfamily called *ICAM-1* and *ICAM-2* on APCs or target cells, and *CD2* on the T cell binds *LFA-3* (*CD58*) and *CD59*, both of which are the receptors on sheep red blood cells that mediate the rosetting phenomenon described above. A surface protein called *B7* on APCs interacts with receptors called *CD28* and *CTLA-4* on T cells. All of these adhesion molecules serve to strengthen the connection between T cells and APCs, between cytotoxic T cells and target cells, and between helper T cells and B cells and to induce the intracellular signals that lead to cell proliferation, generation of antigen recognition specificity and effector responses. For exam-

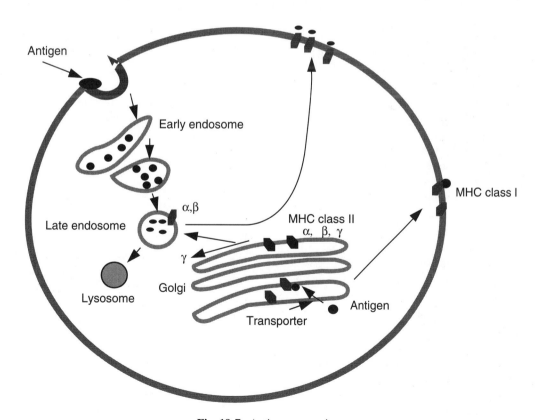

Fig. 19-7. Antigen processing.

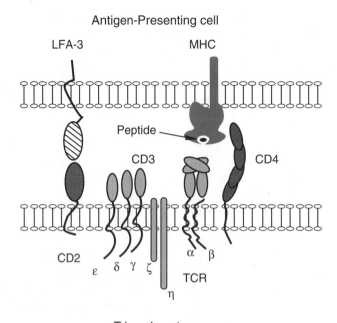

Fig. 19-8. Receptor-mediated interaction between T cells and antigen-presenting cells.

ple, interaction between the T-cell receptor plus CD3 and class II molecules on APCs in the absence of the other paired binding reactions listed, conventionally designated "costimulatory" or "second" signals, leads to loss of specific responsiveness, known as anergy rather than acquisition of immune recognition.

Many of the intracellular signals generated during lymphocyte–APC interactions are similar to those described for platelet (Ch. 14) and phagocyte activation (Ch. 18), namely, rises in intracellular calcium concentration and activation of G-proteins of tyrosine kinases and of phosphoinositide turnover, although cellular activation in lymphoid cells often leads to cellular proliferation, as was described for neoplastic cells in Chapter 19, in contrast to phagocytes and platelets. Also identified as early steps in the signal transduction pathways of lymphoid cells are reactions in which enzymes such as one designated *lck*, which is a member of the *src* oncogene family, catalyze phosphorylation of proteins on tyrosine residues, an event associated with cellular growth control (Ch. 19). Dephosphorylation of

these proteins may be mediated by a membrane protein called *CD45*, which has *protein tyrosine phosphatase* activity. Cellular signalling is also required for antibody *isotype switching*, the conversion by B cells from synthesizing IgM to IgA or IgG; as described in the following chapter, defects in this signalling lead to a failure of the switch.

REACTIVE CHANGES OF LYMPHOID CELLS

Lymphocytes, like phagocytes, respond to infection or inflammation. In many bacterial infections, the lymphocyte count rises, although not usually above 5,000 to 10,000 cells/μl. Responding to the infection, a fraction of the lymphocytes undergoes blast transformation, so that atypical lymphocytes may be common in infection and inflammatory states. Some infections uniquely favor changes in the lymphocyte count. Infections caused by the bacterial species *Bordetella pertussis*, the organism that causes the respiratory disease whooping cough, are associated with extraordinary lymphocytosis, with lymphocyte counts between 20,000 and 80,000/µl. The pertussis microorganism releases a factor that somehow stimulates the increase in blood lymphocytes. However, a reactive lymphocytosis of this degree ordinarily is unusual in adults. Viral infections frequently increase the lymphocyte count and induce substantial atypicality to the morphology of the lymphocytes. Processes affecting the number of peripheral blood lymphocytes frequently can cause proliferation of lymphocytes in the lymph nodes and the spleen. Such enlargements of the lymph nodes and spleen are called, respectively, *lymphadenopathy* and *splenomegaly*.

An infection affecting the lymphoid system frequently encountered in clinical medicine is *infectious mononucleosis*. In infectious mononucleosis there is a fever, sore throat, enlargement of the lymph nodes and spleen, and a lymphocytosis with atypical lymphocytes. The signs and symptoms persist for variable lengths of time, from as short as days to as long as months. The term "mononucleosis" is a meaningless archaic holdover from times of equivocation over the cell type increased in the blood. The most common cause of infectious mononucleosis is an infection with a DNA herpes virus that infects B cells, *the Epstein-Barr virus (EBV)*.

The virus enters the B cell by binding one of its outer membrane glycoproteins, gp350/220, to the receptor for the C3d fragment of complement, complement receptor type 2 (CR2), also designated CD21. The virus is transported to one pole of the cell, a process called *capping*, and then the virus is internalized by receptor-mediated endocytosis and begins replication in the lymphocyte. The atypical lymphocytosis of infectious mononucleosis is a reaction of T cells to the infected B cells. Any and all lymphoid organs can become enlarged in infectious mononucleosis. Although fever and debility are the main clinical problems of infectious mononucleosis, due to elaboration of cytokines by activated lymphoid cells, an occasional serious complication is rupture of the enlarged spleen, which is abnormally susceptible to trauma. Sometimes the enlargement and ulceration of the pharyngeal tonsils can be sufficient to interfere with nutrition. In such instances, brief treatment of the patient with corticosteroids can produce remarkable shrinkage of the lymph nodes and amelioration of the symptoms.

Diseases that affect the normal balance of cells of the lymphoid system can occasionally lead to abnormal immune responses. Rare patients with infectious mononucleosis will develop autoantibodies against their own blood cells or other tissues. Very rarely, the proliferation of atypical T cells can be sufficiently intense as to behave like a malignant neoplasm and progresses to kill the patient by infiltrating vital organs. This catastrophe has occurred within families, and the susceptibility to such a devastating course of EBV mononucleosis is transmitted as an X-linked trait, leading to this condition being named the *X-linked lymphoproliferative syndrome*. Although cancerous in its invasive behavior, this disorder is not an expansion of a single cell clone as occurs in the leukemias. EBV infection is strongly associated with a B-cell neoplasm of Africans called Burkitt's lymphoma and with epithelial neoplasms of the nasopharynx. When normal blood lymphoid cells are cultivated in tissue culture, it appears that it is a chronic infection with EBV that confers immortality on the cells, permitting them to persist under culture conditions. For all these reasons, EBV is suspected as an oncogenic (i.e., cancer-causing) virus. The verdict is not in, however, as it is also possible that these tumors are only susceptible to infection with EBV. Nevertheless, there is no doubt but that EBV causes infectious mononucleosis.

The diagnosis of infectious mononucleosis caused by EBV can be suspected by observation of an atypical lymphocytosis in the setting of appropriate clinical signs and symptoms, usually in a young adult. The diagnosis can be established by observing a rise in antibody titers against EBV several weeks after the onset of the illness. This serological test is rarely necessary, however, because of an unusual immunological phenomenon associated with the disease. Within weeks after the onset of signs and symptoms, the patient's serum contains an IgM antibody that reacts with erythrocytes of various animal species. The reason for the production of this antibody, called *heterophile* (meaning "likes other species"), is unclear, but the presence of heterophile antibody is extremely useful for the diagnosis of EBV infectious mononucleosis. The capacity of a patient's serum to agglutinate sheep or horse erythrocytes establishes the presence of heterophile antibodies. Heterophile antibodies appear in other disorders affecting the immune system, such as serum sickness, but the specificity of the presence of a heterophile antibody for infectious mononucleosis can be established by absorption tests. The heterophile found in EBV infectious mononucleosis will bind to cow but not to guinea pig erythrocytes. Therefore, if the patient's serum persists in agglutinating sheep or horse erythrocytes after exposure to guinea pig erythrocytes, and the loss of this agglutination potential occurs after reaction with beef erythrocytes, the heterophile reaction is specific for EBV infectious mononucleosis.

The clinical picture of infectious mononucleosis can arise in other viral infections such as viral hepatitis and infections with cytomegalovirus or herpes virus. Such infections occur typically in persons who have recently received many blood transfusions. The protozoan *Toxoplasma gondii,* an organism that can be acquired from the ingestion of poorly cooked meat, as well as from house cats, can also cause an illness resembling infectious mononucleosis. Unlike EBV infectious mononucleosis, these other infections do not elicit high EBV or heterophile antibody responses. Some bacterial infections also cause a clinical picture resembling infectious mononucleosis. Typhoid fever, secondary syphilis, and leptospirosis are examples that must be considered in patients with the signs and symptoms of infectious mononucleosis

who fail to demonstrate heterophile antibodies after appropriate absorptions.

Patients with diseases affecting lymphoid cells usually present with generalized signs and symptoms, as well as enlargement of many lymphoid organs, the spleen, and peripheral lymph nodes (Fig. 19-1). The lymph nodes may enlarge up to several centimeters in diameter and may become tender and painful. Usually the lymph nodes are freely movable when probed by the examiner's fingers. Some infections have a predilection to enlarge particular lymph nodes. It is very common for cervical lymph nodes to be enlarged in viral diseases of the respiratory tract and in infectious mononucleosis. In rubella virus infections, the preauricular lymph nodes are uniquely enlarged. Generalized lymphadenopathy is also a manifestation of AIDS or its precursor, AIDS-related complex (ARC) (Ch. 20).

Occasionally the physician encounters enlargement of lymph nodes in a single area with little or no obvious evidence of systemic disease. A first consideration should always be whether an infection or a neoplasm exists in the region providing lymphatic drainage to the involved lymph node. In cases of infections and inflammatory conditions associated with lymph gland enlargement, the lymph node may be actually infected *(lymphadenitis)*, or it may be infiltrated or simply reacting to the infection or some other process in the drainage area *(lymphadenopathy)*. It is common for inguinal lymph nodes to be palpable in adults, probably because of subclinical fungal infections affecting the feet. A biopsy of an enlarged reactive lymph node will usually show normal lymph node architecture as well as increased number and size of germinal follicles. If microorganisms are within the lymph node, they might be visible or possibly can be cultivated. In the case of acute bacterial infection, necrosis and abscess formation with invasion by poly morphonuclear leukocytes will be observed by the pathologist. Infections attributable to tuberculosis or other facultative intracellular parasites can be associated with lymph nodes containing granulomata with or without giant cells. Any infection can lead to reactive enlargement of lymph nodes. Some infections particularly prone to produce lymphadenopathy include anthrax, bubonic plague, tularemia, tuberculosis, and syphilis. *Cat scratch fever* is associated with low grade fever and enlargement of lymph nodes following a contact with a cat. Histologically the nodes contain microabscesses or granulomas. The cause of this self limited reaction is not definitely known, although there is evidence that an unusual bacillary organism called *Rochalimae henselae* is responsible.

The enlargement of lymph nodes in an otherwise asymptomatic patient can herald the presence of a malignant neoplasm. This neoplasm can originate from the lymphoid system itself, in which case the disorder is a lymphoma, or reflect invasion of the lymph nodes by an unrelated cancer. Lymph nodes enlarged by the presence of epithelial malignant neoplasms will frequently feel very hard to the touch because of the extensive fibrosis elicited by the malignant cells. If, because of persistence, large size, or rapid enlargement of a lymph node, the physician decides to have the node surgically excised, the pathologist should be alerted in advance. The pathologist will want to prepare some of the tissue in such a way as to allow for the detection of lymphocyte surface markers as described earlier in this chapter (see also Ch. 20). Once the specimen has been fixed in formalin for routine histological examination, it is possible but more difficult to perform marker studies.

SUGGESTED READINGS

Brown JH, Jardetzky TS, Gorga JC et al (1993) Three-dimensional structure of the human class II histocompatibility antigen HLA-DRI. Nature 364:33

Cooper MD (1987) B lymphocytes. Normal development and function. N Engl J Med 317:1452

Eckhardt LA (1992) Immunoglobulin gene expression only in the right cells at the right time. FASEB J 6:2553

Krensky AM, Weiss A, Crabtree G et al (1990) T-lymphocyte-antigen interactions in transplant rejection. N Engl J Med 322:510

Lieber MR (1992). The mechanism of V(D)J recombination: a balance of diversity, specificity, and stability. Cell 70:873

Margileth AM, Hayden GF (1993) Cat scratch disease. N Engl J Med 329:53

Matsumura M, Fremont DH, Peterson PH, Wilson IA (1992) Emerging principles for the recognition of peptide antigens by MHC class I molecules. Science 257:927

Nepom GT (1989) Structural variation among major histocompatibility complex class-II genes which predispose to autoimmunity. Immunol Res 8:16

Rothbard JB, Gefter ML (1991) Interactions between immunogenic peptides and MHC proteins. Annu Rev Immunol 9:527

Rothenberg EV (1992) The development of functionally responsive T cells. Adv Immunol 51:85

Shinkai Y et al (1992) Rag-2-deficient mice lack mature lymphocytes owing to inability to initiate V(D)J rearrangement. Cell 68:855

Stern LJ, Wiley DC (1992) The human class II protein HLA-DR1 assembles as empty $\alpha\beta$ heterodimers in the absence of antigenic peptides. Cell 68:465

van Noesel CJM, van Lier RAW (1993) Architecture of the human β–cell antigen receptors. Blood 82:363

20

Immunodeficiency and Autoimmunity Caused by Defects of the Lymphoid System

The immense complexity of the lymphoid system renders it highly susceptible to the derangements that impair the immune response. These abnormalities may be hereditary or acquired, transient or permanent, and may affect the sensory (afferent) or effector (efferent) limbs of the system. The clinical consequence of quantitative or qualitative lymphoid deficiency may stem primarily from failure to deal adequately with microorganisms (*immunodeficiency*).

During fetal life, the developing immune system becomes programmed not to react to host antigens. T cells percolating through the thymus that react strongly with cell antigens are deleted by a process called *negative selection*, in contrast to *positive selection*, which encourages T-cell receptor gene rearrangements in postnatal life to produce receptors that bind avidly to target cells. These selection processes result in the death of around 99 percent of the fetal thymocytes! Accordingly, exposure of the fetus even to foreign matter will cause it to fail to react to later contact with that antigen, a state defined as *tolerance*. Instead of a sustained clonal proliferation of specific B or T cells in response to antigens,

the induction of tolerance in utero or postnatally by a complex set of factors in which the timing and dose of antigen; failure of cell–cell interaction; pathological cell–cell interaction, such as excessive T-cell suppression; or blockade of crucial receptors by persistent or excessive antigen or by immune complexes result instead in an abortion or depletion of such clones. Lymphoid system defects, therefore, can also result in a loss of control over the ability to discriminate self from nonself and can manifest as *autoimmune disease*. Immunodeficiency and autoimmunity may coexist in the same instances. Under certain circumstances, clinicians purposely create lymphoid deficiency. This immunosuppression is done to prevent rejection of transplanted organs or to ameliorate the ravages of autoimmune disorders.

GENERAL FEATURES OF IMMUNODEFICIENCY

In disorders in which antibodies are deficient, the patient suffers from recurrent and severe infection caused by high-grade encapsu-

323

lated pathogens, such as *Diplococcus pneumoniae*, *Streptococcus pyogenes*, *Hemophilus influenzae*, and *Neisseria menigitidis*. This susceptibility is the result of impaired opsonization and recognition of these organisms by macrophages. The diagnosis of antibody deficiency is easily established by measuring the serum immunoglobulin concentrations by means of the techniques described in Chapter 17.

If a lymphoid deficiency is primarily a decreased functioning of T cells, the affected person is susceptible to infection with facultative intracellular parasites, such as fungi, viruses, and mycobacteriae. This susceptibility arises from the failure of T cells to arm macrophages to deal with these parasites and from the inability of certain killer T cells to destroy pathogens or pathogen-infected host cells that sustain the microorganisms. Such patients frequently have white patches in the oral cavity, which represent growth of the fungus *Candida albicans*, also called *Monilia* or thrush.

A common virus infection that becomes problematic in the setting of T-cell dysfunction or deficiency is varicella-zoster. Primary exposure to this virus usually causes chickenpox, a self-limited disease characterized by fever and a bullous rash in the normal host. In the T-cell-deficient person, the infection can become fulminant, leading to fatal pneumonia and encephalitis. After the initial infection in the normal host, the virus becomes dormant but persistent in sensory ganglia of the central nervous system (CNS). It can emerge under some circumstances by migrating down the neurons into the skin in regions innervated by the particular ganglion and can cause a painful bullous eruption in that area called *herpes zoster,* or *shingles.* Although localized herpes zoster can occur in normal persons, it arises frequently in T-cell-deficient patients and can disseminate widely over the body. If it affects the trigeminal nerve tract, it can cause a painful ophthalmitis.

Patients with T-cell deficiency can also fall prey to the ravages of a slow virus (lentivirus) that causes *multifocal leukoencephalopathy,* a widespread cerebral degeneration that results in

ANTIBODY DEFICIENCY STATES

Congenital
    X-linked agammaglobulinemia
    X-linked hypogammaglobulinemia with
        elevated IgM levels
    Dysgammaglobulinemia
        Selective IgG subclass deficiency
        IgM deficiency
        IgA deficiency
    Ataxia telangiectasia (IgA hypercatabolism)
    Wiskott-Aldrich syndrome (defective anti-polysaccharide antibody formation)
Acquired
    Common variable hypogammaglobulinemia
    Neoplasm-associated hypogammaglobulinemia
        Chronic lymphatic leukemia
        Thymoma
        Multiple myeloma
    Protein-losing states
        Nephrotic syndrome
        Enteropathy
        Intestinal—lymphatic fistula
    Radiation, chemotherapy and splenectomy, treatment for Hodgkin's disease

motor and sensory dysfunctions and dementia.

An additional complication of severe T-cell deficiency or malfunction is the syndrome called *graft-versus-host disease* (GVHD). This condition arises when the immunoincompetent host receives an infusion of foreign T cells. Such an infusion occurs if the patient receives a transfusion of whole blood or bone marrow in an attempt to reconstitute a failed bone marrow, or occasionally it occurs in utero when maternal lymphocytes gain access to the circulation of an immunodeficient fetus. The deficiency of host T-cell function results in an inability to reject the foreign T cells. However, the infused T cells have no such problem and,

DISORDERS THAT OFTEN LEAD TO RECURRENT OR SEVERE INFECTIONS FROM FACULTATIVE INTRACELLULAR PARASITES

Disorders affecting T lymphocytes
    Congenital thymic aplasia
    Cytotoxic antibodies against T lymphocytes
    Hodgkin's disease
    Sarcoid
    Acquired immunodeficiency syndrome (AIDS)
Disorders affecting all lymphoid cells
    Severe combined immune deficiency, congenital X-linked, and autosomal recessive variants
    Immunosuppressive therapy
        Corticosteroids
        Antimetabolites
        Ionizing irradiation
Pathogenesis unclear
    Wiskott-Aldrich syndrome (thrombocytopenia, eczema, X-linked)
    Protein-calorie malnutrition
    Mucocutaneous candidiasis

if viable and present in sufficient quantities, recognize the new host as foreign and proceed to proliferate and try to kill host cells and tissues. The skin, gastrointestinal tract, and liver are prime targets of this onslaught, so that patients with GVHD can develop jaundice from liver failure, exfoliative dermatitis, diarrhea with fluid and electrolyte depletion, and even frank sloughing of the gut mucosa. The practical issue here is that patients with suspected T-cell deficiency should either not receive whole blood or leukocyte transfusions, or else the blood products to be used should be treated first with ionizing radiation, which prevents the T cells from proliferating.

The diagnosis of T-cell deficiency or malfunction can be established by means of skin tests with antigens that ordinarily elicit cell-mediated immune reactions. An intradermal injection of these antigens (e.g., killed *Candida albicans*, killed mumps virus, or a protein of the *Streptococcus* called streptokinase) normally causes an accumulation of lymphocytes and macrophages manifesting as an area of induration within a few days. For a skin test to give a positive reaction, the subject must have been previously exposed to the antigen as well as have normal T-cell function.

Both T- and B-cell derangements may exist in some lymphoid-deficiency states. Autoimmunity can express itself by the formation of antibodies against blood cells, leading to autoimmune hemolytic anemia, thrombocytopenia, or leukopenia. The presence of autoantibodies against circulating proteins, such as immunoglobulin molecules, leads to immune complex disease in various forms, or organ damage, especially in the joints and kidneys.

DISORDERS OF IMPAIRED B- AND T-CELL FUNCTION

Lymphocyte Depletion

One method used in the laboratory for inducing a profound immunodeficiency state in experimental animals is to cannulate the thoracic duct and drain lymphocytes. Rarely, an equivalent situation occurs in the clinical setting, if a fistula develops between the bowel and the thoracic duct. This event, leading to the indiscriminate loss of T and B lymphocytes, can follow abdominal trauma or as a consequence of cancer of the large bowel. It is also a feature of a congenital disorder called *intestinal lymphangiectasia*, in which lymphoid channels become massively dilated and allow lymphocytes and proteins to drain into the bowel lumen. In these disorders, patients usually have a very low blood lymphocyte count. The patients also have peripheral edema, because of the concomitant loss of lymphatic protein, which leads eventually to a state of plasma protein deficiency with a resulting loss of intravascular osmotic pressure.

Medication-Associated Immunosuppression

Certain pharmacological agents used in medicine are uniquely or particularly toxic to lymphoid cells. Corticosteroids, which are more toxic to T cells than B cells, kill lymphocytes after binding to cytoplasmic receptors. Azathioprine, 6-mercaptopurine, and methotrexate are antimetabolites that interfere with the synthesis of DNA. Cyclophosphamide is converted by the liver to alkylating agents, compounds that cross-link base pairs in DNA. These and other drugs used in cancer chemotherapy (Ch. 19), especially if combined with ionizing radiation therapy delivered to large regions of the body, reduce the number and function of lymphoid cells and lead to varying degrees of immunosuppression.

Ideally physicians would like to have medications with particular specificity for the immune system. One class that comes close binds to intracellular proteins called *immunophilins* and appears to impair the signal transduction processes involved in lymphocyte activation. These drugs (cyclosporine, FK506, and rapamycin), although potent immunosuppressive agents, are not totally specific, however, because they cause renal and hepatic damage. Thalidomide, a drug with sedative and teratogenic effects, has recently been shown also to be immunosuppressive. Under investigation as immunosuppressives are monoclonal antibodies directed against the accessory molecules, CD4, CD8, CD3, CD2, or β-integrins (Ch. 18) to inhibit specific antigen-driven immune responses or even to induce tolerance.

Severe Combined Immune Deficiency

Severe combined immune deficiency is a congenital disorder of profound lymphoid cell dysfunction. In its most virulent form, the disease becomes manifest very early in life. Infants with this disorder rapidly lose T-cell function and, later, B-cell function. Patients commonly manifest a failure to gain weight and have a persistent diarrhea. The ordinary susceptibility of infants to infection is markedly increased. If an attempt is made to immunize the patient with live virus, such as those used against polio or smallpox, even these attenuated viruses cause devastating and even fatal infections. The chronic infections of these patients render them anemic. If a well-meaning physician gives such a patient a blood transfusion, catastrophic GVHD can occur. Unless maintained in a germ-free environment indefinitely, affected patients die of infection. The definitive treatment for the disease is reconstitution of the patient's lymphoid system by infusion of normal lymphoid stem cells from the bone marrow of a histocompatible donor. The stem cells recapitulate the process of development ordinarily occurring in utero, interacting with the thymus and marrow of the recipient and establishing a normal lymphoid immune system.

The inheritance of severe combined immune deficiency is of an autosomal recessive pattern in half the patients and X-linked in the rest. In half the patients showing X-linked inheritance, the disorder can be related to an enzyme deficiency resulting in a metabolic derangement affecting purine metabolism. The lymphoid cells, and in most cases other blood cells of the patients, are deficient in either adenosine deaminase, purine nucleoside phosphorylase, or 5'-nucleotidase. The reactions catalyzed by these enzymes are shown in Figure 20-1. Why these enzyme deficiencies are particularly deleterious to lymphoid cells is unclear, although accumulation of certain nucleosides or their metabolites may be responsible. T cells appear more susceptible than B cells, possibly explaining why T-cell abnormalities appear first. Infusions of normal erythrocytes can produce temporary improvements in immune function in patients with severe combined immune deficiency because of absence of adenosine deaminase. The adenosine deaminase-containing erythrocytes trap and soak up the elevated blood adenosine levels in the patients, thereby acting as an adenosine sink. The transient changes in

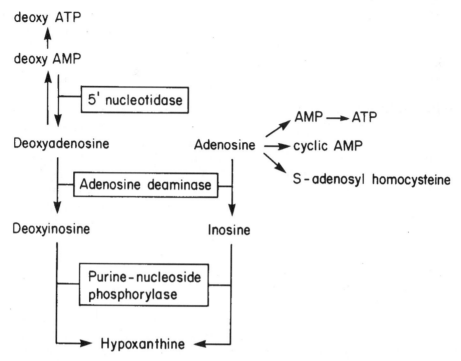

Fig. 20-1. Pathways of purine metabolism affected by enzyme deficiencies associated with genetic severe combined immunodeficiency syndromes.

immune function possibly reflect an abrogation of the presumed toxic effects of the high adenosine concentrations of lymphoid cells. Enzyme replacement therapy using adenosine deaminase conjugated to polyethylene glycol in order to prolong the circulation time of the enzyme has also been clinically effective. Because relatively little active enzyme is required to prevent immunodeficiency and since the affected target cells of this disorder are hematopoietic, adenosine deaminase deficiency causing severe combined immune deficiency is an ideal candidate for treatment by gene replacement using bone marrow cells, and research is under way to realize that goal.

DISORDERS IN WHICH PRINCIPALLY T-CELL FUNCTION IS IMPAIRED

Any infection caused by one organism, especially when severe, can transiently impede the response of T cells to others. This impairment can be diagnosed by the failure of the patient to mount a cell-mediated immune response against an antigen deposited in the skin. This failure to respond is called *anergy.* Inflammatory states not known to be caused by microorganisms also are associated with T-cell hypofunction. These states include sarcoidosis and other idiopathic granulomatous disorders and malignant neoplasms, especially Hodgkin's disease (Ch. 27). Severe protein and calorie malnutrition seriously impedes T-cell function. Measles, ordinarily a self-limited viral disease of childhood, has devastated populations living in regions of endemic malnutrition.

In a rare congenital disorder called *the DiGeorge syndrome*, the patient is born without a functioning thymus or parathyroid gland, probably because of an in utero viral infection that impedes development of the third branchial pouch area. The absence of a thymus in the fetal and neonatal period prevents the normal development of lymphoid cells into T cells; such patients suffer the consequences of absent cell-mediated immunity. Some patients with this disorder have been treated successfully by transplantation of a fetal thymus.

Acquired Immunodeficiency Syndrome

The acquired immunodeficiency syndrome (AIDS) has transformed immunodeficiency from a rather uncommon disorder into a major public health concern. AIDS results from the destruction of the host's helper (CD4) T lymphocytes by a slow-acting retrovirus (lentivirus) named *human immunodeficiency virus, type I (HIV-I)*.

The virus has a glycoprotein on its surface, designated *Gp 160*, which mediates the virus's entry to cells that express the plasma membrane major histocompatibility complex (MHC) accessory molecule designated CD4 (Ch. 19), these cells being helper T lymphocytes, mononuclear phagocytes, and megakaryocytes. Once within the target cell, the virus degrades its glycoprotein coat by a protease and then, like other retroviruses, uses a reverse transcriptase enzyme to copy its genetic material, which is RNA, into DNA, and this DNA integrates with the host-cell DNA. There it may remain dormant for some time, but eventually it programs synthesis of infective virions, often in response to stimuli that elicit lymphocyte or phagocyte activation. The viruses then slowly but inexorably spread from cell to cell by budding from the surface of the infected cell and entering an uninfected one. They also infect by promoting syncytium formation between infected and uninfected cells. Virus production results in killing of the host T cell. Because the reverse transcriptase of HIV-1 is error-prone, it encodes mutations in the resulting DNA, which, if the virus is viable, are better equipped to elude the host's immune system.

Over a period of months to years an increasing number of CD4-bearing cells, especially lymphocytes, are destroyed. Given the central role of helper T lymphocytes in cell-mediated immunity, this destruction renders the afflicted host bereft of defense against facultative intracellular parasites. Monocytes and macrophages are less susceptible to destruction, but may carry the virus throughout the body and, in response to viral infection, may elaborate toxic products that destroy normal host tissues. The incubation period between initial infection and disease can be extremely long, up to 10 years, and this long interval led to early optimism that some infected persons might not develop AIDS. With time, however, it has become apparent that infection dooms the host to die eventually of opportunistic infections or other complications summarized below.

CLINICAL FEATURES

HIV-1 infection may be inapparent for long periods, although some patients may have an acute illness resembling infectious mononucleosis (Ch. 19) during which high levels of HIV-1 virus is detectable in the peripheral blood. When opportunistic infections set in on patients with AIDS, the number of CD4-bearing T lymphocytes has usually fallen to 500/μl or less. The usual manifestation is an infection associated with impaired cellular immunity. Oral moniliasis, cutaneous *herpes zoster* infections, and gastrointestinal *Clostridium difficile, Cryptosporium,* and *Microsporidium* infestations are common. The pathogen *Rochalimaea quintana,* the cause of trench fever, was recently identified as the cause of bacillary angiomatosis, a cutaneous and osseous vasculitis occurring in HIV-1-infected individuals. Cholangitis caused by microsporidia has also been noted in these patients. Particularly important and potentially lethal is lung inflammation caused by the protozoal organism *Pneumocystis carinii.* Cough, fever, and shortness of breath characterize this infection, the treatment of which requires antibiotics and may necessitate ventilatory support. The antibiotics, a combination of trimethoprim and a sulfonamide or pentamidine, interfere with folic acid metabolism of the infecting pathogen.

Unfortunately, these antibiotics frequently elicit allergic reactions in the patients. Mycobacterial infections are often encountered in AIDS. *Mycobacterium tuberculosis* should be containable by appropriate antibiotics, although a frightening development has been the appearance of *M. tuberculosis* strains resistant to all previously efficacious agents. Another mycobacterium, *Avium intracellulare,* ordinarily a saprophyte but devastating to the immunosuppressed AIDS sufferer, has no highly effective therapy, although new antibiotics are being tested. *Toxoplasma gondii,* another protozoal pathogen, viruses (particularly cytomegalovirus), and fungi such as *Cryptococcus neoformans* can invade the central nervous system of AIDS patients.

Another feature of AIDS is the appearance of certain cancers. One such neoplasm is known as *Kaposi's sarcoma,* a proliferation of blood-filled capillaries that has a red-purple appearance. Kaposi's sarcoma was originally described as an indolent neoplasm of elderly Jewish or Mediterranean men and of immunosuppressed Africans, but in AIDS patients it can be a rapidly growing and lethal disease. A second cancer found in AIDS patients is a virulent neoplasm of B lymphocytes, *diffuse histiocytic (large cell) lymphoma* (Ch. 28). The disorder can arise in any body organ, but characteristically it presents in the central nervous system of AIDS victims. The propensity of AIDs patients to develop certain cancers is also seen in other forms of immunodeficiency and may be a result of abnormal immune surveillance against cancer cells or of injury to normal cells caused by uncontrolled action of the intact elements of the immune system. Indeed, AIDS patients also have unusual autoimmune disorders, such as immune thrombocytopenia, and reactions to medications, as mentioned in the previous paragraph.

Cerebral atrophy leading to dementia and wasting are additional attributes of AIDS. Evidence suggests that the HIV-1 virus infests mononuclear phagocytes in the brain, and that somehow this infection results in the destruction of neuronal tissue. Cerebral toxoplasmosis or cerebral lymphoma must be differentiated from this AIDS-associated encephalopathy. The wasting associated with AIDS may arise from chronic infection with various pathogens or from the elaboration of catabolic substances such as interleukin-1 or tumor necrosis factor by HIV-infected mononuclear phagocytes. AIDS patients often suffer from chronic diarrhea due to either intestinal parasites such as *Clostridium difficile, Cryptospiridium,* or shigellosis or possibly to HIV infection of the gastrointestinal epithelial cells, which contributes to inanition.

The varied manifestations of AIDS has caused it to supplant syphilis as "the great imitator." At the present time the "official" diagnosis of AIDS as established by the Centers for Disease Control requires that the patient have suffered from a clear-cut AIDS-related infection or from Kaposi's sarcoma or B-cell lymphoma in the setting of immunodeficiency without there being another explanation for the immunodeficiency. A patient with lymphadenopathy, fever, night sweats, and immunodeficiency, especially if a member of a defined AIDS risk population, in the absence of the "official" criteria is said to have *AIDS-related complex (ARC).*

EPIDEMIOLOGY

Epidemiologists hypothesize that the virus originated in rural central Africa and was carried by infected patients to cities. From there it was transported by Africans traveling to Europe and to the Caribbean basin by Haitians who had worked in Zaire. The residence of the virus in blood cells meant that transmission followed the exchange of blood and blood products. Accordingly, passage of AIDS has been documented by whole blood transfusion, by the infusion of certain blood fractions used as replacement therapy for inherited disorders of blood coagulation, and by blood mixing between infected mothers and their fetuses. By far the major initial mechanism of spread of this disease, however, has been venereal, and the establishment of the virus in homosexual men during the mid-1970s resulted in its widespread dissemination in this population in western countries, whereas heterosexual spread was more common in the Third World. Increasingly, however, the most important vector for blood-borne AIDS virus transmission in developed countries has been contaminated needles used by intravenous drug abusers.

There are some differences in disease manifestations in the different risk groups. Infected neonates develop symptoms more quickly than adults, and Kaposi's sarcoma is more common in male homosexual victims than in other patients. An important point is that abundant evidence indicates that contact with body fluids of AIDS patients other than blood or genital secretions constitutes little risk of infection. The incidence of AIDS has risen exponentially from a handful in 1980 to over a million and a half cases worldwide.

DIAGNOSIS

The discovery of HIV-1 as the probable cause of AIDS and ARC in the early 1980s led to immunological tests for diagnosis of infection, as infected persons generate antibodies to components of the virus. Serological tests for serum antibodies to the AIDS virus are routinely done on blood samples donated for transfusion (Ch. 31). When else to perform this test has been a controversial issue. Presently, physicians may request an antibody test on the serum of patients suffering from signs or symptoms of AIDS, provided that the patient gives consent. Members of risk groups may obtain such tests at so-called alternate test sites, which also provide counseling should the test be positive.

In the most widely used screening test, known as an *enzyme-linked immunosorbent assay (ELISA)*, a series of wells are coated with viral antigen, and test serum samples are added to the wells. If a sample contains antibodies to the viral antigen, they will bind to the antigens on the surface of the well. The well is washed and then reacted with an antibody against immunoglobulins. This "secondary" antibody,

which is linked to an enzyme that generates a colored product from a chromogenic substrate, remains in the well only if antibodies to the AIDS antigen are present. After washing, the substrate is added, and the amount of product is determined colorimetrically. If the serum sample contained antibody, color formation takes place. One problem with ELISA tests, other variations of which are possible, is that a significant number of false-positive results arise. Therefore, a positive test is followed up by another test in which virus is dissolved in the detergent sodium dodecyl sulfate, and the viral components are separated on a gel by electrophoresis. The proteins in the gel are transferred to nitrocellulose paper, which is then reacted with antibodies linked to a color-producing enzyme. This analysis is more rigorous, because proteins migrate in the electric field at a rate inversely proportional to molecular weight. Therefore, detection of antibody-reactive polypeptides of appropriate mobilities increases the rigor of the test. Even this so-called Western blotting technique, however, yields false positives. The problem of false positivity and fear of violation of civil liberties have inhibited the application of these tests to routine screening of healthy people. The armed forces, on the other hand, do screen all volunteers for military service in the United States.

The application of antibody screening has drastically diminished the transmission of AIDS by blood transfusion. In addition, heating of blood concentrates and other purification techniques have decreased the risk for patients with coagulation disorders. Unfortunately, there is a "window" of weeks to months between infection and seroconversion, so some infected blood donations may slip through the screening process in this way. It is also likely that the tests also fail in some instances for technical reasons.

TREATMENT AND PREVENTION

Aside from the management of opportunistic infections and neoplasms, there is presently little in the way of specific treatment. The

AIDS epidemic has forced intensified efforts to develop specific antiviral therapies and expedite their testing in patients. One approach has been to design nucleoside analogue chemicals that inhibit the reverse transcriptase enzyme of the virus. One such agent, a dideoxynucleoside called azidothymidine or zidovudine (abbreviated *AZT*), has been shown to decrease the incidence of infections in AIDS patients, slow the progression of AIDS, and increase survival. Other nucleoside analogues that appear to have similar effects are dideoxyinosine (ddI) and dideoxycytidine (ddC). Regrettably, AZT, which is quite expensive, is not a cure, because the HIV-1 virus develops resistance to it, and some patients experience serious side effects, including bone marrow failure. Patients receiving AZT who develop anemia have been shown to have inappropriately low (> 500 mUnits/ml) erythropoietin levels and to respond to 150 units of the hormone/kg three times a week with rises in hematocrit and reduced transfusion requirements.

A theoretical avenue is to prevent virus dissemination within the body by infusion of soluble CD4 molecules, the cell surface receptors to which the HIV Gp 160 binds to enter cells. Such "bogus" receptors cover the determinants on the free virus that promote cell entry and also prevent cell-to-cell transfer of the virus by syncytium formation. Unfortunately, the affinity of the soluble CD4 constructs for the virus has been low, and no therapeutic efficacy has been demonstrable in AIDS patients treated with this material. Monoclonal antibodies reactive with certain epitopes of Gp 160 may turn out to be more effective. Efforts to produce a vaccine against HIV are hampered by considerable genetic variation between viral isolates and the tendency of the virus in a given individual to undergo mutations. Moreover, because patients with the disorder have demonstrable humoral and cell-mediated immune reactions to the virus, it is unclear whether vaccination will inhibit the disease.

In the absence of effective treatment or a vaccine, *avoidance of infection* remains the most potent weapon against AIDS. Because transmission by casual contact is rare, purging of infected blood from the transfusion pool, prevention of exposure to contaminated hypodermic needles, and use of condoms to minimize exposure to infected genital fluids are highly effective measures.

At an international AIDS conference in July of 1992, reports surfaced describing patients with low levels of CD4-bearing T cells but no evidence of HIV infection. These disclosures raised the specter of a new epidemic of acquired immunodeficiency with no known cause. Subsequent systematic research revealed that this phenomenon is extremely rare, and epidemiologically and clinically different from AIDS. Its cause is probably heterogenous.

DISORDERS OF IMPAIRED B-CELL FUNCTION AND OTHER DISEASES AFFECTING ANTI-BODIES

A family of congenital and acquired disorders, the antibody deficiency syndromes encompass a spectrum of abnormalities ranging from the total absence of B cells to B cells variably incapable of making antibodies. With further research, the antibody deficiency syndromes are being found to be increasingly heterogeneous.

Congenital Diseases

Congenital agammaglobulinemia is X-linked in inheritance. The absence of circulating immunoglobulins results from either the absence or nonfunctioning state of B cells. In X-linked agammaglobulinemia, no B cells mature from lymphoid precursors, and the affected patients are unable to produce any type of antibody. Recently the basis of this disorder has been traced to mutations or deletions of a gene encoding a tyrosine kinase presumably involved in signal transduction required for B-cell differentiation. In a clinically related disorder, X-linked *hypogammaglobulinemia*, B cells make large quantities of IgM, but not IgG or IgA. Curerent evidence links this disease to defects in a gene encoding a cell surface protein, Gp 39, which binds to the CD40 protein on the surface of T cells, thereby promoting B-cell isotype switching required for IgA or IgG synthesis. The *dysgammaglobulinemias* are diseases in which there is a selective inability of B cells to generate certain subclasses of IgG.

One of every 500 persons lacks IgA, both in blood and in secretions. These IgA-deficient people lack B cells capable of producing IgA. It is not absolutely certain that such patients are unusually susceptible to infections. However, they are at risk for making antibodies to IgA, should they receive blood transfusions from normal persons, and may have serious reactions when given multiple transfusions. Another situation associated with IgA deficiency is a rare genetic disease transmitted as an X-linked disorder, called *ataxia telangiectasia.* In this situation, the reason for low IgA levels is not a lack of IgA-producing B cells, but rather an abnormally exuberant breakdown of the protein. Affected patients have tortuous superficial capillaries, the telangiectasias, visible on the skin of the antecubital fossae and on the sclerae of the eye. They have perversions of cerebellar function and mental retardation, responsible for the ataxia. In addition to IgA deficiency, these patients have various subtle anomalies of immune function, including a propensity to develop autoantibodies and malignancies of the lymphoid system.

Another unusual X-linked inherited disease is the *Wiskott-Aldrich syndrome.* Wiskott-Aldrich syndrome appears early in life, with eczema, thrombocytopenia, and repeated infections. The immunological bases of these abnormalities are not clear. They reflect a subtle derangement of the lymphoid system, preventing the normal elaboration of certain antibodies against polysaccharides, which may account for the susceptibility to infection. Improper regulation of immune responses allow autoantibodies to develop, explaining in part the thrombocytopenia, a consequence of antiplatelet autoantibodies. One feature that possibly links the platelet and lymphoid aspects of this disorder is the fact that both cell types fail to express a sialic acid-rich surface glycoprotein, sialophorin or CD15. The gene encoding sialophorin is not on the X chromosome, however, so that its loss is a consequence of the underlying genetic defect. The Wiskott-Aldrich syndrome has been cured by transplantation of bone marrow.

Acquired Disorders

At any time in life, an unexplained event can prevent previously normal B cells from maturing properly or from secreting immunoglobulins. This acquired antibody deficiency, called *common variable hypogammaglobulinemia,* is the most frequent cause of immunoglobulin deficiency encountered in practice. Some infected patients go on to develop lymphoid neoplasms.

Conversely, impairment of antibody formation occurs frequently in the setting of certain neoplasms of the lymphoid system. Often patients with chronic lymphatic leukemia or with tumors of the thymus produce subnormal quantities of immunoglobulins. Furthermore, patients with these diseases may develop autoantibodies against normal blood cells. The basis of the immunoglobulin deficiency in this setting is in part a crowding out of normal B cells in lymphoid organs by overgrowth of malignant clones. Alternatively, the production of autoantibodies against normal B cells may account for the immunoglobulin deficiency. Finally, imbalances in suppressor and helper subsets of T cells caused by the neoplastic process may impair antibody formation.

Another neoplasm associated with impaired antibody production is *multiple myeloma*, a clonal proliferation of plasma cells described in Chapter 29. This tumor, unlike chronic lymphatic leukemia or most of the other lymphoid malignancies, does not primarily involve the lymph nodes or blood, but rather the bone marrow, and is associated with the formation of large amounts of useless immunoglobulins. It is possible that the clonal proliferation of malignant B cells crowds out normal B cells. However, the abnormal immunoglobulins have been shown to stimulate mononuclear phago-cytes to suppress immunoglobulin synthesis by normal B lymphocytes.

If a loss of immunoglobulins exceeds pro-duction, a state of *hypogammaglobulinemia* can result. In general, a protein-losing state such as the nephrotic syndrome, wherein plas-ma protein pours into the urine, or in protein-losing enteropathy, in which the source of plas-ma protein loss is the gastrointestinal tract, the immunoglobulin deficiency can be sufficiently profound to cause recurrent infections.

An immunodeficiency state of particular importance to the hematologist is a conse-quence of multiple insults to the immune sys-tem affecting both phagocytes and lymphoid cells, which can result from aggressive treat-ment of a lymphoid neoplasm, Hodgkin's dis-ease. It is often necessary to remove the spleen of patients with Hodgkin's disease for diagnos-tic purposes. In cases of extensive disease, treatment may require considerable application of ionizing radiation to lymphoid tissue and admixture of systemic chemotherapy that is toxic to lymphoid cells. This therapeutic tour de force, which can actually be curative against the malignancy, wreaks sufficient havoc to the antibody-forming mechanism to prevent the maintenance of normal levels of immunoglo-bulins against high-grade encapsulated pathogens. The combination of antibody deficiency and the absence of a spleen renders the patient extraordinarily susceptible to infec-tions with encapsulated organisms, such as *Pneumococcus, Haemophilus influenzae,* or *Streptococcus,* and these infections can be overwhelming and fatal.

TREATMENT OF IMMUNODEFICIENCY DISORDERS AFFECTING ANTIBODIES

Except in those states in which protein losses or catabolism are excessive, replacement thera-py with human immunoglobulin preparations is possible. The half-time for the clearance of normal immunoglobulin is about 30 days, so

that monthly administrations of immunoglobu-lin are an acceptable treatment of antibody deficiency syndromes. The immunoglobulins are obtained from relatively easy fractionation procedures done on plasma acquired from blood donors. The product, consisting primari-ly of IgG, is usually called γ-globulin. γ -Globulin prepared by classical plasma fraction-ation techniques must be given by intramuscu-lar injections, because the immunoglobulin preparations contain aggregates of IgG that can activate complement and produce anaphylactic reactions, if given intravenously. Recently, more highly purified γ-globulin preparations have become available and are suitable for intravenous administration. The initial dosage for primary immunodeficiency is 200 mg/kg/month, with subsequent adjustments for clinical response. Patients with secondary immune deficiency associated with chronic lymphocytic leukemia require 400 mg/kg every three or four weeks. The drawback of these preparations is their expense; a single dose may cost $1,000. Another problem in the treatment of antibody deficiency is that immunodeficient patients often have a propensity to generate autoantibodies and will produce antibodies against the injected immunoglobulin, resulting in its rapid clearance. Therefore, the plasma immunoglobulin levels of patients receiving γ-globulin should be monitored periodically. The use of immunoglobulin in patients with high concentrations of paraproteins but low normal immunoglobulins presents a special problem. The high endogenous immunoglobulin levels cause all immunoglobulins—endogenous or administered—to be catabolized rapidly. Therefore, more frequent immunoglobulin administration is required in this setting, and such treatment may not be practical.

AUTOIMMUNITY

Autoimmunity is an instance in which toler-ance fails. The process that turns off the immune response when the offending antigen is no longer present, for example, is, in a sense an example of *autoimmunity*. The very novelty of the variable portion of antibody molecules or T-cell antigen receptors generated by the recombination of germline genes to react with specific antigens causes the immune system to see them as "foreign." Hence, the system produces an immune response to the immune response. The resulting cascade of "antibodies against antibodies" or of cell-mediated immunity against activated T cells is known as an *idiotype network,* from the Greek *idios* meaning "unique." This physiological *idiotype response* can become pathological when the antibody–antibody complexes elicit inflammatory responses. Immune complexes of this sort underlie the pathogenesis of disorders such as cryoglobulinemia and certain kinds of vasculitis (see also Ch. 17). Evidence indicates that tolerance is not merely the passive elimination of autoreactive cells, but an active programming of cells renewed by contact with self-antigens. Sequestration of lymphoid cells away from antigens, for example, has been found in experimental settings to lead to expression of autoimmunity to red blood cells. The lymphocytes making antierythrocyte antibodies had homed to the peritoneal cavity where they were out of touch with host erythrocytes. Injection of red cells into the peritoneal cavity resulted in destruction of the lymphocytes and cessation of antibody production.

Another instance of autoimmune disease occurs when the immune response to infectious agents, especially viruses, elicits immunological reactions to host tissues. This process may be facilitated by the binding of viruses to human lymphocyte antigens (HLA) on cell surfaces, in which case the recognition of the foreign pathogen overlaps self-configurations on the HLA molecules. The connection between the HLA system and autoimmunity is strengthened by the epidemiological association between certain host histocompatibility genotypes and autoimmune disorders. The role of HLA type may be direct as regards the binding of antigens to cell surfaces, or indirect, having to do with the innate reactivity of the immune system to all antigens. This innate susceptibility is evidenced by the association between certain autoimmune diseases and possession of particular HLA phenotypes. One example is HLA-B27, which is associated with a high incidence of ankylosing spondylitis.

Other genetic factors clearly are involved in autoimmunity, however, in that certain families express large numbers of autoantibodies that are not definitely associated with histocompatibility type. Additional evidence for an infectious provocation of autoimmunity is the association of autoimmunity with immunodeficiency states—in which the persistence of pathogens may be greater in the host—and its expression following infections, especially in children. Autoimmunity may be highly tissue specific, as, for example, autoimmune thyroiditis, or may be quite generalized, as in systemic lupus erythematosus.

Autoimmunity plays a pathogenetic role in many hematological diseases. Particularly important examples are the immune-mediated cytopenias (autoimmune hemolytic anemia, autoimmune thrombocytopenia, autoimmune neutropenia) and pernicious anemia (autoantibodies to parietal cells or to intrinsic factor).

SUGGESTED READINGS

Aruffo A et al (1993) The CD40 ligand, gp39, is defective in activated T cells from patients with X-linked hyper-IgM syndrome. Cell 71:291

Carson DA (1992) Genetic factors in the etiology and pathogenesis of autoimmunity. FASEB J 6:2800

Daar ES, Moudgil T, Meyer RD, Ho DD (1991) Transient high levels of viremia in patients with primary human immunodeficiency virus type 1 infection. N Engl J Med 324:961

Fauci AS (1993) CD4+ T-lymphocytopenia without HIV infection—no lights, no camera, just facts. N Engl J Med 328:429

Greene W (1991) The molecular biology of human immunodeficiency virus type 1 infection. N Engl J Med 324:308

Henry DH et al (1992) Recombinant human erythropoietin in the treatment of anemia associated with human immunodeficiency virus (HIV) infection and zidovudine therapy. Overview of four clinical trials. Ann Intern Med 117:739

Janeway CA, Jr (1992) Selective elements for the Vβ region of the T cell receptor: Mls and the bacterial toxic mitogens. Adv Immunol 50:1

Koehler JE, Quinn FD, Berger TG et al (1992) Isolation of Rochimalaea species from cutaneous and osseous lesions of bacillary angiomatosis. N Engl J Med 327:1625

Moore RD, Hidalgo MHS, Sugland BW, Chaisson RE (1991) Ziduvidine and the natural history of the acquired immunodeficiency syndrome. N Engl J Med 324:1412

Murakami M, Tsubata T, Okamoto M et al (1992) Antigen-induced apoptotic death of Ly-1 B cells responsible for autoimmune disease in transgenic mice. Nature 357:77

Pantaleo G, Graziosi C, Fauci AS (1993) The immunopathogenesis of human immunodeficiency virus infection. N Engl J Med 328:327

Porter SB, Sande MA (1992) Toxoplasmosis of the central nervous system in the acquired immunodeficiency syndrome. N Engl J Med 327:1643

Robey EA, Ramsdell F, Kloussis D et al (1992) The level of CD8 expression can determine the outcome of thymic selection. Cell 69:1089

Rosen FS, Cooper MD, Wedgewood RJP (1984) The primary immunodeficiencies. N Engl J Med 311:235

Scadden DT, Zon LI, Groopman JE (1989) Pathophysiology and management of HIV-associated hematologic disorders. Blood 74:1455

Shilts R (1987) And the Band Played On. Politics, People and the AIDS Epidemic. St. Martin's Press, New York

Strober W, Erhardt TRO (1993) Chronic intestinal inflammation: an unexpected outcome in cytokine or T cell receptor mutant mice. Cell 75:203

Tsukada S et al (1993) Deficient expression of a B cell cytoplasmic tyrosine kinase in human X-linked agammaglobulinemia. Cell 72:279

Vetrie D et al (1993) The gene involved in X-linked agammaglobulinaemia is a member of the *src* family of protein-tyrosine kinases. Nature 361:226

von Boehmer H, Kisielow P (1991) How the immune system learns about self. Sci Am October:74

Walsh CT, Zydowski LD, McKeon FD (1992) Cyclosporin A, the cyclophilin class of peptidylprolyl isomerases, and blockade of T cell signal transduction. J Biol Chem 267:13115

Wormser GP (1992) AIDS and other Manifestations of HIV Infection. 2nd Ed. Raven Press, New York

21

Pathophysiology of Blood Cell Replication, Neoplasia, and Therapy of Hematological Malignancies

The majority of the disorders described in Chapters 22 to 29 result from abnormalities in differentiation, replication, or both of blood cell precursors induced by acquired genetic changes in the machinery that controls these vital cellular functions. Most of these diseases involve malignant transformation of the affected cells—aplastic anemia, for example, may be a neoplasm (its effects are certainly "malignant"), but one cannot examine cells that aren't there for properties of cancer. When the defects primarily involve very early stem cells, the diseases fall into the category classified as *stem cell diseases*, which include aplastic anemia, the myelodysplastic syndromes, and the myeloproliferative disorders (Ch. 22). The *myeloid leukemias* are disorders of progenitor cells further along the developmental pathways of phagocytic (neutrophilic and monocytic), erythroid, and megakaryocytic lineages. Neoplasia of cells originating from the lymphoid stem cell results in *lymphoid malignancies*, the lymphocytic leukemias, the lymphomas, and the plasma cell neoplasms summarized in Chapters 24 to 29. This chapter reviews general principles of cell growth, neoplasia, and the approach to treatment of neoplastic disease that set the stage for subsequent chapters dealing with specific diseases of blood cell proliferation and differentiation.

Contrary to the commonly held idea, malignant cells do not necessarily engage in wildly rapid multiplication. In fact, the multiplication rate of such cells is often slower than that of normal hematopoietic stem cells. The ill effects of hematologic malignancies stem more from the failure of the neoplastic cells to differentiate and also to enter that inevitable state following normal life—death—than from rapid growth. Such immortal and immature neoplastic cells crowd out and suppress normal bone marrow cells, and, in addition, they may invade normal tissue and impair its function.

CLONAL GROWTH

The continued reproduction of the transformed cell leads to what is termed a *clonal expansion*. The clonal and genetic nature of the neoplastic process was first documented by studying the electrophoretic mobility of the enzyme glucose 6-phosphate-dehydrogenase (G6PD) of tumor cells in persons heterozygous for the A and B isozymes. Recall that these enzymes have different mobilities in an electric field. The body cells of persons inheriting genes for both isoenzymes will be either A or B because of random inactivation of the X chromosome. This means that the dividing bone marrow phagocyte precursors will have an equal chance of making either A or B G6PD isozymes, and their progeny will yield on average an equal mix of these enzymes. On the other hand, a clonal proliferation of a single cell will contain only one or the other enzyme, and the malignant cells of patients with neoplasms are either of the A or B type (Fig. 21-1). Currently, clonality can be documented in dividing cells by detection of uniform cytogenetic changes or in cells irrespective of their proliferative ability by the presence of abnormal gene products that can be measured by highly specific monoclonal antibodies. In addition, clonal messenger RNA transcripts can be recognized by the polymerase chain reaction even when present in only a few cells (see below).

ONCOGENES: RELATION TO NORMAL CELL GROWTH CONTROL AND TO THE MOLECULAR BASIS OF NEOPLASMS

General Features

A major dividend of molecular cloning techniques has been the discovery that changes in the structure or expression of one or more of a limited number of normal cellular genes can cause cells to exhibit the characteristics of malignancy defined above. These genes have therefore been named *oncogenes*. Oncogenes were actually first identified as the parts of the genetic material of certain viruses responsible for malignant transformation of infected cells in animals. Most of these viruses are so-called *retroviruses*, which have RNA as their genetic material and use a reverse transcriptase enzyme to make complementary DNA in infected cells that then integrates into the host DNA. The

integrated DNA either has no effect, programs the synthesis of more virus using the cell's synthetic machinery, or causes the cell to undergo malignant transformation. It is now believed that viruses, requiring actively dividing cells in order to replicate themselves, co-opted genes used by cells to induce division of the host cell. Therefore, oncogenes ultimately influence what is termed the cell growth cycle or simply *the cell cycle*. The normal control of this cycle is depicted in Figure 21-2.

An important aspect of the discovery of cellular oncogenes was the ability to transfer DNA from tumors into nonmalignant cells in tissue cultures, a process called *transfection,* and to observe a change in the target cell from normal to transformed phenotype. Definition of this phenotype included piling up of the transformed cells on the surface of the tissue culture dish and the ability to form tumors in immunodeficient mice. Subsequent study of the transforming DNA revealed the identity between the regions important for transformation, the structure of viral oncogenes, and the presence of similar genes in normal cells.

The nomenclature of oncogenes has arisen from the historical identification of such genes and depends on the source of the genetic material. Cellular genes homologous to viral oncogenes usually bear the name related to the viral system such as *src* (the "sarc" or sarcoma-producing gene of Rous sarcoma virus of fowl), *abl* (the Abelson virus first discovered as a cause of lymphoid tumors in rodents), or *fes* (feline sarcoma virus). The prefix *v* or *c* (e.g., *v-abl* or *c-abl*) denotes whether the gene is viral or cellular. In some cases, more than one related viral oncogene is known, in which instance a prefix denotes the specific viral gene: examples are *ras* genes related to Kirsten murine sarcoma virus *(Ki-ras),* Harvey murine sarcoma virus *(Ha-ras),* or Rasheed rat sarcoma virus *(Ra-ras).*

Oncogenes induce malignant transformation by working through aspects of the normal cellular equipment regulating cell growth and movement. As first introduced in Chapter 1, cell division, including the proliferation of nor-

Normal cells of G6PD
Heterozygote - half A, half B

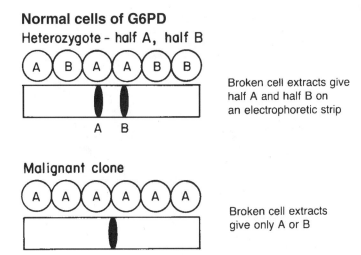

Broken cell extracts give
half A and half B on
an electrophoretic strip

Fig. 21-1. Glucose 6-phosphate dehydrogenase activity in cells as a marker of clonal expansion.

mal hematopoietic precursors, can be triggered by growth factors that bind to receptors on the external surface of the plasma membrane. This binding elicits *signals* in the cytoplasm that interact with cellular factors (transducers) that further react with components in the nucleus that regulate genes controlling cellular proliferation. Therefore, oncogene products can theoretically function at any of these control points inside or outside the cell to induce the malignant phenotype (Fig. 21-3). Cells ordinarily express the products of their own oncogenes under carefully regulated circumstances, but the constitutive expression of these genes following transformation or the expression of altered gene products can result in neoplastic cell behavior. The action of any one oncogene may be indadequate to cause a tumor, and most

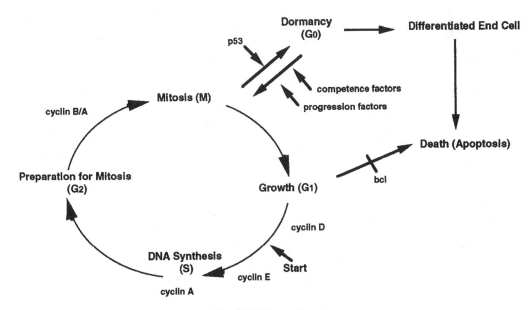

Fig. 21-2. The cell cycle.

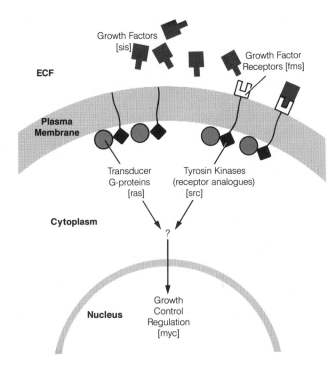

Fig. 21-3. Action of oncogenes.

information concerning the development of human tumors is consistent with the involvement of more than one genetic event; it may require the concerted action of many genes in order to evolve a frank cancer.

One class of oncogenes, for example, programs the synthesis of secreted substances nearly identical to normal factors that elicit cell growth and division. These growth factors chronically stimulate the cell to divide. An example of such an oncogene that acts in this so-called autocrine fashion is *c-sis*, which produces a product resembling platelet-derived growth factor. Another set of oncogenes encodes molecules that act as receptors for growth factors. However, unlike normal receptors, which are active only when ligated by their specific agonist, these oncogene-derived receptors behave as if activated constitutively. Examples of this class are the product of *c-fms*, which resembles the receptor for the phagocyte growth factor granulocyte colony-stimulating factor (G-CSF), *v-* and *c-src*, and the middle T antigen of polyoma virus. Both *c-fms* and middle T, in common with a large class of growth

factor receptors, have enzymatic activity catalyzing phosphorylation of proteins on tyrosine residues. The *tyrosine kinase* activity resides in the portion of the molecules extending into the cytoplasm, and phosphorylation induces changes in target proteins that induce cell proliferation. The human gene for stem cell factor, *c-kit,* is related to a viral oncogene, *v-kit*, and is a member of the tyrosine kinase receptor family. The activation of a growth factor receptor transmits (transduces) a signal to the nucleus that induces cell division. One of the target systems is the cascade of enzymes involved in membrane phosphoinositide turnover (Ch. 18). Another "transducer" oncogene product is a set of guanosine triphosphate (GTP)-binding proteins that interact with plasma membrane (and possibly other) enzymes, the so-called *G-proteins* described in the previous chapter. A different class of oncogenes, the *ras* genes, are also G-proteins that behave as if constitutively in the GTP-bound active state that normally only occurs when the cell is stimulated by activated receptors. The cytokines that induce proliferation of hematopoietic cells, such as interleukin-2 (IL-2), IL-3, IL-5, macrophage (M)-CSF, and stem cell factor, all activate the *c-ras*-related proteins when they bind to their respective receptors.

The ultimate target of signaling for cell division is in the nucleus, and some oncogenes act directly at that site. Examples of such oncogene products are *myc, fos, myb, jun,* and the large T antigen of polyoma virus. Many of the nuclear oncogenes are *transcription factors* that bind to specific DNA sequences in the controlling region of genes, usually "upstream" (in the 5'-direction of the DNA on the chromosome) from the protein coding sequences to regulate mRNA synthesis. Growth control factors including nuclear oncogenes may act directly by binding to these sequences (so-called *cis*-acting factors) or induce synthesis or activation of other DNA-binding (*trans*-acting) factors, which may reside on different genes from the final target genes. The transcription factor-related oncogenes have structural elements identified for normal DNA-binding transcription factors. One class of these elements functions to facilitate the self-association of the transcription factor required for presentation of basic DNA-binding sites. The chemical structures mediating this self-association are the *helix–loop–helix* domain and a leucine-rich domain that creates a so-called *leucine zipper* structure. *c-jun* and *c-fos* contain leucine zippers, and *c-myc* has both helix–loop–helix and leucine zipper domains. Another class, exemplified by a structure generated by histidines and cysteines that is stabilized by zinc atoms (called *zinc finger domains*) bind directly to transcription activation sequences in DNA. Some of the genes that, when modified, cause neoplasia are normally active in hematopoiesis. For example, so-called *homeobox* "master" genes related to genes that program the development of entire segments of organisms control the development of specific blood cell lineages.

Yet another way by which an oncogene can work is exemplified by *Bcl-2. Bcl-2,* associated with certain lymphomas (Ch. 28), appears to work by inhibiting the genetically programmed cell death (apoptosis) that is required for normal growth control. Rearrangements of

one such gene, designated *mll,* are associated with particularly virulent leukemias of infants and young children.

Because oncogenes are indigenous to all cells, some change in their composition or expression is required for neoplastic behavior. *Ras* oncogenes isolated from tumor cells, for example, have single base substitutions that cause them to be constitutively active in signal transduction rather than subject to usual control by regulatory factors. Oncogenic *src* gene products have lost regulatory domains that normally keep them switched off for phosphorylating their substrates on tyrosine residues. In these instances it is the abnormal gene products that presumably affect the cellular phenotype. A more frequent finding is that an oncogene has a normal primary sequence, but its expression is greatly increased. This situation arises from another event common to neoplastic cells, especially in leukemias, the rearrangement of chromosomes. This rearrangement can put DNA sequences that promote or enhance the expression of cellular genes inappropriately in the proximity of oncogenes, causing the oncogenes to be excessively expressed. Fusion genes that include segments of homeobox genes and of other RNA transcription factors have been implicated as oncogenes. Presumably, the causes of and predispositions to genetic damage increase the frequency of point mutations and/or chromosomal rearrangements, leading to the recombinations that express abnormal oncogenes or normal oncogenes inappropriately.

The mirror image of oncogene mutation or overexpression that leads in a dominant fashion to malignant behavior is the loss or inactivation of genes, sometimes called *recessive* or *anti-oncogenes,* that inhibit growth responses. One example of this situation occurs in retinoblastoma; susceptibility can be inherited in association with abnormalities of a gene, *rb,* on chromosome 13. The germline-associated loss of the normal *rb* gene product in combination with somatic mutations accounts for the high incidence of retinoblastoma in families. A similar genetic predisposition, based on a gene on chromosome 11, leads to Wilms tumor. The cytokine paradoxically named tumor growth factor-β, (*TGF-β*), actually inhibits cell proliferation, and some neoplastic cells have been shown to lack receptors for this molecule.

The most prevalent recessive oncogene identified thus far is the *p53* gene on chromosome 17, which is frequently deleted or mutated in many epithelial neoplasms and in some leukemias; transgenic mice in which the *p53* gene is inactivated develop many malignant neoplasms. *p53* is a transcription factor that initiates production of mRNAs for cellular components that either inhibit cell growth or else induce cell death. Agents that injure genes, such as ultraviolet or γ-irradiation or cancer chemotherapeutic agents, described below, induce *p53*, which slows down cell growth while the cell tries to repair the genetic damage. If the repair fails, *p53* may be able to produce cell death. Thus *p53*, and possibly other recessive oncogenes, appear to exercise genetic surveillance and protect cells from neoplastic transformation. p53's role can be undermined, if it is genetically inactivated (as in the transgenic mice) or prevented from exercising its normal function because of overexpression of proteins that bind to it. Examples of such oncogenic proteins are the simian virus 40 (SV40) oncogene called large T and the product of a human oncogene called MDM2, which is amplified in certain sarcomas.

HOW CAN MALIGNANT CELLS BE CONTROLLED?

Treatment of hematological malignancies is directed toward the destruction of malignant stem cells. The goal is to achieve selectivity, that is, the maximal destruction of tumor stem cells with minimal damage to healthy stem cells. Some biological principles are useful in thinking about the development and application of such therapy. When all is said and done, the "best" combination and timing of treatments for a given time and a given disease are usually arrived at by a mixture of theoretical ideas and trial and error. As new therapies become available, the "best" treatments change.

Removal or Killing of Tumor Cells

Surgery is an effective way to remove many localized epithelial and connective tissue tumors but is rarely applicable to hematological malignancies, because the tumor cells are usually disseminated at the time of diagnosis. Surgery is primarily used for obtaining tissue for histological analysis. The killing of dispersed malignant cells requires some agent that can seek them out and then attack their mechanisms for living or their capacity to replicate. Some properties of cells affect their susceptibility to such therapeutic attacks, and these properties vary at different stages in their life cycle. The cell cycle is summarized schematically in Figure 21-2 and Table 21-1. Therefore, the susceptibility of cells to killing by different methods varies with the type of cell and the stage of its life cycle. Most treatments act best on rapidly dividing cells, because the metabolic demands of these cells and a maximal number of structural rearrangements may be occurring. Treating dividing cells is analogous to throwing a wrench into a moving (as opposed to a stationary) machine. The susceptibility to killing by various agents also depends on the ability of the cells to permit the entry of the toxic agents and on whether the cell can destroy the toxins. It is fortunate that some

Table 21-1. The Cell Cycle

Phase of Cell Cycle	Metabolic and Structural Events
All	Maintenance of energy charge for metabolic reactions (ATP synthesis)
	Maintenance of redox potential (to keep components reduced)
	Maintenance of membrane integrity and ion gradients
G1, G2	Synthesis of structural molecules (RNA, protein, lipids, sugars)
S	DNA synthesis
M	Construction and disassembly of chromosomes and mitotic spindle
	Dissolution and restructuring of nuclei
	Formation of cleavage furrow
	Movements for cell separation (cytokinesis)

malignant stem cells are, for various reasons, more susceptible to damage than are normal stem cells. This selectivity can arise from a number of factors:

1. A higher number of the tumor stem cells are in cycle and/or are cycling more rapidly than are normal cells. Agents that are especially toxic to cycling cells then kill more tumor cells than normal cells.

2. The tumor stem cell has a unique, unusually active, or missing metabolic pathway that renders it more susceptible to a toxin than normal cells.

3. The tumor stem cell is less able to protect itself or recover from toxic damage than the normal cell.

The most desired goal of treatment is to achieve the eradication of all tumor stem cells. An observation relevant to this goal made for tumors in experimental animals is that many toxic agents kill a *fixed fraction* of tumor cells rather than a fixed number of cells, and the size of the fraction killed is proportional to the dose of treatment. The major importance of such fractional killing and its dose-dependence is that the treatment by a single agent given once will only be curative when the treatment dose is high and/or the tumor burden is small. For example, even if a treatment kills a high fraction, say 99 percent, of tumor cells, and 10 billion cells were originally present, 100 million cells will still survive the treatment. This phenomenon partly explains why combinations of treatment are more effective than single agents, because each can reduce the tumor cell burden by a fraction until a sufficiently low level of cells is reached below which their survival is no longer possible. Another reason favoring the use of treatment combinations is improved selectivity. A combination of agents acting against tumor stem cells by different mechanisms may be less toxic to normal cells than a higher dose of a single agent. For all of these reasons, it is customary to treat neoplasms beyond the time when obvious tumors have disappeared; such therapy of inapparent disease is called *adjuvant treatment.*

Prolonged survival free of tumor is the ultimate test of whether therapy is successful. Since repetitive and intensive treatment is often a means to this success and is not without cost, surrogate measures of tumor eradication are desirable, but rarely absolutely reliable. A recent addition to tumor-specific markers detectable by biochemical (enzymes and secretory products), cytogenetic (clonal chromosomal rearrangements), and immunochemical (surface antigens) has been the highly sensitive detection of tumor-specific mRNA transcripts by polymerase chain reaction technology.

As our understanding of the *control* of the cell cycle improves, new approaches to treatment may emerge. This control resides in the growth factors, receptors, signal-transducing mechanisms, and gene transcription and translation pathways described above that become deregulated by malignant transformation. These pathways impact on different parts of the cell cycle. For example, certain growth factors such as *abl* and *ras* are designated "*competence factors,*" because their expression is required for cells to progress from G0 to G1; on the other hand, while this progression can be initiated by these oncogenes, it requires the action of other factors such as insulin or insulin-like growth factor type I, which are therefore called "*progression factors.*" Conversely, the anti-oncogene *p53* prevents progression of cells from G0 to G1.

The mitotic process itself is now known to be induced by a complex set of protein cascades, primarily controlled by protein phosphorylation. Studies with yeasts, which are eukaryotic cells like blood cells yet are readily amenable to genetic analysis, have been important sources of knowledge about mitotic pathways. A protein aggregate, *maturation factor,* results in modifications of structural proteins that result in dissolution of the nuclear envelope and construction of the mitotic spindle as well as numerous other cellular changes required for the formidable task of cell division. Maturation factor is in turn regulated by a set of *cyclins,* which the cell produces as it enters and degrades as it leaves the period of mitosis (Fig. 21-2). Other cyclins act at different parts of the cell cycle, and therapies directed at these pathways may be more selective than those presently available.

Differentiation or Suicide of Tumor Cells

Cell differentiation usually takes cells out of the division cycle. Tumor stem cells completely or partially fail to differentiate. Some therapies work by overcoming the differentiation block of malignant cells. An example of such a therapy is the use of all-*trans* retinoic acid in acute promyelocytic leukemia (Ch. 23). As discussed in Chapter 28, one of the causes of lymphoid neoplasia is the rearrangement of the *bcl* gene, which normally contributes to the programming of cell death or *apoptosis*. Apoptosis, in contrast to necrosis, is a mechanism by which cells destroy their DNA and degrade their cytoplasmic contents in an orderly way that does not lead to inflammation or scarring. Apoptosis appears to be a means for organisms to eliminate senescent cells and to weed out autoreactive lymphoid cells during negative selection (Ch. 20). It is possible that some therapies thought to work by cytotoxicity actually induce apoptosis of tumor cells, and a better understanding of what makes cells undergo apoptosis may lead to new antitumor agents.

WHY DO TUMOR STEM CELLS BECOME RESISTANT TO TREATMENT?

First, tumor stem cells sometimes have a growth rate equal to or less than that of normal stem cells. In such cases, treatments active against rapidly growing cells have no selective effect. Second, tumor stem cells can generate protective mechanisms that repel assaults against them. The genetic makeup of tumor stem cells tends to be unstable, and antitumor treatment itself can select for tumor stem cells resistant to the treatment. For example,

enzymes can be induced that inactivate the effects of the treatment. This resistance can evolve along several lines. One that has been elucidated in recent years is the induction by tumor cells of a gene that encodes a transport system also known as *P-glycoprotein* that efficiently pumps a remarkably diverse spectrum of structurally unrelated cytotoxic drugs out of the cell. This gene has been cloned and sequenced and is referred to as the *multidrug resistance* or *mdr1* gene. Alternatively, the cells may increase the content of enzymes that detoxify the drugs or bypass the blocks in key metabolic pathways caused by certain agents. These and other mechanisms explain why cytotoxic drugs may be effective for a while, yet become ineffectual later in time. The use of treatment combinations may block this trend toward resistance. By attacking cells at multiple vulnerable points, it is hoped that the ability of a few cells to survive and develop resistance can possibly be prevented.

THERAPIES USED AGAINST HEMATOLOGICAL MALIGNANCIES

Ionizing Radiation

Ionizing radiation is used for the cure or palliation of hematological tumors. Its curative potential is mainly in localized Hodgkin's disease (stages I–II) and in a few cases of localized non-Hodgkin's lymphomas of the large cell type. Short of cure, ionizing radiation has extensive value in the palliative treatment of lymphoma, leukemia, and multiple myeloma. Tumor masses often melt away in response to radiation. Effects of tumor infiltrates on tissues and organs such as pain, neurological dysfunction, and compression of intestinal, urinary, or airway pipelines, can be rapidly and dramatically reversed. A recent application of radiation therapy in hematology has been its use in bone marrow transplantation (Ch. 32). In the treatment of congenital disease affecting blood cells, ionizing radiation directed at the entire bone marrow, essentially *total-body irradiation*, destroys the genetically abnormal bone marrow stem cells in preparation for engraftment with histocompatible normal cells. In addition, this type of therapy is under evaluation for the treatment of nonlymphocytic and stem cell leukemias. Total-body irradiation is used in this setting in an effort to destroy all leukemic stem cells. Thereafter, normal bone marrow is given.

TYPES OF IONIZING RADIATION

x-Rays and γ-rays are of the electromagnetic wave spectrum and are also considered high-energy photons. x-Rays are emitted when rapidly moving electrons are suddenly decelerated in a vacuum. The energy of x-rays is defined by the voltage used to produce them. Thus, kilovoltage x-rays, used primarily in former years, emerge from devices generating 200 to 400 kv. Modern machines use several million, up to 25 million, volts to produce megavoltage x-rays. Still higher energy x-rays, up to 40 million volts, can be generated by a device called a betatron. γ-Rays arise from changes of energy states during the decay of certain radionuclide elements. A frequently used source of γ-rays is cobalt 60 (^{60}Co). A mass of ^{60}Co used for radiation therapy may be housed in a shielded container; it undergoes about 10^{16} disintegrations per minute. The *curie is* the unit of radioactive decay expressed in disintegrations per minute, 1 curie being equal to 2.2 x 10^{12} disintegrations per minute. Therefore, a clinical ^{60}Co source has several thousand curies. The ^{60}Co emits γ-rays with energies of 1.33 and 1.7 million electron volts.

Electrons are generated with high velocities from a linear accelerator or a betatron. The emitted electrons can have energies from 6 to 18 million electron volts or higher.

Heavy particles, such as protons, neutrons, π-mesons, and α-particles can be produced with a cyclotron. Because of their large masses, these particles can be very destructive to cells; the rate of transmission of energy from the radiation to the cell components per unit distance, the linear energy transfer (LET), is highest for these particles. The LET for the particles is highest when they have slowed to a particular speed, and this state of high-energy transfer is called the *Bragg peak*. Therefore, by adjusting the geometry of the incident beam, it is possible to limit heavy particle damage to a very discrete area.

The therapeutic or toxic dosage of radiation is ultimately determined by the energy transfer from radiation to tissue and is quantified as the amount of energy absorbed per unit mass of tissue. The current standard usage to indicate this sum is the *Gray* (abbreviated Gy), which is equivalent to one joule of energy absorbed per kilogram of tissue. The Gray is equivalent to 100 rad, rad being the unit of dosage used in the past and still frequently encountered. The rad is similar to the roentgen (abbreviated R), which is the amount of radiation able to ionize air.

MECHANISMS OF ACTION OF IONIZING RADIATION

Various types of ionizing radiation damage vital cell components. The mechanism of destruction may be either direct or indirect. Direct damage occurs when the radiation ionizes and thereby breaks bonds in nucleic acids and proteins. Such direct damage is predominant in the action of heavy particles. A significant amount of the cytotoxic effect is indirect in that the radiation ionizes water molecules and oxygen dissolved in the water to yield free radicals that secondarily oxidize and destroy cell components. This indirect damage explains why the capacity of ionizing radiation to kill cells is in part proportional to the oxygen tension of the cell and why the center of large, bulky, and poorly vascularized tumors is relatively resistant to radiation damage. This effect has also encouraged therapists to devise ways to increase the oxygen tension of tumors with hyperbaric oxygen or other techniques and to experiment with chemicals, radiation sensitizers that mimic the effect of oxygen on radiation damage. Metronidazole, a drug originally used to treat infections caused by the protozoan *Trichomonas vaginalis,* is a radiation sensitizer.

The relationship between radiation dose and a cytotoxic effect in experimental cell systems can be shown to fit a curve in which the number of cells surviving falls exponentially as the dose of radiation increases, a finding consistent with a random hit mechanism (Fig. 21-4). The exponential curve is straightened out by plotting the radiation dose against the logarithm of surviving cells. It should be noted that there is a threshold radiation dose below which no killing occurs. Below this dose, the damage is insufficient and/or repair processes are adequate to prevent cell killing. The position of the threshold and the steepness of the slope of the curve depend on the type of radiation involved and on the characteristics and environment of the cells. In general, cells that (1) are dividing rapidly, (2) have a long mitotic phase, and (3) are relatively undifferentiated are most easily damaged by ionizing radiation. Tumor stem cells of hematological malignancies often have these properties, making them highly radioresponsive.

FRACTIONATION

One aspect of selectivity in radiation therapy is the finding that malignant cells are less effective than normal cells in recruiting new cell growth and repairing radiation damage. Therefore, the delivery of a tumoricidal dose of radiation therapy in fractions rather than all at once can kill a tumor, but with less damage to normal tissue. Furthermore, as a tumor shrinks, its oxygenation may improve, enhancing the indirect damaging effect of later radiation fractions.

GENERAL PRINCIPLES OF TREATMENT WITH RADIATION

The technology of radiation therapy is highly sophisticated and currently permits the therapist to select methods that deliver maximal destructive energies to a tumor with minimal damage to other cells. For example, the high-voltage x-rays and γ-rays and heavy particles available can penetrate the body without damaging the skin and superficial tissues. On the other hand, kilovoltage x-rays and electron beams can be used for skin tumors, such as mycosis fungoides or symptomatic cutaneous leukemic infiltrates. The radiation therapist works with a physicist and a technologist to establish the geometry and extent of the dosage applied to the patient. In the process, heavy metal templates may be designed and built for each patient to limit the beams to where they

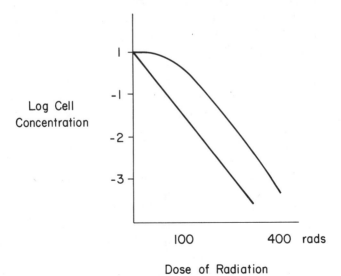

Fig. 21-4. The relationship between radiation dose and cytotoxic effect in experimental cell systems.

are intended by shielding normal tissues. Modern devices can minimize the complications of irradiation to both patient and medical personnel.

COMPLICATIONS OF RADIATION THERAPY

Complications of radiation therapy are the result of cell necrosis and genetic damage. The tissues most susceptible to these effects are those containing cells in rapid turnover, such as the skin, hematopoietic tissue, and the gastrointestinal tract. Therefore, the acceptable dosage of radiation therapy varies inversely with the amount of susceptible tissues exposed: A high dose is acceptable over a small area, but a relatively low dose may be lethal over the entire body. Nevertheless, sufficiently high doses of radiation can damage fibroblasts of connective tissue, bone, and even muscle and nerve cells. Therefore, high amounts of radiation therapy must be carefully directed to minimize the exposure of normal tissues, and only rarely can local doses exceed 50 Gy. In the radiation therapy of lymphoid organs, for the treatment of Hodgkin's disease, for example, the usual dose is 45 Gy given in fractions over 6 weeks.

Despite careful precautions, radiation therapy can lead to certain complications. Irradiation of large areas of the body often causes fatigue and nausea. Irradiation of the pelvis, spine, and long bones can produce transient bone marrow failure, and a total body dose of 4.5 Gy yields permanent bone marrow aplasia. Radiation of the abdomen, by damaging intestinal stem cells, can cause abdominal cramps, watery diarrhea, and gastrointestinal hemorrhage. In children, radiation of growing cartilage and bony epiphyses may result in growth retardation. Pulmonary damage, cardiac fibrosis, premature coronary atherosclerosis leading to acute myocardial infarction, and interstitial nephritis have all been described as late consequences of radiation therapy.

Ionizing radiation is potentially carcinogenic. The development of nonlymphocytic leukemia and of solid tumors (carcinomas and sarcomas) in tissues exposed to radiation is an infrequent but definite complication of this therapy. The mechanism of carcinogenesis is unknown but probably has something to do with damage to the stem cell's genetic material. Cells in tissues exposed to ionizing radiation express various manifestations of such damage, including chromosomal breaks and chromosomal rearrangements. The damage is not sufficient to kill the cell but causes mutations that in some cases lead to malignant behavior.

Chemotherapy

Chemotherapy is defined as the treatment of tumor stem cells by means of medications and hormones. Chemotherapy has the advantages of penetrating many areas and of lodging an active attack against disseminated tumors. Nevertheless, chemotherapy cannot easily infiltrate large, bulky, and poorly vascular tumors, and many drugs do not penetrate the blood–brain barrier. For the treatment of acute lymphatic leukemia, it is necessary to give radiation therapy to the cranium or to inject drugs into the cerebrospinal fluid, or both, in addition to oral and intravenous chemotherapy in order to eradicate malignant cells in the central nervous system.

It is customary to use combinations of drugs having different mechanisms of action to maximize the fractional killing of tumor stem cells and to minimize the ability of the cells to develop resistance to a single form of therapy. Efforts are even made to inhibit resistance by agents such as verapamil, which inhibits the membrane channel encoded by the *mdr* gene. For some diseases, drug therapy is continued after the induction of a remission, with the goal of eradicating, or at least repressing, clinically latent but nonetheless finite numbers of tumor stem cells. This rationale supports the use of maintenance therapy in the acute leukemias and adjuvant therapy after the surgical resection or localized radiation therapy of tumors.

Most chemotherapeutic agents have serious side effects, so that although administration of chemotherapy is technically less complex than radiation therapy, meticulous attention to the preparation of the medications, to the proper dose, and to the route of administration is mandatory, and careful records of what was given when must be maintained. The dosage is usually determined according to the patient's body surface area in meters squared (m^2) rather than weight; convenient nomograms are available for converting height and weight into surface area.

DEVELOPMENT OF CHEMOTHERAPEUTIC AGENTS

Occasionally chemotherapeutic agents are developed by an inductive process, that is, they are synthesized or engineered to inhibit a particular metabolic reaction of tumor cells. More often than not, however, drugs enter the clinical arena by a screening process in which they are found to kill tumors in animals. The usual approach is to try various agents against animal tumors, using an approach that lends itself to rapid, reproducible evaluation. These tumors are usually virulent, that is, small numbers inoculated into the animal will grow rapidly and kill the organism within a short time. One example is a lymphoid neoplasm of mice, called L1210 leukemia. In such a system, the ability of a drug to cure or increase the survival time of the inoculated animals is taken as an index of its effectiveness. Although many effective chemotherapeutic agents are active in these animal models, it is disconcerting that some drugs very active against human cancers occasionally are unimpressive in the animal screening tests.

When new compounds are judged worthy of clinical trial, they are initially given in research institutions to consenting patients with malignant neoplasms, in order to determine the toxicity of the drug. Because the tumors in these patients are usually far advanced, determination of efficacy is not a major goal in such phase I trials. Once the toxicity of the drugs is determined, the drugs are tested for antitumor activity in phase II trials.

If the agents are active, they are then compared in phase III trials against other drugs in patients with a variety of tumors, preferably in a carefully controlled manner. In further phase II trials, dose and schedule adjustments and combinations with other treatments are compared for relative efficacy. Because of the inherent variability in the growth rates and responsiveness of tumors of similar histology, large numbers of patients are needed for evaluation in such studies. Furthermore, because so many factors can influence the natural history of tumors, concurrent controlled trials in which patients are randomly allocated to groups receiving the two treatments being compared are optimal for determining the effectiveness of various treatments.

MECHANISM OF ACTION OF VARIOUS CHEMOTHERAPEUTIC AGENTS

Alkylating Agents

Many drugs used in chemotherapy are alkylating agents (Table 21-2). These are bifunctional or multifunctional compounds with reactive electron-negative groups appropriately spaced to form adducts with macromolecules. Their ultimate toxicity may be mechanical insofar as the alkylating agents cross-link side groups of nucleic acids and proteins, thereby impairing their biological functions, such as transcription, translation, replication, and enzymatic activity. The differences between these drugs in clinical terms largely rest in their routes of administration, rates and onset of action, and mechanisms of elimination, which, in some instances, influence their toxicity. For example, cyclophosphamide itself is not an alkylating agent, but it is converted by the liver microsomal system into phosphoramide mustard, an alkylating compound. Also, unlike other alkylating agents, the alkylating agents derived from cyclophosphamide are excreted in the urine. Contact of these compounds with the bladder can cause a hemorrhagic cystitis and possibly bladder cancer. Co-administration with cyclophosphamide of sodium-2-mercap-

Table 21-2. Alkylating Agents

Alkylating Agent	Route of Administration	Usual Use	Unique Toxicity
Mechlorethamine	IV	Hodgkin's disease	
Chlorambucil	Oral	Chronic lymphatic leukemia	
Cyclophosphamide	Oral or IV	Non-Hodgkin's lymphomas, solid tumors	Hemorrhagic cystitis
Melphalan	Oral	Multiple myeloma	
Nitrosoureas	Oral or IV	Lymphomas, solid tumors	Renal damage
Busulfan	Oral	Chronic granulocytic leukemia	Pulmonary fibrosis
Procarbazine	Oral	Lymphomas	
Cisplatin	IV	Solid tumors, lymphomas	Auditory nerve damage

toethane sulfonate (MESNA) limits bladder damage, because MESNA accumulates in the urinary bladder where it locally reactivates the alkylating agent. In contrast to other alkylating agents, cyclophosphamide is relatively selective in its bone marrow toxicity and does not suppress megakaryocyte turnover to the degree obtained with other alkylating agents.

The general toxicity of alkylating agents for normal cells involves inhibition of growth of relatively rapidly dividing stem cells in the bone marrow, skin (especially the hair follicles), and gastrointestinal tract. Not surprisingly, their principal side effects are pancytopenia, hair loss, and ulceration of mucous membranes. Some alkylating agents have particular side effects. Different alkylating agents are used to treat different diseases. When rapid tumor destruction is not necessary, as for example in a patient with multiple myeloma without life-threatening pancytopenia or renal

failure (Ch. 29), the convenience of oral administration of medication is a factor in the selection of melphalan as the treatment of choice. Once a malignancy becomes resistant to the action of a particular alkylating agent, others may be active, despite similar biochemical mechanisms for cytotoxic effects.

Antimetabolites

Chemicals that inhibit specific enzymes required for the survival of tumor stem cells are antimetabolites (Table 21-3). The relevant metabolic pathways are dedicated to the synthesis of RNA and DNA, and the compounds used are generally analogues of normal substrates of these pathways. The toxic complications of antimetabolites are generally very similar to those of alkylating agents.

Folic acid is a methyl group donor for the conversion of deoxyuridine-5′-phosphate (dUMP) to thymidine-5′-phosphate (dTMP), a

Table 21-3. Antimetabolites

Antimetabolites	Route of Administration	Mechanism of Action	Usual Use	Usual Toxicity
Methotrexate	Oral or IV	Inhibition of tetrahydrofolate reductase	Lymphatic leukemias, solid tumors	Hepatic cirrhosis (rare)
6-Mercaptopurine	Oral or IV	Inhibition of DNA synthesis	Acute leukemias	Hepatic
6-Thioguanine	Oral or IV	Inhibition of DNA synthesis	Acute leukemias	Hepatic
6-Azacytidine	Oral or IV	Inhibition of DNA synthesis	Acute nonlymphocytic leukemias	Hepatic
Azathioprine	Oral	Converted to GMP in vivo	Immunosuppression	Hepatic
5-Fluorouracil	IV	Inhibition of thymidylate synthase	Solid tumors	
Cytosine arabinoside	Continuous IV infusion	DNA polymerase	Acute nonlymphocytic leukemias	

precursor of thymidine triphosphate (TTP) and the thymine base of DNA. The chemotherapeutic antimetabolite methotrexate (MTX) is a folic acid analogue that binds competitively to the enzyme tetrahydrofolate reductase. Inhibition of this enzyme prevents the conversion of folic acid to tetrahydrafolic acid, the active form of the vitamin. One feature of methotrexate treatment is that it is possible within a few hours after administration of the drug to give formyl tetrahydrofolate, also known as folinic acid or citrovorum factor. This compound is distal to the metabolic block and can reverse the toxic effects of the methotrexate. Rescue with citrovorum factor has been used after administration of very large doses of methotrexate. This strategy, which uses grams of intravenous methotrexate (the usual dose being measured in milligrams), followed by orally administered folinic acid, is effective against some neoplasms. Most methotrexate given in this way is excreted by the kidneys and, because of the high concentrations involved, can precipitate in the nephrons, especially at acid pH, causing renal damage. Therefore, renal function must be normal before attempting such treatment, and vigorous hydration and alkalinization of the urine with sodium bicarbonate should be attempted.

Purine and pyrimidine bases containing sulfhydryl groups or other substituents can be incorporated into and lead to the formation of abnormal DNA or RNA, which are ineffective for cell survival. Cytosine arabinoside (ARA-C), 6-mercaptopurine (6-MP), and 6-thioguanine (6-TG) are examples of this class of antimetabolites and are used in the treatment of acute leukemia. 5-Fluorouracil (5-FU) is an agent used in the treatment of solid tumors, and azathioprine is an antimetabolite used for immunosuppression in the treatment of autoimmune disorders and for organ transplantation.

The efficacy of purine antagonists depends on the uptake and phosphorylation of the analogues. Resistance to these agents may in part derive from the induction in tumor stem cells of phosphatases, which dephosphorylate the base analogues, thereby preventing their incorporation into DNA. Cytosine arabinoside is rapidly deaminated and must therefore be infused rapidly or continuously. Another interaction of importance is the inactivation of 6-MP by the enzyme xanthine oxidase. Allopurinol, a xanthine oxidase inhibitor, is often given to patients with neoplasms to prevent urate overproduction resulting from cell lysis and release of purines. Allopurinol can therefore delay inactivation of 6-MP, causing a normal dose to become toxic. Methotrexate is a competitive inhibitor of tetrahydrofolate reductase; therefore, a mechanism of resistance of tumor stem cells is the production of greater amounts of the enzyme. Indeed, in cultured cells resistant to methotrexate, it is possible to document the presence of reduplicated DNA segments coding for the tetrahydrofolic acid reductase enzyme.

Inhibitors of the enzyme adenosine deaminase have demonstrated efficacy in the treatment of lymphoid neoplasms, especially chronic lymphocytic leukemia (Ch. 24) and hairy cell leukemia (Ch. 27). The specific compounds are 2-deoxyadenosine, fludarabine (fluoro-ara-adenosine monophosphate), and deoxycoformycin.

Antibiotics

Compounds with antitumor actions originally extracted from living organisms are classified as antibiotics. These compounds act as cell toxins by diverse methods.

Vinca Alkaloids and Taxol. The vinca alkaloids are compounds isolated from the periwinkle plant. The active principles are vincristine and vinblastine. The known biochemical actions of these agents are that they bind with very high affinity to the cell protein tubulin and inhibit the assembly of this protein into microtubules, one of the cell's important fiber systems that in particular forms the mitotic spindle. Because these compounds bind to the ends of preformed microtubules, substoichiometric quantities can profoundly affect the balance between assembled and unpolymerized tubulin in cells. The toxicity of the two vinca alkaloids used in practice differs. Vinblastine is primarily suppressive to the bone marrow, whereas vincristine produces a dose-dependent neuropathy. This neuropathy is both sensory and motor and may be manifested initially by paresthesias in the toes, followed by loss of deep tendon reflexes in the ankles and then difficulty with gait. Autonomic neuropathy may occur, leading to constipation and even ileus. The neuropathy is reversed after cessation of treatment, although the remission of symptoms may be slow. Taxol has the opposite biochemical effect from vinca alkaloids in that it stabilizes microtubules against depolymerization.

Anthracycline Compounds. These antibiotics are brightly colored multiple-ring chemicals with conjugated sugars. They have two known effects: (1) they bind directly to cellular DNA; and (2) they appear to generate toxic oxygen metabolites, and may thereby damage cells by a process analogous to the microbicidal effect of activated phagocytes or the indirect effects of radiation therapy. The anthracyclines are toxic to rapidly growing cells, especially the bone marrow and hair follicles. Anthracyclines, like nitrogen mustard, are very toxic to subcutaneous tissues and cause extensive necrosis if extravasation occurs during an intravenous infusion. The most troublesome toxicity unique to anthracyclines is damage to the heart. The mechanism for this relatively specific toxicity has not been established. This toxicity is expressed as heart failure, which occurs when a critical cumulative dose is exceeded. Although the critical dose can be approximated below which cardiac failure is rare ($450 \ mg/m^2$), the threshold for a given patient is impossible to predict. Furthermore, there is no simple test that currently permits the physician to predict that congestive heart failure is impending in a given patient. Therefore, the dose of anthracyclines must be restricted to the population threshold for most patients and reduced further or avoided for patients with preexisting cardiac disease. Because anthracyclines are highly effective broad-spectrum chemotherapeutic agents, this cardiac damage is frustrating.

Bleomycin. A mixture of sulfur-containing polypeptides, bleomycin has been shown to sever DNA strands. Its principal advantage is its lack of bone marrow toxicity; it has been used for the treatment of lymphomas. It causes allergic reactions and skin and pulmonary toxicity.

Etoposide and Teniposide. These agents are semisynthetic analogues of a natural product, podophyllotoxin, used in the treatment of common warts. The drugs promote the degradation of nuclear DNA, and are inhibitors of the DNA repair enzyme topoisomerase II. Teniposide is active against acute lymphoblastic leukemia. The principal side effects of these agents are hypersensitivity reactions and secondary leukemias.

HORMONES USED IN THE TREATMENT OF HEMATOLOGICAL DISEASES

Corticosteroids

Natural and synthetic glucocorticoids are used in the treatment of leukemias, Hodgkin's disease, and non-Hodgkin's lymphomas. They are also frequently used in hematology for immunosuppression of autoimmune disorders. Glucocorticoids have many actions on many organ systems. Their ability to kill lymphoid cells appears to be associated with their binding to cytoplasmic receptors, which then go into the nucleus. Beyond this, their mode of action is unknown. The limiting factor in corticosteroid therapy is the myriad of side effects (Table 21-4) associated with Cushing's syndrome, the name granted to the endogenous overproduction of glucocorticoids.

Enzymes

Theoretically, a selective nutritional requirement of tumor stem cells could be exploited by depriving the system of that nutrient. Acute lymphoid leukemia cells, unlike normal cells, have a requirement for the amino acid asparagine. Because infusion of the bacterial enzyme asparaginase can effectively starve acute lymphatic leukemia cells, it is used in the treatment of human acute lymphatic leukemia. Such enzyme preparations, if contaminated with other bacterial substances, can lead to allergic reactions and other toxic effects, including acute pancreatitis and disorders of the coagulation system.

TOXICITY OF CHEMOTHERAPEUTIC DRUGS

Side effects of chemotherapy are listed in Tables 21-2 through 21-4. Certain common toxic manifestations of chemotherapy deserve elaboration.

Bone Marrow Failure

The willingness to accept bone marrow failure during chemotherapy is a relative matter. In an attempt to induce a complete remission in the acute leukemias, total bone marrow failure is a planned integral part of the treatment, and the risk of bleeding and infection and the supportive measures directed against these risks are usually acceptable. In contrast, for other hematological malignancies, such profound bone marrow suppression is not warranted; the physician monitors the numbers of peripheral red blood cells, platelets, and granulocytes to ascertain whether an occasional patient is having an extraordinarily profound bone marrow effect from the treatment. This effect may occur in patients receiving chemotherapy who have previously received radiation therapy to large areas of the bone marrow. It may be necessary in such cases to reduce dosages of drugs. Hematopoietic hormones such as GM-CSF and G-CSF (Chs. 1 and 22) shorten the duration of chemotherapy-induced bone marrow failure by increasing the rate of repopulation of normal blood cell progenitors. A theo-

retical concern that these growth factors might stimulate neoplastic cell proliferation has not yet been borne out.

In disorders such as the acute leukemias and aggressive (high-grade) lymphomas, it is possible, at least initially, to prevent bleeding complications by platelet transfusions (Ch. 31). When patients have had multiple platelet transfusions, however, alloimmunization against foreign platelet antigens may become a problem. A widespread but controversial practice is to give platelet transfusions when the platelet count falls below 20,000/μl even in the absence of overt bleeding. When sepsis or the requirement for surgical interventions increase the bleeding risk, prophylactic platelet transfusions may be more readily justified.

Infectious complications due to therapy-related leukopenia are less easily avoidable, and common pathogens include *Streptococcus viridans*, *Staphylococcus aureus*, *Escherichia coli*, *Klebsiella* species, and *Pseudomonas aeruginosa*. Sites of these infections are the skin, the gastrointestinal tract, the respiratory tree, and also large-bore catheters routinely placed in the subclavian vein to provide easy access for chemotherapeutic agents, blood products, and antibiotics. The infections may present only with fever, since reduced white blood cell counts damp localized signs of inflammation. Because of the vulnerability of the patient in this setting, the physician will usually begin empiric broad-spectrum antibiot-

Table 21-4. Hormones

Hormone	Use in Hematology	Side Effects
Glucocorticosteroids	Therapy of lymphoid neoplasms Immunosuppression Therapy of hypercalcemia Therapy of malignant disease	Fluid retention Hypokalemia Osteoporosis Myopathy Aseptic necrosis of the femoral head Protein catabolism Hirsutism Dental atrophy and purpura Mental alterations Neutrophilia caused by inhibition of phagocyte function Suppression of lymphoid function
G-CSF	Therapy of bone marrow failure caused by chemotherapy	Fever

ic therapy without waiting for the results of blood and orofical cultures. The choice of antibiotics may be guided by knowledge of microorganisms prevalent in a particular treatment center. Persistent fever in a patient receiving antibacterial antibiotics is suggestive of fungal infection requiring the addition of antifungal agents.

Carcinogenesis

Certain chemotherapeutic agents have the property of inflicting sublethal damage on normal stem cells, eventually causing evolution to a malignant state. Acute nonlymphocytic leukemia is the most frequent neoplasm to arise after chemotherapy. Alkylating agents are especially active in this regard, and risk of chemotherapy increases if ionizing radiation was included in the treatment. The increasing effectiveness of chemotherapy in the treatment of certain cancers has allowed more patients to live long enough to manifest the carcinogenic complication of their earlier therapy. Recognition of this complication of chemotherapy has led therapists to try to establish the minimal treatment required to eradicate malignant disease and minimize the carcinogenic risk.

Metabolic Effects of Tumor Killing

When chemotherapy or radiation therapy work effectively against a large mass of tumor cells, the body may be exposed to the debris released by the dead and dying cancer cells. One troublesome component is uric acid, which accumulates as a result of breakdown of tumor cell nucleic acids. Uric acid can deposit in the joints and other tissues, producing gout or causing renal stones and even urinary outflow obstruction. Treatment of this complication includes liberal administration of fluids in order to maintain urine flow and dilute the uric acid concentration. Maintenance of an alkaline urinary pH level by means of sodium bicarbonate can also minimize precipitation of the uric acid. However, uric acid accumulation can be prevented by priming patients with allopurinol before instituting chemotherapy.

Allopurinol functions as an inhibitor of xanthine oxidase—the enzyme responsible for converting purines to uric acid (at the steps where hypoxanthine is changed to xanthine, and subseguently to uric acid). In the occasional case of excessive tumor lysis, cellular destruction can lead to hyperkalemia, hyperphosphatemia, and hypocalcemia.

Nausea and Vomiting

Both chemotherapy and radiation therapy can cause nausea and vomiting. The cause of this disagreeable side effect is multifactorial. Direct damage to the gastrointestinal mucosa can play a role. Perturbation of certain areas of the brain stem—one being called the chemoreceptor trigger zone—and of the vestibular system may be involved. Finally, a conditioning effect takes place once patients come to dread the nausea and vomiting of treatment: They may actually begin to retch at the thought of an appointment with the physician. Unfortunately, there are no foolproof answers to these problems. Antihistamines, phenothiazines, anticholinergic antiemetics, corticosteroids, and butyrophenones are useful in some patients.

Sedation with barbiturates and minor tranquilizers such as lorazepam may reduce the agony and the memory of nausea and vomiting, especially in the case of drugs showing a high incidence of this complaint. The alkylating agents, especially nitrogen mustard, nitrosoureas, cisplatin, and procarbazine, are particularly problematic in this regard. Care must be taken not to oversedate; otherwise the patient runs the risk of aspirating gastric contents into the lungs while vomiting. Some patients, particularly young people, may obtain relief from nausea and vomiting if given tetrahydrocannabinol, the active principle of the marijuana plant. Older persons tend to find the cerebral effects of this drug unpleasant. Psychiatric assistance and hypnosis can be useful in dealing with the conditioning aspects of nausea and vomiting. Recently a novel serotonin receptor antagonist, ondansetron, has become available that is very effective either alone or in combination with dopamine D_2

inhibitors, in controlling emetic effects of chemotherapy. A problem with this medication is that it is expensive.

Malnutrition

Patients with cancer are very concerned with nutrition, having been conditioned about the wasting caused by the disease. Alimentation can be disturbed by the nausea and vomiting associated with therapy, by problems with chewing and swallowing resulting from cases in which radiotherapy has been delivered to the head and neck, and from anxiety. In addition, there is considerable speculation as to the nutritional aspects of cancer. A very vocal and persuasive group has promoted the idea that nutritional imbalances and deficiencies are of great importance in the causation and spread of malignancies. Although these theories currently have debatable scientific merit, patients with neoplasms are often aware of these ideas and are concerned about them. Therefore, the physician should be sympathetic to the patient's nutritional concerns. A nutritionist is a valuable ally in the treatment team and can advise the physician and the patient about types of feeding useful for a given patient. In some cases the use of total parenteral nutrition, the infusion of needed calories and vitamins by the intravenous route, may be appropriate.

Immunotherapy

It would be helpful if the immune system could deal with tumor stem cells as well as it handles microorganisms. Immune destruction of tumor cells would have the advantage over most current anticancer treatments of not requiring that the target cells be especially active or in cycle.

Unfortunately, human cancer cells appear to be too much a version of self to be perceived as foreign and disposed of by immunological defenses. This ability of tumors to avoid detection by the immune system exists despite the fact that many tumor cells do have unique sur-

face antigens. In an effort to make use of these antigens, attempts were made to stimulate the immune system in a general way by administering relatively nontoxic microbial products such as the bacillus Calmette-Guérin (BCG). It was hoped that the "angry" immune system consisting of lymphocytes and macrophages activated by the microbial materials would now eliminate tumor cells. This nonspecific immunotherapy seemed beneficial in a few cases, but on the whole was not very successful.

Monoclonal antibodies have the theoretical advantage of very great specificity for unique tumor antigens. The antibodies could then target tumor cells for killing by the body's immunological effector mechanisms. Alternatively, these antibodies can be tagged with chemotherapeutic agents or toxins. This approach takes advantage of a limitation of "straight" antibody therapy—the problem of antigenic modulation (Ch. 30). Tumor cells, like lymphocytes and phagocytes, can internalize surface antigens reacted with antibodies, thereby removing from their surfaces the signals needed for immunological destruction. However, if the surface-bound antibodies contain toxins, these entities could be brought into the cell like Trojan horses. Unfortunately, the theoretically appealing elements of monoclonal antibodies as antitumor agents have only rarely been realized at the practical level.

Other Biological Therapies

Reference has been made in other chapters to the responsiveness of certain neoplasms to "natural" products of the body. These include hairy cell leukemia, which can remit during therapy with α-interferon; chronic granulocytic leukemia, which can be controlled by either recombinant α- or γ-interferons; and a very few cases of non-Hodgkin's lymphoma, which have responded to human leukocyte-derived interferons. The mechanisms by which these antiviral agents affect neoplasms are unknown. The interferons can be shown to inhibit the growth of cells in tissue culture, and such antiproliferative effects may be one of their antineoplastic actions. On the other hand, they also activate mononuclear phagocytes, and it may be that they enhance other aspects of host responses to the tumor. Another "biological response modifier" under study is IL-2. This lymphokine (Ch. 1), among other effects, activates natural killer cells to increased cytotoxicity against a variety of tumors in tissue culture and has caused some striking regressions of solid tumors, notably renal cell cancers and melanomas. Unfortunately, IL-2 is very toxic, causing, among other effects, impressive capillary permeability leading to serious body fluid shifts, such that intensive nursing care has been required to care for patients receiving this agent.

OVERVIEW

The treatment of the hematological malignancies—the leukemias and lymphomas, and, when specialists act as medical oncologists, the solid tumors—is in a continuing state of evolution. Improved therapeutic strategies are best sought in well-designed controlled therapy trials in which large numbers of patients are enrolled. Although only a few large medical centers will have enough patients to test hypotheses regarding treatment, cooperative treatment groups have been organized to include participation of physicians with relatively small practices in such studies. Participating physicians must be willing to take the time required to obtain laboratory data and record results of therapy. They must also be sufficiently motivated to convince a patient to enter the protocol, pointing out that the patient's individual interests, as well as posterity, are well served and dispelling the notion that the patient is merely a guinea pig. Patients and physicians alike are understandably desirous of the "best" treatment, but both must be made to understand that it takes therapeutic trials to establish the "best" therapy as fact rather than opinion. Few therapies can be considered routine. The treatment plan against

lymphomas, solid tumors, and occasionally the leukemias may require surgery to make the diagnosis, and, in the case of solid tumors, as treatment. Radiation therapy will often be required in the treatment plan. Nursing and social service personnel are part of the team as well. This interdisciplinary approach requires intensive cross-consultation among members of the therapeutic unit to arrive at an integrative treatment that is best for a given patient.

In this consortium of expertise, however, someone must act as the primary physician to guide the discussion and keep very close track of the patient and his or her family. In the case of hematological malignancies, the hematologist or hematologist–oncologist will often have this role, although an internist or other generalist may take it on with assistance from specialists. The treatment of a localized or of a slowly evolving malignancy may be relatively straightforward and create little morbidity, but the therapy of many hematological malignancies constitutes an extreme physical, emotional, and economic strain on the patient and the patient's family. The physician must mobilize all necessary resources to deal with the problems that arise. The physician has to use all measures of support to anticipate and deal with the physical complications of the diseases and treatment. The primary physician must also be prepared to manage patiently the patient's anxieties and those of the patient's family. The patient must be encouraged occasionally to bear up when appropriate and forge ahead with the sometimes grueling and disagreeable aspects of therapy. Sometimes assistance from social service personnel and from patient support groups may be helpful in dealing with economic problems and in minimizing the disruptive effects of the disease on the family. For example, with help from visiting nursing services, it may be possible to avoid repeated visits to the medical center. Honestly appraised, the practice of hematology is no more depressing than that of many other specialties of internal medicine. Nevertheless, experience has shown that it is helpful for members of the treatment team to discuss their feelings about some of the very ill patients and about the terminal illnesses of patients with each other and with mental health professionals.

Patients with malignancy especially fear pain. There is no excuse in nearly all cases for this fear to become a reality. Pain often arises from the infiltration and disruption of normal tissues by malignant cells and from penetration of nerve roots. Both processes can be amplified by anxiety. Pain medication should not be withheld or limited out of fear of addiction. Medication should usually be given by a regular schedule to control pain rather than "as needed," because the patient may be too frightened, concerned about addiction, or incapable of making the appropriate requests. Many patients whose mental status allows can determine their own schedule and dose of medications that best control their pain without undue obtundation. The effectiveness of opiates and other pain medications can be enhanced by the appropriate use of tranquilizing drugs.

Despite advances in the management of hematological malignancies and the increasing proportion of "cures," many patients will die as a result of their disease. The goal of the physician should be to make the patient's remaining life as useful and comfortable as possible. The administration of appropriate paliative treatment and of supporting care should be as challenging and rewarding to the physician as the achievement of cures.

SUGGESTED READINGS

Aronson SA (1991) Growth factors and cancer. Science 254:1146

Bishop JM (1991) Molecular themes in oncogenesis. Cell 64:235

Bolen JB, Rowley RB, Spana C, Tsygankov AB (1992) The Src family of tyrosine protein kinases in hemopoietic signal transduction. FASEB J 6:3403

Chen P-L, Chen Y, Bookstein R, Lee W-H (1990) Genetic mechanisms of tumor suppression by the human p53 gene. Science 250:1576

Committee on the Biological Effects of Ionizing Radiations (1990) Health Effects of Exposure to Low Levels of Ionizing Radiation. National Academy Press, Washington, DC

DeVita VT, Jr, Hellman S, Rosenberg SA (1989) Cancer. Principles & Practice of Oncology. 3rd Ed. JB Lippincott, Philadelphia

Drugs of choice for cancer chemotherapy (1993) The Medical Letter 35:43

Farmer G, Bargonetti J, Zhu H et al (1992) Wild-type p53 activates transcription in vitro. Nature 358:83

Fong C, Brodeur GM (1987) Down's syndrome and leukemia: epidemiology, genetics, cytogenetics and mechanisms of leukemogenesis. Cancer Genet Cytogenet 28:55

Grossbard ML, Press OW, Appelbaum FR et al (1992) Monoclonal antibody-based therapeutic therapies of leukemia and lymphoma. Blood 80:863

Herrstedt J, Sigsgaard T, Boesgaard M et al (1993) Ondansetron plus metopimazine compared with Ondansetron alone in patients receiving moderately emetogenic chemotherapy. N Engl J Med 328:1076

Hockenbery DM, Oltvai ZN, Yin X-m et al (1993) Bcl-2 Functions in an antioxidant pathway to prevent apoptosis. Cell 75:241

Hollstein M, Sidransky D, Vogelstein B, Harris CC (1991) p53 mutations in human cancers. Science 253:49

Hughes WT et al (1990) Guidelines for the use of antimicrobial agents in neutropenic patients with unexplained fever. J Infect Dis 161:381

Hunter T, Pines J (1991) Cyclins and cancer. Cell 66:1071

Lawrence HJ, Largman C (1992) Homeobox genes in normal hematopoiesis and leukemia. Blood 80:2445

Löwenberg B, Touw IP (1993) Hematopoietic growth factors and their receptors in acute leukemia. Blood 81:281

Massagué J (1992) Receptors for the TGF-b family. Cell 69:1067

McMahon SB, Monroe JG (1992) Role of primary response genes in generating cellular responses to growth factors. FASEB J 6:2707

Moore MAS (1992) Does stem cell exhaustion result from combining hematopoietic growth factors with chemotherapy? If so, how do we prevent it? Blood 80:3

Nichols J, Nimer SD (1992) Transcription factors, translocations, and leukemia. Blood 80:2953

Norbury C, Nurse P (1992) Animal cell cycles and their control. Annu Rev Biochem 61:441

Pastan I, Gottesman MM (1991) Multidrug resistance. Annu Rev Med 42:277

Rous P (1911) Transmission of a malignant new growth by means of a cell-free filtrate. JAMA 56:198

Sato T, Nakafuku M, Kaziro Y (1992) Function of *ras* as a molecular switch in signal transduction. J Biol Chem 267:24149

Sherr CJ (1993) Mammalian G_1 cyclins. Cell 73:1059

Thirman MJ, Gill HJ, Burnett RC et al (1993) Rearrangement of the *MLL* gene in acute lymphoblastic and acute myeloid leukemias with 11q23 chromasomal translocation. N Engl J Med 329:909

Vogelstein B, Kinzler KW (1992) p53 function and dysfunction. Cell 70:523

22

Stem Cell Disorders

Diseases affecting the pluripotent stem cell fall into four main categories (Table 22-1): (1) reversible or permanent stem cell *proliferation failure*—the *aplasias*; (2) qualitative abnormalities of stem cells in which there is *impaired differentiation*—the *myelodysplasias*; (3) *uncontrolled proliferation* of stem cells—the *myeloproliferative disorders*; and (4) overt *malignant transformation* of the stem cells—*chronic myelogenous leukemia*. The diseases described in this section overlap each other, as well as the acute myelogenous leukemias described in the next chapter. The prefix "*myelo-*," literally meaning "of the bone marrow," in reference to stem cell diseases has come to encompass primarily those cell lineages distinct from the lymphoid, i.e. granulocytic, monocytic, erythroid, and megakaryocytic, because failure of differentiation or overproduction of these lines characterizes the disorders. However, chronic myelogenous leukemia can also involve lymphoid cells late in its evolution, and, as explained in the next chapter, acute leukemias can sometimes have myeloid and lymphoid features in common.

Most acquired stem cell diseases are disorders exhibiting abnormal stem cell clones. These clones may manifest as increased, decreased, or qualitatively altered production of peripheral blood cells, and in almost all cases involve the entire bone marrow. Yet at some time the clone must have arisen from one area of the bone marrow, another factor in support of the idea that stem cells leave the bone marrow and return to it in other locations.

APLASTIC ANEMIA

A large number of disease processes can interfere temporarily or permanently with the viability of the pluripotent stem cell. The end result is a single clinical syndrome somewhat incompletely designated aplastic anemia, because the patient has leukopenia and thrombocytopenia as well as anemia, that is, pancytopenia.

The consequences of pancytopenia are grimly straightforward: weakness and pallor due to anemia, infection as a result of leukopenia, and bleeding from thrombocytopenia. The erythrocyte morphology is usually normal, and the anemia is therefore classifiable as normocytic and normochromic, but often, for unexplained reasons, the mean corpuscular volume may be abnormally high. Usually, the reticulocyte count is low, especially in the face of the anemia, indicating a failure of an erythroid response to the low circulating hemoglobin concentration. All the leukocyte forms are reduced in concentration, but especially the phagocytes, the polymorphonuclear leukocytes, and monocytes, leaving the differential white blood cell count a monotonous picture of typical and a few atypical lymphocytes. Even the total lymphocyte count will be reduced, and the lymphocytes remaining presumably are long-

Table 22-1. Stem Cell Disorders

Initial Disorder	Evolutionary Disorder
Bone marrow failure	
Aplastic anemia	Acute nonlymphocytic leukemia
Bone marrow dysplasia	
Paroxysmal nocturnal hemoglobinuria	Aplastic anemia or acute nonlymphocytic leukemia
Myelodysplasia	
Cyclic neutropenia	
Chronic idiopathic neutropenia	
Bone marrow hyperplasia	
Polycythemia vera	Myelofibrosis or acute nonlymphocytic leukemia
Myeloid metaplasia	Myelofibrosis
Bone marrow neoplasia	
Chronic granulocytic leukemia	Blast crisis
Essential thrombocythemia	Acute nonlymphocytic leukemia
Erythroleukemia	

lived memory cells. Few platelets will be seen on the blood smear, and the actual count confirms the presence of thrombocytopenia.

The known causes of aplastic anemia are physical, chemical, and biological agents capable of attacking the pluripotent stem cell in the bone marrow. These various insults presumably damage the genetic material of the pluripotent stem cell with sufficient vigor to cause cell death.

Physical Agents

Ionizing radiation directed against the entire bone marrow above a dose of 7 Gray will destroy all bone marrow stem cells and induce permanent pancytopenia. External radiation must be of the γ-ray or x-ray type capable of penetrating the body and gaining access to bone marrow cells. Lower doses of ionizing radiation are progressively less damaging, but reduce the reserve capacity of the bone marrow to respond to demands imposed by bleeding or infection. Radiation is most destructive to rapidly dividing cells, the mitotic compartment described in Chapter 1. It is evident from the

rates of maturation of erythrocytes and granulocytes that basophilic normoblasts, myeloblasts, promyelocytes, and myelocytes turn over rapidly and are therefore susceptible to irradiation damage and other genetic insults. However, the fact that the bone marrow can recover from sublethal damage indicates that a portion of the stem cells are in a dormant or nondividing state at the time of exposure and are recruited into differentiation and replication after bone marrow aplasia. Indeed, one can show that the total number of granulocyte–macrophage colony-forming units (GM-CFU) in culture falls in the bone marrow of patients receiving cytotoxic chemotherapy or radiation toxic to the bone marrow.

Chemical Agents

Chemicals and drugs are frequently suspect in the causation of bone marrow failure, although only a few agents can be implicated definitively. Since the early 1900s, a frequent association of industrial exposures to benzene and benzene derivatives has made these organic solvents the prime culprits responsible for bone marrow damage and even leukemia. The mechanism of this effect is unknown. The extensive use of these chemicals for multiple uses in modern society creates the problem that an exposure to such chemical agents cannot always be identified. Certain medications are implicated as stem cell toxins. The most clearcut examples are drugs used in cancer chemotherapy that are designed to kill tumor stem cells.

Acute damage to the bone marrow stem cells by toxins or drugs may be manifested primarily by neutropenia. The basis of this fact is the short life span of the neutrophil. About 7 days after the differentiation of stem cells is impaired, the bone marrow reserve of mature neutrophils will be depleted. Within 6 to 12 hours, the last blood neutrophil will leave the circulation; the profound neutropenia that results is commonly called *agranulocytosis*. The longer life span of reticulocytes and erythrocytes (120 days) and of platelets (7 days) buffers the impairment of production of these cells, and the resumption of stem cell activity will replenish erythrocytes and platelets faster than neutrophils, the generation time of erythrocytes and platelets being 4 days and 5 days, respectively, in contrast to 7 days for neutrophils. Drugs frequently associated with acute agranulocytosis are listed below.

Chloramphenicol, an antibiotic with a broad antibacterial spectrum, causes two types of bone marrow failure. The first is a dose- and time-dependent phenomenon in which the drug induces bone marrow suppression that is reversible after the medication is discontinued. Most, if not all, patients receiving chloramphenicol are subject to this effect, which manifests initially by a decrease in the reticulocyte count and a concomitant rise in serum iron, a result of cessation of erythropoiesis. Examination of the bone marrow at this time indicates vacuolation of the normoblasts. Subsequently, the white blood count, mainly the polymorphonuclear leukocyte count, falls, ultimately followed by a drop in the platelet count. This common and reversible toxicity of chloramphenicol on the bone marrow is overshadowed by the devastating permanent destructive effect of chloramphenicol on the bone marrow of the occasional patient.

Ethanol is also toxic to the bone marrow, although its direct effects on hematopoiesis are usually only apparent in the setting of heavy alcoholism, with or without concomitant vitamin (folic acid) deficiency. In the absence of folate deficiency, the anemia, leukopenia, and thrombocytopenia of alcohol are self-limited and rapidly reversible. Chronic alcoholism, however, can precipitate serious pancytopenia and complications thereof when associated with hepatic cirrhosis. Spur cell anemia and, more commonly, congestive splenomegaly can contribute to anemia. Hypersplenism together with alcoholic bone marrow suppression may aggravate thrombocytopenia, which together with coagulation factor deficiency resulting from the failing liver predisposes to bleeding. The development of aplastic anemia in patients receiving a large variety of drugs commonly used in clinical medicine has raised the suspicion that these medications have a causal role, although proof thereof is hard to document. Nevertheless, a first step in the evaluation of a patient with pancytopenia should be to determine whether there has been an exposure to solvents or drugs and, whenever possible, to discontinue the exposure.

Biological Agents

Biological agents are also capable of causing the clinical picture of aplastic anemia. In disseminated tuberculosis, a granulomatous inflammatory infiltrate can replace the bone marrow. Neoplasms such as metastatic cancer, acute leukemia, multiple myeloma, and the lymphomas are capable of producing similar effects. Neutropenia, thrombocytopenia, or pancytopenia are concomitants of certain rare inborn errors of amino acid metabolism associated with accumulation of ketone bodies and glycine in the blood and urine. These disorders, grouped under the designation of *ketotic hyperglycinemias,* are methylmalonic acidemia, propionic acidemia, and isovaleric acidemia. It is presumed that one of the organic acids that accumulates in these disorders is toxic to the bone marrow stem cells.

A genetic disorder predisposes to the development of aplastic anemia. Patients with *Fanconi's anemia*, an uncommon autosomal recessive disorder, are found to have breaks in their chromosomes as well as various skeletal abnormalities. At about 5 to 7 years of age, progressive bone marrow failure occurs. The pluripotent stem cells in these patients are unusually susceptible to DNA damage. Genes capable of correcting (complementing) this defect have been identified, although their specific functions in DNA repair are not yet known. The diagnosis of Fanconi's anemia is made by demonstrating induction of chromosomal breaks in cultured lymphoid cells treated with DNA cross-linking agents such as diepoxybutane.

Viruses have long been suspected as a cause of bone marrow failure, but few specific examples have been definitely established. Because bone marrow aplasia occasionally accompanies acute viral hepatitis, the hepatotoxic viruses have been implicated for some patients, although the known varieties (hepatitis A, B, and C) do not appear clearly involved in the causation. On the other hand, there is good evidence that a *parvovirus*, a DNA virus that infects many animals and birds, is the cause of transient inhibition of erythropoiesis that becomes clinically manifest in patients with congenital and acquired hemolytic disorders. The evidence for the role of this virus is the presence of viral particles in bone marrow specimens of patients with sickle cell anemia, thalassemia major, or other congenital hemolytic anemias who develop pancytopenia, so-called *aplastic crises*, followed by the appearance of antibodies against the virus. Individuals with normal bone marrow function may have transient suppression of red blood cell production, but without the demand imposed by peripheral blood cell destruction, the steady-state levels of blood cells do not decline markedly.

In most cases of aplastic anemia, none of the aforementioned causes can be identified, and the aplastic anemia is said to be of unknown cause, that is, *idiopathic*. Idiosyncratic reactions to unidentified toxins are difficult to rule out.

Because many diseases including blood disorders are attributable to autoimmunity, it is appealing to speculate that autoimmunity against hematopoietic stem cells accounts for aplastic anemia. The fact that some patients suffering from aplastic anemia have a response or even remission induced by immunosuppressive therapy lends support to this idea (see below).

The success of bone marrow transplantation in reconstituting normal stem cell function in many patients with idiopathic aplastic anemia (Ch. 32) is evidence that whatever it was that destroyed the bone marrow is no longer present; otherwise, it would destroy the engrafted stem cells. The success of engraftment with bone marrow from identical twins, a setting in which no immunosuppression is required to prevent rejection of the donated bone marrow

graft by the recipient's immune system, argues further against an important role of autoimmunity in the pathogenesis of many cases of idiopathic aplastic anemia.

The failure of hematopoiesis is not demonstrably attributable to lack of the erythropoietic or other hormones that stimulate blood cell synthesis, because the levels of these factors that can be measured are markedly elevated in patients with aplastic anemia.

Diagnosis and Management

Pancytopenia is an indication for examination of the bone marrow by both aspiration and biopsy. The biopsy is essential because infiltration of the bone marrow with granulomas or cancer cells can produce fibrosis, which in turn can result in an inability to aspirate marrow cells. Because bone marrow aplasia yields the same dry aspirate encountered in these other diseases, a diagnosis of aplastic anemia might be made in error, whereas a bone marrow biopsy would indicate the presence of tuberculosis, cancer, or fibrosis. The approach to the management of these various diseases differs considerably; hence a correct diagnosis is essential.

The biopsy specimen in aplastic anemia shows bone spicules; fat; marrow stromal cells, including fibroblasts, mast cells, and macrophages; some lymphocytes; and either a reduction or absence of normal hematopoietic cells, that is, cells of the erythroid, granulocytic, or megakaryocytic lineages (Fig. 22-1). Occasionally, a bone marrow biopsy specimen of a patient with pancytopenia will have only slightly reduced normal or even increased numbers of hematopoietic cells. This finding may simply mean that the sample obtained is not representative of the total bone marrow mass. Alternatively, the observation of normal or increased hematopoietic cells in the face of pancytopenia can be a reflection of ineffective hematopoiesis. This finding is characteristic of a preleukemic syndrome. There is no completely reliable method for evaluating the hematopoietic activity of the total bone marrow. Ferrokinetic studies yield a characteristic

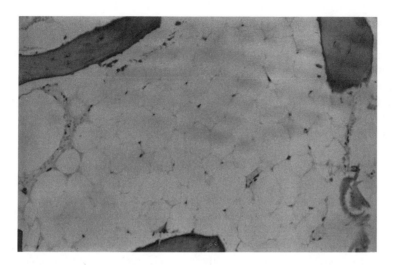

Fig. 22-1. "Empty" bone marrow of a patient with aplastic anemia. Biopsy specimen.

picture in bone marrow failure. After injection of radioactive iron, the uptake of the iron into the bone marrow from the plasma is delayed or nonexistent. This pattern contrasts with that in ineffective erythropoiesis, in which the iron rapidly enters the bone marrow but, as in aplastic anemia, fails to appear in peripheral red blood cells.

Treatment of Stem Cell Failure

The first management principle is supportive care of the patient with pancytopenia; if, however, a remediable cause of the bone marrow failure is detectable, treatment should be begun as soon as possible. The approach to supportive treatment is essentially identical to that outlined for the patient with acute leukemia. Anemia is treated with transfusions of packed erythrocytes and thrombocytopenia with platelet transfusions. Infection must be diagnosed early with appropriate cultures of body fluids and excreta and must be treated vigorously with appropriate antibiotics.

Supportive care can maintain a reasonable existence for long periods of time in some patients with pancytopenia. However, for the profoundly thrombocytopenic patient, transfusions of platelets are needed at least weekly, and the supportive care becomes both expen-

sive and tedious. Long-term transfusions with erythrocytes can lead to iron overload and the organ damage characteristic of hemochromatosis. Eventually, the development of antibodies against transfused erythrocytes and platelets limits the effectiveness of transfusion support. Moreover, the state of the art of phagocyte transfusion is not up to that of erythrocyte and platelet transfusions (Ch. 31). Therefore, the patient with severe bone marrow depression is at high risk for overwhelming sepsis with low-grade pathogens.

It is possible to minimize infections in the pancytopenic patient by literally sterilizing the patient and the environment. The patient's skin is bathed with antiseptic solutions. Food is autoclaved, and the patient ingests nonabsorbable broad-spectrum antibiotics to remove microorganisms from the gastrointestinal tract. The patient is placed in a meticulously cleaned room the air intake of which is filtered to clear out microorganisms. These heroic measures can be effective, but their expense, effort, and negative psychological impact limit their utility.

Idiopathic aplastic anemia is probably the final common denouement of different pathological processes. The relative rarity of idiopathic aplastic anemia—fewer than 1500 cases in the United States per year—makes it difficult to establish definitive prognostic and therapeutic guidelines. Left untreated, most patients with profound pancytopenia and very empty marrows as shown by aspirate and biopsy are condemned to a permanent state of aplasia. However, some patients, especially those with some evidence of residual bone marrow cellularity, may show transient or even long-standing improvement in their hematopoiesis with time.

In the minority of patients who have a residual population of stem cells, cytokines, such as erythropoietin, granulocyte colony-stimulating factor (G-CSF) and granulocyte–macrophage (GM)-CSF, and others, may improve peripheral blood counts with the exception of platelets.

The treatment of choice for patients with severe aplastic anemia is now bone marrow transplantation, the repletion of stem cells by infusion of bone marrow from a histocompatible donor, usually a sibling (Ch. 32). Therefore, an early step in the evaluation of a patient with aplastic anemia is to establish whether suitable bone marrow donors are available and to begin histocompatibility testing procedures as soon as possible. The urgency is based on the premise that (1) infection can set in at any time and either kill the patient or compromise the success of transplantation; and (2) the more transfusions the patient receives for support, the greater the risk of sensitization against antigenic determinants on the cells of the potential bone marrow donor.

For the patient who lacks a potential bone marrow donor, it is reasonable to arrange for a program of supportive care and a trial of immunosuppressive therapy. In particular, anti-lymphocyte antibodies have produced therapeutic responses in about half of treated patients, and these patients have had longer survivals than patients given supportive care alone. Other immunosuppressive agents, especially cyclosporin, increase the response rates and induce hematopoietic responses in some patients who have failed treatment with anti-lymphocyte antibodies, although they do not clearly prolong overall survival. There are even case reports of patients with aplastic anemia responding to intravenous high-dose immunoglobulin therapy. Unfortunately, a high proportion, about half, of the patients who have

responded to immunosuppressants have gone on to develop clonal hematopoietic disorders such as myelodysplastic syndromes (described below) and leukemias, implying that the underlying cause of the stem cell failure was genetic damage rather than autoimmunity—further evidence that aplastic anemia is a clonal, neoplastic disease.

MYELODYSPLASIA

The myelodysplastic syndromes form a group of interrelated stem cell diseases ranging from what is designated *refractory anemia*, a chronic anemia unresponsive to iron, vitamins, or other measures without other blood cell abnormalities to a blatantly "preleukemic" state with anemia, rising percentage of blasts in the bone marrow, thrombocytopenia, and bizzare myeloid and erythroid maturation. The cause and pathogenesis of the refractory anemias are unknown, but all evidence points to their being manifestations of acquired genetic changes in the pluripotent stem cell that programs a wide variety of phenotypic abnormalities in blood cell maturation, morphology, and function—all related to impairment of blood cell maturation. The refractory anemias may be chronic and stable or may evolve to either pancytopenia or leukemia.

The anemias are refractory in that most do not respond to treatment of the patient with iron, folic acid, vitamin B_{12}, or pyridoxine, agents that would be expected to be effective against deficiency disorders involving these compounds and that present with similar erythroid morphology. The erythrocytes are frequently macrocytic. Ringed sideroblasts may be prominent in the bone marrow along with varying degrees of megaloblastic maturation (Fig. 22-2A). The anemias are of variable severity, and some patients require frequent red cell transfusions. Numerous deficiencies of enzyme activities involved in heme synthetic pathways have been observed in the bone marrow cells of such patients.

Thrombocytopenia, a neutrophilic leukocytosis, and monocytosis sometimes may be present. Abnormalities of neutrophilic polymorphonuclear leukocyte maturation reminiscent of the myelodysplastic changes seen in the maturation pattern in acute myeloid leukemia (Ch. 23) are frequently encountered. These aberrations include giant pink or azure granules coexisting in the same granulocytic cells, the Pelger-Hüet anomaly of the nuclei of neutrophils, or marked nuclear hypersegmentation of the neutrophils (Fig. 22-2B).

That myelodysplasia has a neoplastic aspect is strengthened by the fact that these disorders are one of the complications of the treatment of cancer and leukemia with mutagenizing thera-

py. Furthermore, the bone marrow cells from a majority of patients with myelodysplasia have discernable chromosomal abnormalities, particularly hypoploidy and loss of specific chromosomal segments. The most common finding is monosomy or partial loss of the long arm of chromosome 7 ($7q^-$). Alterations of chromosomes 3 and 5 are also frequent findings. In addition, between 10 and 40 percent of patients with myelodysplasia have transforming *ras* mutations in their bone marrow cells.

The classification of the myelodysplastic syndromes (Table 22-2) depends on the mor-

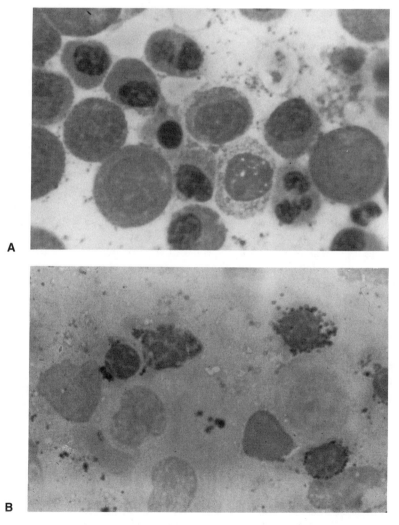

Fig. 22-2. (**A**) Ringed sideroblasts revealed by Prussian blue stain in the bone marrow of a patient with refractory anemia. (**B**) Pelger-Hüet neutrophils and dysplastic blasts in the bone marrow of a patient with a myelodysplastic syndrome.

Table 22-2. French-American-British (FAB) Classification of the Myelodysplastic Syndromes

Classification	Characteristics
Refractory anemia (RA)	Anemia unresponsive to iron. 15% progress to acute nonlymphocytic leukemia (ANLL)
Refractory anemia with ringed sidero-blasts	>15% of marrow erythroblasts are ringed sideroblasts; 15% progress to ANLL
Refractory anemia with excess blasts (RAEB)	5–20% of nucleated marrow cells are blasts; dysplastic features are prominent, and thrombocytopenia is common; 30% progress to ANLL
Chronic myelomonocytic leukemia (CMML)	Refractory anemia, thrombocytopenia, monocytosis, 5–20% bone marrow blasts, 40% progression to ANLL
RAEB "in transformation"	20–30% bone marrow blasts, anemia, thrombocytopenia, invariable progression to ANLL

phology and course of the refractory anemias. The propensity of the disorder to progress to frank leukemia is related to the number of affected cell lines and the degree of immaturity and dysplasia of the bone marrow. The presence of chromosomal abnormalities, especially complex changes, is associated with increased risk of leukemic progression. The most important discriminator in prognosis of these diseases, however, is the number of blasts detected in the bone marrow: patients whose marrows have less than 5 percent blasts have a significantly longer survival than patients whose marrows contain greater than 5 percent blasts. The patients whose myelodysplasia arises in the setting of previous chemotherapy or radiotherapy are more likely to fall into this category. Since 30 percent bone marrow blasts define acute leukemia, the patients with blast percentages between 5 and 30 can be considered to have *oligoblastic leukemia*.

Treatment

Since myelodysplasia is a disease of impaired blood cell differentiation, investigators have tried various therapies to induce differentiation. A variety of chemicals, notably retinoids, vitamin D analogues, polar planar compounds such as dimethylsulfoxide (DMSO), and hexamethylene bisacetamide (HMBA) stimulate differentiation of certain leukemic cell lines in tissue culture, and a number of these agents have been tested in humans. Blood cell counts in a minority (up to a third)

of patients with myelodysplasia have improved with the use of 13-cis retinoic acid, although mucocutaneous irritation and itching has been a significant side effect that may have masked greater efficacy. Recent evidence suggests that alpha-tocopherol therapy can counteract this toxicity, however, and better results due to longer administration of the drug may be forthcoming. Low doses of cytotoxic agents, such as cytosine arabinoside, have had limited effectiveness. They probably work by killing malignant blast cells. Hematopoietic growth factors have had relatively little success thus far, although GM-CSF therapy has not led to widespread acceleration of frank acute leukemic evolution of myelodysplasia, a hypothetical side effect. Combination therapy trials with old and new growth factors together with diffentiation agents are currently in progress. A very important consideration before treating a patient with an experimental drug is to define a clear end point such as reduction of transfusion requirements or improvement in leukopenia or thrombocytopenia, since it is not clear that new agents are free of risk.

MYELOPROLIFERATIVE DISORDERS

Polycythemia Vera

Polycythemia vera is the name historically given to a chronic myeloproliferative disorder in which the production of erythrocytes, phagocytes, and platelets is increased and in which the accumulation of erythrocytes is the dominant feature. The erythrocyte mass may increase to very high levels. In patients who have two glucose 6-phosphate-dehydrogenase (G6PD) isoenzymes in addition to polycythemia vera, the erythrocytes contain a single G6PD isoenzyme. This feature indicates that polycythemia vera is a disorder of a pluripotent clone stem cell that acquires a selective advantage through a reduction in control over its proliferation. Erythropoietin levels are low in the urine of patients with polycythemia vera, further illustrating that the blood proliferation that occurs in this disease is autonomous. The neutrophil and platelet counts are often elevated but to levels less than 25,000/µl and 800,000/µl, respectively. Leukocyte alkaline phosphatase activity is usually elevated. The basophil count is frequently increased and may be responsible for elevations in blood and urinary histamine in patients with polycythemia vera. The peripheral blood morphology is usually normal.

The main clinical manifestation of the increased hematopoiesis of polycythemia vera is ascribable to the effects of the elevated red blood cell concentration on blood flow. The relationship between blood flow and erythrocyte concentration is complex and depends on cardiac output, blood vessel size, and the hematocrit. A relatively small hematocrit elevation above the normal range can cause blood flow in an organ to fall by one-third to one-half. Therefore, symptoms of polycythemia vera are often those of deficient cerebral blood flow, such as headaches, dizziness, and abnormalities of vision. Engorgement of skin blood vessels can cause a ruddy color, and, for reasons that are unclear, patients with polycythemia vera suffer from itching of the skin after a warm bath. Some patients with polycythemia vera have abnormally activated platelets that aggregate spontaneously or after minimal stimulation. This platelet hyperactivity, in some instances combined with elevated platelet counts, can contribute to vascular insufficiency by promoting coagulation in engorged capillaries with slow blood flow.

Both arterial and venous *thromboses*, particularly hepatic and portal vein thromboses, may occur. Paradoxically, the hyperactive platelets may not function properly in hemostasis, and a bleeding tendency can result as well. The increased cell turnover in polycythemia vera can lead to *hyperuricemia*.

DIAGNOSIS AND MANAGEMENT

First, erythrocytosis must be diagnosed by showing that the patient actually has an elevated red cell mass. An elevated hematocrit, the usual presenting finding, only suggests the presence of erythrocytosis; it does not establish it. The distinction between an elevated hematocrit and erythrocytosis is important; in fact, the combination of a modest elevation in the hematocrit and a normal red cell mass is common. Known as Gaisbock's syndrome or stress erythrocytosis, this combination is typically seen in hard-driving middle-aged men who tend to be smokers, overweight, and hypertensive. The red cell mass in these patients is generally on the high side of normal, whereas plasma volumes are in the low–normal range, leading to a high hematocrit without an increase in red cell mass. Stress erythrocytosis is important to diagnose, because patients with this condition may be at risk for heart attacks and other vascular occlusive disease.

The red cell mass can be measured by labeling a known quantity of the patient's red cells with ^{51}Cr, reinjecting them, and after sufficient time for complete mixing, determining by what factor the tagged cells were diluted by the patient's own circulating red cells.

The second task is to differentiate polycythemia vera from the various causes of secondary polycythemia (described in Ch. 12), which are physiological responses to tissue hypoxemia. These diseases can be diagnosed by measurements of arterial oxygen saturation or the hemoglobin oxygen dissociation curve. Certain clinical features are helpful in pointing to a diagnosis of polycythemia vera. Patients with polycythemia vera tend to be middle-aged or elderly men with elevations in the granulocyte and platelet counts as well as the hematocrit, absence of pulmonary disease, and moderate splenic enlargement. The serum uric acid level is often elevated in conditions of accelerated myelopoiesis. Uric acid is a breakdown product of purine metabolism. The bone marrow examination shows an excessive number of normal red cell precursors.

The goal in the treatment of polycythemia is to reduce the red cell mass. This reduction can be easily achieved in many patients by means of monthly phlebotomies. Unfortunately, bleeding promotes platelet production, and, when the abnormal platelets of polycythemia increase in number, the bleeding and thrombotic manifestations of the disease become more of a problem. Therefore, treatment is often directed at the abnormal stem cell. In the past, radioactive phosphorus, ^{32}P-phosphoric acid, was a widely used therapy. Injected into the circulation, ^{32}P incorporates into the DNA of the bone marrow stem cells. The β-radiation emitted by the radionuclide kills some of these cells. The treatment is sufficient to reduce the proliferation of polycythemia vera bone marrow for prolonged periods of time. The relative permanence of the treatment and the control of platelet production are offset by the carcinogenic risk of ionizing radiation. Carcinogenesis as well as pulmonary and gonadal fibrosis also complicate the administration of alkylating agents, such as busulfan, formerly given to suppress the proliferation of the bone marrow. The treatment of choice today for control of polycythemia is hydroxyurea, a suppressive agent with much lower transforming potential, and polycythemia vera can be managed successfully with hydroxyurea for long periods of time. The disease may evolve slowly over a period of years into acute myelogenous leukemia. Alternatively, it may enter a "burntout" phase wherein the bone marrow proliferation returns to normal. Thereafter, the bone marrow may even begin to develop fibrosis, and pancytopenia may ensue. Until hydroxyurea has lowered the blood counts, an orally administered agent, anagrelide, can prevent thrombotic complications associated with polycythemia and other myeloproliferative disorders, and hyperuricemia is responsive to the purine synthesis inhibitor allopurinol.

Idiopathic Myelofibrosis

Although focal fibrosis of the bone marrow can be an accompaniment of inflammatory disease and of metastatic cancer, a distinct disease entity is idiopathic myelofibrosis. In this disorder, a progressive fibrosis of the bone marrow is accompanied to a variable degree by evidence of increased proliferation of granulocytes and by the development of myeloid metaplasia, that is, foci of hematopoiesis in the liver and spleen. This extramedullary hematopoiesis differs from the extraosseous blood cell development associated with severe hemolytic anemias, in which the bone marrow expands by direct extension into neighboring tissues. In idiopathic myelofibrosis with myeloid metaplasia, the bone marrow develops in the organs of hematopoiesis of fetal life: the liver and spleen. It is not known why myeloid metaplasia occurs in response to idiopathic myelofibrosis and why it is unusual in other diseases that infiltrate the bone marrow, such as lymphomas and solid tumors. Idiopathic myelofibrosis is sometimes the sequel of long-standing polycythemia vera.

Studies of G6PD isoenzymes in idiopathic myelofibrosis have indicated that the granulocyte proliferation reflects the expansion of a single clone of stem cells, whereas the fibroblasts populating the bone marrow are not of a single clonal origin. From this work it is concluded that the bone marrow fibrosis represents a reaction to some stimulus elaborated by the clonal disorder. To some extent, the accumulation of granulocytes in the blood is itself a reaction to the fibrosis. The peripheral blood picture is usually initially that of a leukoerythroblastic reaction with immature granulocytes and erythrocytes in the peripheral blood. The erythrocyte morphology is abnormal, featuring misshapen red cells, especially teardrop forms.

The cause of idiopathic myelofibrosis is unknown. The clonality of the disorder implies an acquired genetic disease resembling cancer or leukemia. In addition, chromosomal abnormalities are frequent in idiopathic myelofibrosis, particularly deletions of the long arm of chromosome 13 (13q⁻) and t[1;13] translocations. One hypothesis relates the frequent presence of morphologically abnormal and dysfunctional platelets in idiopathic myelofibrosis (Ch. 14) to the fibrotic process. Platelets contain a growth factor called platelet-derived growth factor (PDGF), which is mitogenic for a variety of cells including fibroblasts. Interestingly, one of the two polypeptides comprising PDGF is highly homologous to an oncogene product of the acute transforming primate retrovirus, the simian sarcoma virus *c-sis*. It is proposed that elaboration of PDGF or PDGF-related peptides by the aberrant megakaryocytes in idiopathic myelofibrosis stimulates fibroblastic proliferation, resulting in a net increase in collagen deposition in the bone marrow. In support of the idea that aberrau cytokines can cause cell proliferations leading to disease, it has recently been shown that elaboration of a soluble focus of mast cell growth factor (*c-kit* ligand) leads to hyperpigmentation and cutaneous proliferation of mast cells.

The clinical manifestations of idiopathic myelofibrosis are initially the effects of splenomegaly, which can become massive. The enlarged spleen can impair digestion and appetite by compressing the stomach and can create an unpleasant feeling of heaviness in the left upper quadrant. The enlarged spleen can also sequester and destroy peripheral blood cells. The enlarged spleen may become infarcted, resulting in acute left upper quadrant pain radiating into the left shoulder. A friction rub may be audible in the left upper quadrant when the patient respires in such cases. The spleen can even rupture after minimum trauma in this area, causing an acute abdomen and possible death from hemorrhage.

Later in the course of idiopathic myelofibrosis, bone marrow failure and pancytopenia become dominant, as the myeloid metaplasia cannot compensate for the loss of bone marrow function incurred by the myelofibrosis. The liver may fail from compromised parenchymal function caused by progressive myeloid metaplasia within the organ. The patient eventually dies of liver failure, hemorrhage, or infection. The usual treatment for idiopathic myelofibrosis is palliative, involving support for the progressive pancytopenia, packed erythrocyte transfusions for the anemia, and platelet infusions for thrombocytopenia. Splenectomy can alleviate the symptoms of massive splenomegaly and occasionally lead to an improvement in peripheral blood counts when splenic sequestration of cells dominates splenic hematopoiesis.

The rate of progression of idiopathic myelofibrosis is variable. In some cases the course may be relatively slow and stable. Patients who present without large spleens, severe anemia, or thrombocytopenia may have a median survival of 10 years. Others with these findings, however, may succumb within a year or two.

Intensive cytotoxic treatment followed by allogeneic bone marrow transplantation (Ch. 32) has led to the cure of a few patients with idiopathic myelofibrosis. This outcome is not only of importance for the patients eligible for such therapy but also because it demonstrates that the primary disorder resides in the hematopoietic stem cell, not the fibrous stroma that proliferates. Also remarkable is the fact that the normal transplanted hematopoietic cells engrafted in the fibrotic bone marrow space and that the fibrosis resolved following transplantation.

Essential Thrombocythemia

There is no definitive diagnostic marker for this disease, which is established by exclusion from other causes of elevated platelet counts. Patients may be recognized by incidental platelet counts or else by symptoms of either bleeding or thrombosis. Bleeding occurs at mucosal surfaces and on the skin, and thrombosis may be either arterial or venous. An unusual manifestation of this disease is *erythromelalgia*, characterized by pain and burning of the toes, palms, or soles. Aspirin therapy, which evidently inhibits abnormal platelet aggregation in small vessels, provides relief. The newer antiplatelet agent anagrelide may also be effective. Essential thrombocythemia does not usually evolve into other myeloproliferative states or to leukemia and is compatible with a normal life expectancy, provided that hemorrhagic and thrombotic complications are appropriately managed. Hydroxyurea provides effective therapy, administered at a dosage that would keep the platelet count less than 500,000/μl.

Chronic Myelogenous Leukemia

Chronic myelogenous leukemia, also called chronic granulocytic leukemia, is a disease characterized by a proliferation of a malignant clone of pluripotent stem cells usually expressed as an exuberant production of cells in the granulocyte lineage, especially neutrophils and basophils. This aspect of chronic myelogenous leukemia, called the *chronic phase,* may persist, causing relatively little morbidity to many patients for a variable duration averaging 2 to 3 years. After this time, the malignant nature of the process becomes more striking. The proliferating cells become predominantly immature blasts that manifest the malignant propensity to invade organs, and the disease comes to behave like an acute leukemia. The acute leukemic phase of chronic myelogenous leukemia is designated chronic granulocytic leukemia in blastic crisis. The incidence of chronic myelogenous leukemia is highest in middle-aged persons, and affects males more than females, but it may occur in childhood.

In the chronic phase of chronic myelogenous leukemia, the peripheral blood contains granulocytes, predominantly neutrophilic, usually 15,000/μl and often up to 100,000/μl; the granulocytes are at all stages of maturation. The increased granulocyte mass is also evident in the bone marrow and spleen, and the latter can often be massively enlarged. The crowding effect of the proliferative process in the bone marrow can produce a leukoerythroblastic picture such that misshapen erythrocytes and teardrop forms appear in the peripheral blood. Chronic granulocytic leukemia in the chronic phase is easily distinguished from other myeloproliferative disorders and leukemoid reactions, which may also express leukoerythroblastic pictures in the peripheral blood, as well as splenomegaly by the presence of two phenomena unique to chronic myelogenous leukemia.

The first is a chromosomal aberration wherein a translocation of genetic material takes place between the long arms of the 22nd and 9th chromosomes t(9;22)(q34;q11). This translocation is most evident from the short-legged appearance of chromosome 22 in karyotypic analyses (Fig. 22-3). This chromosome is called the *Philadelphia chromosome* (abbreviated Ph) after the city in which it was first observed. The presence of the Philadelphia chromosome is not only diagnostic of chronic myelogenous leukemia, but has also provided the evidence, in addition to G6PD isoenzyme typing of erythrocytes and leukocytes, for the clonal origin of chronic myelogenous leukemia. Furthermore, the abnormal chromosome can be found in dividing cells of lymphocytic as well as granulocytic lineage, indicating that chronic myelogenous leukemia is a disorder of the pluripotent stem cell.

The second feature of chronic myelogenous leukemia, which is only slightly less specific for the disease than the Philadelphia chromosome, is a low level of activity of the enzyme *alkaline phosphatase* in the mature-appearing polymorphonuclear leukocytes. Only occasionally is a low alkaline phosphatase score found in other disorders, including some cases of the myeloproliferative diseases and paroxysmal nocturnal hemoglobinuria.

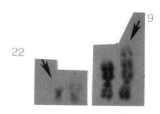

Fig. 22-3. Balanced t[9;22] translocation: origin of the Philadelphia chromosome.

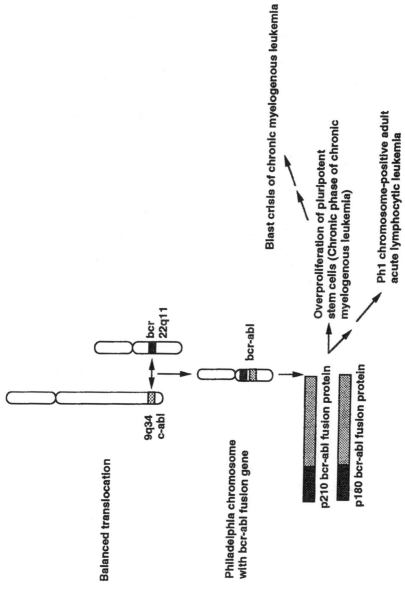

Balanced translocation

9q34
c-abl

bcr
22q11

**Philadelphia chromosome
with bcr-abl fusion gene**

bcr-abl

p210 bcr-abl fusion protein

p180 bcr-abl fusion protein

Overproliferation of pluripotent
stem cells (Chronic phase of chronic
myelogenous leukemia)

Blast crisis of chronic myelogenous leukemia

Ph1 chromosome-positive adult
acute lymphocytic leukemia

Fig. 22-4. Schematic rendition of the t[9;22] translocation and the pathogenesis of chronic myelogenous leukemia and other Philadelphia chromosome syndromes.

MOLECULAR PATHOGENESIS

Chronic myelogenous leukemia was the first example of a consistent genetic abnormality associated with neoplastic disease. The key event in the balanced translocation between chromosomes 9 and 22 is the placement of an oncogene, usually on chromosome 9 to chromosome 22. The oncogene is *c-abl*, which is related to the transforming gene *v-abl* of the Abelson virus, a retrovirus that produces a lymphoid neoplasm in mice. The *abl* oncogene is a representative of the class described in Chapter 21 that has tyrosine kinase activity believed to be involved in the stimulation of cell division. The region on chromosome 22 where *c-abl* lands is called the *bcr cluster gene*. What then happens is that a fusion product of the 5′ portion of *bcr* and the 3′ portion of *c-abl* is produced constitutively that has tyrosine kinase activity greater than that of the normal *c-abl* gene product (Fig. 22-4). The situation is more complex, however, in that the protein transcribed by *bcr* is a guanosine triphosphate (GTP)ase related to the *ras* family of transforming oncogenes. The translocation between chromosomes 9 and 22, moreover, is under some form of control, as evidenced by the phenomenon of *genomic imprinting*, wherein there is a parent-determined bias in the origin of the chromosomal fragment. In most cases examined, the origin of the chromosome 9 fragment is paternal and that of chromosome 22 is maternal.

In a minority (~5 percent) of patients with chronic myelogenous leukemia, the stem cells have more complex translocations involving at least three chromosomes, two being chromosomes 9 and 22. The clinical course of disease of patients with these complex translocations does not differ from the usual type of chronic myelogenous leukemia. On the other hand, *abl* is not the whole story in the neoplastic behavior of chronic granulocytic leukemia. The *bcr/abl* fusion gene product does not by itself transform fibroblasts in transfection assays, and mutant oncogenes, which include *myc*, *p53,* and *ras*, can be expressed in chronic gran-ulocytic leukemia cells. Moreover, once chronic myelogenous leukemia goes into blast crisis, the *bcr/abl* gene may be deleted without alteration in the progress of the disease.

CLINICAL FEATURES

The initial effects of chronic myelogenous leukemia on the patient are manifestations of the enlarged granulocyte mass. The enlarged spleen may cause a feeling of discomfort in the left upper quadrant or even impair the patient's appetite and digestion by compressing the stomach. When the granulocytic proliferation becomes extensive, the patient begins to suffer from loss of appetite and weight loss. Anemia and thrombocytopenia have been ascribed to "crowding" of the bone marrow by the granulocytic proliferation, although another possibility is that as the disease evolves, differentiation failure of the erythroid and megakaryocytic lineages occurs. Occasionally, a plethora of granulocytes in the peripheral blood can cause obstruction of the blood circulation with signs and symptoms of cerebral hypoxia or organ infarction. Nevertheless, in many patients with chronic myelogenous leukemia in the chronic phase, the disease may present relatively few problems.

The onset of blast crisis is heralded by progressive immaturity of the peripheral blood granulocytes, by increases in the basophil count in the peripheral blood, and by the appearance of chromosomal abnormalities in addition to the Philadelphia chromosome. Treatment of the chronic phase does not influence the time of onset of blast crisis in chronic myelogenous leukemia.

The blasts in blast crisis chronic myelogenous leukemia may resemble myeloblasts or lymphoblasts, a variability reflecting the pluripotent stem cell origin of the leukemic process. When the lymphoblastic morphology is evident, an event seen in one-third of cases, the blasts contain the thymocyte enzyme, terminal deoxyribonucleotide transferase (Ch. 19), also a marker of lymphoblasts in acute lymphoblastic leukemia (Ch. 25) and also may express clonal immunoglobulin gene rearrangements characteristic of B-cell maturation.

TREATMENT

The goal of therapy of the chronic phase of chronic myelogenous leukemia is to keep the granulocyte count from rising above 25,000/µl, an end relatively easily accomplished by small doses of alkylating agents or with hydroxyurea (Ch. 21). Following these treatments, the white blood cell count falls, the hematocrit may rise, and the spleen may decrease in size. A recent addition to the therapeutic armamentarium has been the recombinant lymphokines, α and γ-interferon. Although the responses to these agents are less reliable than those to chemotherapeutic agents, they are potentially less toxic. Either low-dose alkylating agents or α-interferon represent suppressive and not curative treatment. The Philadelphia chromosome persists in the setting of normal blood counts, indicating the lingering specter of the malignant clone.

Stable-phase chronic myelogenous leukemia invariably progresses to the blast phase, and the blasts have proved extremely resistant to chemotherapy. Vincristine and prednisone, drugs useful in the treatment of acute lymphoblastic leukemia, can yield responses when the blastic phase of chronic myelogenous leukemia is lymphoid in appearance and markers, but the responses are transient. To avoid an inevitably fatal outcome, therefore, it is necessary to replace the malignant stem cell with allogenic bone marrow transplantation. This approach is theoretically the treatment of choice for patients with suitable marrow donors (Ch. 32). About 50 percent of patients thus transplanted have had prolonged leukemia-free survival. Preferably this approach would be taken long before the emergence of blasts resistant to cytotoxic agents used to ablate the host bone marrow before transplantation. Unfortunately, bone marrow transplantation is not uniformly successful and risk-free, and its failures and risks must be balanced against the median survival of relatively asymptomatic patients with chronic myelogenous leukemia.

These uncertainties have encouraged investigators to stratify patients in the chronic phase according to features that may predict the duration of this phase. In general, patients with relatively low white blood counts, low percentages of blasts, small spleens, lack of anemia and thrombocytopenia, and relatively few chromosomal abnormalities can expect longer survival. Researchers are determining whether it is possible to prolong the chronic phase of chronic myelogenous leukemia in patients not eligible for bone marrow transplantation by administration of combinations of chemotherapeutic agents with or without autologous bone marrow transplantation. To reduce the number of Philadelphia chromosome-expressing chronic myelogenous leukemia blasts coexisting with normal stem cells in the patient's bone marrow, investigators are studying the effects of treating the bone marrow with drugs that might kill the malignant blast cells such as α-interferon prior to infusing the marrow back into the patient.

OTHER STEM CELL DISORDERS

Paroxysmal Nocturnal Hemoglobinuria

Paroxysmal nocturnal hemoglobinuria is an acquired clonal disorder of the pluripotent stem cell. The disease has a variety of clinical manifestations. The abnormal pluripotent stem cell clone coexists to a variable degree with the normal stem cells and yields progeny having altered surface membranes. These alterations in membrane structures on the external surfaces of erythrocytes, phagocytes, and platelets cause the membranes under certain circumstances to appear foreign to the components of the alternative pathway of complement activation (Ch. 17). The sequential attachment of alternative complement pathway proteins, C3, followed by the late-acting complement components to the membrane of the erythrocyte leads to its lysis.

Although the fundamental defect in the paroxysmal nocturnal hemoglobinuria cell membrane is unknown, it has recently become evident that a number of phenomena related to these cells can be explained by a common abnormality, the failure to synthesize or retain a class of membrane proteins normally bound to the lipid bilayer by a phosphatidylinositolpeptidoglycan (PIG) linkage. One such protein is the enzyme acetylcholinesterase, long known to be deficient on paroxysmal nocturnal hemoglobinuria cells. Others are surface receptors including the class III Fcγ receptor that is normally present on polymorphonuclear leukocytes and macrophages (but not monocytes) (Ch. 18) and the lymphocyte adhesion molecule LFA-I. More pertinent to the functional abnormalities of the disorder is the fact that *decay-accelerating factor (DAF)*, an entity that inhibits the propagation of complement action by participating in the inactivation of C3 on the cell surface, *C8-binding protein*, and *CD59*, which block the membrane attack complex (C5 to C9) are three such sugar-lipid-linked proteins. Their deficiency on paroxysmal nocturnal hemoglobinuria cells can explain at least in part the complement sensitivity of those cells.

The significance of the hemolysis in a given patient depends on the size of the abnormal stem cell clone and on the circumstances alluded to above. If the abnormal clone is small, a small number of complement-sensitive erythrocytes may turn over rapidly; the only clinical evidence of the disease will be a small increase in the reticulocyte count and possibly evidence of hemosiderin in the urine. At the other extreme, the patient may have massive intravascular hemolysis, and chronic brisk hemolysis can lead to iron deficiency from iron loss as hemosiderin into the urine.

In the test tube, the binding of complement components to erythrocytes is promoted by increasing the hydrogen ion concentration or by decreasing the ionic strength of the medium. The latter is accomplished by diluting the blood with a sucrose solution adjusted for a physiological osmotic strength. Paroxysmal nocturnal hemoglobinuria, but not normal erythrocytes, binds complement components in this medium of low ionic strength; after centrifugation of the erythrocytes, the supernatant fluid over the normal erythrocytes is colorless, whereas that over the paroxysmal nocturnal hemobglobinuria cells is red. This procedure is the *sucrose hemolysis* test (or sugar water test), which is used to diagnose paroxysmal nocturnal hemoglobinuria.

The factors that determine the degree of complement fixation and hemolysis in the patient with paroxysmal nocturnal hemoglobinuria are unclear. The nocturnal exacerbation of hemolysis sometimes observed in which hemoglobulin appears in the urine at night—hence the name of the disease—has been ascribed to lowering of the blood pH by alveolar hypoventilation during sleep. Whether true or not, hemolysis in paroxysmal nocturnal hemoglobinuria can be quite variable in severity and can occur at any time.

Another clinical problem of paroxysmal nocturnal hemoglobinuria is arterial and venous thrombosis and the attendant infarction of organs, the circulation of which becomes compromised. Paroxysmal nocturnal hemoglobinuria is one cause of a hypercoagulable state possibly because platelets and granulocytes fix complement and aggregate. Platelets and granulocytes are more resistant to complement-mediated lysis than are erythrocytes, hence neutropenia and thrombocytopenia in paroxysmal nocturnal hemoglobinuria cannot be ascribed to direct complement-mediated destruction. However, the membrane perturbations inflicted by complement deposition on these cells render them "sticky," leading to their inappropriate aggregation in the vasculature.

Because hypoplasia of the bone marrow and pancytopenia are manifestations of paroxysmal nocturnal hemoglobinuria, this disease is one cause of the clinical spectrum of aplastic anemia. Although paroxysmal nocturnal hemoglobinuria is a rare disease, a sufficient number of cases have evolved after variable periods of time into acute myelogenous or myelomonocytic leukemia to merit consideration of paroxysmal nocturnal hemoglobinuria as yet another clonal preneoplastic disorder.

The treatment of paroxysmal nocturnal hemoglobinuria in its hemolytic phase is the same as that of any chronic hemolytic anemia of comparable severity. The treatment of paroxysmal nocturnal hemoglobinuria-associated bone marrow hypoplasia is similar to that of bone marrow failures in general. Because children and adolescents with paroxysmal nocturnal hemoglobinuria are more likely than adults to develop bone marrow failure, they should be considered as candidates for bone marrow transplantation (Ch. 32).

Cyclic Neutropenia

Cyclic neutropenia is a genetically inherited disease in which the activity of the pluripotent stem cell oscillates with a regular periodicity to create cyclic hematopoiesis. The principal expression of this intermittent hematopoiesis is a cyclic fluctuation in the peripheral blood neutrophil and monocyte counts, although subtle variations in reticulocyte, erythrocyte, and platelet counts can be detected. The reciprocal variations between neutrophil and monocyte counts reflect the shorter bone marrow maturation time of the monocyte compared with that of the neutrophil. The reason for the waxing and waning of the stem cell differentiation is unknown. Patients with cyclic neutropenia may become symptomatic when the granulocyte count is at its nadir. Such patients develop mouth ulcers and fevers at this time and, rarely, life-threatening infections. Cyclic neutropenia also exists in a strain of gray collie dogs. The disease can be cured by bone marrow transplantation from normal dogs, indicating that the disease process resides in the stem cell.

Congenital Neutropenia

Neutropenia in the newborn can arise from severe infection, from the presence of maternal isoantibodies against neutrophils, or as a genetically inherited trait. Inherited neutropenia, a rare condition, may be transmitted as a dominant recessive trait and when severe is sometimes designated Kestmann Syndrome. The manifestations of inherited neutropenia are variable. For example, in some families affected members show depressed monocyte, lymphocyte, and neutrophil counts, whereas in other families affected members show elevated monocyte, lymphocyte, or eosinophil counts. The tendency of the affected person to acquire bacterial infections is inversely related to the average neutrophil count (Ch. 18). Kestmann syndrome responds to therapy with G-CSF. For patients who manage to survive beyond early childhood with congenital neutropenia, the infection rate may decrease as other defenses become better developed. It is likely that many cases of congenital neutropenia are the result of an inborn defect in the stem cell. However, an interesting observation is that bone marrow from some of these neutropenic patients yields many mature neutrophils in tissue culture, suggesting some environmental insults in the patient's bone marrow.

SUGGESTED READINGS

Baumeleu E, Guiguel m, Macy JY et al (1993) Epidemiology of aplastic anemia in France: a case control study. Blood 81:1471

Bennett JM, Catovsky D, Daniel MT et al (1982) Proposals for the classification of the myelodysplastic syndromes. Br J Haematol 51:189

Berk PD (1986) Therapeutic recommendations in polycythemia vera based on Polycythemia Vera Study Group protocols. Semin Hematol 23:132

Besa EC et al (1990) Treatment of 13-cis retinoic acid in transfusion-dependent patients with myelodysplastic syndrome and decreased toxicity with addition of alpha tocopherol. Am J Med 89:739

Cheson BD (1990) The myelodysplastic syndromes: current approaches to therapy. Ann Intern Med 112:932

Dunbar CE, Stewart FM (1992) Separating the wheat from the chaff: selection of benign hematopoietic cells in chronic myeloid leukemia. Blood 79:1107

Gillie AP, Gabrilove JL (1993) Cytokine treatment of inherited bone marrow failure syndromes. Blood 81:1669

Holguin MH, Wilcox LA, Bernshaw NJ et al (1989) Relationship between the membrane inhibitor of reactive lysis and the erythrocyte phenotypes of paroxysmal nocturnal hemoglobinuria. J Clin Invest 84:1387

Jocié G, Hency-Amap M, Bacipalupo A et al (1993) Malignant tumors occurring after treatment of aplastic anemia. N Engl J Med 329:1152

Kantarjian HM, Deisscoth A, Kurzrock R et al (1993) Chronic myelogenous leukemia: a concise update. Blood 82:691

Longley BJ, Morgauoth GS, Tyrell L et al (1993) Altered metabolism of mast-cell growth factor (*c-kit* ligand) in cutaneous mastocytosis. N Engl J Med 328:1382

Low MG, Ferguson MAJ, Futerman AH, Silman I (1986) Covalently attached phosphatidylinositol as a hydrophobic anchor for membrane proteins. Trends Biochem Sci 11:212

Marmont AM (1991) Autoimmune myelopathies. Semin Hematol 28:275

Mitus AJ, Barbui T, Shulman LN et al (1990) Hemostatic complications in young patients with essential thrombocythemia. Am J Med 88:371

Ohnor, Naoe T, Hirano M et al (1993) Treatment of myelodysplastic syndromes with all-*trans* cetinoic acid. Blood 81:1152

Reik W (1992) Imprinting in leukaemia. Nature 359:362

Strathdee CA, Gavish H, Shannon WR, Buchwald M (1992) Cloning of cDNAs for Fanconi's anaemia by functional complementation. Nature 356:763

Thomas ED, Clift R (1989) Indications for marrow transplantation in chronic myelogeous leukemia. Blood 73:861

Tichelli A, Gratwohl A, Wursch A et al (1988) Late haematologic complications in severe aplastic anaemia. Br J Haematol 69:413

Ward HP, Block MH (1971) The natural history of agnogenic myeloid metaplasia (AMM) and a critical evaluation of its relationship with the myeloproliferative syndrome. Medicine 50:357

Young NS, Alter BP (1993) Aplastic Anemia in Adults and Children. WB Saunders, Philadelphia

Young N, Harrison M, Moore J, Mortimer P, Humphries RK (1984) Direct demonstration of the human parvovirus in erythroid progenitor cells infected in vitro. J Clin Invest 74:2024

23

Acute Myelogenous Leukemias

The acute myelogenous leukemias, synonyms for which are acute *granulocytic* or acute *nonlymphocytic* leukemias, represent part of the spectrum of neoplasms affecting "myeloid" cell precursors discussed in the previous chapter. The specific names of the disorders depend on the predominant neoplastic cell type, usually determined by its appearance (Fig. 23-1). Most of the acute myelogenous neoplasms are first diagnosed when extensive infiltration of the bone marrow with leukemic cells has occurred, and they tend to be rapidly fatal when untreated. Therefore, these disorders came to be called the *acute* leukemias, in contrast to chronic myelogenous leukemia (see previous chapter) and chronic lymphatic leukemia (Ch. 26) in times when no effective therapy was available for the diseases.

CAUSES OF AND PREDISPOSITION TO ACUTE MYELOGENOUS LEUKEMIA

As described in Chapter 21, various forms of injury to immature, dividing bone marrow precursors predispose to the development of neoplasia by causing mutations in the *genetic makeup of the dividing cells*. The kinds of injury include those known to produce alterations in genes, such as ionizing radiation, exposure to organic solvents, and alkylating chemicals used in cancer chemotherapy. Variations, which may also be genetically determined, in the underlying susceptibilty of hematopoietic precursors to somatic damage affect the likelihood of whether these injuries lead to neoplastic transformation. An important consequence of this tranformation is acquisition of autonomous growth released from the usual regulation imposed by cytokines.

It is important to put these risks in perspective. One factor is the intensity of exposure to injurious agents. Although the degree of exposure imposed by ionizing radiation and chemotherapy during treatment of malignant tumors is sufficient to increase the risk of subsequent leukemia, the risk is relatively small and usually justified, if the treatment significantly improves immediate survival such as in Hodgkin's disease (Ch. 27). The normal cell has a capacity to resist and repair genetic damage; this accounts for why this kind of injury does not invariably lead to neoplasia. However, in some genetic conditions, the resistance to such injury may be reduced, predisposing to a higher-than-normal incidence of acute leukemia.

In two rare autosomal recessive diseases—Bloom syndrome and Fanconi's anemia—bone marrow failure occurs early in life (Ch. 22), and the affected patients have a high probabili-

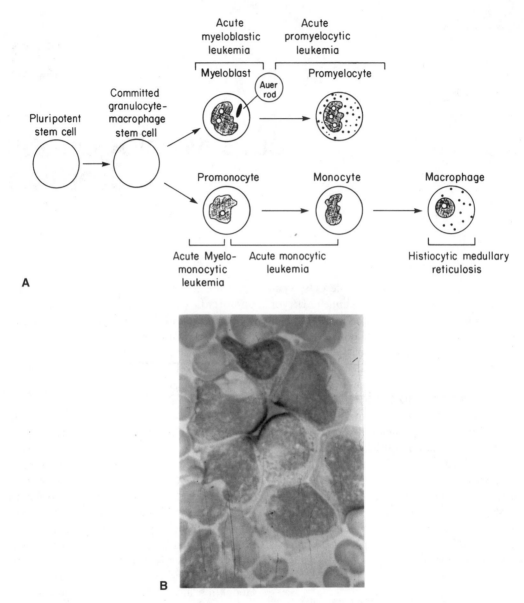

Fig. 23-1. (**A**) Developmental origin of acute (nonlymphocytic) leukemias of the phagocyte lineage. (**B**) Leukemic myeloblasts, two of which contain Auer rods.

ty of developing acute leukemia. The incidence of acute leukemia is also elevated in trisomy 21, also known as Down syndrome, a common congenital disorder caused by abnormalities in the separation of chromosomes after fertilization of the ovum. All cells of affected persons have an extra chromosome number 21, which is somehow associated with mental retardation. The connection between the genetic disorder and the predisposition to the development of acute leukemia (which can be lymphocytic as well as myelogenous) is not understood, but presents another association between a known genetic abnormality and the leukemic process. A small number of patients who develop certain types of myelogenous leukemias described below also are afflicted with nonseminomatous germ cell tumors, suggesting that fundamental genetic abnormalities in early embryonal cells predispose the patient to hematological malignancies. Finally, in acute myelogenous leukemias, the neoplastic cells have aberrations in their chromosomal architecture, another finding indicative of genetic damage.

Although viruses can cause granulocytic leukemias in animals and are implicated in the causation of at least one lymphoid neoplasm in humans, there is no evidence that viruses produce acute granulocytic leukemia in humans.

CLASSIFICATION OF THE ACUTE MYELOGENOUS LEUKEMIAS

As fine a classification as is possible is important with diseases in general and in neoplastic diseases in particular. The better the classification of the disease, the more accurately can physicians evaluate the prognosis and response to therapy. An indolent disorder, for example, might appear to be more responsive to treatment than an aggressive one, whereas the differential responses reside in the intrinsic nature of the two diseases rather than the effectiveness of the therapy.

The hallmark of acute myelogenous leukemia is a relatively monotonous infiltration of the bone marrow and sometimes the blood with a population comprising at least 30 percent immature phagocytes. The appearance of the predominant cell type on Wright-stained smears was for many years the basis of the classification of the acute leukemia. A predominance of myeloblasts defined acute myeloblastic leukemia; promyelocytes, acute promyelocytic leukemia; and monocytes, acute monocytic leukemia, respectively. Although in comparison with the heterogeneity of normal bone marrow, the morphology of leukemic cells is relatively uniform, often the appearance of the leukemic cells is bizarre and variable, reflecting abnormal differentiation. The cells may have features of both myeloblasts and monocytes, defining the entity *myelomonocytic*

leukemia. Even in what was called acute myelogenous leukemia, myeloblasts may vary in size and shape, may demonstrate partial differentiation to form strange promyelocytes, or may look like monocytes or macrophages. The peculiarities in the morphology of differentiation are defined as myelodysplastic changes and consist of oddities in nuclear morphology, including large size and marked variation in the aggregation state of the chromatin and alterations in the size and shape of cytoplasmic granules. One may occasionally see large basophilic and eosinophilic granules in the same cell, a highly unusual occurrence in normal granulocytopoiesis. In one particular configuration, granules form elongated needles called Auer rods (see Fig. 23-1). Because these granules are all azurophilic, they contain the enzyme peroxidase. Therefore, the peroxidase stain will sometimes help detect granules in leukemic cells, where they are sparse, identifying such cells as being of the granulocytic lineage. Occasionally, no granules can be discerned at all, and the cells do not resemble either lymphoid or phagocyte origin by morphological criteria. The disease in this case was called acute undifferentiated leukemia and may be a neoplasm derived from stem cells.

The variability in morphology of leukemic cell populations meant that earlier efforts at classification were fairly crude. One important event in the classification of acute nonlymphocytic leukemias was the coming together of experts in the 1970s to achieve a consensus relating the morphology and clinical behavior of the leukemias with the markers available at the time, for the most part histochemical enzyme reactions. This classification was called the *French-American-British* or *FAB classification* and divided the acute granulocytic leukemias into six classes, M1 through M6 (Table 23-1). Classes M1 through M3 represent leukemias in which cells of the neutrophilic lineage with different degrees of maturation prevail and in which the enzyme myeloperoxidase can be detected. M4 and M5 have monocytic cells of differing maturity that express a nonspecific esterase. M6 is a leukemia with

Table 23-1. Classification of Acute Nonlymphocytic Leukemias

FAB Designation	Characteristics
M1	Myeloblastic (immature neutrophilic) lineage detected by > 3% blasts with azurophilic granules, Auer rods, or staining with peroxidase histochemical reaction; no further maturation noted; surface antigens reactive with neutrophil-specific lineage markers may be present
M2	> 50% of bone marrow cells are myeloblasts or promyelocytes; neutrophil-lineage-specific surface antigens present
M3	Most cells are promyelocytes with many azurophilic granules and/or aggregated Auer rods; neutrophil-lineage-specific surface antigens present
M4	> 20% of marrow cells are myeloblasts or promyelocytes in addition to which > 20% are promonocytes and monocytes; both monocyte- and neutrophil-lineage-specific markers present
M5	> 90% of the phagocyte lineage cells are monocytes of variable maturity; monocyte-lineage-specific surface markers present
M6	Hallmarks of acute nonlymphocytic leukemia (myeloblasts and promyelocytes with or without Auer rods) plus easily detectable numbers of bizarre erythroid precursors
M7	Pleomorphic blasts with markers for platelet peroxidase, platelet glycoproteins, and factor-8-related antigen; frequent fibrosis of the bone marrow

immature cells with erythroid features, and its incidence is associated with patients who have received therapy with alkylating agents (Ch. 21). The discrimination of granulocytic leukemias from lymphocytic leukemias was markedly improved by the introduction of monoclonal antibodies (Ch. 19) reactive against surface antigens such as CD14, CD13, and CD33 of phagocytes. M0 and M7 classes have been added to the original FAB list. In M0 leukemia the malignant cells have surface antigens characteristic of phagocytes but completely lack myeloperoxidase-containing granules or staining for sudan black B. M7 leukemia expresses markers associated with megakaryocytes and platelets and is therefore called *acute megakaryoblastic leukemia.*

Further evidence in support of the importance of genetic alterations in leukemia has come from leukemic cell chromosomal analysis (or karyotypes). Clonal chromosomal defects are detected by cultivating cells in the presence of a DNA synthesis inhibitor that synchronizes the cells so as to permit analysis of a large number of metaphases. The fine structure of the chromosomes is then visualized by means of fluorescent dyes that bring out a band pattern in the chromosomal arms. These high-resolution techniques have shown that a majority of phagocytic cell lineage leukemias demonstrate chromosomal abnormalities. This information has provided further evidence for

the clonality of acute granulocytic leukemias and has also defined additional syndromes of acute granulocytic leukemia that are characterized by distinct chromosomal abnormalities.

A variant of M4 leukemia, for example, is the finding of an admixture of myelomonocytic blasts and eosinophils. Distinctive for this variant is a cytogenetic abnormality consisting of inversion, translocation, or sometimes deletion of the long arm of chromosome number 16. The most common aberration is an inversion between the short and long arms, designated [inv(16)(pl3;q22)] where p and q indicate the short and long arms, respectively, and the numbers the specific bands involved. This disorder accounts for about 5 percent of acute granulocytic leukemias and may be somewhat more responsive to therapy than the other types. Another syndrome with a characteristic chromosomal aberration is an M2 variant with frequent Auer rods in which mature neutrophils may express the Pelger-Hüet anomaly (see Fig. 18-4). The cytogenetic finding is a translocation from the long arm of chromosome 21 to the long arm of chromosome 8 [t(8;21) (q22;q22)]. A monoblastic leukemic syndrome is associated with the translocation of a segment of chromosome 11 to the chromosome 9 [t(9;11) (p22;q23)]. Two oncogenes, *can* and *dec*, have been associated with breakpoints in t(6;9)(p23;q34) translocations respectively found in a small fraction of M2 cases. About

70 percent of acute myelogenous leukemias arising in persons previously exposed to chemotherapy or radiation (Ch. 19) demonstrate deletions of the long arm of chromosomes 5 or 7 (5q⁻) or (7q⁻). Finally, a rare variant in which elevated platelet counts are encountered expresses inversions or translocations on chromosome 3 [t(3;3)(q21;q26.2)] or [inv(3;3)(q21;q26.2)].

Promyelocytic (M3) leukemia is nearly always accompanied by a translocation between chromosome 15 and 17 [t(15;17)(q22;q21)], and the leukemic cells express a transcript of fusion-derived mRNA containing *RAR-α* and a region of chromosome 15 called *pml* or *myl*. This reciprocal t(15;17) translocation in acute promyelocytic leukemia is of particular interest. The *RAR-α* gene encodes a cellular receptor for retinoic acid, a chemical well known to induce differentiation of undifferentiated cells, and the sequence of the *pml* gene is consistent with a zinc finger type of DNA-binding transcription control factor (Ch. 19). The expression of this gene in fusion products with the *myl/pml* locus on chromosome 15 (*RAR/PML* or *PML/RAR*) accounts for the responsiveness of a high proportion of patients with acute promyelocytic leukemia to treatment with all-*trans* retinoic acid (Fig. 23-2). This therapy works by inducing differentiation of the malignant cells rather than killing them.

PATHOGENESIS OF ACUTE MYELOGENOUS LEUKEMIA

The most frequently detected oncogene abnormality in this disease is the presence of N-*ras* mutations, which have been detected in about a third of the cases examined thus far. A type of cell called HL-60, which resembles the promyelocyte, was originally isolated from a patient with acute leukemia. HL-60 cells grow in tissue culture and have, in addition to a N-

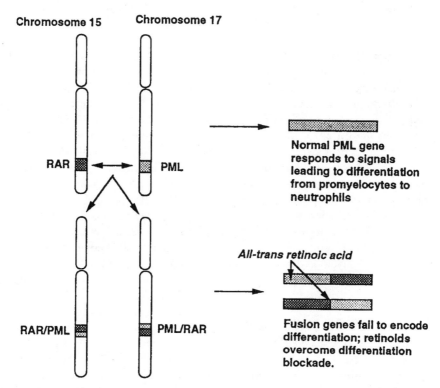

Fig. 23-2. The 15–17 chromosome translocation and retinoic acid-responsive acute promyelocytic (M3) leukemia.

ras mutation, marked hyperexpression of *c-myc*, a transforming oncogene (especially when combined with N-*ras* mutations) encoding a nuclear protein. The HL-60 cells can be induced to differentiate into mature neutrophils by a variety of agents. One of the first events accompanying differentiation and loss of the capacity to divide is a marked decrease in expression of the *c-myc* gene product. *p53* mutations (see Ch. 21) have also been detected in leukemic cells.

Oncogenes or possible oncogenes reside at or near points of chromosomal abnormalities in certain acute granulocytic leukemias. The oncogene *c-ets 1*, a homologue of an avian viral leukemia oncogene, resides on chromosome 22, which translocates to chromosome 9 in the M5 variant described above. The genes for hematopoietic growth factors granulocyte–macrophage colony-stimulating factor (GM-CSF) and M-CSF and also the receptors for M-CSF (which is also an oncogene *c-fms*) and for platelet-derived growth factor (PDGF) all reside on the long arm of chromosome 5 (5q), which is deleted (5q⁻) or otherwise abnormal in a number of acute granulocytic leukemias. A loss of differentiating factors or their receptors that drive phagocyte progenitors to mature and lose proliferative potential might predispose such cells to malignant transformation. Finally, the myeloperoxidase gene (Ch.18) is located on chromosome 17; this gene is transcriptionally activated early in neutrophil development. It is possible that this makes this region of the chromosome susceptible to mutation or else that myeloperoxidase promoter elements contribute to the expression of other factors contributing to the leukemic state. Furthermore, the myeloperoxidase gene is rearranged in the t(15;17) translocation.

CONSEQUENCES OF THE ACUTE MYELOGENOUS LEUKEMIAS

The major clinical problem engendered by acute leukemia is bone marrow failure. Indeed, the pathological definition of acute leukemia requires that more than 30 percent of the bone marrow nucleated cells be malignant "blasts." With further clonal expansion of the neoplastic cells, the normal marrow elements diminish in number, possibly because some leukemic cells release inhibitors of normal hematopoiesis or simply because of evolving faillure of differentiation. The consequences of bone marrow failure are anemia, hemorrhage, and infection because of diminution in the numbers of normal erythrocytes, platelets, and phagocytes, respectively.

Although "leukemia" means "white blood," implying the presence of large numbers of malignant leukocytes in the blood, this "leukemia" only occurs in a few cases of acute leukemias of phagocytes at the time of diagnosis. In most patients the total white blood cell count is initially decreased and the bone marrow is packed with leukemic cells. A "leukemia" with high peripheral blood white cell concentrations is more prevalent in leukemias with monocytic and myelomonocytic morphology (M4 and M5), but these are a few of the total cases encountered. The presence of large numbers of immature phagocytes in the blood does not invariably indicate a diagnosis of acute granulocytic leukemia, as reactions to stress or other processes irritating the bone marrow can cause a reactive phagocytic leukocytosis in the blood. In contrast to a *leukemoid reaction*, however, in which all stages of neutrophil maturation populate the blood, the leukemic disorders exhibit mature polymorphonuclear leukocytes and very immature cells with an absence of maturational stages in between. This phenomenon is called the *leukemic hiatus*. When the leukemic cell count in the blood becomes very high (greater than 100,000 cells/ml), a leukemic sludge can actually impair blood circulation, causing pulmonary insufficiency and neurological symptoms because of defective tissue oxygenation.

The neoplastic cells have a propensity to invade normal tissues. The most frequently ravaged organs are those that come into intimate contact with the circulation, such as the spleen, liver, bone, and lymph nodes; these organs are often enlarged and painful in the acute leukemias. Actually, no organ is immune to infiltration. The central nervous system and other sites can serve as sanctuaries when invaded where leukemic cells lie clinically inapparent for a time, relatively protected from antileukemic agents that do not readily cross the blood–brain barrier. Leukemic cells can cause organ dysfunction by diffuse infiltration of a given organ or can establish a solid tumor mass called a *chloroma*. The term chloroma arises from the greenish color these lesions sometimes have. The green hue is caused by the presence of the enzyme peroxidase in the malignant cells.

The metabolic effect of leukemic proliferation takes its toll on the organism in terms of inanition, presumably because the leukemic cell burden robs the host of nutrients and elaborates substances that derange metabolic regulatory mechanisms.

In addition to the general effects of leukemic proliferation, specific subtypes of acute granulocytic leukemias are associated with special clinical features. In acute promyelocytic leukemia (M3), the patient is invaded by a large burden of malignant cells bearing azurophilic granules. Apparently the contents of these granules leak into the circulation and nonspecifically activate the coagulation system, causing disseminated intravascular coagulation, which results in generalized bleeding (Ch. 15). The malignant cells in acute myelomonocyte and monocytic leukemia (M4 and M5) are uniquely invasive of body tissues. Patients with this disorder have considerable organ enlargement, including painful enlargement of the gums. Presumably the cells are capable of responding to chemotactic factors in the bacteria-rich milieu of the oral cavity. Another feature of acute monocytic leukemia is that the malignant cells release large quantities of the enzyme lysozyme.

Mature macrophages have a limited capacity to proliferate. It is therefore not surprising that neoplasms of this cell line are relatively rare. *Histiocytic medullary reticulosis* is a disorder in which macrophages appear to undergo a malignant transformation. Unlike most other forms of malignant transformation of phagocytes, the cells in histiocytic medullary

reticulosis are quite capable of phagocytosis. In some cases, this phagocytosis is uncontrolled, and the malignant macrophages engulf normal blood cells. Therefore, some of the anemia, thrombocytopenia, and neutropenia associated with this disease may be attributable to abnormal clearance of these cells by the malignant macrophages.

TREATMENT OF ACUTE MYELOGENOUS LEUKEMIA

Treatment for these disorders is designed to destroy, suppress, or induce differentiation of the malignant clone. This principle, first introduced here, is applicable to the systemic treatment of many other hematological malignancies (Ch. 21). Chemotherapeutic agents are used for this purpose, with the strategy of achieving some selective toxicity against the leukemic cells without destroying all the normal stem cells. That such selectivity is possible is evidenced by the fact that various combinations of drugs temporarily restore the bone marrow and blood of patients with acute leukemia to a normal state. This normalization by means of chemotherapy is called *induction of a complete remission.* Some of the drugs used and their mechanisms of action are described in Chapter 21. As discussed in that chapter, combinations of drugs are employed to kill many leukemic cells rapidly before resistance to the antileukemic agents can emerge.

Many drug regimens with complex dosing schedules are used in researching ever more effective approaches, but the mainstays of chemotherapy for this group of leukemias are the purine analogue cytosine arabinoside, and an anthracycline. A standard approach to treatment would be 100 mg/m^2/day of cytosine arabinoside for 7 days, during 3 of which daunorubicin, 45 mg/m^2 is also administered. During the early part of remission induction, allopurinol is administered to prevent uric acid toxicity resulting from purine accumulation following death of a large number of leukemic cells.

Initial efforts to induce complete remissions are successful in about two-thirds of all patients with acute myelogenous leukemia and close to 90 percent of young patients in good health who can tolerate intensive treatment. Patients over 60 years of age tolerate the treatment less well. Since the best quality of life is achieved by complete remission, however, standard induction therapy is now advocated even in elderly patients unless serious additional medical problems preclude this approach. In the patients who do not reach complete remission, either the leukemic cells do not disappear at all in response to the drugs or do not completely disappear. The latter situation is called a *partial remission.* Unfortunately, the induction of a complete remission in these diseases is usually preceded by a period in which the production of normal blood cells is totally suppressed. This temporary aplasia of the marrow results from the effect of the preexisting leukemia and of the chemotherapy on the bone marrow stem cells. For 2 to 3 weeks after completion of chemotherapy, the patient suffers from progressive anemia and profound thrombocytopenia and granulocytopenia and is subject to hemorrhage and infection. Therefore, during the period of bone marrow aplasia, the patient requires supportive care in the form of erythrocyte, platelet, and occasionally white blood cell transfusions and treatment of infections with appropriate antibiotics. Unfortunately, some patients otherwise destined to achieve a complete remission may die in this interval because of infection or hemorrhage. It is now possible to shorten this dangerous period of pancytopenia by administering the phagocyte growth factor G-CSF to stimulate recovery of the normal bone marrow as well as stem cells harvested from peripheral blood that serve as targets for the growth factors. There has been some concern that the enhancement of hematopoiesis with pharmacologic doses of cytokines might "exhaust" bone marrow stem cells, especially in the setting of cytotoxic chemotherapy, and research is under way to identify combinations of hematopoietic hormones and other therapies and their timing to avoid this theoretical complication if it

exists. What is particularly exciting about the ability of all-*trans* retinoic acid to induce differentiation of leukemic blast cells in acute promyelocytic leukemia is the fact that this approach avoids the side effects of cytotoxic chemotherapy, and it is hoped that future research might reveal similar strategies in other leukemias. Unfortunately, leukemia can become resistant to retinoic acid therapy as to other forms of antileukemic treatment.

After the period of bone marrow suppression, abetted by infusions of G-CSF and of stem cells, the surviving and infused normal stem cells regenerate populations of erythrocytes, polymorphonuclear leukocytes, monocytes, and platelets. The state of remission lasts for a variable length of time, usually months to several years for patients treated with "standard" chemotherapy regimens developed in the 1970s, but goes on for many years in a minority of cases, suggesting that long-term remission equivalent to cure is possible.

The reappearance of leukemic cells in bone marrow or blood heralds the onset of *relapse.* Possible reasons for relapse are that (1) not all leukemic cells were killed but are present in numbers too small to be visible in the bone marrow sample viewed during the complete remission; (2) dormant leukemic cells are resistant to the chemotherapy and become active; (3) leukemic cells are protected from the drugs because they hide in tissues such as the brain and testis, which are poorly penetrated by the chemotherapeutic drugs; and (4) whatever damaged the bone marrow stem cells causing the development of leukemia in the first place also transforms the remaining normal cells, and they eventually become malignant. In other words, even after the first leukemic clone is eradicated, a new one emerges.

To combat the first possibility, researchers have tried different combinations of drugs that are more effective in killing leukemic cells. Another approach has been to follow induction of a complete remission with one or more courses of combination chemotherapy. This *intensification* strategy, frequently employing very high doses of cytosine arabinoside with or without an anthracycline, is intended to kill small numbers of residual leukemic cells. Very high doses of cytosine arabinoside (~3 g/m^2/day) with or without an anthracycline (e.g., daunorubicin, 45 mg/m^2) are typical drugs used in intensification regimens. Intensification appears to be superior to long-term treatment with lower doses of chemotherapy (*maintenance therapy*), and, in contrast to acute lymphocytic leukemia (Ch. 24), maintenance therapy is not generally used.

Against the second possibility, ionizing radiation may be directed at the apparent sanctuaries where leukemic cells are believed to hide. One strategy to prevent relapse is the complete ablation of the marrow and its replacement with completely normal stem cells. This approach, using allogeneic bone marrow transplantation, is described in Chapter 32; it is increasingly being shown to produce long-term remissions, equivalent to cures in about two-thirds of appropriately selected patients. These individuals are relatively young patients with histocompatible bone marrow donors. With standard antileukemic therapy or with bone marrow transplantation when histocompatibility is less than optimal, the long-term remission rate is much lower, on the order of 10 to 20 percent.

The fourth reason for relapse, inherent damage to the bone marrow, appears to account for the poor responsiveness to treatment of acute myelogenous leukemias arising after cytotoxic treatment of lymphomas and myelomas (Chs. 24 to 29), solid tumors, or even leukemias. These secondary leukemias and other hematopoietic disorders include the *myelodysplastic syndromes*, discussed in the previous chapter, and are the consequence of genetically altered stem cells.

After relapse, it is possible to induce additional remissions with repetitive chemotherapeutic treatment. However, the probability of complete remission becomes progressively lower with successive attempts at induction,

and the duration of the remissions becomes shorter. Eventually resistant to all therapy, patients die of complications of bone marrow failure or of tissue infiltration with leukemic cells.

Eosinophilic "Leukemia": Hypereosinophilic Syndrome

The blood eosinophil count very rarely becomes elevated above its normal low level (less than 200/µl) in the absence of infections or allergic disorders. When this elevation occurs, and especially if the eosinophil count becomes very high, the patient is said to have the *hypereosinophilic syndrome*. The blood contains mature eosinophils, and the bone marrow has eosinophils in all stages of maturation. Usually the neutrophil, lymphocyte, and platelet counts are normal, although moderate anemia may be present. Extensive invasion of tissues by eosinophils does not usually occur. This picture clearly differs from acute nonlymphocytic leukemias. Indeed, it is not always certain whether the eosinophil proliferation is a normal response to an unknown stimulus or a primary neoplastic disorder of eosinophil production. This ignorance underlies the use of the noncommittal term hypereosinophilic syndrome in those patients. Changes observed in the chromosomal structure of eosinophils of some patients with this disorder are consistent with a malignant basis of the disease.

The major disability inflicted by the accumulation of eosinophils in some patients is the development of cardiac damage. This damage is expressed as arrhythmias, progressive fibrosis of the endocardium, and eventually heart failure. The basis of this insult to the heart is unknown, but is possibly a toxic effect of substances released from eosinophils.

The rarity and variable severity of this disease has prevented the development of a consensus regarding treatment. In patients with cardiac toxicity, corticosteroids, cytotoxic chemotherapy, and leukopheresis, the removal of eosinophils by attaching the patient to an extracorporeal continuous flow centrifuge has been employed with variable success.

Langerhans Cell Histiocytosis

This uncommon disorder, formerly known as *histocytosis X*, affects mainly children and young adults and is caused by the growth of atypical cells believed to be transformed mononuclear phagocytes of the Langerhans cell type (Ch. 18). The proliferation of these cells can occur in any organ, but most frequently takes place in bone. The growth may appear as an isolated lesion affecting one site, or it may involve multiple organs and progress. Often solitary growths contain eosinophils as well as macrophagelike cells; such lesions have been termed *eosinophilic granulomas*. When the process is more widespread and progressive, bones of the skull are often involved, leading to a constellation of complications including exophthalmos (caused by orbital infiltration), endocrine hormone deficiencies (because of destruction of the pituitary gland after invasion of the sella turcica), and necrotic skin lesions. This progressive form of Langerhans histiocytosis also carries the eponym *Hand-Schüller-Christian disease*. In its most aggressive form, Langerhans histiocytosis rapidly evolves to cause extensive organ dysfunction and constitutional deterioration with high fever and prostration and frequently death. Bone marrow infiltration by this process can produce bone marrow failure. This variant has the eponym *Letterer-Siwe disease*. The progressive variants of Langerhans histiocytosis, with their attendant poorer prognoses, are more common in children younger than age 3.

Therapy for Langerhans histiocytosis is highly effective for localized disease and involves surgical excision of small lesions or radiotherapy of larger ones. For Langerhans histiocytosis of intermediate severity, this treatment together with supportive care, such as endocrine hormone replacement, can prevent death and limit

morbidity. Various forms of chemotherapy employed against progressive disease are only marginally successful.

SUGGESTED READINGS

Bennett JM, Catovsky D, Daniel MT (1976) Proposals for the classification of the acute leukemias: French-American-British (FAB) Cooperative Group. Br J Haematol 33:451

Cassileth PA et al (1992) Varying intensity of postremission therapy in acute myeloid leukemia. Blood 79:1924

DeThé H, Chomienne C, Lanotte M et al (1990) The t(15:17) translocation of acute promyelocytic leukaemia fuses the retinoic acid receptor α gene to a novel transcribed locus. Nature 347:558

Flaum M, Scholey RT, Fauci AS (1981) A clinico-pathologic correlation of the idiopathic hypereosinophilic syndrome. 1. Hematologic manifestations. Blood 58:1012

Fong C, Brodeur GM (1987) Down's syndrome and leukemia: epidemiology, genetics, cytogenetics and mechanisms of leukemogenesis. Cancer Genet Cytogenet 28:55

Longmore GD, Lodish HF (1991) An activating mutation in the murine erythropoietin receptor induces erythroleukemia in mice: a cytokine receptor superfamily oncogene. Cell 67:1089

Löwenberg B, van Putten WLJ, Touw IP et al (1993) Autonomous proliferations of leukemic cells in vitro as a determinant of prognosis in adult acute myeloid leukemia. N Engl J Med 328:614

Nimer S, Golde DW (1987) The 5q⁻ abnormality. Blood 70:1705

Tilley H et al (1990) Low-dose cytarabine versus intensive chemotherapy in the treatment of acute nonlymphocytic leukemia in the elderly. J Clin Oncol 8:272

Warrell RP, Jr, (1993) Retinoid resistance in acute promyelocytic leukemia: new mechanisms, strategies, and implications. Blood 82:1949

Warrel RP, Jr, de Thé Hr, Wang Z-Y et al (1993) Acute promyelocytic leukemia. N Engl J Med 329:177

Yunis LL, Brunning RD, Howe RB, Lobell M (1984) High resolution chromosomes as an independent prognostic indicator in adult acute nonlymphocytic leukemia. N Engl J Med 311:812

24

Lymphoid Neoplasms: Overview

Lymphoid neoplasms are composed of transformed lymphoid cells that exhibit uncontrolled growth and invasion. Together with leukemias, lymphomas account for 40,000 to 60,000 deaths annually in the United States. The incidence rate of these disorders approaches that of colon and breast cancers.

Compared with the classification for neoplasms of "myeloid" cells, that for lymphoid neoplasms is much more complex. This complexity arises from the great biological diversity of lymphoid cells that is not readily apparent from their morphology. The current understanding of the biology of lymphoid cells, summarized in Chapter 19, is becoming increasingly helpful in the diagnosis and treatment of lymphoid neoplasms. However, the classification of lymphoid neoplasms is still often based on more archaic anatomical and histological considerations.

ETIOLOGY AND PATHOGENESIS OF LYMPHOID NEOPLASMS

As was described for neoplasms of myeloid cells, mutations in the genetic material of susceptible lymphoid cells may lead to the proliferation of malignant clones. Mutagenic agents are possible causes of this genetic change. Exposure to ionizing radiation increases the incidence of acute, but not chronic lymphatic leukemias. In contrast to the granulocytic leukemias, there is more evidence linking viruses with lymphoid neoplasia in humans. Human T-cell leukemia virus type 1 (HTLV-1), a retrovirus, is the cause of one variant of a human T-cell leukemia that is endemic in southern Japan and in the Caribbean basin (Ch. 28). Epstein-Barr virus (EBV) infection, which causes the atypical lymphocytes of infectious mononucleosis (Ch. 20), is associated with the neoplastic cells in a minority of cases of two human lymphoid tumors, Hodgkin's disease (Ch. 27) and Burkitt's lymphoma (Ch. 28). EBV infection is also implicated in the pathogenesis of the 1 percent incidence of non-Hodgkin's lymphomas arising in organ transplant recipients who have undergone immunosuppression. Nevertheless, a causal relationship between viruses and most lymphoid neoplasms in humans is far from established.

Another condition associated with the development of lymphoid neoplasia, usually of one particular type, is immunodeficiency. Occasionally, congenital or acquired antibody deficiency states precede the development of this lymphoid neoplasm. Patients with acquired immunodeficiency syndrome (AIDS) or receiving immunosuppressive treatment to prevent the rejection of engrafted organs, usually the kidney, have a relatively high incidence of this type of lymphoid neoplasm. Because immunodeficiency and immunosuppression dispose to recurrent or chronic infections, one may speculate that it is the infection rather than the immunodeficiency per se that is most closely related to the development of the lymphoid malignancy. For example, there is an epidemiological relationship between chronic malarial infestation in the development of Burkitt's lymphoma. The injection of pristane into the peritoneal cavity of a certain strain of mice causes a large proportion of these mice to develop a malignant neoplasm of B cells. However, the carcinogenic effect of the oil is limited to that particular genetic strain. Therefore, the effect of inflammation or infection in producing lymphoid malignancy is dependent on a particular feature of the host that is genetically programmed, possibly a subtle form of immunodeficiency or an imbalance in the numbers or functions of lymphoid cells.

The evidence for such a relationship between imbalances in the immune system and the development of lymphoid neoplasms is the epidemiological association between certain autoimmune disorders and lymphoid neoplasms. It has been reported that patients with lymphoid malignancies have more autoimmune disorders, such as systemic lupus erythematosus (SLE), among their blood relations. Furthermore, certain lymphoid neoplasms develop in patients with some autoimmune diseases. One example is Sjögren syndrome, which is characterized by salivary and lacrimal gland impairment caused by the invasion of these glands by lymphocytes. Another example is celiac disease, in which there is a degeneration of the epithelial lining of the small intestine and lymphoid cell infiltrates in the intestinal submucosa.

As described in Chapter 21, a unifying principle behind the multiple routes to neoplasia is the abnormal expression of cellular oncogenes or the incorporation of viral oncogenes into mammalian cells. Oncogenes have been identified in a variety of animal and human lymphoid neoplasms, and some possible mechanisms of their expression have been identified.

Some of the cellular oncogenes of lymphoid cells become activated by being brought into association with the immunoglobulin and T-cell receptor regions of the genome that undergo rearrangement in the course of normal lymphoid cell maturation (Chapter 19), suggesting how chronic immune stimulation might predispose to lymphoid neoplasia, and a number of these associations are described in the following chapters. One predisposing factor, therefore, to lymphoid neoplasia could be overactivity of the V-D-J recombining activity of lymphoid precursors, and there is evidence that such overactivity occurs in the X-linked genetic disorder *ataxia telangiectasia*, which features mental retardation, cerebellar ataxia, telangiectasias in the antecubetal fossae, and a predilection to lymphoid and other malignancies. Cells derived from patients with this disease also fail to show induction of the tumor suppressor gene *p53* following ionizing radiation. An appreciable frequency of mutations in the *p53* gene predicted to lead to neoplasia have been found in patients with some of the lymphoid neoplasms discussed in ensuing chapters, specifically Burkitt's lymphoma, B-cell acute lymphocytic leukemia, and multiple myeloma.

The indicators of clonal lymphoid proliferation in lymphoid neoplasms include surface immunoglobulins with predominantly λ or κ light chains, detectable by fluorescence-activated sorting of peripheral blood or lymph node cells, or nonrandomly rearranged T-cell or immunoglobulin genes that can be very sensitively monitored by the polymerase chain reaction; these indicators are useful for monitoring the extent of the disease and its response to treatment.

In certain disorders characterized by the proliferation and invasion of tissues (operationally "malignant" behavior) by lymphoid cells, however, it has not been possible to identify with certainty a clonally malignant cell population. Hodgkin's disease, described in Chapter 27, is one example. Another is the unusual situation described in Chapter 20, in which patients with infectious mononucleosis die from an apparently malignant proliferation of lymphoid cells. Still another example is *angioimmunoblastic adenopathy*, a disorder characterized by lymphadenopathy. Patients have a systemic disease characterized by manifestations of inflammation, including polymorphonuclear leukocytosis, monocytosis, elevation in the concentration of the plasma acute-phase reactants, and immunoglobulins, with resulting rouleau formation and high erythrocyte sedimentation rates. Many of these patients have associated autoimmune phenomena, such as rheumatoid arthritis, immune complex inflammatory disease, or autoimmune blood cell destruction. The lymph node enlargement is characteristic in that the number of cells ordinarily found in lymph nodes increases, accompanied by a proliferation of capillaries that branch at perpendicular angles. This histology is what gives this disease the name angioimmunoblastic adenopathy. In some cases, angioimmunoblastic adenopathy occurs in patients who have been receiving various types of medication, suggesting a reactive response. The natural history of angioimmunoblastic adenopathy is variable. Some patients undergo spontaneous remissions, whereas others succumb to progressive debilitation, eventually leading to death. Destructive organ infiltration by the lymphoid process may be a feature in this relentless course. There is no evidence that treatment affects the outcome of angioimmunoblastic adenopathy.

ANATOMY: LYMPHOMA, LEUKEMIA, AND MIXTURES OF THE TWO

If the expression of the malignant lymphoid proliferation takes place predominantly in the bone marrow and peripheral blood, the disorder is defined as a *lymphatic leukemia. Acute lymphatic leukemia* (ALL) describes an aggressive and rapidly destructive process in which immature lymphoid cells take over the bone marrow and eventually can invade peripheral tissues. *Chronic lymphatic leukemia* (CLL), on the

other hand, is a relatively indolent disorder in which the lymphocytes in the bone marrow and blood appear more mature and grow more slowly. The term *lymphoma* encompasses a family of diseases representing tumors of lymphoid cells of variable maturity in which the primary expression of the malignant process is in the tissues, usually in the lymph nodes, spleen, and other lymphoid organs, but occasionally in extralymphatic tissue sites. Depending on the type and stage of evolution of the lymphoma, neoplastic lymphocytes can appear in the peripheral blood, and some lymphomas are closely related to leukemias in biological and clinical behavior. Therefore, there can be considerable overlap between lymphomas and leukemias.

For lymphomas there is a staging system for analyzing the extent of involvement of the body by the malignant process (Table 24-1). This staging system is particularly useful in the evaluation of patients with Hodgkin's disease (Ch. 27). Stage I refers to involvement of a single region of lymph nodes, for example, a group of cervical lymph nodes, the left or right axillary lymph nodes, or the left or right inguinal lymph nodes. Stage II defines involvement of two or more regions of lymph nodes, but restricts the involvement to one or the other

Table 24-1. Staging: Extent of Disease[a]

Stage	Definition
I	Involvement of a single lymph node region
II	Involvement of two or more lymph node regions on the same side of the diaphragm (II), which may be accompanied by localized involvement of an extralymphatic organ or site (II$_E$)
III	Involvement of lymph node regions on both sides of the diaphragm (III), which may also be accompanied by involvement of the spleen (III$_S$) or by localized involvement of an extralymphatic organ or site (III$_E$)
IV	Diffuse or disseminated involvement of one or more extralymphatic organs or tissues, with or without associated lymph node involvement

[a]The presence or absence of fever, night sweats, and/or unexplained loss of 10 percent or more of body weight in the preceding 6 months is denoted by the suffix letters B and A, respectively.

side of the diaphragm. For example, a stage II lymphoma might involve the right or left axillary and right or left cervical lymph nodes on one side of the body, or mediastinal and cervical lymph nodes. Stage III lymphoma is present when two or more lymph node-bearing regions are involved on both sides of the diaphragm. Involvement of para-aortic and mediastinal lymph nodes would be an example of a stage III lesion. For stages I through III, the subscript S designates that the spleen is involved. The subscript E denotes extension of the disease from the lymph node into contiguous tissues. For example, involvement of the parenchyma of the lung by direct extension of disease arising in mediastinal lymph nodes with involvement of cervical lymph nodes would represent stage II_E. Disease encompassing the mediastinum, the para-aortic region, and the spleen would be classified as stage III_S. Stage IV represents extranodal lymphoma, possibly involving the liver, the bone marrow, or other nonlymphoid organs.

Lymphomas are often first recognized by the painless enlargement of one or more of the peripheral lymph nodes. Alternatively, the enlargement of internal lymph nodes or growth of lymphoma in an extralymphatic location such as the intestine, bone, or nasopharynx causes symptoms by encroaching on internal organs. Compression of the tracheobronchial tree by lymphoma can produce respiratory difficulties, such as cough, wheezing, or dyspnea. More widespread growth of the neoplasm can obstruct lymphatic drainage in the chest, resulting in pleural effusions with dyspnea. The narrowing of the superior vena cava or other major veins returning to the heart can lead to superior vena cava syndrome. In this condition there is flushing and edema of the face. Because of the generalized distribution of lymphoid tissue in the body, practically any organ system can become impaired should lymphoma arise in or near it.

The initial evaluation of the extent of lymphoma is done by means of physical examination of the patient and by radiographic examinations routinely used in clinical practice. This approach is called *clinical staging*. To evaluate the extent of disease in the abdomen, it is sometimes necessary and desirable to subject the patient to an exploratory laparotomy or to use an endoscopic procedure called a *laparoscopy*, in which an endoscope is inserted into the peritoneal cavity. This more invasive approach is called *pathological staging*. The usefulness of this staging classification and the necessity for precise evaluation of the extent of disease depend on the type of lymphoma and the age and condition of the patient.

HISTOLOGY

Hematologists and pathologists have attempted to classify lymphoid neoplasms according to the histological appearance of cells obtained from the blood, bone marrow, or lymphoid organs. In this pursuit, cell size, cell-staining characteristics, nuclear shape, and the appearance of cells forming nodules that resemble lymphoid follicles or diffuse sheets have all been taken into account. The morphology of lymphoid neoplasms has correlated somewhat with their biological behavior, thereby providing a relatively useful classification for the clinician. The microscopic appearance of lymphoid neoplasms is described in the chapters that follow.

IMMUNOBIOLOGY

In recent years, it has become possible to supplement the histological analysis of lymphoid neoplasms with the type of marker analysis that defines the lineage and stage of maturation of lymphoid cells (Fig. 24-1). This approach has permitted definition of the likely cell of origin of many lymphoid neoplasms, and in some cases it has sorted out malignancies that appeared very similar on histological examination but that were very different in clinical behavior. Unfortunately, some lymphoid neoplasms still escape definition by currently available techniques.

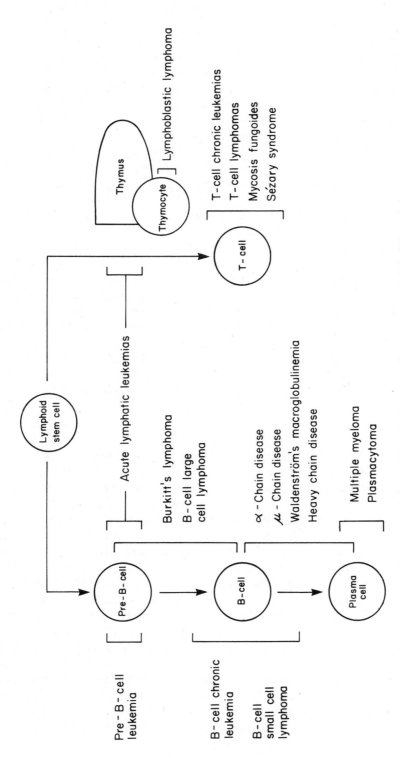

Fig. 24-1. Lymphoid neoplasms: Origins according to immunological differentiation.

The development of monoclonal antibodies reacting with cell surface antigens characteristic for B cells and T cells for particular stages of maturation of lymphoid cells and in some cases indicative of clonality of the cells has been an important step in advancing the classification of lymphoid neoplasms (Ch. 19). It is commonplace, therefore, for samples of peripheral white blood cells or of gently dispersed lymph nodes or tumor masses to be reacted with a panel of monoclonal antibodies such as the ones listed in Table 19-1 and then analyzed by immunofluorescence microscopy or by flow cytometry in a fluorescence-activated cell sorter. The latter technique has the advantage of automation and the ability through application of different fluorophores and wavelengths to detect simultaneously the reactivity of several different antibodies. It can also determine cell size by the extent to which the cell scatters incident light and can document nuclear ploidy from reactivity of the cells with fluorescent DNA-binding dyes. The application of a panel of varying specificity of antibodies helps add confidence to straightforward diagnostic cases and may help clarify more difficult instances. This approach was initially especially useful for the diagnosis and classification of B-cell neoplasms, as these are the most frequent lymphoid malignancies. The ability, for example, to detect surface expression of immunoglobulins of one or another (λ or κ) light chain class by monoclonal antibody reactivity is a simple diagnostic test for clonality of a B-cell population. Although individual B lymphocytes produce either λ or κ light chains, a mixture of normal B lymphocytes expresses both types of light chain, whereas a clone of B cells will show one or the other exclusively. The monoclonal antibodies reactive with T cells are useful for identifying a neoplasm as being of T-cell origin as well as helping to pinpoint its maturational stage. They do not, however, prove clonality of the T-cell proliferation.

A refinement in the classification of B-cell neoplasms and a handle on the clonality of T-cell tumors has arisen from molecular genetics, specifically from the ability to detect clonal populations of cells with rearranged genes. As explained in Chapter 19, B and T cells establish a repertoire of immunoglobulins and T-cell antigen receptors, respectively, by putting mRNA-translating parts of these molecules together in different combinations. Because each cell expresses a particular rearranged gene, samples of normal B cells and T cells represent populations with multiple gene rearrangements. A single clone of B cells, however, demonstrates only a unique pattern of immunoglobulin gene rearrangements, as detected by the technique known as *Southern blotting* (named for its originator, E. M. Southern) (Fig. 24-2).

DNA is isolated from the cells to be tested and partially digested into fragments by bacterial *restriction enzymes* that recognize particular nucleotide base sequences. The fragments are then subjected to electrophoresis through a porous gel that separates them according to length, the shorter segments moving faster in the electrical field. The gel is then overlaid with nitrocellulose paper, and fluid convection is used to transfer the DNA fragments in the gel onto the filter to which they adhere in a position replicating where they traveled in the gel. Radioactively labeled genomic or cDNA probes encoding a region of the gene of interest, for example, the J region of the T-cell receptor DNA or the J region of the immunoglobulin gene, bind to the particular DNA fragments on the paper that have the appropriate complementary sequences. The paper is apposed to an x-ray film, and the location of these complexes on the paper is then detected by radioautography. In most lymphoid cell preparations the probes will react slightly with fragments containing unrearranged germline genes. The variation in restriction enzyme targets in normal cell populations presents so many different-sized reactive fragments that the probes do not bind with sufficient density to be detected. In clonal cell populations, on the other hand, the probe recognizes the fragment containing the single

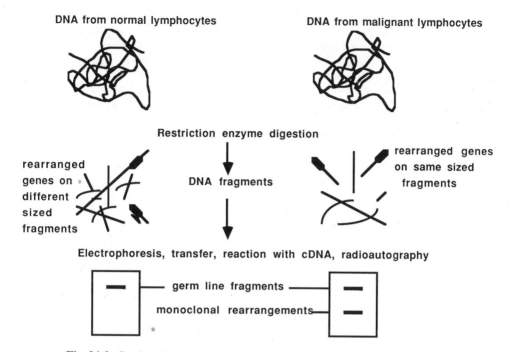

DNA from normal lymphocytes

DNA from malignant lymphocytes

Restriction enzyme digestion

rearranged
genes on
different
sized
fragments

DNA fragments

rearranged genes
on same sized
fragments

Electrophoresis, transfer, reaction with cDNA, radioautography

germ line fragments

monoclonal rearrangements

Fig. 24-2. Southern blotting for restriction fragment analysis of tumor clonality.

rearranged sequence in addition to the germline sequence-containing fragment, and an additional band appears on the autoradiogram.

In summary, then, surface antigens, gene rearrangements, chromosomal aberrations, and expression of specific oncogenes complement histological, anatomical, and clinical classification of the lymphoid malignancies.

Why is the classification of lymphoid neoplasms so important? Lymphoid neoplasms are a heterogeneous group of diseases having variable rates of progression. The diseases vary in responsiveness to different treatments. Some are more responsive than others, and a few have a potential for cure. Therefore, knowledge of when to treat a given disease with what modalities, and how vigorously, is of profound practical importance. We often lack the information on which to make decisions pertinent to these points. Therefore it is hoped that a more precise classification of lymphoid neoplasms will relieve the frustrations that beset our current abilities to predict the natural history of lymphoid tumors and to treat them.

Meantime it is necessary to use anatomical, histological, and immunological approaches. Consult Figure 24-1 when reading Chapters 25 through 29, which describe the various lymphoid neoplasms.

SUGGESTED READINGS

Davis TH, Morton CC, Miller-Cassman R, Balk SP, Kadin ME (1992) Hodgkin's disease, lymphomatoid papulosis, and cutaneous T-cell lymphoma derived from a common T-cell clone. N Engl J Med 326:1115

Foon KA, Todd RF, III (1986) Immunologic classification of leukemia and lymphoma. Blood 68:1

Hartwell L (1992) Defects in a cell cycle checkpoint may be responsible for the genomic instability of cancer cells. Cell 71:543

Höllsberg P, Hafler DA (1993) Pathogenesis of diseases induced by human lymphotropic virus type I infection. N Engl J Med 328:1173

Kastan MB, Zhan Q, Ed-Deiry WS et al (1992) A mammalian cell cycle checkpoint pathway utilizing p53 and *GADD45* is defective in ataxia telangiectasia. Cell 71:587

Klein G (1992) Epstein-Barr virus-carrying cells in Hodgkin's disease. Blood 80:299

Korsmeyer SJ (1992) Bcl-2 initiates a new category of oncogenes: regulators of cell death. Blood 80:879

Penn I (1991) The changing pattern of posttransplant malignancies. Transplant Proc 23:1101

Randhawa PS et al (1992) Expression of Epstein-Barr virus-encoded small RNA (by the EBER-1 gene) in liver specimens from transplant recipients with post-transplantation lymphoproliferative disease. N Engl J Med 327:1710

Showe LC, Croce CM (1987) The role of chromosomal translocations in B- and T-cell neoplasia. Annu Rev Immunol 5:253

Swerdlow SH (1992) Biopsy Interpretation of Lymph Nodes. New York, Raven Press.

Weiss LM, Movahed LA, Warnke RA, Sklar J (1989) Detection of Epstein-Barr viral genomes in Reed-Sternberg cells of Hodgkin's disease. N Engl J Med 320:502

25

Acute Lymphocytic Leukemia

Acute lymphocytic (sometimes called lymphatic) leukemia is the expansion of a clone of malignant cells, which if left untreated rapidly leads to death. Acute lymphocytic leukemia initially arises in the bone marrow, but it progresses to involve the blood and peripheral tissues. The morphology of the bone marrow in acute lymphatic leukemia is characterized by a monotonous infiltrate of lymphoid cells called *lymphoblasts*. Like typical lymphocytes, the lymphoid blasts in acute lymphatic leukemia tend to have a high nuclear:cytoplasm ratio, and the nuclei have coarse chromatin and indistinct nucleoli (Fig. 25-1). The cells may vary in size from that of typical lymphocytes to cells three to four times that volume. The cytoplasm ordinarily has no granules (Fig. 25-1). As with myelogenous leukemia, there is a French-American British classification of the morphology for acute lymphatic leukemia (Table 25-1).

In nearly all cases of acute lymphatic leukemia, the cells contain the thymocyte enzyme terminal deoxyribonucleotide transferase (Tdt) and, to a variable extent, express other markers indicating different expressions of lymphoid differentiation. Two-thirds of affected patients have cells bearing an antigen, CD10, on the outer surface of the membrane. This antigen was originally called the *common acute lymphocytic leukemia antigen (CALLA)*. Despite lacking immunological markers of B cells and expressing a thymocyte enzyme, the malignant cells of "common" acute lymphocytic leukemia show immunoglobulin gene rearrangements characteristic of B cells at a very early (pre-B) stage of development.

In about 15 percent of cases of acute lymphocytic leukemia, the lymphoid blasts bear surface markers characteristic of T cells (CD2, CD3, CD1, CD5, and CD7). The indefinite border between leukemia and lymphoma is exemplified by what was formerly classified L3 acute lymphocytic leukemia. In these cases, which are uncommon, the cells contain cytoplasmic immunoglobulin, a feature of more mature pre-B cells than the phenotype in "common" acute lymphocytic leukemia. The lymphoid blasts may also have surface immunoglobulin, complement receptors, and CD9, CD24, CD19, and CD20, surface markers distinct for B cells. The neoplastic cells have a characteristic chromosomal abnormality in which there is a translocation of genetic material between chromosomes 8 and 14 [t(8;14)(q24;q32)], and in this translocation, the *myc* oncogene is associated with the immunoglobulin locus. As explained in Chapter 28, all of these features are characteristic of small non-cleaved cell lymphoma.

Translocations involving chromosome 11 band q23 also appear in about 12 percent of acute lymphocytic leukemia patients, and some

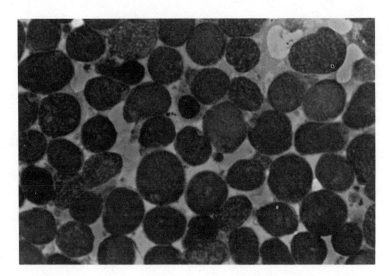

Fig. 25-1. Malignant lymphoblasts in acute lymphocytic leukemia.

of the patients' cells have markers of both B cells and phagocytic (myeloid) cell lineages, a finding sometimes called "biphenotypic." The cells with t(4;11) translocations express oncogenic fusion proteins encoded by the juxtaposition of part of a gene, *ALL-1* on chromosome 11, with a gene on chromosome 4. *ALL-1* is similar in sequence to a so-called homeotic gene, *trithorax*, that programs the embryonic development of the fruit fly, *Drosophila melanogaster*.

The division of cases of acute lymphatic leukemia into immunobiological categories has implications for prognosis of the disease and its responses to treatment. The "common" pre-B cell variety of the disease has the best prognosis, the more mature pre-B cell variety has the worst prognosis, and the T-cell variety has an intermediate prognosis. A number of oncogenes have been identified in the regions of chromosomal breaks occurring in cases of acute T-cell leukemia with cytogenetic abnormalities. In about a quarter of cases of B-cell acute lymphatic leukemia and a fifth of T-cell acute lymphocytic leukemia, the cells also have detectable granulocyte lineage surface antigens CD13, CD14, or CD33, and these cases have a 30 percent poorer three-year survival following diagnosis and treatment.

Acute lymphocytic leukemia is the principal neoplasm of children aged 2 to 8. It may be that this predisposition for the young reflects acquisition of immune responsiveness to environmental antigens during that time. The active recombination of immunoglobulin genes then increases the risk that an aberrant splice will occur leading to activation of an oncogene. A significant number, about one-third, of adults with what by all other criteria is acute lymphocytic leukemia actually have a variant of chronic myelogenous leukemia, a stem cell disorder described in Chapter 22. These patients' malignant stem cells carry a balanced 9:22 chromosomal translocation called Philadelphia chromosome; the cells differentiate into relatively immature lymphocytes. There is also a distinct biological difference between childhood and

Table 25-1. French-American British Classification

Type	Morphology
L1	Small cells of uniform size; round nucleus; nucleoli not prominent
L2	Large cells, variable in size; irregular nucleus with prominent nucleoli
L3	Large cells uniform in size, vacuolated cytoplasm, round nucleus with prominent nucleoli; this class is now grouped with the small non-cleaved cell type of lymphoma (Ch. 28)

adult lymphatic leukemia with respect to the outcome of treatment. The prognosis for children, who more frequently have the L1 type, is much better than for adults who are more likely to have the L2 variant and Philadelphia chromosome-positive neoplastic cells.

EFFECTS OF ACUTE LYMPHOCYTIC LEUKEMIA ON THE HOST

As in acute myelogenous leukemia, the initial and most important manifestation of acute lymphocytic leukemia is bone marrow failure. Suppression of normal bone marrow elements leads to anemia, thrombocytopenia, and neutropenia, which predispose to weakness and pallor, bleeding, and serious bacterial infections, respectively. Occasionally the bone marrow infiltration with the neoplasm can cause thinning of the bones and bone pain. The latter symptom has sometimes resulted in an incorrect diagnosis of arthritis in cases of acute lymphatic leukemia in which the symptoms in the bones preceded the development of overt bone marrow failure manifested by reduction in the peripheral blood counts. Invasion of other organs by the leukemic process generally occurs first in organs contiguous with the blood and lymphatic system, the lymph nodes, spleen, and liver. However, any tissues are susceptible to invasion, including the central nervous system. In cases of acute lymphatic leukemia in which the blast cells bear T-cell markers, masses of leukemic infiltration are often observed in the mediastinum. This phenomenon possibly represents a homing propensity by the malignant T cells toward the thymus gland.

TREATMENT

Following acute management of any hemorrhagic or infectious complications of the leukemic process, therapy is immediately directed toward complete eradication of the leukemic cells by means of cytotoxic drugs. The principles of induction of a remission in addition to the maintenance of that remission are similar to the treatment described for acute myelogenous leukemia (Ch. 23). In practice, however, the approach to therapy and the expected results, especially in childhood acute lymphocytic leukemia, differ somewhat from the approach to acute myelogenous leukemia.

The leukemic blast cells of most cases of acute lymphocytic leukemia are highly susceptible to killing by cytotoxic drugs, especially by corticosteroids, reflecting the sensitivity of lymphoid cells to this agent. Indeed, a combination of the corticosteroid prednisone and the drug vincristine, which prevents the assembly of microtubules, is sufficient to induce a complete remission in most cases of the childhood form of acute lymphatic leukemia. As neither of these drugs is particularly toxic to other bone marrow cells, it is theoretically possible to induce a remission in acute lymphocytic leukemia without causing the patient to endure the dangerous 3 weeks or so of complete bone marrow failure that patients with acute myelogenous leukemia must undergo during remission induction. Although mature pre-B-cell markers, high leukemic blast concentration in the blood, infiltration of organs with blasts, and male sex suggest a worse prognosis, it is not currently possible to identify with certainty which patients will respond satisfactorily to a mild regimen. It is therefore necessary to subject nearly all patients to more vigorous treatment, and therefore to additional side effects.

As is the case with acute myelogenous leukemias, the therapy of acute lymphocytic leukemia involves different regimens for *induction* of a remission and *consolidation* of the remission (intensification); supportive care for complications of the disease and of the treatment plays an important role in the overall management of the patient. Unlike acute myelogenous leukemia, however, acute lymphocytic leukemia treatment includes *maintenance therapy*. Current regimens for the induction of a remission in the common childhood form of acute lymphocytic leukemia include an anthracycline, asparaginase, vincristine, and prednisone (Ch. 21). Allopurinol is given during the phase of major cytoreduction. Intensification therapy may involve use of a single agent such as asparaginase or methotrexate at high doses or alternatively a repetition in the course of the drugs used to induce remission.

In the development of treatment of children with acute lymphocytic leukemia, the incidence of complete remissions became sufficiently frequent and duration sufficiently long that it was possible to discern that some relapses resulted from the persistence of leukemic cells in certain sanctuaries, such as the central nervous system, where the drugs could not easily penetrate because of the blood–brain barrier. It was found that treatment of the brain and spinal cord either with radiation alone or in combination with chemotherapy delivered to the cerebrospinal fluid by the administration of drugs through a needle into the lumbar cistern could prevent such relapses in most cases. The use of *maintenance therapy* with drugs other than those employed to induce remissions, daily 6-mercaptopurine and weekly methotrexate for example, further reduces the incidence of relapse. Maintenance therapy for 2 to 5 years after induction of remission and intensification treatment currently permits about 85 percent of children with acute lymphatic leukemia in the best prognostic category to enjoy sufficiently long, complete remissions as to use the term "cure." Considering that only 20 years ago a diagnosis of acute lymphatic leukemia in children was virtually a death sentence, the degree of success in treatment of acute lymphatic leukemia was spectacular. However, a significant fraction of children and nearly all adults with acute lymphocytic leukemia still suffer relapse when treated with the regimens found so successful in other children. This problem has led hematologists to apply more aggressive chemotherapy regimens against acute lymphocytic leukemia, more akin to those used in acute granulocytic leukemia. The problem with this approach is that the short-term bone marrow and long-term immunosuppressive effects of the chemotherapy

can erode some of the possible beneficial effects of increased tumoricidal potentials of more drugs. It is hoped that a more precise cytological classification of acute lymphocytic leukemia will succeed in sorting out those patients who require more aggressive treatment from those who do not. At present, it is only possible to say that the neoplasms bearing T-cell characteristics or Philadelphia chromosomal translocations are clearly less favorable than the common null cell types of acute lymphocytic leukemia and that the presence of granulocytic antigens worsens the prognosis.

Another issue in the treatment of acute lymphocytic leukemia is knowing when the leukemic cells have actually been eradicated. In the immediate post-treatment period, cells may persist but be incapable of further growth and will eventually die. Later on, however, detection of leukemic cells is a prediction of relapse. The polymerase chain reaction, which can detect the presence of the clonal nonrandom chromosome translocations of the leukemic clone in 1 in 100,000 nucleated cells, allows for such evaluation and prediction of relapse several months before it becomes apparent by standard bone marrow aspiration, but even this sensitive molecular method does not identify potential relapsers when it does not yield a positive result.

Adults with acute lymphatic leukemia do not fare as well as most children between the ages of 2 and 8. Although a high proportion of complete remission can be achieved in adults with acute lymphatic leukemia, the inevitability of eventual relapse is high, with only a small fraction of patients enjoying complete remissions that last more than several years. Therefore, bone marrow transplantation is being assessed as therapy for young adult patients with acute lymphocytic leukemia following the induction of a complete remission. The question as to why the "childhood" variant of acute lymphatic leukemia is so much more amenable to cure by chemotherapy is of great practical importance to hematologists.

Nevertheless, the cure of acute lymphatic leukemia by cytotoxic treatments bears a price. Surviving children have detectable losses of cognitive function, retardation of growth, and evidence of gonadal damage (although puberty develops normally in males and slightly early in females), and over half have evidence of cardiac dysfunction, particularly left ventricular contractility, which may be a liability in later life. When alkylating agents (Ch. 21) are used in the treatment that leads to cure, there is also a small but definite risk of subsequently developing acute granulocytic leukemia or solid tumors, particularly neoplasms of the central nervous system.

SUGGESTED READINGS

Barrett AJ et al (1992) Bone marrow transplantation for Philadelphia chromosome-positive acute lymphoblastic leukemia. Blood 79:3067

Lipschultz SE, Colan SD, Gelber RD et al (1991) Late cardiac effects of doxorubicin therapy for acute lymphoblastic leukemia in childhood. N Engl J Med 324:808

Mahmoud HH, Rivera GK, Hancock ML et al (1993) Low leukocyte count with blast cells in cerebrospinal fluid of children with newly diagnosed acute lymphoblastic leukemia. N Engl J Med 329:314

Melo JV, Gordon DE, Tuszynski A et al (1993) Expression of *ABC-BCR* fusion gene in Philadelphia-positive acute lymphoblastic leukemia. Blood 81:2488

Neglia JP, Meadows AT, Robison LL et al (1991) Second neoplasms after acute lymphoblastic leukemia in childhood. N Engl J Med 325:1330

Niemeyer CM, Sallan SE (1992) Acute lymphoblastic leukemia. p. 1247. In Nathan DG, Oski FA (eds): Hematology of Infancy and Childhood. 4th Ed. WB Saunders, Philadelphia

Pui C-H, Behm F, Crist WM (1993) Clinical and biological relevance of immunolgic marker studies in childhood acute lymphoblastic leukemia. Blood 82:343

Wiersma SR, Ortega J, Sobel E, Weinberg KI (1991) Clinical importance of myeloid antigen expression in acute lymphoblastic leukemia of childhood. N Engl J Med 324:800

26

Chronic
Lymphocytic Leukemia

Chronic lymphocytic leukemia is a neoplasm characterized by the proliferation of a clone of B-lymphoid cells that circulates in the blood and infiltrates the bone marrow and, to a variable extent, other tissues. In contrast to what occurs in acute lymphocytic leukemia, the deleterious effects of malignancy on the organism develop slowly or not at all. Other lymphoid neoplasms associated with circulating malignant lymphocytes are considered leukemic variants of lymphomas and are described in Chapter 28. Chronic lymphocytic leukemia overlaps most closely with a lymphoma called small cell lymphoma. The distinction between these two diseases is fuzzy and relatively arbitrary; if blood lymphocytosis is the predominant feature, clinicians will usually call the disorder chronic lymphocytic leukemia, whereas if lymphadenopathy is the major manifestation, the patient has small cell lymphocytic lymphoma.

GENERAL FEATURES

The diagnosis of *chronic lymphocytic leukemia* is very likely when the blood of an adult, usually a man, consistently contains more than 10×10^6 lymphocytes/μl, or when more than 30 percent of the nucleated cells in the bone marrow are lymphocytes. These lymphocytes may be typical or atypical, but ordinarily they are not as bizarre as the blasts seen in acute lymphatic leukemia (Fig. 26-1). The lymphocyte count in the blood may be extremely high, exceeding 100,000 cells/μl.

Chronic lymphocytic leukemia represents a clonal proliferation of relatively mature-looking B cells. Like normal B cells, the malignant cells have complement receptors and immunoglobulins on the external surfaces of their plasma membranes. The clonal nature of the proliferation can be demonstrated by measurement of glucose-6-phosphate dehydrogenase isoenzymes, as described for acute myelogenous leukemia (Ch. 23), and by the fact that the surface immunoglobulin on the malignant B cells is of only one light chain class (i.e. , κ or λ). The cells ordinarily have surface immunoglobulins with μ or δ heavy chains, that is, the surface immunoglobulins are of the IgM and IgD classes, as is the case for normal B cells. The leukemic B lymphocytes differ quantitatively from normal B cells in that the former express less immunoglobulin on their membranes than the latter. In addition, the cells have nonrandomly rearranged immunoglobulin genes, as expected for a clonally expanded B-cell population.

The B-cell chronic lymphatic leukemia cells may have cytogenetic abnormalities, although the low proliferative activity of the leukemic B

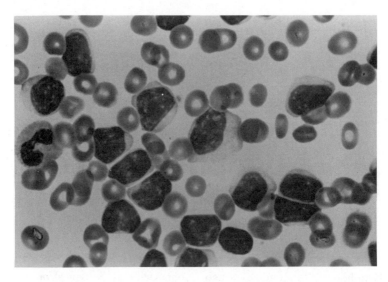

Fig. 26-1. Accumulation of malignant lymphocytes in the peripheral blood of a patient with chronic lymphocytic leukemia.

cell in this disease makes detection of chromosomal aberration difficult. The most frequent findings are trisomy 12 and structural abnormalities of chromosomes 13q and 14, which are observed respectively in about 15 percent of cases. A possible oncogene, *bcl-3*, has been identified in the breakpoint associated with t(14;19)q32;q13.1) translocations, and the chromosome 13 aberration is in the region where the retinoblastoma (*rb*) gene, a recessive oncogene, resides (Ch. 21). As amplified below, cytogenetic changes indicate a worse prognosis.

The leukemic B cells also perform less well than normal cells in tests of B-cell function such as proliferation in response to mitogens or in induction of immunoglobulin synthesis. B-cell chronic lymphatic leukemia cells express, in addition to surface immunoglobulin molecules, receptors for IgG (Fc receptors), C3 receptors, the histocompatibility antigen HLA-DR (Ia), and a variety of B-cell antigens (CD19, CD20, CD21). In the majority (about 85 percent) of cases, the malignant cells also express a T-cell antigen, CD5, implicated in the polyclonal expansion of lymphocytes causing various autoimmune disorders.

Prolymphocytic leukemia is a variant of B-cell chronic lymphatic leukemia. The cells are larger and more immature in appearance than the usual B-cell chronic lymphocytic leukemia cells and have prominent nucleoli. The cells tend to have more surface immunoglobulin and less CD5 antigen. The morphology and surface phenotype of prolymphocytic leukemia is associated with higher leukemic cell counts and more pronounced splenomegaly. Prolymphocytic leukemia may therefore represent a progression to greater malignancy of B-cell chronic lymphocytic leukemia.

In a minority of cases of chronic lymphocytic leukemia, the lymphoid cells in the blood have additional T-cell markers, and these cells may exhibit suppressor or helper functions. T-cell chronic lymphatic leukemia cells have clonally rearranged T-cell receptor genes and may also have cytogenetic abnormalities, the most usual being an inversion of chromosome 14, inv(14) (q1 1q13).

EFFECTS OF CHRONIC LYMPHATIC LEUKEMIA ON THE PATIENT

Chronic lymphatic leukemia is often an indolent disease that tends to affect elderly men, who may die of other causes and infrequently need specific treatment for the disorder. The median overall survival with this disease is in the range of 15 years for patients without cytogenetic abnormalities and half as long for patients who have such defects. The disease can affect patients adversely in a number of ways, elaborated below, and several staging systems have been devised to classify the progression of the leukemia (Table 26-1).

Organ Infiltration

The lymph nodes and the spleen are most susceptible to enlargement because of infiltration by chronic lymphatic leukemia cells. When the lymph nodes, bone marrow, and spleen become intensely infiltrated, chronic lymphocytic leukemia truly becomes indistinguishable from small cell lymphocytic lymphoma in that the architecture of these organs is replaced with sheets of small lymphocytes. However, the concentration of surface immunoglobulin is higher in lymphocytes of patients with diffuse well-differentiated lymphoma than in the cells of patients with chronic lymphatic leukemia. Late in the evolution of chronic lymphatic leukemia or in atypical cases or variants of chronic lymphatic leukemia, infiltrations of other organs, including the lung, kidneys, and skin, can occur. The enlargement of lymph nodes and the spleen can become sufficient to cause pain or compromised function of contiguous organs, and proliferation of leukemic cells in the bone marrow can result in anemia or thrombocytopenia.

Advanced chronic lymphatic leukemia can cause anemia, thrombocytopenia, and occasionally granulocytopenia because of replacement of the bone marrow by the malignant infiltrate. The deficiency of normal peripheral blood cells may be exacerbated by enlargement of the spleen, which sequesters and clears the erythrocytes, granulocytes, and platelets from the blood. In some cases, this clearance is accelerated because of the elaboration of autoantibodies against the normal blood cells.

Immunodeficiency and Autoimmunity

Most patients with typical B-cell chronic lymphatic leukemia have reduced levels of normal polyclonal serum immunoglobulin. The cause of this reduction is partly a reflection of the failure of the chronic lymphatic leukemia clone to differentiate into normal plasma cells capable of secreting antibodies. In addition, a general imbalance in lymphoid cells may also lead to an excess of suppressor activity, which may result in decreased immunoglobulin production. Some patients have a sufficient hypogammaglobulinemia to become susceptible to infection with encapsulated bacteria. The derangements in lymphoid cell balance incurred by the lymphoid proliferation can lead to elaboration of autoantibodies against normal blood cells and other host tissues (Ch. 30). Therefore, 10 to 20 percent of patients with B-cell chronic lymphatic leukemia will have autoimmune hemolytic anemia, autoimmune thrombocytopenia, or rheumatoid arthritis.

Paraprotein Production

In most cases of typical B-cell chronic lymphatic leukemia, the malignant cells have small amounts of surface immunoglobulin and are incapable of differentiation into plasma cells. In a small percentage of cases of chronic lym-

Table 26-1. Staging Sytems for Chronic Lymphatic Leukemia

Rai System			Binet System		
Stage	Clinical Features	Avg. Survival (years)	Stage	Clinical Features	Avge Survival (years)
0	None	> 10	A	< Three areas involved	>10
I	Lymphadenopathy	8	B	> Three areas involved	5
II	Hepato/splenomegaly	6	C	Anemia and thrombocytopenia	2–3
III	Anemia	2–3			
IV	Thrombocytopenia	2–3			

phatic leukemia, patients may express a monoclonal gammopathy, usually with an M component of the IgM class. Monoclonal gammopathies associated with lymphoid neoplasms are described in more detail below and in Chapter 17.

TRANSFORMATION

At some point in the course of chronic lymphocytic leukemia, the lymphoid cells become more primitive in appearance, acquiring the features described for prolymphocytic leukemia above or of the cells seen in large cell lymphomas described in Chapter 28. The patient now has a more aggressive lymphoid neoplasm that grows more rapidly and invades lymphoid and other organs more actively. The patient whose disease has evolved to a large cell lymphoma is said to have *Richter syndrome*. The patient may have high fever, weight loss, enlarging lymph nodes, and hepatosplenomegaly. In some of these transformed cases it is possible to document that the morphologically changed neoplasm represents a metamorphosis in the phenotype of the original leukemic clone. In others the disease appears to be an entirely new tumor. Hodgkin's disease (Ch. 27) has also emerged in patients with chronic lymphocytic leukemia.

TREATMENT

B-cell chronic lymphocytic leukemia may progress slowly or not at all. Because most patients are elderly, they often die of other causes. When treatment is needed, it is because of the complications of more aggressive evolution of the disease enumerated above, that is, significant organ impairment or the ravages of immune dysfunction. Knowing precisely in a given patient when the benefits of treatment outweigh the risks is sometimes difficult. Features that lead physicians to earlier treatment include evidence of aggressiveness of the disease such as bulky lymphadenopathy or splenomegaly, constitutional symptoms, anemia, thrombocytopenia, or symptomatic autoimmune disorders. Laboratory signs pointing to emergence of these criteria for treatment include a lymphocyte count greater than 50 x $10^6/\mu l$, doubling of the lymphocyte count in a year's time, diffuse infiltration of the bone marrow by lymphocytes, or the appearance of autoantibodies.

Because of the basic benignity of chronic lymphatic leukemia, treatment, when needed, can often be mild, consisting of radiation of enlarged or impaired organs or small doses of chemotherapy with alkylating agents such as *chlorambucil* or *cyclophosphamide* or with a-interferon (see below and Ch. 21). Aggressive phases of chronic lymphatic leukemia characterized by marked splenic enlargements, pancytopenia, painful enlargement of lymph nodes, fever, weight loss, or autoimmune cell destruction may require higher doses of the drugs or combinations of them with corticosteroids, vinca alkaloids, and other agents such as adenosine deaminase inhibitors. As explained in Chapter 20, adenosine deaminase deficiency lead to immune deficiency, because the metabolic effects of the enzyme defect leads to accumulation of metabolites that kill lymphocytes. Taking advantage of this phenomenon, investigators have designed adenosine deaminase inhibitors that are effective in the treatment of chronic lymphocytic leukemia. These include *deoxycoformycin*, *2-chloroadenosine*, and *fludarabine*. The latter two drugs appear, despite similarities in structure, not to lead to cross-resistance. Although these agents primarily kill T lymphocytes, they are highly effective in inducing remissions in chronic lymphocytic leukemia and small cell lymphocytic lymphoma.

Patients with hypogammaglobulinemia secondary to chronic lymphocytic leukemia may benefit from intravenous immunoglobulin replacement therapy in terms of having fewer pyogenic infections, although the general cost effectiveness of this expensive treatment has been questioned, since the incidence of infection may be low.

SUGGESTED READINGS

Brecher M, Banks PM (1990) Hodgkin's disease variant of Richter's syndrome: a report of 8 cases. Am J Clin Path 93:333

Foon KA, Rai KR, Gale RP (1990) Chronic lymphocytic leukemia: new insights into biology and therapy. Ann Intern Med 113:525

Ghani AM, Krause JR, Brody JP (1986) Prolymphocytic transformation of chronic lymphocytic leukemia. Report of three cases and a review of the literature. Cancer 57:75

Juliusson G, Elmhorn-Rosenborg A, Liliemark J (1992) Response to 2-chlorodeoxyadenosine in patients with B-cell chronic lymphocytic leukemia resistant to fludarabine. N Engl J Med 327:1056

Kipps TJ, Carson DA (1993) Autoantibodies in chronic lymphocytic leukemia and related systemic autoimmune diseases. Blood 81:2475

Lee JS, Dixon DO, Kantarjian HM et al (1987) Prognosis of chronic lymphocytic leukemia: a multivariate regression analysis of 325 untreated patients. Blood 69:929

Piro LD, Carrera CJ, Carson DA, Beutler E (1990) Lasting remissions in hairy-cell leukemia induced by a single infusion of 1-chloloroadenosine. N Engl J Med 322:1117

Robertson LE, Huh YO, Butler J et al (1992) Response assessment in chronic lymphocytic leukemia after fludarabine plus prednisone: clinical, pathological, immunophenotypic, and molecular analysis. Blood 80:29

27

Hodgkin's Lymphoma

When in 1832 Thomas Hodgkin published a paper entitled "On Some Morbid Appearances of the Absorbent Glands and Spleen," he was reporting the first description of malignant lymphoma. Today Hodgkin's disease, or Hodgkin's lymphoma, is viewed as a malignant disorder affecting lymphoid tissue, the morphological appearance of which can be quite variable, but which has one consistent feature: the presence of a large cell with two nuclei called the *Reed-Sternberg cell*, after its initial describers. Hodgkin's disease was also the first lymphoid neoplasm to be cured, first by radiation therapy and subsequently by combination chemotherapy.

Hodgkin's disease ordinarily presents as a painless enlargement of one or more of the lymph node regions. In distinct contrast to the non-Hodgkin's lymphomas, which are generally widely disseminated at the time of diagnosis, Hodgkin's disease is often localized and may spread slowly through the lymphatic channels to contiguous lymph node regions. The indolent and contiguous route of spread of many cases of Hodgkin's disease has implications for therapy. If the disorder is untreated or if treatment fails, Hodgkin's disease eventually spreads widely and invades normal organs, killing the patient by interfering with the functioning of these organs.

The constant finding of Reed-Sternberg cells implies that these cells represent the malignant proliferation underlying Hodgkin's disease. Their large size and bizarre appearance (Fig. 27-1) are consistent with malignant neoplasia. The presence on these cells of Ki-1 (CD30), a cell surface antigen associated with the activation of B- and T-cell blasts, suggests they are of lymphoid origin as is a case report describing a t(8;9) chromosomal translocation in the Reed-Sternberg cells of a patient. This patient had previously had a benign skin eruption called lymphomatoid papulosis, which consists of T cells that morphologically resemble Reed-Sternberg cells and that in about one-fifth of cases evolve into cutaneous lymphoma (Ch. 28); the T cells of the patient had the same chromosomal translocation. The molecular cloning of CD30 revealed it to be similar in structure to a nerve growth factor receptor. In a minority of cases of Hodgkin's disease, biopsy specimens have the t(14;18) chromosomal rearrangement frequently observed in non-Hodgkin's lymphoma (Ch. 24), suggesting that these cases may be of B-cell origin. Other cases, however, have had a chromosomal translocation and monoclonal T-cell receptor rearrangements indicative of a T-cell malignancy. In some respects, Hodgkin's disease behaves as if it were an infection or inflammatory disease. The lymph node architecture becomes replaced by normal inflammatory cells; these cells ordinarily outnumber the Reed-Sternberg cells. Furthermore, patients

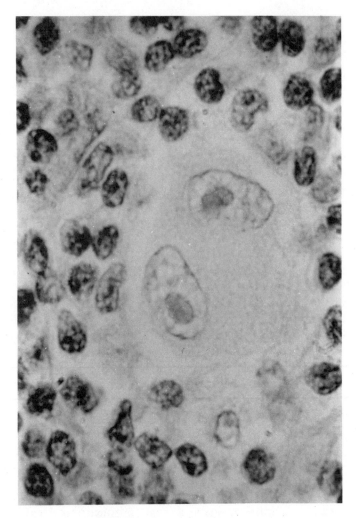

Fig. 27-1. Reed-Sternberg cell.

with Hodgkin's disease frequently manifest signs and symptoms associated with inflammation, such as fever, weight loss, polyclonal hypergammaglobulinemia, changes in acute-phase reactant proteins, monocytosis, eosinophilia, and soaking night sweats. It is possible that these diverse manifestations of Hodgkin's disease represent secretion of different cytokines by malignant Reed-Sternberg or other lymphoid cells.

When describing a patient with Hodgkin's disease, the staging system of lymphoma also takes into account whether a patient has systemic symptoms that can be ascribed to neoplasm. The symptoms are (1) an unexplained loss of more than 10 percent in body weight, (2) soaking night sweats, and (3) fever. The absence of these features designates a patient as stage A (e.g., stage IA or IIA), and the presence of the symptoms indicates stage B (e.g., IIIB or IVB). An unusual systemic manifestation of Hodgkin's disease is periodic fever that is present for some days, remits, and then returns. This symptom has been named *Pel-*

Ebstein fever after the physician who first described it. Some patients diagnosed as having Hodgkin's disease complain of pain in affected lymph nodes after ingesting alcohol. Hodgkin's disease patients may occasionally suffer from severe, generalized itching of the skin. As is the case for many inflammatory conditions and some neoplasms, patients with Hodgkin's disease may express anergy.

The histology of Hodgkin's disease is classified according to the cells surrounding the Reed-Sternberg cells. A uniform infiltrate of normal-appearing typical lymphocytes in the presence of Reed-Sternberg cells defines what is called *lymphocyte-predominant* Hodgkin's disease. If the surrounding infiltrate consists of macrophages, lymphocytes, and eosinophils, the entity is called *mixed cellularity* Hodgkin's disease. *Nodular sclerosis* Hodgkin's disease is said to be present when the lymph node contains large bands of collagen. The Reed-Sternberg cells reside in lacunae evident throughout the fibrotic matrix. Lymphocyte predominance, mixed cellularity, and nodular sclerosis are the histologies usually found in young adults, the age population in which Hodgkin's disease most frequently occurs.

A second peak of incidence of Hodgkin's disease occurs in elderly persons. These patients frequently manifest a histological pattern composed of large numbers of extremely bizarre Reed-Sternberg cells and a minimal inflammatory infiltrate. This category of Hodgkin's disease is called *lymphocyte-depleted* Hodgkin's disease.

To some extent, the histological pattern predicts the pace of the disease and response to treatment. Lymphocyte-predominant Hodgkin's disease has the most favorable prognosis, whereas lymphocyte-depleted Hodgkin's disease is most virulent and least responsive to therapy. The histological pattern does not influence treatment. The nodular sclerosis pattern is most often seen in the younger age group of patients affected. Lymphocyte depletion Hodgkin's disease is most often seen in elderly patients with advanced stages of disease.

DIAGNOSIS AND MANAGEMENT

The progressive enlargement of one or more lymph nodes that cannot be explained by a localized or generalized infection requires that the lymph node be excised surgically and examined by a pathologist. Whenever possible, the lymph node of choice for pathological examination should not be an inguinal lymph node, because these lymph glands are so often involved in a reaction to chronic fungal infections of the feet. If a pathologist arrives at a diagnosis of Hodgkin's disease because of the histological pattern of the lymph node, the clinician has the responsibility to evaluate the extent of involvement of the disease, the procedure defined as staging. Staging is especially important in Hodgkin's disease because it determines the approach to treatment. The system of staging for Hodgkin's disease follows the numerical outline described in Table 24-1.

Considerable staging can be obtained by a careful physical examination and simple laboratory information, such as x-ray films of the chest. These techniques enable the physician to identify superficial lymph node involvement, the presenting sign of Hodgkin's disease in by far most cases, to determine whether mediastinal lymph nodes are involved and, if so, whether the disease has extended to involve the lung parenchyma. More elaborate tests such as computed tomography, magnetic resonance imaging, and radioactive gallium scanning are required to evaluate whether the disease involves lymphoid tissue in the abdomen as well.

The test most frequently employed, however, is the *lymphangiogram*. Radiopaque contrast material is injected into the lymphatics of the foot in the webbing between the first and second toes. The dye courses up the lymphatic channels of the legs, enters the pelvic system, converges in the channel surrounding the aorta, then into the mediastinum, and eventually into the thoracic duct. A series of x-ray films of the pelvis and abdomen taken over a period of hours reveals in the normal case opacification of lymph nodes encountered by the path of the contrast dye. Lymph nodes showing tumor involvement are recognized by enlargement and by regions within them that do not opacify with the dye. Aberrant flow of the dye is also observed, an indication of obstruction of the lymphatic channel by the Hodgkin's disease.

The neoplastic proliferation that characterizes Hodgkin's disease can be eradicated by means of sufficient doses of ionizing radiation. Furthermore, when localized, the disease spreads by regional extension to adjacent lymph node regions. Therefore, radiation directed at involved lymph nodes and others surrounding it can cure the localized Hodgkin's disease in a large proportion of cases. Following the initial cures of Hodgkin's disease with radiation therapy, investigators wanted to establish with greater certainty whether abdominal lymph nodes were involved and to determine whether Hodgkin's disease had invaded the spleen in order to plan optimal treatment. An exploratory laporatomy was used to obtain this information. During the operation, the surgeon palpated the para-aortic and pelvic lymph node regions and removed any palpable lymph nodes for biopsy. The surgeon then excised the spleen and a sample of liver for histological examination. The spleen was cut into multiple sections and examined by the pathologist for gross and microscopic foci of Hodgkin's disease. For Hodgkin's disease arising in cervical lymph nodes and shown by the staging procedures not to involve the abdomen or mediastinum, radiation would customarily be delivered to both sides of the neck, the axillae, and the mediastinum. This radiation field, called an upper mantle (Fig. 27-2), would serve to treat the obvious disease and the regions to which it most likely would have spread. Even when Hodgkin's disease was more widespread, for example, in stages II or III disease, more extended radiation fields involving the upper mantle and the para-aortic and pelvic nodal regions were potentially sufficient to be curative in a substantial number of cases.

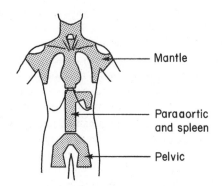

Fig. 27-2. Radiation fields.

In addition to being susceptible to radiation, Hodgkin's disease will melt away dramatically, and often permanently, in response to a variety of chemotherapeutic agents (Ch. 21). The chemotherapy regimen called MOPP, the acronym for six cycles of a combination of *m*echlorethamine (nitrogen mustard) 6 mg/m^2 intravenous, days 1 and 8, vincristine (*O*ncovin) 1.4 mg/m^2 intravenous, days 1 and 8, *p*rocarbazine 100 mg/m^2 orally, days 1 through 14, and *p*rednisone 40 mg/m^2 orally, days 1 through 14 for the first and fourth treatment cycles, was the first to induce cures of a lymphoproliferative malignancy. MOPP and other combinations of drugs, such as ABVD for doxorubicin (*A*driamycin) 25 mg/m^2 intravenous, *b*leomycin 10 mg/m^2 intravenous, *v*inblastine 6 mg/m^2 intravenous, and *d*acarbazine 375 mg/m^2 intravenous, all on days 1 and 15, can induce complete remissions, and even cures, in more than one-half the patients whose disease recurs after radiation therapy. They can also be used with curative outcome in patients in whom the disease is too widespread (for example, in stage IV) for radiation to be useful, and they can be used repeatedly to salvage patients whose disease has relapsed. Current research is directed toward identifying optimal regimens and doses of these combinations.

In light of the foregoing, one may well ask why it is necessary to resort to complex staging procedures. Why not simply deliver radiation to all node-bearing areas and treat with chemotherapy? The answer to this question lies in the toxicity of the treatment, which is proportional to the amount of treatment given. The side effects of anticancer therapy are described in Chapter 21. However, the most problematic complications of the treatment of Hodgkin's disease are derangements in immunological function and, especially, leukemogenesis. The susceptibility to infection with high-grade encapsulated organisms of patients subjected to staging splenectomy and a combination of chemotherapy and radiation for Hodgkin's disease is well known. Both ionizing radiation and anticancer drugs, especially alkylating agents, have the capacity to induce leukemia. The incidence of acute leukemia, usually of the acute granulocytic type, is disturbingly high in patients treated for Hodgkin's disease with chemotherapy. The incidence of leukemia and other neoplasms begins at about 5 years after completion of treatment, is proportional to the amount of chemotherapy given, and is higher in patients with more advanced stages. Interestingly, patients who undergo splenectomy have a higher risk of secondary neoplasms than patients with intact spleens. Other complications of treatment for Hodgkin's disease include infertility, accelerated osteoporosis in hypogonadal female patients, and thyroid diseases, such as Graves hyperthyroidism, thyroid ophthalmopathy, hypothyroidism, and thyroid cancer.

It can be appreciated, therefore, that the clinician is faced with some difficult decisions concerning the managment of Hodgkin's disease. The staging laparotomy remains useful for verifying that patients who by physical examination and radiographic analyses seem to have minimal disease and are candidates for cure by radiation therapy alone really have early stage disease. The laparotomy, however, is now recommended for relatively few patients. For example, certain subsets of patients with clinically apparent minimal disease rarely have positive laparotomies. These include patients with disease limited to above the cricoid cartilage, patients with clinical stage I disease and lymphocyte-predominant

histology, patients with clinical stage 1A nodular disease with nodular sclerosis histology, and patients with isolated inguinal or iliac Hodgkin's disease. Conversely, for patients who have large mediastinal adenopathy (large being defined as occupying more than a third of the thoracic volume), hilar adenopathy, or B symptoms, the chance of more widespread disease is sufficiently great that many clinicians advocate chemotherapy with radiation to the large disease masses, and the laparatomy adds nothing to the management.

It is somewhat controversial just how much treatment to deliver to a Hodgkin's disease patient with stage III or with bulky stage I or II disease. Chemotherapy is obviously required for stage IV lesions. The treatment guidelines ordinarily dictated by the anatomical extent of Hodgkin's disease may be modified by the histological pattern of a given case. Mixed cellularity or nodular sclerosis morphologies are considered more aggressive than the lymphocyte-predominant morphology. Radiation therapy combined with intensive chemotherapy regimens is very hard on patients, although as in the treatment of acute leukemia, hematopoietic growth factors and stem cells are helping to ameliorate the resulting bone marrow suppression. Clinical researchers are continuously evaluating new combinations to obtain the most effective approach with the fewest complications. Precisely definable treatment recommendations are not available for all situations and are modified as more experience is obtained with different combinations of treatment.

Another challenge in the management of Hodgkin's disease is the treatment of relapsed disease or of patients who do not achieve complete remissions following initial therapy. Approaches to these problems include the use of very high doses of cytotoxic drugs active against Hodgkin's disease with or without localized or total body irradiation followed in some cases by autologous bone marrow transplantation (Ch. 32). Once again, cytokines that stimulate the bone marrow and infusions of stem cells help to reduce the toxicity of such treatment, although damage to various organs and a small incidence of veno-occlusive disease remain serious problems.

SUGGESTED READINGS

Bookman MA, Longo DL (1986) Concomitant illness in patients treated for Hodgkin's disease. Cancer Treat Rev 13:77

Cannellos GP, Anderson JF, Propert KJ et al (1992) Chemotherapy of advanced Hodgkin's disease with MOPP, ABVD, or MOPP alternating with ABVD. N Engl J Med 327:1478

Desch CE et al (1992) The optimal timing of autologous bone marrow transplantation in Hodgkin's disease patients after a chemotherapy relapse. J Clin Oncol 10:200

DeVita VT, Jr, Hubbard JM (1993) Hodgkin's disease. N Engl J Med 328:560

Dürkop H, Latza U, Hummel M et al (1992) Molecular cloning and expression of a new member of the nerve growth factor receptor family that is characteristic for Hodgkin's disease. Cell 68:421

Hagemeister FB et al (1990) NOVP: a novel chemotherapeutic regimen with minimal toxicity for treatment of Hodgkin's disease. Semin Oncol 17:34

Hancock SL, Cox RS, McDougall IR (1991) Thyroid diseases after treatment of Hodgkin's disease. N Engl J Med 325:599

Hodgkin T (1832) On some morbid appearances of the absorbent glands and spleen. Tr Med Chir Soc Glasgow Vol XVII.

Urba WJ, Longo DL (1992) Hodgkin's disease. N Engl J Med 326:678

Levitt SH et al (1992) The role of radiation therapy in Hodgkin's disease: experience and controversy. Cancer 70:693

Tourani JM et al (1992) High-dose salvage chemotherapy without bone marrow transplantation for adult patients with refractory Hodgkin's disease. J Clin Oncol 10:1086

28

Non-Hodgkin's Lymphomas

The non-Hodgkin's lymphomas are a group of diseases resulting from the clonal proliferation of lymphoid cells as solid tumors in lymphoid organs and other tissues. Most of these diseases at some point in their evolution have malignant cells in the peripheral blood or bone marrow causing them to overlap in definition with acute and chronic lymphocytic leukemias.

The classification of these disorders is difficult because anatomical, histological, and immunological characterizations do not always pigeonhole these disorders into clinically useful terms. The dominant approach today is to define non-Hodgkin's lymphoma according to its histological appearance and its clinical features and, whenever possible, to supplement this information by identifying the type of lymphocyte involved in terms of its immunological phenotype (e.g., B cell or T cell), by detection of chromosomal translocations characteristic of certain lymphoma types, and by the expression of oncogenes or fusion genes that can be sensitively assayed by the polymerase chain reaction.

Histology is the mainstay of the initial diagnosis, and therefore it is essential that the pathologist have a generous and well-preserved tissue specimen, preferably obtained by surgical biopsy. In examining lymph node biopsy specimens, the pathologist looks for effacement of the normal architecture of the lymph node by a monotonous infiltrate of cells. The cell size is noted, and the lymphoma is broadly grouped into a *small cell* or *large cell* class. When the cells of the lymphoid neoplasm are very large and have vacuolated nuclei with multiple large nucleoli, the lesion is said to be a large cell lymphoma.

The pathologist notes whether the cells have a tendency to form nodules reminiscent of germinal follicles in the normal lymph nodes or the white pulp of the spleen; if this is the case, the lesion is called *nodular* or *follicular* lymphoma (Fig. 28-1A). If the cells do not arrange to form such nodules, the pattern is described as *diffuse* lymphoma (Fig. 28-1B). The pathologist further describes the morphology of the neoplasm in terms of its *differentiation*. When the neoplastic cells look somewhat like typical small lymphocytes, the pathologist refers to them as *well-differentiated* lymphocytic cells. When the morphology of the lymphocytes departs from this basic description, the lesion is said to be *poorly differentiated*. The nuclei of the lymphocytes of some lymphomas have predominant infoldings and cleavages, and the descriptive terms *cleaved* or *uncleaved* accompany the diagnosis. Additional morphological features of the neoplastic cells, such as the presence of fine projections, can also be important.

Most non-Hodgkin's lymphomas are B-cell malignancies. This conclusion is based on the detection of homogeneous immunoglobulin on the outer surface of the membranes of the neo-

413

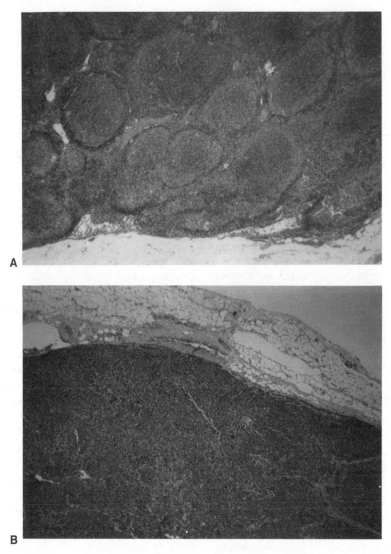

Fig. 28-1. (**A**) Nodular non-Hodgkin's lymphoma. (**B**) Diffuse non-Hodgkin's lymphoma, intermediate grade.

plastic cells, and these immunoglobulins bear either all κ or all λ light chains. The surface immunoglobulin is usually of the IgM and IgG classes. The staining of surface immunoglobulins is greater on cells of the lymphomas than it is on the cells found in chronic lymphocytic leukemia. As described in Chapter 24, B-cell lymphomas express clonal immunoglobulin gene rearrangements.

Over the years, several systems for classifying non-Hodgkin's lymphoma have been pro-

posed, and some bear the names of their founding pathologists, such as Rappaport or Lukes and Collins, or where the classification was made, as in the Kiel (Germany) classification. To varying degrees, the classifications use the morphological characteristics such as cell size, differentiation, and nuclear cleavage described above. This chapter follows a classification arising from a U.S. National Cancer Institute panel called the *Working Formulation for Clinical Usage.* A comparison of this approach with the older systems appears in Table 28-1.

In general, the degree of malignancy, defined as rapidity of growth and lethality, also termed *grade,* increases from the top to the bottom of the table. It is worth noting that the identification of tumor types in general and lymphomas in particular from histological specimens can be difficult. When pathologists experienced in lymphoma diagnosis were given each other's specimens to re-examine, they agreed concerning the specific classification in about 75 percent of cases; this 25 percent of non-concordance was even documented when the pathologists looked at slides they themselves had previously diagnosed! Therefore, if a lymphoma does not behave clinically as it should according to its classification, it may be misclassified.

TYPES OF LYMPHOMA ACCORDING TO THE WORKING FORMULATION

Low-Grade Non-Hodgkin's Lymphoma

The neoplastic cells of these diseases either have the morphology of small "mature" lymphocytes (*small lymphocytic* or *plasmacytoid cell lymphoma*) or else tend to aggregate into nodules resembling the follicles of lymph nodes (*follicular small cleaved cell lymphoma*). The nodule-forming tumors presumably originated in normal germinal follicles, whereas the diffuse lesions may arise from B lymphocytes residing in the medullary regions of lymph nodes. The surface markers of the small lymphocytic variety of disease resemble those found on B-cell chronic lymphatic leukemia cells, namely, weak expression of surface immunoglobulin, C3 and Fc receptors; class II major histocompatibility complex (MHC) antigens; B-cell antigens CDI9, 20, and 21; and the T-cell marker CD5. The other two variants of low-grade non-Hodgkin's lymphoma express larger amounts of surface immunoglobulin as well as Ia, CD19, and CD20 antigens. Unlike the small lymphocytic type, however, the common acute lymphoblastic leukemia antigen (CALLA) is usually expressed and CD5 is not.

Chromosomal anomalies are frequent in low-grade lymphomas. One of the most common is a t(14;18) [q32q21] translocation. Because the gene encoding the immunoglobulin heavy chain resides in the affected region of chromosome 14, it is presumed that the neoplastic transformation is somehow associated

Table 28-1. Classification Schemes for Non-Hodgkin's Lymphoma Cell Types

Working Formulation	Lukes/Collins Classification	Rappaport Classification
Low-grade lymphomas		
Small lymphocytic	Small lymphocytic	Difffuse well-differentiated
Follicular small cleaved	Small cleaved follicular center cell	Nodular poorly differentiated
Follicular, mixed small and large cleaved	Small and large cleaved follicular center cell	Nodular mixed
Intermediate-grade lymphomas		
Follicular large	Large/small cleaved follicular	Nodular histiocytic
Diffuse small cleaved	Small, cleaved, diffuse follicular center	Diffuse poorly differentiated
Diffuse mixed small and large	Small, large, cleaved, noncleaved, follicular center, diffuse	Diffuse mixed
Diffuse large	Large, cleaved, noncleaved, follicular center diffuse	Diffuse histiocytic
High-grade lymphomas		
Large, immunoblastic	Immunoblastic sarcoma	Diffuse histiocytic
Lymphoblastic	Convoluted T-cell	Lymphoblastic
Small, noncleaved	Small, noncleaved follicular center	Diffuse undifferentiated Burkitt's
Small, noncleaved	Small, noncleaved follicular center	Diffuse undifferentiated non-Burkitt's

with the rearrangements occurring in this gene during normal B-cell development. In the translocation a locus known as *bcl-2* moves into the Ig heavy chain locus, and the gene product of *bcl-2* is produced in much larger amounts in neoplastic B cells than in normal mature B cells. The protein encoded by *bcl-2* in cells resides at the inner membrane of mitochondria and somehow prolongs the life of the cell.

The low-grade lymphocytic lymphomas, like Hodgkin's disease, tend to arise in lymph nodes and can be slow in growth. They differ from Hodgkin's disease, however, in that they are nearly disseminated at the time of diagnosis. In other words, staging workup procedures will frequently detect disease in areas beyond the region of initial presentation. Like B-cell chronic lymphatic leukemia, low-grade B-cell lymphomas can transform from an indolent to a more aggressive state, resembling the large cell lymphoma described below. This evolution presumably is an expression of the inherent genetic instability of cancerous cells and represents the outgrowth of a cell clone that proliferates more rapidly and is more invasive than the tumor from which it originated. Interestingly, transgenic mice expressing a *bcl-2* gene overexpressing *bcl-2*, in the way the human lymphoma cells with t(14;18) translocation do, had hyperplastic lymphoid follicles and after 7 to 14 months developed high-grade lymphomas.

Intermediate Grade Non-Hodgkin's Lymphoma

The intermediate grade lymphomas progress more rapidly than the low-grade neoplasms. *Follicular large cell lymphomas* express many of the markers associated with the low-grade neoplasms, although surface immunoglobulin is found in only 65 percent of cases. The *diffuse small cleaved cell lymphoma* variant resembles the follicular counterpart in having large amounts of surface immunoglobulins, MHC class II, CD19, CD20, and CD2 antigens. The *diffuse mixed* and *diffuse large cell lymphomas* are more heterogenous. Ninety percent

of the diffuse large cell neoplasms bear some B-cell markers, but in various combinations. In addition, 10 percent have only T-cell markers. Some cases have been observed to have a chromosomal translocation involving chromosome 10 t(10;14)(q24;q32) in which the immunoglobulin gene locus transposes to a gene called *lyt-10*, which encodes a protein that resembles a transcription factor NF-κB originally shown to enhance immunoglobulin κ light chain production. Since other oncogenes are homologous with NF-κB, *lyt-10* may be the oncogene responsible for these types of lymphoma.

High-Grade Non-Hodgkin's Lymphoma

The *large cell immunoblastic lymphomas* are a partial exception to the rule that the non-Hodgkin's lymphomas are usually disseminated at the time of presentation. Up to 40 percent of these tumors may be localized at initial diagnosis; they are also the type most frequently found outside of lymph nodes, such as in the bones, central nervous system, and gastrointestinal tract. This is also the lymphoma type that most often arises in patients who are immunosuppressed, for instance in patients with acquired immunodeficiency syndrome (AIDS) or who are pharmacologically immunocompromised following organ transplantation. The lymphomas of these patients have the *myc* oncogene associated with the immunoglobulin gene locus. Patients with large cell lymphomas whose cells show duplications of chromosome 3p and who lack *bcl-2* rearrangements have the best prognosis. The tumor cells of AIDS patients with large cell lymphoma also usually express Epstein-Barr virus (EBV) proteins, and it has been suggested that this infection preceded the clonal expansion of the tumor cells, implicating the infection in the pathogenesis of the lymphoma.

The *T-cell immunoblastic lymphomas* are distinguishable from the B-cell large cell lymphomas described in the previous paragraph in having markers and clinical behavior more closely resembling the T-cell acute lymphatic

leukemias. The cells express terminal deoxynu-
cleotidyltransferase activity and a variety of T-
cell markers, although the marker phenotype
tends to be more mature than that found in T-
cell acute lymphatic leukemia, and the common acute lymphoblastic leukemia surface
antigen is only found in 40 percent of cases.
The lymphoblastic lymphoma also mimics T-
cell acute leukemia in presenting as mediastinal adenopathy.

The disorders grouped in the Working
Formulation as *small non-cleaved lymphomas*,
often called *Burkitt's lymphomas*, are among
the most aggressive and the most interesting.
The tumors are proliferations of relatively
small cells with round or oval nuclei and multiple prominent nucleoli. Macrophages are often
seen within the monotonous background of
malignant cells, giving the overall histological
picture an appearance described as a starry sky
when seen at low power. The cells have monoclonal immunoglobulin, usually of the IgM
type, on their surfaces, indicating a B-cell origin. It has been speculated that these cells arise
from the sites possibly of cells ordinarily found
in germinal centers of normal lymph nodes.
This disease was first described by the British
surgeon Dennis Burkitt as a tumor of the jaw of
African children living in areas endemic for
malaria. This association between malaria and
the lymphoma led Burkitt to suspect an infectious basis for the pathogenesis of the disorder.
This speculation became more intriguing when
it was learned that the affected children had
very high titers of antibody in their serum
against EBV, which, it will be recalled, infests
B cells as the causative agent of infectious
mononucleosis. This association led to the
speculation that Burkitt's lymphoma was the
result of chronic immunological stimulation by
malarial infection coupled with transforming
effects of the EBV infection.

This lymphoma is encountered infrequently
in parts of the world other than the endemic
region in Africa. The nonendemic disease is
histologically identical to the African variant,
but occurs in somewhat older children and
young adults and usually presents in the
abdominal lymph nodes rather than in the jaw.

Moreover, the association between high EBV
antibody titers is less constant. Burkitt's lymphoma is an extremely rapidly growing neoplasm; left untreated, it is fulminant and fatal.
However, as amplified below, it is sometimes
gratifyingly responsive to therapy.

The differences between the so-called
endemic (African) and sporadic varieties of
this disease are reflected in molecular terms.
First, the tumor cells in the African disease
almost invariably express C3 receptors, whereas the cells of the sporadic type do not. At the
genetic level, both varieties have a t[8,14]
translocation in which the *c-myc* oncogene on
chromosome 8 usually relocates to the heavy
chain immunoglobulin locus on chromosome
14. This dislocation of *c-myc* results in its overexpression, strongly implicating this oncogene
in the pathogenesis of the malignant process. In
a minority (20 percent) of cases *c-myc* moves
to the κ or λ light chain loci on chromosomes 2
or 22, respectively, instead of (t[2;8] and
t[8;22]). Although there is heterogeneity in the
position of the break in chromosome 8 associated with these translocations, the general organization of the breaks is characteristic for either
the endemic or sporadic types of the disease. In
the endemic variety of this lymphoma, the so-
called class III break point on chromosome 8 is
quite distant from the coding region of the *c-
myc* locus; in the sporadic variety, the break
point is either within (class I) or just upstream
(class II) of the *c-myc* locus. In the class I and
II breaks, it is the disruption of the *c-myc* gene
per se that prevents a regulatory part of the
gene from controlling its expression. In the
class III rearrangement, enhancing elements in
the immunoglobulin gene may drive the transcription of the *c-myc* gene.

OTHER LYMPHOMAS NOT ENCOMPASSED IN THE WORKING FORMULATION

Anaplastic Large Cell Lymphoma

Anaplastic large cell lymphoma is an agres-
sive disorder in which the malignant cells

express the Ki-1 (CD30) surface antigen and frequently have t(2,5) chromosomal translocations. This disease, previously called "malignant histiocytosis," is treated like large cell lymphoma in the Working Formulation.

Diffuse Intermediate Lymphoma

Diffuse intermediate (mantle zone) lymphoma has malignant cells that tend to surround the normal follicles of lymph nodes. The cells express CD5 and frequently have t(11,14) chromosomal translocations. The disease is managed like follicular or diffuse small cell lymphoma.

MALToma

MALToma is an acronym for lymphomatous accumulations of small malignant B cells in mucosal surfaces of the gastrointestinal tract, the salivary glands, and the orbit. T cells infiltrate the lesions as well. This disease has a relatively good prognosis.

Splenic Lymphoma

In *splenic lymphoma with villous lymphocytes*, malignant B cells with spiny projections collect in the white pulp of the spleen, causing splenomegaly. This disorder is frequently associated with monoclonal gammopathies and is treated like diffuse small cell lymphomas.

Human T-Cell Leukemia/Lymphoma

Human T-cell leukemia/lymphoma virus lymphoma is endemic in southern Japan and in the Caribbean area, although sporadic cases arise elsewhere. The malignant cells are found in enlarged lymph nodes and circulate in large numbers in the blood, explaining the designation leukemia/lymphoma. An additional characteristic of this neoplasm is a propensity to produce lytic bone lesions and hypercalcemia.

The tumor is very malignant and fairly unresponsive to treatment. The cells are histologically of the large cell or "histiocytic" type and are diffusely oriented in lymph nodes. Immunologically they are T cells of the helper cell subset. It is this condition in which the evidence for a viral cause of human lymphoid neoplasia is strongest. Proviral DNA sequences of the c-type human T-cell leukemia virus (HTLV-l) have been identified in the malignant T cells. Antibodies against proteins of this virus are found in the serum of patients and in the serum of persons in endemic areas. Most importantly, the virus causes the malignant transformation of cultured human T cells. The disease is extremely aggressive and relatively resistant to antineoplastic therapy.

Hairy Cell Leukemia

Hairy cell leukemia, an uncommon lymphatic neoplasm, is characterized by the proliferation of cells having long cytoplasmic projections (Fig. 28-2). These cells are called *hairy cells*. The proliferation of cells primarily occurs within the spleen and bone marrow, causing bone marrow failure and sequestration and clearance of normal blood by the enlarged

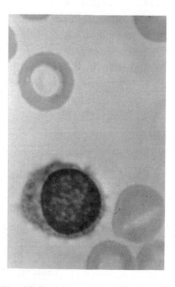

Fig. 28-2. Appearance of hairy cell.

spleen. In contrast to splenic lymphoma with villous lymphocytes, the hairy cell infiltrates reside in the red pulp of the spleen. The major manifestation of the disease is pancytopenia. Only in one-half of cases are significant numbers of hairy cells seen in the blood—so the disease is more a lymphoma than a leukemia. The cells are of B-lymphoid origin, since they express surface immunoglobulin of variable class and the surface antigen CD19. The leukemia cells in 95 percent of cases contain an enzyme that hydrolyzes phosphate esters at an acid pH, an acid phosphatase, that is resistant to inhibition by sodium tartrate. This *tartrate-resistant acid phosphatase* can be detected by a histochemical procedure; its presence is strongly suggestive of the diagnosis.

Cutaneous Lymphomas

In the *Sézary syndrome* diffuse infiltration of the skin by malignant lymphocytes occurs, leading to generalized reddening and thickening and scaling (erythroderma). Cells in the Sézary syndrome have characteristic convoluted nuclei, unusual in classic B-cell chronic lymphatic leukemia (Fig. 28-3). These *Sézary cells,* as they are called, have T-cell markers

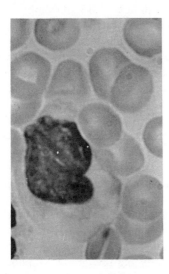

Fig. 28-3. Appearance of Sézary cell.

and T-cell functions. They lack terminal deoxyribonucleotide transferase, indicating a more mature cell structure than that of acute lymphocytic leukemia. The virus causing human T-cell lymphoma/leukemia described above was actually first isolated from a patient with Sézary syndrome. Following further study it has become evident that the association of this virus with the Sézary syndrome is unusual.

Mycosis Fungoides

Just as diffuse well-differentiated lymphoma is analogous to chronic lymphatic leukemia, there is a form of T-cell lymphoma that invades the skin but does not express a blood lymphocytosis. This disease, called *mycosis fungoides*, presents as patches of scaly nodular and ulcerative lesions on the skin. The skin lesions have a purplish hue indicative of invasion by cells in addition to the inflammatory process. Both mycosis fungoides and Sézary syndrome eventually evolve to invade the lymphoid organs and other tissues.

EFFECTS OF LYMPHOMA ON THE PATIENT

Organ Infiltration

The low-grade lymphomas tend to arise in lymph nodes and to grow slowly. Like chronic lymphatic leukemia, initially they may cause relatively few problems for the patient. Difficulties, when they occur, sometimes not for 5 to 10 years after onset of obvious disease, arise from painful enlargement of the lymph nodes and spleen or from impingement of these enlarged organs and other structures or from extension of the process directly into other organs. When the bone marrow is extensively involved, bone marrow failure can be a major difficulty. These complications emerge earlier in the intermediate- and high-grade lymphomas, consistent with the more aggressive evolution of these neoplasms. Some of the lymphomas have particular predispositions to arise in certain organs. African Burkitt's lymphoma presents as tumor of the jaw, whereas the American variant more commonly involves the abdomen. Large cell lymphoma has a greater tendency than small cleaved cell lymphoma to originate in extranodal tissues.

Paraprotein Elaboration

Some low-grade B-cell lymphomas in the spectrum ranging from chronic lymphatic leukemia to diffuse small cell lymphocytic lymphoma will express sufficient maturation toward the plasma cell to secrete monoclonal immunoglobulins. The cells sometimes, but not invariably, may have features resembling mature plasma cells. These *plasmacytoid lymphocytes* have a round, eccentric nucleus with clumps of chromatin around their periphery. The predominant immunoglobulin secreted is IgM; when significant quantities of IgM accumulate in the serum, the disease is designated *Waldenström's macroglobulinemia*. If there is a significant accumulation of excess IgM, the hyperviscosity syndrome described in Chapter 17 can arise. A principal clinical problem of patients with Waldenström's macroglobulinemia can be the presence of the IgM paraprotein, requiring treatment with plasmapheresis if the underlying neoplasm is not responsive to chemotherapy.

Some lymphoid neoplasms may generate immunoglobulin heavy chains of the μ, α, or γ class or fragments thereof without producing light chains. The neoplasms secreting μ heavy chains usually occur in elderly men and often involve nasopharyngeal lymph nodes, the liver, and the spleen. The infiltration of lymphoid tissue in the oropharynx causes a swelling of the uvula. This disease is called *μ heavy chain disease*. *α Heavy chain disease* occurs in association with abdominal or, less frequently, respiratory lymphoid proliferation, which varies in degree of differentiation and malignant appearance. The intestinal involvement causes gastrointestinal symptoms and a malabsorption

syndrome. This disorder is most frequently observed in young persons residing in the Mediterranean area and the Near East. Secretion of γ heavy chains occurs very rarely and is associated with chronic lymphatic leukemia. Other complications of non-Hodgkin's lymphomas can cause hypercalcemia mediated by elaboration of the vitamin D-related product calcitriol.

MANAGEMENT

The fundamental paradox of non-Hodgkin's lymphoma today is that the low-grade lymphomas are indolent and compatible with survival with disease for decades, yet currently these diseases are not clearly curable. In contrast, many of the high-grade lymphomas are highly aggressive, producing disability and death in months if not successfully managed, yet about half of these disorders are potentially susceptible to cure.

Knowing when and how much to treat the patient with non-Hodgkin's lymphoma remains a major challenge for clinicians. The initial staging of the patient following establishment of the diagnosis by biopsy of a lymph node or tissue infiltrate consists of bone marrow examination, computerized axial tomographic (CAT) scanning of the chest, abdomen, pelvis, and (in patients with large cell lymphoma) the brain, a [67]gallium scan, which may identify deposits of disease, and other tests as indicated by the patient's signs and symptoms. These procedures establish the extent of disease, which may determine the need for treatment or a baseline from which progression will indicate that need and provide something to monitor response to the treatments. Predilections of certain lymphomas to appear in particular organs should lead the clinician to examine those areas. Lymphoma in the epidural space implies disease in the central nervous system as well. Lymphoma in Waldeyer's ring is usually associated with gastrointestinal infiltration, and vice versa.

Generally the low-grade lymphomas, like chronic lymphatic leukemia, require relatively little treatment for long periods of time, as they cause little difficulty for the patient. When treatment is necessary, the low-grade non-Hodgkin's lymphomas are initially very sensitive to ionizing radiation and a variety of cytotoxic drugs, including corticosteroids, alkylating agents, antitubulins, anthracyclines, antimetabolites, and others such as α-interferon, as described in Chapter 21. The drugs, however, do not seem to cure the disease or even clearly alter the natural history of the diseases, which may permit the patient to live for 10 or more years. Therefore, because of the short- and long-term toxicities of the chemotherapy and radiation therapy, one common approach has been to subject patients with indolent varieties of non-Hodgkin's lymphoma to as little treatment as possible. As in the case of chronic lymphocytic leukemia, reasons for treatment include development of bulky lymphadenopathy, painful splenomegaly, anemia or thrombocytopenia, and compromise of vital organs such as airways or blood vessels. If the lymphoma is a paraprotein-secreting B-cell neoplasm causing the hyperviscosity syndrome or other complications, chemotherapy can be helpful in reducing the accumulation of the abnormal protein. Some hematologists prefer to treat patients with low-grade non-Hodgkin's lymphoma, especially younger individuals, with more aggressive combination chemotherapy and eradicate all evidence for disease; the remissions induced by such treatment can last for many years, although it is inevitable that the disease will recur.

At present, researchers are testing the hypothesis that extremely aggressive antitumor therapy directed at the "incurable" non-Hodgkin's lymphomas, such as the diffuse small cell lymphomas and even the nodular lymphomas, might in fact lead to cures. The strategies often employ allogeneic or autologous bone marrow transplantation (Ch. 32) as part of the treatment approach, which trades off the risk of treatment toxicity (including death) against the hope of long-term cure. Because of the indolent natural history of the low-grade lymphomas, it will take a long time to assess the value of this experimental treatment. Another experimental approach to the therapy of B-cell lymphomas that can be extended to B-cell leukemias as well is to take advantage of the unique structures encoded by rearranged immunoglobulin genes and expressed on the surface of the neoplastic lymphocytes to prepare tumor-specific "vaccines." Since the rearrangement-derived idiotypes are unique to the expanded neoplastic clone, they are potentially specific targets for cell-mediated immune destruction. Another innovative experimental treatment is using antibodies to B-cell antigens tagged with radioactive iodine in hopes that the radioactive "bullet" will kill the neoplastic cells.

Patients with intermediate and high-grade lymphomas often require treatment at the time of diagnosis; treatment can definitely affect the natural history of the more aggressive forms of this disease. As with the low-grade lymphomas, standard chemotherapy or radiation therapy does not appear to "cure" patients with many variants of the high-grade lymphomas, although combinations of antitumor drugs can produce durable complete remissions in a majority of cases.

In contrast to the low-grade lymphomas, the large cell, the mixed large and small cell, and the small noncleaved cell lymphomas are potentially curable with chemotherapy. Even patients with human immunodeficiency virus (HIV) disease in whom large cell lymphomas arise frequently can be cured, provided that they are not already debilitated by AIDS. In some instances, particularly when there is localized disease or extremely bulky tumors, radiation therapy is also utilized. As in the treatment of many hematological neoplasms, combinations of antineoplastic drugs are employed. A regimen named CHOP, consisting of the alkylating agent cyclophosphamide, the anthracycline doxorubicin, the antitubulin vincristine, and the corticosteroid prednisone, for example, can induce complete remissions of sufficient duration to justify the term "cure" in about half of appropriately selected patients. Presumably this favorable outcome occurs in part because highly malignant neoplasms may

Table 28-2. Correlation of Number of Risk Factors with Survival

Number of Risk Factors	Complete Response Rate (%)	5-Year Survival (%)
0, 1	87	71
2	67	50
3	55	43
4, 5	44	26

have a large fraction of dividing cells that are particularly sensitive to the treatment. If the treatment is not completely successful, the disease progresses. Patients with small non-cleaved cell lymphoma and with lymphoblastic lymphoma should also receive intrathecal chemotherapy, because these tumors frequently invade the central nervous system.

By analyzing the outcome of a large number of patients with intermediate and high-grade lymphomas treated with anthracycline-containing regimens, a prognostic index has been generated. The study determined adverse risk factors, namely age greater than 60 years, stage III or IV disease, involvement of two or more extranodal sites, elevated serum lactate dehydrogenase (LDH) levels, and physical debility and correlated the number of these factors with the frequency of complete response to therapy and the probability of survival at 5 years from diagnosis (Table 28-2).

The most important factor in survival is whether initial therapy leads to a complete remission. Patients achieving complete remission who subsequently relapse have a good chance of responding to subsequent therapy. To determine how best to obtain durable remissions, researchers are offering selected patients intensive chemotherapy regimens featuring high doses of antineoplastic drugs and autologous bone marrow transplantation in which tumor cells are removed ("purged") with monoclonal antibodies. Growth factors and stem cells that maintain adequate levels of phagocytes allow patients to endure these intensive regimens.

As discussed above, low-grade non-Hodgkin's lymphomas can undergo transformation into higher grade. Rapid growth of lymph nodes, emergence of new symptoms, and appearance of malignant cells in the blood

(Fig. 28-4) are harbingers of such transformation. Application of therapies directed against de novo high-grade lymphomas to the transformed disease can in some cases eradicate the cell clone that has undergone evolution and restore the disease to its original more indolent course.

Hairy cell leukemia is responsive to a spectrum of treatments. Some patients with spleens enlarged by leukemic infiltration react to splenectomy with a marked and prolonged rise in peripheral blood counts and a fall in the number of circulating hairy cells. Hairy cell leukemia was one of the first diseases shown to be highly responsive to therapy with α-interferon. The mechanism of action of α-interferon in this instance is not clear, that is, whether it has a direct cytotoxic effect on the hairy cells, enhances host immunological reactions against the hairy cells, or promotes the differentiation of the hairy cells. Subsequently α-interferon

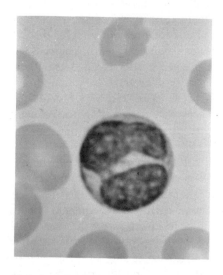

Fig. 28-4. Peripheral blood malignant cell in a non-Hodgkin's case of lymphoma in transformation.

was shown to be effective in other types of chronic lymphocytic leukemia and in other chronic leukemias. Treatment of most patients with hairy cell leukemia, in particular with adenosine deaminase inhibitors used in the therapy of chronic lymphocytic leukemia, can result in complete and sustained remissions. A circulating form of the interleukin-2 receptor shed by the malignant cells has proved to be a useful marker of response to treatment and of relapse in some cases of hairy cell leukemia.

SUGGESTED READINGS

Armitage JO (1993) Treatment of non-Hodgkin's lymphoma. N Engl J Med 328:1023

Blayney DW, Jaffe ES, Fisher RS et al (1983) The human T-cell leukemia/lymphoma virus, lymphoma; lytic bone lesions, and hypercalcemia. Ann Intern Med 98:144

Dalla-Favera R (1991) Chromosomal translocations involving the *c-myc* oncogene and their role in the pathogenesis of B cell neoplasia. In Brugge J, Curran T, Harlow E, McCormick F (eds): Origins of Human Cancer: A Comprehensive Review. Cold Spring Harbor Laboratory, Cold Spring Harbor, NY

Fisher RI, Gaynor ER, Dahlberg S et al (1993) Comparison of a standard regimen (CHOP) with three intensive chemotherapy regimens for advanced non-Hodgkin's lymphoma. N Engl J Med 328:1002

Gordon LI et al (1992) Comparison of a second-generation combination chemotherapeutic regimen (m-BACOD) with a standard regimen (CHOP) for advanced diffuse non-Hodgkin's lymphoma. N Engl J Med 327:1342

The International non-Hodgkin's lymphoma prognostic factors project (1993) A predictive model for aggressive non-Hodgkin's lymphoma. N Engl J Med 329:987

Jones SE, Miller TP, Connors JM (1989) Long term followup and analysis of prognostic factors for patients with limited stage diffuse large cell lymphoma treated with initial chemotherapy with or without adjuvant radiotherapy. J Clin Oncol 7:1186

Kaminski MS, Zasdny KR, Francis IR et al (1993) Radioimmunotherapy of B-cell lymphoma with $[^{125}I]$ anti B1 (anti .CD 20) antibody. N Engl J Med 329:459

Kwaak LW, Campbell MJ, Czerwinski DK et al (1992) Induction of immune responses in patients with B-cell lymphoma against the surface immunoglobulin idiotype expressed by their tumors. N Engl J Med 327:1209

Levine AM (1992) Acquired immunodeficiency syndrome-related lymphoma. Blood 80:8

McDonnell TJ, Korsmeyer SJ (1991) Progression from lymphoid hyperplasia to high-grade malignant lymphoma in mice transgenic for the t(14;18). Nature 349:254

Neri A, Barriga F, Inghirami G et al (1991) Epstein-Barr virus infection precedes clonal expansion in Burkitt's and acquired immunodeficiency syndrome-associated lymphoma. Blood 77:1092

Press OW, Eary JF, Appelbaum et al (1993) Radiolabeled antibody of B-cell lymphoma with autologous bone marrow support. N Engl J Med 329:1219

Saven A, Piro LD (1992) Treatment of hairy cell leukemia. Blood 79:1111

Seymour JF, Gagel RF (1993) Calcitriol: the major humoral mediater of hypercalcemia in Hodgkin's disease and non-Hodgkin's lymphomas. Blood 82:1383

Smalley RV, Andersen JW, Hawkins MJ et al (1992) Interferon alpha combined with cytotoxic chemotherapy for patients with non-Hodgkin's lymphoma. N Engl J Med 327:1336

29

Plasma Cell Neoplasms

Plasma cell neoplasms are B-cell tumors in which the predominant neoplastic cell has the morphology of plasma cells (Fig. 29-1). Although plasma cell tumors are lymphoid neoplasms, and plasma cells ordinarily exist in lymph nodes and other lymphoid organs, plasma cell neoplasia leads principally to a spectrum of diseases of the bone marrow. The spectrum ranges from an indolent plasma cell proliferation detectable only by its secreted products, monoclonal immunoglobulins or fragments thereof, a condition termed *monoclonal gammopathy of uncertain significance*, abbreviated *MGUS*, to a progressive lethal disorder called *multiple myeloma*. Approximately a quarter of patients with MGUS, some aspects of which are described in Chapter 17, eventually develop multiple myeloma. Twenty percent of plasma cell neoplasms arise in extraosseous nonlymphoid tissues, especially the upper airways, as *solitary plasmacytomas*, although a third of patients with these lesions have progression to systemic disease when followed over 20 or more years. Solitary plasmacytomas of bone also progress in 50 percent of cases followed over long periods of time. A few cases of plasma cell neoplasms progress very slowly, and these cases have been designated *"smoldering myeloma."* Only very rarely do plasma cell neoplasms involve the peripheral blood as a plasma cell leukemia, although with fluorescence-activated flow cytometry, it is possible to detect circulating neoplastic plasma cells in many patients with disseminated myelomatosis.

BIOLOGY OF PLASMA CELL NEOPLASMS

About half the cases of plasma cell neoplasms have chromosome abnormalities, including trisomy 3, 5, 9, and 15 and monosomy 13 and 16, and 80 percent of plasma cell neoplasms are aneuploid. In addition to B-cell characteristics, malignant plasma cells also express markers associated with other hematopoietic lines. The growth rates of myeloma cells in vivo are slow, and only a small fraction of cells actively divide at a given time. It has been difficult to culture malignant plasma cells. When culture has been successful, it was found that interleukin-6 is an important growth factor for the cells, and some evidence also indicates that interleukins-4 and -5 also stimulate proliferation. Further evidence for a role of interleukin-6 in the pathogenesis of multiple myeloma comes from the findings that patients with the disorder have high plasma levels of the cytokine, and that mice made to overexpress interleukin-6 developed a myeloma-like neoplastic disorder. No one genetic abnormality accounts for the neoplastic transformation of plasma cells, although high mRNA expression of H-*ras* is detectable in a majority of cases of multiple myeloma. A few other instances have high expression of *c-myc*, and *p53* mutations have been found in cases of advanced or aggressive multiple myeloma.

MULTIPLE MYELOMA

The median age of patients presenting with multiple myeloma is 62 years, although about a fifth of cases are under 50 years of age. In 99 percent of cases of multiple myeloma, the malignant cells secrete either immunoglobulins or isolated light chains; in either case, the light chains are either of the κ or λ type. The paraprotein is detectable as a serum or urine M component. Two-thirds of multiple myelomas that secrete intact immunoglobulin molecules secrete IgG; a third secretes IgA. A smaller fraction of multiple myelomas produces immunoglobulin subunits, generally light chains. Multiple myeloma is a disease of adults over age 40 with a predominance of males; the population it affects is generally younger than that affected by the paraprotein-secreting non-Hodgkin's lymphomas. It has a higher incidence in blacks than in whites.

Effects of Multiple Myeloma on the Patient

DESTRUCTION OF BONE AND BONE MARROW FAILURE

In contrast to the acute leukemias, multiple myeloma frequently causes local and generalized bone destruction evident on radiographs of the skeleton as diffuse osteopenia or as multiple lytic lesions. Lytic bone disease is particularly associated with plasma cell neoplasms that have deletions of the long arm of chromosome 6 (6q−). An x-ray film of the skull in disseminated multiple myeloma frequently exhibits what look like multiple bullet holes in the calvarium (Fig. 29-2). The bone erosion may cause the patient to suffer from back and chest pain, which becomes excruciating when the weakened bones fracture, especially the vertebrae and femurs. Vertebral fractures can lead to spinal compression and severe neurological damage. The mechanism of bone destruction appears to be elaboration by the malignant plasma cells of tumor necrosis factor, interleukin-1, and especially interleukin-6. These cytokines recruit osteoblasts and osteoclasts and uncouple the balance between bone resorption and deposition in favor of the former.

Growth of the malignant plasma cells throughout the bone marrow of multiple bones causes pancytopenia, presumably by crowding out normal hematopoietic precursors. In addition, it has been shown that hyperviscosity associated with the monoclonal gammopathies of patients with plasma cell neoplasms inhibits normal renal erythropoietin formation.

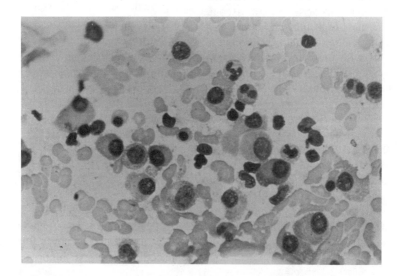

Fig. 29-1. Plasma cells in bone marrow of a patient with multiple myeloma.

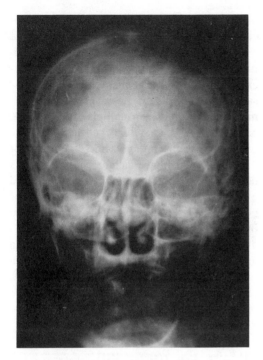

Fig. 29-2. Radiograph of the skull of a patient with multiple myeloma showing lytic bone lesions.

IMMUNODEFICIENCY

The bone marrow failure of multiple myeloma causes neutropenia, which predisposes the patient to infections with low-grade pathogens. The impairment of normal immunoglobulin production in multiple myeloma, resulting from either crowding out or suppression of normal B cells, predisposes the multiple myeloma patient to infection with high-grade encapsulated pathogens as well. Not surprisingly, bacterial infections are a frequent complication of multiple myeloma.

RENAL AND METABOLIC DERANGEMENTS

The paraprotein of multiple myeloma—particularly where the neoplasm secretes light chains that enter the urine (Bence Jones proteinuria) can damage the kidneys, leading to uremia and renal tubular acidosis (Ch. 17). Myeloma paraproteins can directly damage the renal tubules, because light chains precipitate in the tubular lumen to generate tubular casts or else are reabsorbed and accumulate within the tubular cells and impair their function. Indirect kidney damage arises by accumulation of paraprotein-derived amyloid polymers (Ch. 17). Susceptibility of patients with multiple myeloma to infection may also lead to renal damage as a result of infections in the kidney. The renal failure and the serum protein abnormalities of myeloma can cause metabolic and serum electrolyte abnormalities, such as hypercalcemia, hyperphosphatemia, an anion gap, and hyperuricemia. The destruction of bone leads to hypercalcemia; this condition is exacerbated when the patient becomes immobilized because of pain, as well as when the patient has significant renal failure. Because hypercalcemia itself can damage the renal tubules, a vicious cycle ensues. In an effort to evaluate the cause of renal failure in patients with myeloma, the kidney disease has sometimes been made worse by infusions of radiologically opaque dyes for intravenous pyelography or other contrast studies. Relative dehydration of the patient to improve the contrast effect and the high osmolarity of the dye can lead to acute tubular necrosis. Uremia impairs platelet function and red blood cell formation. Thus the renal complications of multiple myeloma can exacerbate the effects of bone marrow failure in causing anemia and hemorrhage.

As described in Chapter 17, immunoglobulins, especially IgM and IgA, can produce a hyperviscosity syndrome. Patients with multiple myeloma can have this problem, although it is more prevalent in Waldenström's macroglobulinemia. A minority of myeloma paraproteins are associated with effects related to specific binding to antigens. Most often, the antigen is a normal immunoglobulin variable domain, in which case the paraprotein can be considered anti-idiotypic. Cases have been described in which the myeloma protein reacted with riboflavin, resulting in yellowing of the skin, with peripheral nerve myelin, causing neuropathy, with insulin resulting in hypoglycemia, or with myocytes to induce muscle hypertrophy. When hyperviscosity is present, it can contribute to cardiac ischemia. In addition, a high-output cardiac failure syndrome has been described in patients with multiple myeloma, and the basis of this complication is not understood. The rare POEMS syndrome, described in Chapter 17, in which polyneuropathy, endocrine failure, hepatosplenomegaly, lymphadenopathy, peripheral edema, and skin and eye changes are associated with a monoclonal gammopathy, arises in the setting of plasma cell neoplasia. Unlike multiple myeloma, however, the plasma cell process associated with POEMS syndrome or with peripheral neuropathy alone usually has osteosclerotic rather than osteolytic bone changes. The prognosis with treatment (see below) is better for these diseases than for multiple myeloma.

Diagnosis

Suspicion of a diagnosis of frank multiple myeloma is raised by the symptoms of bone pain, pallor, and possible bacterial infections in a middle-aged or elderly person. The findings of anemia, rouleau formation, proteinuria, hypercalcemia, uremia, lytic bone lesions, and pathological fractures are highly suggestive of the diagnosis. Magnetic resonance imaging may detect bone marrow infiltrates not visualized by other radiographic procedures. Solitary plasmacytomas may present as soft tissue masses in the upper airway or in bone, where they can cause pathological fractures.

Distinguishing overt multiple myeloma from monoclonal gammopathy of uncertain significance can be difficult. Table 29-1 lists major and minor criteria of multiple myeloma: One major and one minor criterion or three minor criteria, one of which must be increased

plasma cells in the bone marrow and a monoclonal globulin spike, establish a diagnosis of multiple myeloma. Since the plasma cell infiltration of the bone marrow can be patchy, several examinations of the marrow may be necessary to solidify the diagnosis. In isolated plasmacytomas or indolent multiple myeloma, the paraprotein may be present, but the bone marrow sample can be normal. Other indications of disseminated myeloma include circulating cells bearing cytoplasmic immunoglobulins detected by fluorescence-activated cell sorting of peripheral blood, detectable β_2-microglobulin in the plasma, and elevations of lactate dehydrogenase (LDH). The levels of paraprotein and β_2-microglobulin in the patient give a rough idea of the mass of tumor present, and changes in these levels are indications of the progression of the disease.

Treatment

Indolent multiple myeloma or monoclonal gammopathy of uncertain significance requires no treatment. About half of patients with localized disease, as evidenced by negative radiographic studies (computerized axial tomography, magnetic resonance imaging, and radiographs of the skeleton), absence of circulating cells containing cytoplasmic immunoglobulins, and normal immunoglobulin levels can be cured by local radiation therapy alone, and the rest may have long periods without evidence of new lesions. Patients with slowly progressive or smoldering myeloma do not benefit from early treatment. Rapidly rising serum or uri-

Table 29-1. Diagnostic Criteria

Major
1. Tissue plasmacytoma
2. > 30% plasma cells in bone marrow
3. > 3.5 g/dl IgG or > 2 g/dl IgA monoclonal M components; > Ig/24-h excretion of λ or κ light chains in the urine

Minor
A. 10–30% plasma cells in bone marrow
B. Monoclonal M component or urinary light chain excretion at lower levels
C. Skeletal lytic lesions
D. Serum (normal polyclonal) IgM < 50 mg/dl, IgA < 100 mg/dl, IgG < 600 mg/dl

nary paraprotein levels and the onset of signs and symptoms caused by the neoplasm are indications for therapy. Symptomatic myeloma generally means that the tumor mass consists of 10^{11} to 10^{12} malignant cells.

Treatment is directed against the diffuse disease, against local lesions that are troublesome, and toward supportive medical care. Staging of the disease is important for determining prognosis and for identifying patients who might benefit from experimental therapies. Factors associated with poor responsiveness to chemotherapy, rapidity of relapse, or short survival include dense plasma cell infiltration in the bone marrow, high circulating paraprotein (IgG > 70 g/L, IgA > 50 g/L, or > 12 g light chain excretion in the urine/24 hr), high LDH and β_2-microglobulin levels (> 6 mg/L), marked anemia (hemoglobin < 85 g/L), low serum albumin level (< 30 g/L), hypercalcemia (> 3 mM), renal failure, and overexpression by the malignant cells of c-H-*ras*.

Only chemotherapy can influence the progression of disseminated multiple myeloma. A standard chemotherapeutic regimen for this disorder is a combination of an alkylating agent, usually phenylalanine mustard (melphalan) 9 mg/m^2 with a corticosteroid (prednisone) 80 mg, both by mouth for 4 successive days every 28 days until a desired clinical response has been achieved. Over half the patients treated in this manner have a partial remission lasting months to even years. Remission is indicated by partial or complete healing of bone lesions, by improvement in anemia and other manifestations of bone marrow failure, and by diminution or disappearance of the paraprotein. The last-named is an especially useful marker for evaluating the effectiveness of treatment and for heralding the onset of relapse. These effects of treatment certainly improve the quality of life of myeloma sufferers, but the therapy does not arguably affect overall survival. Since multiple myeloma also responds to the other chemotherapeutic agents described in Chapter 19, investigators have attempted to induce more robust remissions and possibly cures with more aggressive regimens than the standard

approach mentioned above; relatively little improvement in remission rates and survival has emerged. Intensive corticosteroid therapy in the form of high doses of dexamethasone is an example of this approach. One justification to apply more intensive treatment, which may reduce the tumor mass more rapidly than standard therapy, is life-threatening pancytopenia or renal disease. Young patients with suitable bone marrow donors have been cured by bone marrow transplantation (Ch. 32), but this modality is currently only appropriate for a minority of patients with this disease. The evidence for involvement of interleukin-6 in the biology of multiple myeloma has led investigators to treat a few patients with advanced disease with monoclonal antibodies against this cytokine. Responses were observed, suggesting that this approach deserves further research.

When chemotherapy is not effective, radiation can be helpful to reduce tumor masses in painful bone lesions and in palliating pathological fractures. General medical measures such as red cell transfusions for anemia, antibiotics for infection, and maintenance of adequate hydration to maximize renal function are important. In patients in whom renal damage is severe or permanent, but in whom chemotherapy is expected to yield a reasonable life expectancy, manifestations of kidney failure can be controlled by means of dialysis therapy. Infusions of recombinant erythropoietin reduce the requirement for red blood cell transfusions in patients anemic because of chemotherapy.

Hypercalcemia can be an especially troubling complication of multiple myeloma, especially because it causes obtundation and even coma and because it predisposes to and exacerbates renal disease. The management of hypercalcemia begins with hydration and diuretics, which may enhance calcium excretion sufficiently to control the metabolic problem. More resistant hypercalcemia may respond to corticosteroids and the hypocalcemia-producing hormone calcitonin or the antitumor antibiotic mithramycin, which may act by inhibiting osteoclast function. Mithramycin, however, must be used cautiously because it causes thrombocytopenia. Diphosphonate compounds are being investigated for a role in the control of hypercalcemia as well as for reduction of osteopenia associated with multiple myeloma.

SUGGESTED READING

Barlogie B (1992) Multiple myeloma. Hematol Clin North Am 6 (2)

Barlogie B, Epstein J, Selvanayagam P, Alexanian R (1989) Plasma cell myeloma—new biological insights and advances in therapy. Blood 73:865

Battaile R, Sany J (1981) Solitary myeloma: clinical and prognostic features of a review of 114 cases. Cancer 48:845

Cavo M, Galieni P, Zuffa E et al (1989) Prognostic variables and clinical staging in multiple myeloma. Blood 74:1774

Cohen DJ, Sherman WH, Osserman EF, Appel GB (1984) Acute renal failure in patients with multiple myeloma. Am J Med 76:247

Farhangi M (1986) Plasma cell myeloma and myeloma proteins. Semin Oncol 13:1

Gahrton G et al (1991) Allogeneic bone marrow transplantation in multiple myeloma. N Engl J Med 325:1267

Klein B et al (1991) Murine anti-interleukin-6 monoclonal antibody therapy for a patient with plasma cell leukemia. Blood 78:1198

Kyle RA (1975) Multiple myeloma: review of 869 cases. Mayo Clin Proc 50:29

Miralles GD, O'Fallon JR, Talley NJ (1992) Plasma-cell dyscrasia with polyneuropathy. The spectrum of POEMS syndrome. N Engl J Med 327:1919

Neri A, Baldini L, Troca D et al (1992) *p53* gene mutations in multiple myeloma are associated with advanced forms of malignancy. Blood 81:128

Osterberg A, Björkholm M, Björeman M et al (1993) Natural interferon-α in combination with melphalan/prednisone versus melphalan/prednisone in the treatment of multiple myeloma Stages II and III. Blood 81:1428

Singh A et al (1993) Increased plasma viscosity as a reason for inappropriate erythropoietin formation. J Clin Invest 91:251

Suematsu S et al (1989) IgG1 plasmacytosis in interleukin 6 transgenic mice. Proc Natl Acad Sci USA 86:7547

30

Immune Destruction
of Blood Cells

GENERAL PRINCIPLES

The destructive potential of the immune system is ordinarily directed against foreign microorganisms. When blood cells from one person are purposefully or accidentally infused into another genetically unrelated person, components on the cell surface, antigens, may be recognized as foreign and fall prey to the immune mechanisms. Such immune reactions generated by humans against other humans are called *isoimmune* reactions; the antibodies produced by humans against the blood cells of other humans are called *isoantibodies*. Isoantibodies limit the survival of transfused blood cells, and the destruction of transfused blood cells can produce systemic symptoms, called a transfusion reaction.

Isoantibodies may also arise from the sensitization of a mother by the blood cells of her fetus. Isoantibodies of the IgG class cross the placenta and can destroy the blood cells of the fetus. The immune system can occasionally become perverse and active against itself. This general pathological process is called *autoimmunity* (Ch. 20). Autoimmunity, or autoaggression as it was first called, can be viewed as a loss of the tolerance ordinarily possessed by the immune system for self-antigens. Blood cells are susceptible to autoimmune destruction, and the immunological reactions may be active against stem cells, erythroid cells,

platelets, lymphoid cells, phagocytes, or combinations of blood cells.

All the effector mechanisms of the immune system—antibody and complement-mediated cell lysis, antibody and complement-mediated opsonization, and lymphoid cell-mediated cell destruction—may be operative in the attack on normal blood cells. Antibodies directed against self-antigens are called *autoantibodies*. Autoimmune blood cell destruction is said to be primary if it occurs in the absence of other diseases known to affect the immune system. Otherwise, the autoimmune disorder is designated secondary. Clearly there must be some reason for the onset of autoimmunity in the primary setting, but the predisposing causation is simply not obvious. Frequently the onset of antibody-mediated blood cell destruction follows a viral infection, especially in children. In this setting, the autoimmune reaction may be the result of immune complexes composed of virus antigens and antibodies against these antigens. The autoimmune disorder of this type frequently remits permanently after a period of months. In older patients, in whom the onset of autoimmune blood cell destruction is less frequently preceded by an obvious infection, the disease tends to be chronic, although variable, in severity. Disorders predisposing to secondary autoimmune blood cell destruction include the congenital and acquired immunodeficiency states, collagen-vascular diseases such as systemic lupus erythematosus, and malignant lymphoid neoplasms, especially of the B-cell variety. Medications, some of which are used frequently in medical practice, are capable of inciting immune-mediated blood cell destruction by a variety of mechanisms.

MECHANISMS

Agglutination

IgM antibodies activate complement and agglutinate cells. It is possible that agglutinated blood cells become trapped in capillaries of organs rich in mononuclear phagocytes such as the liver, lungs, and particularly the spleen, where their exposure to the phagocytes and lymphoid cells that can destroy them is maximized. Agglutination is probably not a major mechanism of blood cell destruction but is a useful phenomenon for identifying the presence of IgM antibodies directed against certain blood cells.

Complement-Mediated Cytolysis

IgM and IgG antibodies can activate complement components, leading to the deposition of complement components C1 to C9, the production of membrane lesions, and loss of cytoplasmic components (Ch. 17).

Opsonization

Opsonization of blood cells leading to recognition by phagocytes is the principal and most prevalent mechanism in operation in immune-mediated blood cell destruction. The Fab region of IgG molecules binds to surface antigens of blood cells, leaving the Fc regions exposed to interact with receptors on phagocytes and lymphoid cells. The phagocytes can bind and either partially or totally engulf the antibody-coated blood cells. Total phagocytosis clears the opsonized cells from the circulation. Partial phagocytosis removes membrane

from the blood cells, reducing their volume as well as their capacity to cope with osmotic stresses.

IgG or IgM antibodies against blood cell surface antigens can bind to these antigens and activate complement, leading to the deposition of C3b, the opsonic fragment of C3 on the blood cell surface. This deposition sets the cell up for total or partial engulfment by phagocytes as well. It will be recalled that C3b is attacked by an enzyme complex, the C3b inactivator and β1H. The balance between the rates of deposition of C3b on the cell and of the rate of C3b inactivation determines, among other factors, whether the cells are susceptible to attack by phagocytes.

The phagocytes primarily involved in the destruction of blood cells are the fixed phagocytes; these macrophages of the mononuclear phagocyte system are located in the organs of clearance, where they come into intimate contact with the opsonized blood cells. The removal of blood cells by phagocytes is most efficient in the spleen, because of its sluggish flow and sievelike structure. Therefore, lightly opsonized blood cells may be destroyed primarily in the spleen, although more heavily coated cells can be removed by the Kupffer cells of the liver. Cytotoxic lymphocytes can also recognize antibody-coated target cells and lyse them.

Role of Temperature

Antibody reactions against blood cell reactions are sensitive to the ambient temperature. IgG antibody molecules against blood cell antigens almost always bind to the blood cells at 37°C, normal body temperature; they have been historically designated *warm-reacting antibodies*. IgM antibody molecules directed against blood cells often bind to the antigens better at lower temperatures; they have been historically termed *cold-reactive antibodies*. Because IgM antibodies agglutinate cells, cold-reactive antibodies have also been termed cold agglutinins. The thermal amplitude of the antibody reaction can be determined by incubating blood cells with a variety of dilutions of antibody-containing serum at different temperatures and observing the maximal dilution or titer of serum that agglutinates the cells.

Cold-reactive IgM antibodies can arise during infections. Viral infections associated with such antibodies include infectious mononucleosis caused by the Epstein-Barr virus, bacterial infections including syphilis, and infections caused by *Mycoplasma*. Occasionally, antibody-secreting lymphoid neoplasms produce monoclonal IgM antibodies in large quantities that react with blood cells at low temperatures. The practical importance of the thermal amplitude of cold-reactive antibodies is that blood cell destruction may be initiated or exacerbated by exposure of the patient to cold temperatures. The presence of antibody molecules or complement components on the surface of blood cells is a necessary condition, but it is not sufficient to cause immune-mediated blood cell destruction. Destruction of blood cells by immunoproteins requires either that the entire complement sequence leads to membrane lysis or that the Fc region of the immunoglobulin molecule, with or without participation of the third component of complement, causes the blood cell to be recognized as foreign by phagocytes or lymphocytes. Therefore, these molecules must be oriented on the blood cell surface so as to engender such recognition. When the Fab domains of IgG antibody molecules bind to blood-cell surface antigens, the Fc portions of the antibody molecules are oriented appropriately to interact with phagocyte Fc receptors or with Cl for complement activation. On the other hand, it will be recalled that B lymphocytes contain surface immunoglobulin. This immunoglobulin is presumably oriented with its Fc region buried within the plasma membrane, and therefore it will not elicit either complement fixation or recognition by phagocytes. However, the surface immunoglobulin can be detected by another antibody molecule specific for immunoglobulin. In a similar fashion, IgG antibodies bound to Fc receptors on cells also have their Fc regions masked. Therefore, only antibodies with the Fab domains apposed to blood cell surface antigens would be expected to have Fc portions free to interact with complement or phagocytic receptors. Even correctly oriented immunoglobulin molecules on blood cell membranes may fail to result in destruction of the blood cells.

Depending on the class of antibody, the propensity for destruction varies. For example, IgM usually has no direct opsonic effect but requires complement deposition for destruction of the target. The effect of complement fixation will depend on the relative rates of complement addition and inactivation. If inactivation of C3b exceeds its deposition, C3 fragments remain on the membrane of the target cell, but the fragments are incapable of fixing later complement components or of expressing opsonic activity. Finally, aggregated immunoglobulins are much more effective than dispersed immunoglobulins in eliciting complement fixation or recognition by phagocytes. Therefore, the antigen density and mobility on the blood cell surface that will influence the aggregation state of the surface molecules can determine whether or not destruction occurs. This factor explains in part why certain red blood cell antigens are more important in the transfusion setting than others.

TREATMENT

Some cases of secondary immune blood cell destruction caused by medications, neoplasms, or collagen-vascular disorders can be successfully managed by treating the underlying condition. In other cases, treatment involves the use of immunosuppressive therapy designed to reduce the concentration of immunoproteins directed against the target blood cells or to interfere with the destructive mechanisms aimed at the coated cells. There are a number of problems with such therapy, however. Initial treatment is usually the administration of corticosteroids, which impair the clearance of opsonized blood cells by mononuclear phagocytes. Even if corticosteroids are effective, their continued use is hazardous because of their potent side effects, which include excessive weight gain, causation of a diabetic state in susceptible patients, and osteoporosis.

Splenectomy is another treatment for autoimmune blood destruction. Many cases treated with splenectomy respond well to a markedly reduced dose of corticosteroids, thereby minimizing or eliminating harmful side effects. In other cases the drug can even be discontinued after surgical removal of the spleen. However, the absence of this most efficient clearance organ may permit the bone marrow production of blood cells to outstrip the rate of clearance. In this situation, instead of being cured of the autoimmune process, the patient is in a compensated state wherein the concentration of affected blood cells is maintained by a greater rate of production than normal. This elevation in blood cell turnover with its increased demand on bone marrow productivity raises the patient's requirement for folic acid and can lead to a folic acid deficiency; such patients should receive supplemental folic acid therapy. Recall that splenectomy puts people at risk for bacterial sepsis (Ch. 18).

When splenectomy and corticosteroids fail to control immunological destruction, more potent immunosuppressive drugs and other radical therapies are enlisted. The therapies include the specific immunosuppressive and more general antineoplastic agents described in Chapter 21. The ones used most frequently in addition to corticosteroids are the vinca alkaloid vincristine and the alkylating agent cyclophosphamide. Immunosuppressive drugs include cyclosporin and related compounds and antilymphocyte globulin. For reasons that are unclear, danazol, an androgenic compound with minimal virilizing activity, can diminish autoimmune blood cell destruction in some cases. Other treatments aim at saturating the clearance capacity of the mononuclear phagocyte system. In one, gamma globulin is administered intravenously in amounts sufficient to increase significantly the total plasma IgG concentration. This maneuver has been shown in some cases to decrease by mass action the binding of specific antibody-coated blood cells to macrophages and thereby to diminish the clearance of the coated cells. The amounts of pooled gamma globulin required make this

treatment very expensive. A variation of this approach is to infuse Rh-positive erythrocytes (see below) coated with anti-Rh antibodies. Although the injected red cells are gradually hemolyzed in the patient, the interaction between the iatrogenically coated cells and the mononuclear phagocyte system diverts the latter from binding and clearing the patient's own cells. In the future, monoclonal antibodies of peptides that inhibit macrophage Fc receptor binding of sensitized platelets may be useful.

SPECIFIC DISEASES OF IMMUNE-MEDIATED BLOOD CELL DESTRUCTION

Immune-Mediated Stem Cell Destruction

In a small number of cases of bone marrow failure, the pancytopenia appears to be the result of cell-mediated or antibody-mediated autoimmunity against pluripotent stem cells. The recovery of a subset of patients with aplastic anemia after immunosuppressive therapy is consistent with this hypothesis (Ch. 22), although such recovery does not rule out the possibility that the medications work directly on affected stem cells. Serum or lymphoid cells from some patients with bone marrow failure have prevented the outgrowth of erythroid or granulocyte–macrophage colonies in cultures of normal bone marrow, suggesting the presence of immunological factors capable of inhibiting hematopoiesis. The antigens on the stem cells that might be targets of immune-mediated stem cell destruction are unknown.

Immune-Mediated Red Blood Cell Destruction

PURE RED CELL APLASIA

Anemia, an absence of reticulocytes, and normal concentrations of platelets and leukocytes in the peripheral blood characterize pure red cell aplasia. This disorder displays an absence or marked diminution of red blood cell precursors in the bone marrow, yet normal numbers of megakaryocytes and granulocyte precursors. Pure red cell aplasia occurs mainly in adults and is frequently associated with neoplasms of the thymus. It is possible to document the presence of circulating complement-fixing antibodies against erythroid cells by permitting bone marrow erythroid cells to incorporate radioactive iron, mixing the bone marrow with a patient's immunoglobulin and complement, and assessing release of the radioactive iron caused by complement-mediated cell lysis. Pure red cell aplasia may respond to treatment with immunosuppressive medication, such as cyclosporin, and, when associated with thymoma, to removal of the thymic tumor.

IMMUNE HEMOLYSIS

Red Blood Cell Antigens Involved in Immune Hemolysis

The red blood cell membrane surface has more than 300 components capable of producing antibodies when injected into animals. Such antigens are designated *blood groups*. A catalog of a patient's red blood cell antigens defines the individual blood type. Only a small number of these antigens are important in immune-mediated red blood cell destruction. The most important blood groups from the standpoint of immune-mediated red cell destruction are in the *ABO system*. The antigens of this system are polysaccharides attached to red blood cell membrane lipids and proteins; each particular antigen is defined by the sugar residing at the end of the carbohydrate chain; the unmodified chain defines a weak antigen called type H. Genes that modify H to program the A and B antigens reside on the long arm of the ninth chromosome and encode for glycosyltransferase enzymes, which attach the specific terminal sugars to the oligosaccharide chains. In the case of type A, a specific enzyme puts N-acetyl-D-galactosamine on the chain; the type B transferase, which differs by only a few amino acids from the type A variant, adds D-galactose instead (Fig. 30-1). The person who has a transferase that again varies only by a small extent of structure is unable to modify the H chain and builds red cell surface glycolipids and glycoproteins containing a terminal fucose residue. This structure is the foundation on which the sugars of the A and B antigens reside in persons possessing the requisite genes. A person lacking these genes is said to have red blood cell type O. The expression of the A and B blood group genes is co-dominant, so that per-

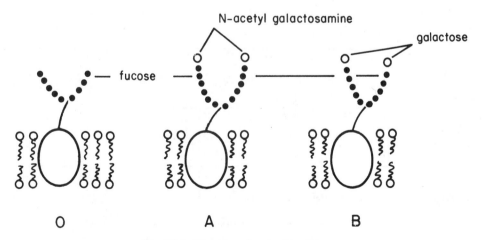

Fig. 30-1. Structure of major blood groups.

sons with the genotype AA or AO both have A antigens on their red blood cells. Similarly, persons with the genotype BB or BO express the B antigen, and those with the genotype AB possess both A and B red blood cell antigens.

The A and B red blood cell antigens are extremely effective in eliciting antibodies; the antigens are so richly endowed on the red blood cell surface that the destructive capacity of such antibodies is great. Furthermore, carbohydrate sequences identical to those found on the red blood cell antigens are widespread in nature, existing on the surface of enteric bacteria and on a variety of plant seeds and pollen. Thus, most people have antibodies in their plasma against either the A or B blood group antigens, whichever is not expressed on their own red blood cells. For example, a person who is red blood cell type A has anti-B antibodies, a person who is red blood cell type B has anti-A antibodies, and a person who is red blood cell type O has both A and B antibodies. Only the person whose red blood type is AB lacks serum antibodies against these antigens (Fig. 30-2). For this reason, persons with red blood cell types A, B, or O will not tolerate red blood cell transfusions that are not matched for these antigens. Type AB persons can theoretically accept red blood cells from persons of any type in this system, although unmatched transfusions are rarely given in practice.

About two-thirds of the population synthesize the A and B carbohydrate sequences on various body secretions. The body fluids of these secretors contain the A and B substances as well as their red blood cells. In rare circumstances an individual's ABO antigens may change. Clearly bone marrow transplantation (Ch. 32) with engraftment of cells of a different ABO type is one such instance. In other cases such as infection or malignant tumors, activities of microbial or neoplastic glycosyltransferases may be responsible. A change in ABO type has also been observed after liver transplantation, and the cause is unknown.

The next most important red blood cell antigen system is called the *Rhesus (Rh) system.* The genes coding for the expression of Rh antigens are located in the first chromosome and program a set of antigens designated C, D, E; the absence of expression of a set of these antigens (which does not mean that the protein is missing, just that it is not antigenic) is termed by convention c, d, e. The inheritance of the antigens occurs in sets, such as CDe, cde, and eDE. The Rh proteins are transmembrane lipoproteins that serve as water channels.

The D antigen is the most active of the Rh antigens in inciting antibodies. A single infusion of erythrocytes containing the D determinant into a patient who does not have this antigen (i.e., whose red cells are defined as Rh negative) is associated with a 50 percent probability that red blood cells in a subsequent infusion of this type will be destroyed.

Plasma Antibody	Anti B	Anti A	None	Anti A & B
Cell Antigens	A	B	AB	O
Genotype	AA or AO	BB or BO	AB	OO

Fig. 29-2. Blood group antigen and antibody profiles.

A variety of other antigens are occasionally of importance for immune-mediated red blood cell destruction. The structural definition of many of these antigens is unknown. Of the various red cell antigens, the *Lewis system* differs from others in that it is not produced by developing red blood cells during maturation; rather, it is taken up as glycolipid molecules from the plasma. The *Ii* system is of interest because the i antigen is expressed on fetal red blood cells. During the first year of life, its expression is reduced and is replaced by the I antigen. Autoantibodies against I or i antigens arise in certain infectious diseases and in malignant lymphoid neoplasms. The *Duffy blood group* is named for the patient in whom antibodies to it were first discovered. It is relatively commonly found on the red cells of whites but is rare in blacks. A possible basis for this difference in distribution is the finding that the Duffy antigen is the receptor to which the malaria parasite *Plasmodium vivax* binds in order to enter the red cell.

Isoimmune hemolysis in adults nearly always arises from the transfusion of imperfectly matched red blood cells. Antibodies against the A and B antigens fix complement, thereby leading to massive intravascular hemolysis and the most serious transfusion reactions. Such reactions may be associated with hypotension caused by the release of vasoactive complement fragments, as well as manifestations of serious hemolysis, hemoglobinuria, hemoglobinemia, and renal failure (Ch. 8). In such cases, the blood transfusion must be stopped immediately, blood and urine samples obtained to verify the presence of hemolysis and the specific incompatibilities, and proper supportive care to prevent and/or manage acute renal failure instituted. The principal effect of isoantibodies directed against other erythrocyte antigens is to compromise the survival of the transfused red cells. The manifestations of such reactions include fall in hematocrit and a rise in serum bilirubin levels.

Isoimmune red blood cell destruction can usually be avoided by carefully matched donors with recipients of blood transfusions.

However, such matching may be difficult when the potential recipient has an unusual blood type or requires long-term transfusion support. The latter class of patients is likely to begin to produce antibodies against antigens that are ordinarily of minor importance.

NEONATAL ISOIMMUNE HEMOLYSIS

Fetal erythrocytes that carry paternal cell surface antigens not found on the maternal erythrocytes can leak across the placenta to enter the maternal circulation; the mother is thus sensitized, causing her to produce antibodies to the paternal and fetal antigens. IgG antibodies directed against these antigens can then cross the placenta in the other direction and begin to destroy the fetal erythrocytes. All fetal erythrocyte antigens have the potential to elicit isoantibodies, but the Rh system, particularly the D antigen, is most important in this regard. The Rh antigens are highly antigenic, because antibodies against them are very destructive to erythrocytes and because, unlike some other antigens, they are not found on other body tissues that could soak up the isoantibodies and divert them from the attack on erythrocytes. The severity of hemolysis in the fetus is variable, but tends to become worse as sensitization occurs with successive pregnancies. The peripheral blood of the fetus and neonate with isoimmune hemolytic anemia shows reticulocytosis, spherocytes, and nucleated erythrocytes, explaining the name historically given this disease: *erythroblastosis fetalis*. In severe cases, the liver and spleen are enlarged and contain foci of extramedullary hematopoiesis. If the hemolysis is sufficiently serious to cause fetal hypoxia and death, the dead fetus is edematous and is said to have died of hydrops fetalis. Presumably, the principal mode of erythrocyte destruction in this setting is IgG-mediated opsonization and clearance by the mononuclear phagocyte system. Partial destruction and symmetrical membrane removal from the erythrocytes by the phagocytes are responsible for the spherocytosis that ensues. Excessive erythrocyte destruction leads to hyperbilirubinemia. In contrast to the adult, who can tolerate large quantities of unconjugated bilirubin, in the fetus and the neonate the brain, especially the basal ganglia, is damaged when the plasma bilirubin level exceeds 20 g/L for any period of time. In fatal cases, the basal ganglia are stained a brownish yellow color called *kernicterus*. Neonatal isoimmune hemolysis with kernicterus was previously a common cause of mental retardation in those infants who survived.

A mandatory element of present-day prenatal care is to check the Rh type of the maternal red blood cells. If the mother's red blood cells are negative for the presence of the RhD antigen, she is at risk for Rh isosensitization by the fetus. It is then necessary to test the mother for the development of anti-RhD antibodies during the pregnancy, although it is unusual for the anti-RhD titer to rise in a first pregnancy. A recent refinement in this management strategy is the ability to determine with safety the RhD genotype of the fetus by DNA amplification of amniotic cells.

In previous years, a rapidly rising maternal anti-RhD titer required amniocentesis, the removal of amniotic fluid by means of a needle inserted through the abdomen, and measurement of bilirubin in the fluid. A sufficiently high amniotic fluid bilirubin level might require the infusion of Rh-negative erythrocytes by a needle into the amniotic cavity. These cells would find their way into the fetal circulation and replace hemolyzed Rh-positive fetal cells. Clearly, this was a risky and invasive treatment. For infants born with erythroblastosis fetalis, a bilirubin rising to levels associated with the danger of kernicterus required the exchange of the fetal erythrocytes with RhD-negative cells by means of catheters inserted into the umbilical vessels.

Since the mid-1960s, it has been standard practice to administer an intramuscular injection of anti-Rh IgG to all Rh-negative women giving birth to Rh-positive infants. Anti-Rh IgG is prepared by injecting normal male volunteers with Rh-antigen-bearing erythrocytes. This passive immunization with anti-Rh antibodies prevents the maternal immune system from mounting an active response against any Rh-bearing erythrocytes that enter the maternal circulation. The routine immunization of mothers at risk with anti-Rh IgG has virtually eliminated isoimmune neonatal hemolytic anemia in the United States.

The erythrocyte antigens of the ABO system can also react with maternal antibodies directed against them. For example, a fetus with type B erythrocyte antigens can sensitize a mother with type A erythrocyte antigens. However, these antibodies are less problematic than anti-Rh antibodies in this setting because (1) the antibodies are usually of the IgM class, which do not cross the placenta; and (2) the carbohydrate components of the A and B antigens are present in secretions of most persons. These secretory molecules soak up IgG antibodies crossing the placenta directed against A or B sequences, thereby lowering the impact against erythrocytes. Nevertheless, mild to moderate neonatal hemolysis is occasionally ascribable to isoimmune reactions involving A and B antigens.

AUTOIMMUNE HEMOLYTIC ANEMIA

In autoimmune hemolytic anemia, the development of autoantibodies against the erythrocyte surface leads to increased erythrocyte clearance and shortened erythrocyte survival. Sometimes the antibodies are directed against the Rh antigens on the erythrocyte, but usually they attack undefined surface constituents present on all erythrocytes. All cells are coated with the autoantibodies, irrespective of cell age. Therefore, the hemolysis is persistent, and the disappearance curve of cells labeled with a marker such as radioactive chromium is exponential in nature. The shortened erythrocyte survival causes anemia and pallor. The hemolysis results in hyperbilirubinemia and attendant jaundice. The anemia and resulting hypoxia stimulate increased erythrocyte production, expressed as increased erythroid cells in the bone marrow, and a rise in the peripheral blood reticulocyte count. The destructive effect of the autoantibodies in conjunction with the mononuclear phagocytes is to remove membrane in a symmetrical fashion from the red cells, thereby resulting in the production of spherocytes. Prolonged autoimmune hemolysis is associated with the hypertrophy of macrophages in the spleen that, along with the sequestration of antibody-coated erythrocytes in the spleen, leads to splenomegaly.

Serological Procedures in Autoimmune Hemolysis

Because erythrocytes lack Fc receptors and do not synthesize immunoglobulin, antibodies on the surface of erythrocytes are nearly always oriented with their Fab regions bound to the erythrocyte-surface antigens. This positioning leaves the Fc region of the molecules available to interact with complement components or with Fc receptors on mononuclear phagocytes in the spleen or elsewhere. Therefore, the detection of IgG antibodies on the erythrocytes usually indicates that hemolysis is taking place. The presence of complement alone on erythrocytes indicates usually that IgM binding to the erythrocytes resulted in the fixation of the third component of complement. Customarily, laboratories test for the presence of IgG or C3 on erythrocytes using specific antibodies against these proteins. The erythrocytes are washed free of serum and suspended at 37°C in an isotonic salt solution to which rabbit antihuman IgG or anti-C3 is added. If the erythrocytes are coated with IgG or C3 molecules, the respective antibodies complex with them. Because the added antibodies are divalent, they have two binding sites for the antigens. They can therefore bridge the molecules coating adjacent erythrocytes and stick the red cells together. A positive reaction is therefore recognized by agglutination of the erythrocytes. The antiglobulin agglutination test is named for its originator, R.A.F. Coombs. The aggregation of a patient's erythrocytes by anti-IgG or anti-C3 is called a positive *direct Coombs test*. If the patient's serum is reacted with normal erythrocytes and agglutination is observed after the cells are washed and incubated with the anti-IgG or anti-C3, the result is a positive *indirect Coombs* test. For an indirect

test to be positive, free antierythrocyte antibodies must have been present in the patient's serum. This situation is observed in about two-thirds of cases of autoimmune hemolytic anemia.

Most cases of autoimmune hemolytic anemia are caused by IgG warm-reactive antibodies. Some of these cases follow viral infections, whereas others occur in the setting of systemic lupus erythematosus (SLE), immunodeficiency disorders, or B-cell neoplasms.

IgM cold-reactive autoantibodies are usually encountered in two settings. In patients with EBV or *Mycoplasma* infections, IgM antibodies are directed against the erythrocyte's I antigen. In this setting of infection, the antibodies may be present without overt hemolysis, or the hemolysis may be mild to moderate. The antibodies disappear once the infection is controlled. On the other hand, other patients, many of whom have, or subsequently develop, B-cell neoplasms, acquire high concentrations of IgM cold-reactive antibodies often directed against the i antigen. Hemolysis in this setting may be relatively severe and exacerbated if the patient becomes chilled. Cold-reactive antibodies are detected by reducing the temperature of a blood sample below 37°C to room temperature or less. Because IgM antibodies can agglutinate the targets with which they react, clumping of the erythrocytes at the lowered temperature reveals the presence of the autoantibodies. Blood containing cold-reactive red cell autoantibodies may show overt erythrocyte agglutination when refrigerated and is said to have *cold agglutinins*. In a rare disorder called *paroxysmal cold hemoglobinuria*, IgM cold-reactive antibodies are directed against the erythrocyte surface antigen designated P_1. Chilling of the patient is associated with severe hemolysis. Paroxysmal cold hemoglobinuria is observed as a complication of syphilis and other infectious diseases.

The treatment of autoimmune hemolytic anemia entails interference with the pathological removal of antibody-sensitized erythrocytes by inhibiting the clearance function of the mononuclear phagocytes. Corticosteroids are effective in this regard and will control the disorder in two-thirds of cases. The remaining patients require more aggressive treatment, such as splenectomy. If splenectomy proves ineffective, immunosuppressive medications may also be needed. The increased erythroid cell turnover may deplete the patient's stores of folic acid, and it is wise to give the patient folic acid supplements. As for treatment of immune-mediated blood cell destruction in general, there are a number of problems with the use of high-dose corticosteroids and splenectomy.

DRUG-INDUCED IMMUNE HEMOLYSIS

A variety of medications result in conditions that produce positive direct Coombs tests and occasionally overimmune hemolysis. Such drugs are known to act by at least three mechanisms.

In the first mechanism, a medication or its metabolites react with antibody against itself, and the medication–antibody combination binds to the erythrocyte surface. The complex sensitizes the erythrocyte to immunological destruction, usually by initiating the participation of complement. The erythrocyte has been called an innocent bystander in this reaction. The antibodies are often of the IgM class. Quinidine and quinine are examples of drugs that act in this fashion.

In the second mechanism, the medication or its metabolites bind first to the erythrocyte. The antimedication antibody, usually IgG, reacts with the cell-bound medication and sensitizes the cell for clearance. Penicillin is a drug that has this effect.

The third mechanism is a case wherein the medication or its metabolites somehow cause the patient to generate antibodies directed against erythrocyte antigens. The drug is required to generate and maintain the antibody, but it need not be present in order for the antibodies, usually of the IgG class, to bind to erythrocytes and sensitize them for immune destruction. How the medication causes the immune system to look at erythrocytes as nonself in such circumstances is unclear. Erythrocyte autoantibodies arising in the setting of treatment with alpha methyldopa, used as an antihypertension drug, is the prototype of such reactions.

Medication-associated antibodies reacting with erythrocytes need not lead invariably to hemolysis. When erythrocyte destruction is a problem, the clinical manifestations are identical to those described for autoimmune hemolytic anemia. Treatment, which is invariably effective, is to withdraw the offending medication.

Immune-Mediated White Blood Cell Destruction

The understanding of the principle that the dominant mechanism by which iso- or autoantibodies destroy blood cells is that the Fab domain of the antibody molecule binds to an antigen on the target cell surface and that the Fc region of the antigen-bound antibody then initiates a variety of effects arose primarily from laboratory studies employing red blood cells as targets of antibodies and in the clinical setting of antibody-mediated erythrocyte hemolytic disorders. Besides the ready availability of cells to study and the susceptibility of erythrocytes to complement-mediated lysis, the red cell was a suitable subject because it lacks Fc receptors. Therefore, antibodies do not ordinarily bind to erythrocytes, and the mere presence of antibody molecules on the red cell surface, detectable by the Coombs test, is strongly suggestive of a potentially destructive state. This is not the case with white blood cells that have membrane Fc receptors. White blood cells, therefore, ordinarily have immunoglobulins bound to their surfaces, and a Coombs type of assay would always report these antibodies. The detection of pathogenetically relevant immunoproteins on the white cell surface has thus depended on tests designed to bring out functions such as opsonic expression of Fc domains of cell-bound immunoglobulins or else on the ability to measure amounts of immunoglobulin above background quantities.

The complexity of the interaction between immunoproteins and erythrocytes is further compounded in the case of living white blood cells, which can process or modulate cell surface antibodies in ways that erythrocytes cannot. As shown in Figure 30-3, white blood cells reacted with antibodies against their cell surface antigens can aggregate the antigen–antibody complexes into patches. The patches coalesce to form a protuberance, or *cap*, at one pole of the cell. The cell may then either internalize the antigen–antibody complexes by endocytosis or release them into the extracellular space, a process called *shedding*. Hence, white blood cells may be capable of cleaning antibodies from their surfaces, and thereby escape immunological destruction.

A few patients with lymphopenia or subnormal immune function have been shown to possess circulating antilymphocyte antibodies. Some of these patients had SLE. Antibodies against antigens on polymorphonuclear leukocytes have been detected in the serum of neonates with neutropenia and in the serum of their mothers. The antibodies disappear from the infants' bloodstream after about 4 weeks of age, the time it takes for the infant to clear IgG, and the neutrophil counts rise at that time. This disorder, *neonatal isoimmune neutropenia*, is the equivalent of erythroblastosis fetalis. The antigen responsible for immunization in neonatal immune neutropenia is an Fc receptor that is genetically polymorphic. Some infants with neonatal isoimmune neutropenia acquire bacterial infections because of the reduction in phagocytic activity.

Autoantibodies against polymorphonuclear leukocytes can cause neutropenia. *Autoimmune neutropenia* has variable manifestations, depending on the severity of the condition. The destructive effect of antibodies may be directed against both peripheral blood granulocytes and granulocyte precursors in the bone marrow when neutropenia is profound. A wide variety of medications can cause neutropenia by means of antibodies. Some medications frequently associated with immune-mediated leukopenia are semisynthetic penicillins, sulfonamides, and thiourea antithyroid drugs.

Isoantibodies against white blood cells, sometimes called "*febrile agglutinins,*" are often invoked as a cause of febrile reactions occurring during blood transfusions that are treated with antipyretic agents, although the responsible antigens on the cells are unknown.

Immune-Mediated Platelet Destruction

DESTRUCTION OF TRANSFUSED PLATELETS

Antibodies directed against platelet surface antigens that are epitopes on platelet membrane glycoprotein IIb/IIIa (formerly known as the PLA$_1$ system) are very destructive to the platelets. However, these antigens, designated HPA 1-5, are present on platelets of more than 98 percent of persons. Therefore, antibodies against HPA antigens only rarely are a problem in platelet transfusion therapy. However, persons who lack the HPA antigen on their platelets and also receive transfusions of HPA-

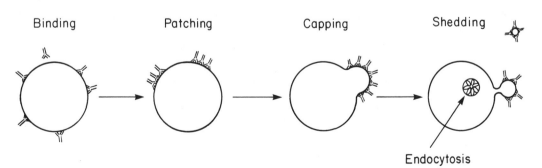

Fig. 30-3. Modulation of cell-bound antibodies by leukocytes.

bearing platelets may develop a condition called *post-transfusion purpura*. The platelets contained in whole blood transfusions are sufficient to elicit this disorder. At some time following the transfusion, the patient generates anti-HPA antibodies. These antibodies are believed to bind HPA antigen released from the transfused platelets, and the antigen–antibody complex then binds to the patient's own HPA-negative platelet. The binding of these complexes causes the destruction of the patient's platelets. The disorder is usually self-limited and remits completely, but it can occasionally be a profound and persistent cause of abnormal bleeding.

HPA-positive infants of HPA-negative mothers can sensitize the mother, and the resulting anti-HPA antibodies cause thrombocytopenia and hemorrhage in the first weeks of life. Infants with *neonatal isoimmune thrombocytopenia* can be treated with transfusions of HPA-negative maternal platelets until the anti-HPA antibodies disappear after 4 to 6 weeks of age. Administration of high-dose intravenous immunoglobulin to the mother pre-partum raises the platelet count of the newborn and reduces the incidence of bleeding.

Thrombocytopenia caused by bone marrow failure is a common problem in hematology. It is treated with supportive care with platelet transfusions. However, platelet surfaces have histocompatibility (HLA) antigens (Chs. 20 and 32), and anti-HLA antibodies arise in many patients and become a limiting factor in the effectiveness of platelet support therapy. The time of detection of anti-HLA antibodies against infused platelets correlates with the onset of refractoriness to the hemostatic effectiveness of the transfusions; the platelet count in the recipient no longer rises in response to such transfusions from the donor to whose platelet antigens the recipient is sensitized. Judicious HLA antigen matching of donors with recipients can prevent such isosensitization and eventually find platelets that will survive in a sensitized recipient. Unfortunately, HLA matching is a somewhat laborious and expensive procedure.

AUTOIMMUNE THROMBOCYTOPENIA

IgG autoantibodies against platelets, sometimes together with C3b, can sensitize the platelets for destruction, leading to autoimmune thrombocytopenia, sometimes called *idiopathic thrombocytopenic purpura (ITP)*. One of the antigens against which some of these antibodies are directed is the glycoprotein β3 integrin GpIIb/IIIa, which on activated platelets binds fibrin, fibrinogen, and fibronectin. Since the autoantibodies have been shown to sensitize platelets from unrelated persons, the antigens are not polymorphic. Platelet autoantibodies may arise in the setting of SLE, immunodeficiency disorders, or B-lymphocyte neoplasms. In such cases the autoimmune thrombocytopenia is defined as *secondary*, whereas if no other illness is evident, the disorder is *idiopathic*. The onset of idiopathic autoimmune thrombocytopenia in adults is usually insidious, not clearly related to another illness, and takes a chronic and intermittent course. The bone marrow examination shows normal or increased numbers of megakaryocytes, and splenomegaly is not present. Since the antibodies are of the IgG class, they cross the placenta, and preterm fetuses of mothers with autoimmune thrombocytopenia can be thrombocytopenic and at risk for bleeding during birth. The incidence of neonatal thrombocytopenia, however, is low in this setting if the mother did not have autoimmune thrombocytopenia prior to the pregancy.

Analogous to the situation with immune leukopenias, the lack of a foolproof serological test confounds the laboratory definition of autoimmune thrombocytopenia. Platelets, like certain leukocytes, have Fc receptors for IgG; in addition, large platelets that accompany many thrombocytopenic states can trap greater than normal amounts of IgG in the open canalicular system. Therefore, the detection of increased IgG associated with platelets does not prove that the antibody is pathogenic. Furthermore, there is evidence that the IgG antibody associated with what is clinically defined as autoimmune thrombocytopenia does not react with platelet antigens directly by binding with its antigen-combining site but rather binds by a different mechanism. Platelet turnover studies, employing autologous radiolabeled platelets (if the thrombocytopenia is sufficiently moderate to permit collection of sufficient platelets), can document whether platelet production or survival account for reduction in the steady-state platelet concentration. Although it is not practical to perform this test routinely, it has given results consistent with increased platelet turnover in "typical" cases of autoimmune thrombocytopenia. In other cases, however, clinically indistinguishable from "typical" autoimmune thrombocytopenia, platelet production has been impaired rather than destruction increased. A defect in production rather than peripheral clearance, however, could still result from an immunological mechanism directed at the megakaryocyte rather than at the mature platelet, and thrombocytopenia in human immunodeficiency virus (HIV) infection may be an example of this pathogenesis. Thrombocytopenia can be the first sign of HIV infection and is found in about 10 percent of patients with acquired immunodeficiency syndrome (AIDS). The presence of HIV-1 in megakaryocytes has been documented, suggesting that this and other viruses may contribute to the pathogenesis of the disease by acting as immunogens together with platelet surface proteins and by inhibiting platelet production. In some patients an antibody has been detected with crossreactivity between GpIIb/IIIa and the HIV-1 surface glycoprotein, Gp160. In children, acute autoimmune thrombocytopenia often follows a viral infection, implying an infectious agent in the initiation of the autoimmune process. Childhood autoimmune thrombocytopenia usually remits spontaneously, again consistent with a different mechanism than that causing adult autoimmune thrombocytopenia.

Patients with autoimmune thrombocytopenia are customarily treated with corticosteroids, which are thought to reduce the clearance of sensitized platelets. If thrombocytopenia persists despite corticosteroid therapy or if prolonged corticosteroid therapy is required to maintain the platelet count, splenectomy is usually performed. About two-thirds of the patients respond to splenectomy, but occasionally more potent immunosuppressive therapy (vinca alkaloids, danazol, or intravenous gammaglobulin or antibody-coated erythrocyte infusion) is required. Accessory spleens have been identified in some patients who failed to benefit from splenectomy. Despite the underlying immunosuppression and possibly a different mechanism for thrombocytopenia, patients with AIDS and autoimmune thrombocytopenia respond to the same treatments as other patients with relatively little additional morbidity. Treatment of the HIV-1 infection with antiviral therapy sometimes relieves the thrombocytopenia.

Because of the rapid clearance of platelets in autoimmune thrombocytopenia, platelet transfusions are of little benefit in the long-term management of this disease. If a patient bleeds massively, has evidence of intracranial hemorrhage, or is going to have an emergency splenectomy, transfusion of 6 to 8 units of platelets every 4 hours or even a continuous infusion of 1 to 2 units per hour may be necessary to control hemorrhage before and during splenectomy.

MEDICATION-ASSOCIATED IMMUNE PLATELET DESTRUCTION

Medications can induce immune-mediated platelet destruction. Penicillin, quinidine, and quinine elicit antibodies that cause reactions resembling the hemolytic disorders produced by these drugs. The surface glycoprotein Gp1b has been implicated as the antigen that binds quinidine-induced antibodies. Antibodies against the anticoagulant heparin may produce thrombocytopenia, possibly because the heparin–antibody complexes bind to the platelets and activate them. In some cases, switching from bovine to porcine heparin alleviates the thrombocytopenia. Although the incidence of this complication of heparin is low, the large-scale use of the anticoagulant in clinical medicine makes the problem familiar to most physicians. Direct-acting antithrombins such as hirudin analogues are being investigated for safety and efficacy and may soon be available to replace heparin in sensitized patients.

SUGGESTED READINGS

Ballem PJ et al (1992) Kinetic studies of the mechanism of thrombocytopenia in patients with human immunodeficiency virus infection. N Engl J Med 327:1779

Bennett PR, Kim CLV, Colin Y et al (1993) Prenatal determination of fetal RhD type by DNA amplification. N Engl J Med 329:607

Berchthold P, McMillan R (1989) Therapy of chronic idiopathic thrombocytopenic purpura in adults. Blood 74:2309

Berchthold P, McMillan R, Tani P et al (1989) Autoantibodies against platelet membrane glycoproteins in children with acute and chronic immune thrombocytopenic purpura. Blood 74:1600

Berchthold P, Wenger M (1993) Autoantibodies against platelet glycoprotein in autoimmune thrombocytopenic purpura their clinical significance and response to treatment. Blood 81:1246

Bettaieb A, Fromont P, Louache F et al (1992) Presence of cross-reactive antibody between human immunodeficiency virus (HIV) and platelet glycoproteins in HIV-related immune thrombocytopenic purpura. Blood 80:162

Boussel J, Abboud M (1987) Autoimmune neutropenia of childhood. Crit Rev Oncol Hematol 7:37

Comenzo RL, Malachowski ME, Rohrer RJ et al (1992) Anomalous ABO phenotype in a child after an ABO-incompatible liver transplantation. N Engl J Med 326:867

de Vetten MP, Agre P (1988) The Rh polypeptide is a major fatty acid-acylated erythrocyte membrane protein. J Biol Chem 263:18193

Doan CA, Bouroncle BA (1960) Idiopathic and secondary thrombocytopenic purpura: clinical study and evaluation of 381 cases over a period of 28 years. Ann Intern Med 53:861

Figueroa M, Gehlsen J, Hammard D et al (1993) Combination chemotherapy in refractory immune thrombocytopenic purpura. N Engl J Med 328:1226

Hayward CPM, Kelton JG (1993) Immune thrombocytopenia. Curr Opin Hematol 1:265

Issit PD (1985) Applied Blood Group Serology. 3rd Ed. Montgomery Scientific Publications, Miami

Karpatkin S, Xia J, Thorbecke GJ (1992) Serum platelet-reactive IgG of autoimmune thrombocytopenic purpura patients is not $F(ab')_2$ mediated and a function of storage. Blood 80:3164

Kunicki TJ, Newman PJ (1992) The molecular immunology of human platelet proteins. Blood 80:1386

Louache F, Bettaieb A, Henri A et al (1991) Infection of megakaryocytes by human immunodeficiency virus in seropositive patients with immune thrombocytopenic purpura. Blood 78:1697

Müller-Eckhardt C (1992) Autoimmune diseases of blood cells. Semin Hematol 29:1

Okseuhendler E, Bierling P, Chevret S et al (1993) Splenectomy is safe and effective in human immunodeficiency virus-related immune thrombocytepenia. Blood 82:29

Petz LD, Garratty G (1980) Acquired Immune Hemolytic Anemias. Churchill Livingstone, New York

Pisciotta PT (1989) Blood Transfusion Therapy. A Physician's Handbook. American Association of Blood Banks, Arlington, VA

Samuels P, Bussel JB, Braitman L et al (1990) Estimation of the risk of thrombocytopenia in the offspring of pregnant women with presumed immune thrombocytopenic purpura. N Engl J Med 323:229

Swisher S (1976) Autoimmune hemolytic disorders. Semin Hematol 13:247

Yamamoto F-I, Clausen H, White T et al (1990) Molecular genetic basis of the histo-blood ABO system. Nature 345:229

Zucker-Franklin DA, Cao YZ (1989) Megakaryocytes of human immunodeficiency virus infected individuals express viral RNA. Proc Natl Acad Sci USA 86:5595

31

Blood Transfusion Therapy

A significant accomplishment of modern biomedical technology has been the development of blood transfusion therapy. The initial successes of blood transfusion therapy were in the realm of whole blood transfusions and were directed at red blood cell and plasma replacement. In recent years the trend has progressively evolved toward transfusion of blood components. There have been several reasons for this tendency. First, frequently only one component of blood is required by a patient, for example, red blood cells, plasma, individual plasma proteins, or platelets. Second, many components, especially plasma, can be stored indefinitely, whereas whole blood cannot be kept for very long time intervals. Third, each component of a whole blood transfusion has the capacity to exert toxic effects. By restricting the transfusion to fewer components, the total toxicity of the transfusion can be minimized. The technology for selective transfusion of erythrocytes, plasma, and, to a lesser extent, platelets has evolved to a high degree. Transfusion of blood phagocytes, principally neutrophils, is possible but lags behind in its technology.

PROCUREMENT OF WHOLE BLOOD AND PLASMA

The usual procedure for obtaining whole blood is to bleed (phlebotomize) a 450-ml unit of blood from a donor. This amount of blood loss is inconsequential to a healthy adult weighing more than 50 kg, and the blood is replaced within 6 weeks, after which the individual can donate again. Increasingly, persons scheduled for elective surgical procedures are encouraged to donate their own blood as a safe and ultimately compatible product for themselves that is also potentially useful for others. The number of such patients who can donate and the number of units obtainable (from 3 to 6 units within 3 weeks) can be increased by having such patients take iron by mouth along with twice weekly administration of intravenous erythropoietin.

The phlebotomy technique is to insert a needle into a suitable vein in the donor's antecubital fossa. To the needle is attached a length of plastic tubing that inserts into a plastic phlebotomy bag containing 40 ml of an anticoagulant and preservative solution. The bag is kept below the level of the needle, and the venous pressure of the donor, enhanced by a tourniquet on the upper arm, is sufficient to maintain flow of blood until 450 ml of blood is in the bag. At that point, blood flow stops because of the increase in pressure in the bag. In addition, the bag may be suspended on a balance beam at the opposite end of a counterweight; when filled, the bag tips the beam, signaling the phlebotomist that the bag is filled.

Before phlebotomy, appropriate selection and screening measures establish that the donor is sufficiently healthy for the procedure. These measures include inquiry as to the donor's state of general health and as to whether there is a history of diseases transmissable by blood transfusion (see below). The donor must have a normal body temperature and blood pressure and adequate weight, all of which are examined before donation. Certainly the donor should not be anemic. A simple test for anemia is to obtain a drop of blood by means of a finger prick and allow it to fall into a copper sulfate solution of defined density. If the red blood cell hemoglobin concentration is below about 13 g/dl, the drop of red blood will not sink into the blue copper sulfate solution. If the red blood cell mass is above this level, the drop sinks to the bottom.

With modern equipment, the entire phlebotomy and subsequent fractionation of whole blood can be done without ever exposing the blood to the air. At the end of the phlebotomy, the tubing leading to the phlebotomy bag is clamped and tied, the needle is cut off distal to the knot, and the bag is then available for transfusion or storage.

The complications of phlebotomy are minimal. The major problem is fainting of inexperienced donors. In many blood banks donors lie supine in special chairs that can be adjusted to lower the donor's head during phlebotomy, a measure that relieves the symptoms of a fainting reaction. Verbal reassurance is also very helpful in this situation.

WHOLE BLOOD AND WHOLE BLOOD FRACTIONS AND THEIR USES

Whole Blood

Whole blood contains all the cells and plasma proteins of the blood. Platelets, phagocytes, and many plasma proteins rapidly become inactivated during storage, so that for practical purposes, whole blood can be considered to consist of erythrocytes and plasma. Fresh whole blood may be indicated for patients suffering from massive hemorrhage. In this circumstance, all blood components are being rapidly lost. Even in this situation, not all com-

ponents need to be replaced to an equivalent extent. In other words, the principal danger to the hemorrhaging patient is loss of blood volume and oxygen-carrying capacity. However, in the circumstance of massive hemorrhage, platelets and clotting factors may be lost to the degree that the hemorrhagic problem is compounded by impaired hemostasis. Therefore, in this circumstance about 1 of every 8 units of transfused blood should be fresh.

Theoretically, whole blood is indicated when a patient needs both erythrocytes for anemia and plasma protein for replacement of intravenous volume. In point of fact, it is recommended in such cases that erythrocytes and plasma be given as separate components, because the plasma for purposes of colloid replacement can be stored indefinitely. It is therefore less wasteful to keep plasma than whole blood, because the erythrocytes and plasma would have to be discarded once the whole blood passed the expiration date during storage. Viewed in this way, there are very few indications for the administration of whole blood, and it has been estimated that the practice of blood fractionation has prevented serious shortages in the supply of blood available for transfusion.

Separation of Packed Erythrocytes and Plasma

The whole blood in its plastic bag is spun in a centrifuge that drives the erythrocytes to the bottom. The transfusion bag has several outlets to which plastic tubing can be attached for fractionation. By rolling up the bottom of the packet, the supernatant plasma can be expressed into the exit tubing, which is attached to a transfer pack. This tubing is then clamped, sealed, tied, and cut, as was done after phlebotomy, when the transfer is completed. The plasma is available for transfusion and storage as are the packed erythrocytes. This procedure can also be used in plasmapheresis to remove abnormal plasma from patients with paraproteinemias. During plasmapheresis, the plasma can be discarded and the packed erythrocytes returned to the patient. Conversely, when patients with polycythemia are subjected to therapeutic phlebotomy, the erythrocytes are discarded and the plasma may be returned to the patient. Packed erythrocytes are the treatment of choice for most chronic anemias requiring blood transfusions. Whole plasma is given to patients requiring intravascular volume, especially if depleted of plasma proteins. Fresh plasma or plasma frozen immediately after separation and stored at –20°C (fresh frozen plasma) is needed for certain coagulation disorders (Ch. 13).

Plasma Fractionation

The chemical separation of plasma proteins was initiated during the 1940s. The classic methods involve addition of salts or solvents to the whole plasma, the addition of which causes the major component proteins, albumin and the immunoglobulins, to precipitate differentially. The precipitates are removed from the liquid by centrifugation and redissolved in water. Albumin can be used to provide this plasma component in patients with liver disease who are unable to synthesize it or in patients with protein-losing disorders. Immunoglobulin is used in the treatment of antibody deficiency diseases.

During the 1960s, procedures for precipitating coagulation factor VIII along with fibrinogen by subjecting plasma to low temperatures revolutionized the treatment of classic hemophilia. In recent years, the isolation of plasma proteins has become increasingly sophisticated and has provided plasma protein fractions of high purity as well as complexes of coagulation factors in varying states of activation. The great advantage of many plasma fractions is their longevity during storage. Many of the fractions can be kept almost indefinitely in a dried state and reconstituted with sterile water or salt solution. The principal problem with such fractions is that they are rather expensive to prepare.

Storage of Whole Blood and Packed Erythrocytes

The problem of erythrocyte preservation is related to factors determining erythrocyte survival. It is necessary to maintain the red blood cell's redox potential, energy charge, and ultimately its membrane integrity. Through trial and error, conditions have evolved for the optimal storage of erythrocytes. The anticoagulant solutions contain glucose as a substrate for glycolysis and citric acid as an anticoagulant to chelate the calcium. In addition to preventing fibrin formation during phlebotomy, the low calcium concentration prevents the slow leak of calcium into red cells, associated with stiffening of the membrane skeleton. The citrate anticoagulant is buffered with sodium citrate and citric acid or, more commonly, sodium phosphate to maintain the blood pH at about 6. The inclusion of adenine in the preservative mixtures helps maintain the adenosine triphosphate (ATP) level of the stored red cells. In such solutions, the cells remain viable for about 21 days at 4°C. The incubation at low temperature slows the glycolytic rate of the cells to a level that sustains viability but that does not lead to a depletion of glucose or an accumulation of waste lactic acid to a toxic level. Under these conditions, the erythrocyte membrane remains able to retain cytoplasmic constituents and to maintain the gradients of sodium and potassium at nearly normal levels, that is, 100 mEq/L of potassium inside and 100 mEq/L of sodium outside. Glucose fuels the reduction of the redox potential to prevent oxidation of glutathione, hemoglobin, and membrane components. If one considers that about 11 million units of blood are transfused per year in the United States, the importance of improving storage conditions can be appreciated. A 1 percent lengthening of the preservation of blood is equivalent to providing 100,000 units that would otherwise have to be procured.

Some changes do take place in erythrocytes during storage. In particular, the high glucose and phosphate concentration in the medium raises the 2,3-diphosphoglycerate concentration of the erythrocytes. The cells also lose some potassium ions and accumulate sodium ions from the medium. The pH of the suspending solution continues to fall because of accumulation of lactic acid. Nevertheless, these storage lesions are reversed when the erythrocytes are infused into the recipient's circulation. The 2,3-diphosphoglycerate falls, and the potassium:sodium ratio rises. The reversibility of the lesions persists until 20 days of storage. Beyond that time, the cells begin to leak increasing quantities of hemoglobin, and the number of irreversibly damaged cells becomes intolerably high.

PROCEDURES INVOLVED IN RED BLOOD CELL TRANSFUSION

Cross-Matching

When a whole blood or packed or red blood cell transfusion is contemplated for a patient, the first priority is to obtain a small sample of blood from the patient. The sample is allowed to clot in a glass tube and is taken to the blood bank, where the serum is separated from the clot by centrifugation. Both the serum and the erythrocytes in the clot are used for the process of *cross-matching,* which is the determination of the blood product most suitable immunologically for the recipient.

The cells are checked for agglutination by serum from type B and type A persons, sera containing anti-A and anti-B IgM antibodies, respectively. Anti-A serum agglutinates erythrocytes containing A antigens, whereas anti-B serum agglutinates erythrocytes containing B antigens. Both will agglutinate erythrocytes from a person with the AB phenotype, as the erythrocytes have both A and B antigens. Neither antiserum reacts with erythrocytes of a person with type O, whose erythrocytes have

neither A nor B antigens. To be doubly sure of the ABO cross-match, as this procedure is called, the ability of the patient's serum to agglutinate known type A and B cells is checked. The result should be symmetrical with the test on the patient's cells. If the cells were found to be type A, the serum should agglutinate only type B cells. If type B cells were found, the serum should agglutinate type A cells. If the cells were type O, the serum should agglutinate both type A and B erythrocytes. If the cells were type AB, the serum should not agglutinate any cells. The cross-match for ABO compatibility is particularly important, because immunological reactions involving this system elicit complement-mediated intravascular hemolysis and inflict serious toxicity on the recipient.

Cross-matching for Rh compatibility is performed by reacting the potential recipient's cells with anti-D antisera in a medium containing a high albumin content, which allows these antibodies, usually of the IgG class, to cause agglutination. The tendency of the IgG antibodies to aggregate after being bound to erythrocytes is enhanced in this protein-rich medium. At this point in the cross-match it is possible to identify the recipient's major blood group and Rh status (for example, A Rh-positive, B Rh-negative, O Rh-positive, AB Rh-positive) and, in theory, to select a suitable unit of whole blood or packed erythrocytes for infusion. However, if feasible, a further cross-match procedure is often carried out that determines whether the recipient has antibodies against other erythrocyte antigens. This matching is done by means of an indirect antiglobulin or *Coombs test* (named after the originator of this important and widely used procedure).

The Coombs test is done by mixing the recipient's serum with erythrocytes from the donor. After the first incubation, the cells are washed free of the recipient's serum by centrifugation and are then suspended in a solution of rabbit anti-human IgG antibody. If the recipient's serum contains any IgG antibodies that react against one or more of the antigens on the donor's red cells, the anti-IgG will now cause those cells to agglutinate. A positive reaction in the pool test then requires that the procedure be repeated against a panel of cells of defined antigenic composition in order to identify the antigen(s) involved. Thereafter, erythrocytes containing this antigen can be avoided in transfusions.

Erythrocytes matched for ABO and Rh blood groups, or even in extreme circumstances, unmatched type O Rh-negative erythrocytes alone, can be used in emergencies. However, it is advantageous whenever possible to take the cross-match one step further, especially when patients have had previous transfusions. Furthermore, the procedure must be repeated when a patient requires additional transfusions.

The Infusion of Packed Erythrocytes or Whole Blood

Blood taken right out of the blood bank is cold, has relatively low pH, and has high citrate, lactate, and potassium contents. If the blood is given rapidly and in large amounts, these properties can be toxic. Of special concern are the ability of citrate to sequester calcium and the effect of the potassium ion on suppressing neuromuscular function. If possible, the blood should be warmed (not burned) and infused as slowly as possible; some recommend that calcium infusions be given when massive transfusions are delivered. The recipient's serum potassium concentration should be monitored if massive transfusion therapy is in progress, especially if there is a question as to the patient's renal function.

FROZEN ERYTHROCYTES

The 21-day storage limit for the whole blood and packed red blood cells is adequate for most transfusions. However, certain circumstances make longer storage desirable. First, if anemic patients requiring repeated transfusions have an unusual red blood cell antigen profile, they will eventually develop antibodies against most erythrocytes in the general population. It may not be possible to

phlebotomize persons with compatible blood types as frequently as the recipient needs the cells. However, if a supply of an unusual type of erythrocytes can be collected over a long time and stockpiled in a frozen state, the problem may be solved. Second, frozen blood can be transported to remote locations and stored wherever freezer facilities are available.

The major problem in frozen storage, cryopreservation, is to avoid damage to cell constituents, especially membranes, by ice crystals that form during freezing. This problem is approached by means of colligative compounds that can both lower the freezing point of water and penetrate the cell's membrane to prevent intracellular as well as extracellular freezing. Cryoprotective agents of this type include glycerol and dimethylsulfoxide. In addition to the use of cryoprotective agents, the temperature must be lowered slowly to prevent ice formation and abrupt phase transitions in cellular components. Therefore, freezing of blood cells requires technology for addition of cryopreservative agents, controlled freezing, frozen storage (usually at $-20°C$ or lower), controlled thawing, and, finally, removal of the cryopreservative. Removal of the cryopreservative is accomplished by extensive washing of the cells. Therefore, an additional advantage of frozen blood is the fact that it is extensively washed free of plasma, a process that reduces its risk of transmitting diseases. After freezing and thawing, about 10 to 15 percent of erythrocytes are lysed. An additional 10 to 15 percent have a short survival after infusion. The rest have a survival nearly equivalent to that of conventionally stored erythrocytes. However, the thawed cells deteriorate rapidly on further storage and must therefore be transfused within 24 hours after thawing. Moreover, a point worth noting is that the frozen and thawed erythrocytes have almost entirely lost their potassium content to the extracellular fluid. The cell will normalize this ionic imbalance after infusion into the circulation by pumping sodium ions out and potassium ions in. Because the initial infusion medium is very rich in potassium, a transient increase in serum potassium can occur in the recipient. On the other hand, if enough frozen and thawed erythrocytes are infused into a recipient, the cells act as potassium traps and can actually pump enough potassium out of the plasma into themselves to cause a transient hypokalemia. Despite the advantages of frozen erythrocytes, the expense and logistical problems caused by the complex technical procedures involved and the additional requirements for freezer space limit the practicality of freezing as a routine method for erythrocyte processing and preservation at the present time.

PLATELET TRANSFUSIONS

Procurement of Platelets

The size and shape of platelets are sufficiently different from those of erythrocytes to allow them to be relatively easily separated from the whole blood. The simplest procedure for this separation, called *plateletpheresis*, is to remove a unit of whole blood, to centrifuge it gently at about 500 times gravity, and to express the platelet-rich plasma into a special platelet storage container (see below) and return the packed red cells to the donor (or keep them for transfusion purposes). The platelets are then concentrated by centrifugation, and excess plasma expressed into a separate plasma container. The final platelet concentrate has a volume of about 50 ml and contains on the order of 10^{11} platelets. The centrifugation procedures partially activate the platelets so that they aggregate, but after standing at room temperature for a short time the cells calm down and can be separated by gentle agitation.

Despite the ease of this procedure, the usual thrombocytopenic patient requires more than 10^{11} platelets. A rule of thumb is that an infusion of a unit of platelets, that is, the platelets derived from a unit of whole blood, will increase the platelet count of a 70-kg person by 10,000 platelets/μl of blood. To increase the yield of platelets from a donor, it is possible to process up to 1,200 ml of plasma from a single donor per week. A more efficient approach, albeit time-consuming for the donor, is to remove blood from one antecubital vein of a donor by means of a pump and to drive the blood into a centrifuge. The blood, depleted of platelet-rich plasma, is pumped back into the antecubital vein in the donor's other arm. The centrifuge device separates platelet-rich plasma from the erythrocytes in the whole blood. The blood flow from the patient into the machine and back may be continuous or intermittent, depending on the technology used. The more platelets that can be obtained from a single donor, the lower the risk of sensitization of the recipient against different HLA antigens on the infused platelets.

Platelet cross-matching for immunological reasons is not routine because of its expense, but in some instances it is indicated and required when prolonged platelet support is necessary.

Storage of Platelets

A curious feature of platelets is that they undergo shape changes resembling agonist-induced activation when chilled to refrigerator temperatures. Hence, platelets stored in the cold (4°C) have a shorter average survival time in a recipient's circulation than do platelets stored at room temperature. Therefore, platelets obtained for transfusion are routinely maintained at room temperature, and because of concerns over bacterial growth, can only be kept for 5 days. In addition, since platelet metabolism is active at room temperature, the platelet concentrates must be agitated continuously in gas-permeable containers, so that CO_2 evolved by respiration of the cells can diffuse out of the bag; otherwise accumulation of CO_2 would lower the pH, and platelets become nonviable when the pH drops below 6.0. Cold-induced activation is also an impediment to freezing of platelet-rich plasma. Although frozen platelets have been shown to function to some extent for hemostasis, they are not widely employed.

Phagocyte (Neutrophil) Transfusions

The turnover rate of blood phagocytes, predominantly neutrophils, is on the order of 10^{10} per day under normal circumstances and up to 10 times that value in states of bacterial infection. If we consider that a 450-ml unit of whole blood contains about 2×10^9 neutrophils, it is obvious that five or preferably more units of whole blood need to be processed and gleaned of neutrophils if the turnover in a recipient is to be approximated. Several technical procedures have been developed to try to accomplish this feat. The procedures involve extracorporeal centrifugation of multiple units of blood in a manner described for plateletpheresis. Blood is centrifuged in a cylindrical container to yield erythrocytes and plasma. However, instead of removing platelet-rich plasma, the devices skim off a neutrophil-enriched buffy coat at the plasma–erythrocyte interface. Unfortunately, this leukopheresis procedure can routinely generate on the order of only 10^{10} neutrophils from an acceptable volume of whole blood. To increase this amount two to three times, a viscous polymer, hydroxyethyl starch, that coats erythrocytes, causing them to separate more efficiently from neutrophils, is added during the procedure. In addition, donors are often given corticosteroids before leukopheresis to increase their concentration of circulating neutrophils.

The technological feat of obtaining phagocytes in large numbers has unfortunately not in and of itself solved the problem of phagocyte support for patients with phagocyte deficiency who are susceptible to bacterial and fungal infection. First, even the impressive numbers of neutrophils acquired are at the theoretical lower limit of maintaining the required neutrophil turnover. Second, it is not clear that the neutrophils obtained are either totally functional or, on the other hand, completely nontoxic. There is some evidence that damaged neutrophils aggregate and collect in the lungs, where they have the potential to injure pulmonary capillary endothelium and produce edema and inflammation. The resulting reaction may destroy lung substance and block the pulmonary microcirculation, both effects resulting in hypoxemia. In addition, neutrophils have a very short survival in the living organism and deteriorate even more rapidly during conditions of storage that have been tried. Another problem is that there is relatively little information concerning the antigens of neutrophils, a deficiency that limits the practicality of cross-matching. Finally, the technology associated with neutrophil transfusion is not only expensive but also potentially hazardous to the healthy blood donor. This hazard results from the need to treat the donor with hydroxyethyl starch, corticosteroids, and anticoagulants. For all these reasons, phagocyte transfusion must be considered of limited utility at present. With the recent availability of growth factors, such as granulocyte colony-stimulating factor (G-CSF) and granulocyte–marcrophage (GM)-CF, which increase peripheral blood phagocyte counts, it may become more feasible to procure leukocytes suitable for transfusion in the future.

COMPLICATIONS OF BLOOD TRANSFUSION THERAPY

Immunological Reactions

As described in Chapter 30, the infusion of ABO-incompatible erythrocytes leads to various hemolytic reactions mediated by the natural IgM isoantibodies directed against A and B antigens and the interaction of these antibodies with the complement system. These types of reactions lead not only to immediate intravascular destruction of the infused cells, but to circulatory instability and possibly serious renal damage as well. Transfusions of Rh-incompatible blood cause generally less serious and delayed hemolytic reactions. In addition, such a transfusion in women of childbearing age sensitizes the Rh-negative mother against an Rh-positive fetus and sets that fetus up for erythroblastosis fetalis. Immunological reactions against other erythrocyte antigens cause variable degrees of delayed hemolysis of the transfused blood. The major consequence of immunological reactions against infused platelets and white blood cells appears to be the short survival of those cells and limitation of their usefulness. However, antibodies against white cells may also damage them and cause them to produce pulmonary and other tissue damage as discussed above. Occasionally immunological reactions occur against plasma components.

Genetically determined plasma IgA deficiency is fairly common. IgA-deficient persons receiving whole plasma may produce anti-IgA antibodies. When blood or plasma containing IgA is subsequently infused into the IgA-deficient recipient, various types of immunological reactions such as urticaria, anaphylactic shock, or serum sickness may occur.

One uncommon immunological consequence of transfusion is the passive transfer of IgE antibodies from an allergic donor to a recipient. Exposure of the previously nonallergic recipient to the antigen to which the donor was allergic results in an allergic reaction in the recipient.

Transfusions of whole blood introduce long-lived lymphocytes into the recipient, and sensitive analyses using the polymerase chain reaction for donor DNA sequences have detected circulating donor white blood cells for several days following transfusion. These infused white blood cells may be responsible for sensitization against histocompatibility antigens, transmission of viral diseases, and other complications the most dangerous of which is graft-versus-host disease (GVHD) (see also Chs. 22 and 32). Most cases of GVHD have occurred in infants with congenital immunodeficiency syndromes and with erythroblastosis fetalis and in adults with immunosuppressing neoplasms such as Hodgkin's disease. Very rare cases of GVHD in transfused individuals without these underlying diseases have occurred, some in the setting of a recipient sharing an HLA haplotype with the donor who is homozygous for that HLA type. If patients with known immune deficiency are to receive transfusions, it may be worthwhile to irradiate the blood to kill lymphocytes present, although the rarity of this complication makes routine irradiation of blood products unnecessary.

Cardiovascular Overload

If through miscalculation or some other reason more blood product is given to the intravascular space than the cardiovascular system can tolerate, pulmonary edema can occur. This complication may arise following a blood transfusion into an anemic person who either because of severe anemia or underlying cardiac disease is in borderline cardiac failure. This complication can sometimes be avoided by giving blood transfusions slowly to patients with underlying cardiovascular disease. The volume of blood coagulation factor infusions can be minimized by employing concentrated coagulation factor fractions presently available. However, some of these preparations contain high concentrations of fibrinogen, and relatively small increments in plasma fibrinogen can cause large increases in blood viscosity.

Infectious Complications Associated with Transfusion Therapy

With modern technology the overt contamination of blood products with microbes as a result of procurement and storage techniques is unusual. On the other hand, the need to store platelets at room temperature rather than under refrigeration increases the risk of bacterial overgrowth. The major infectious complication of blood transfusion therapy, however, is the spread of diseases that are latent in the donor. In theory, any infection in which the offending organism circulates in the blood can be transmitted by blood transfusion therapy. The infections caused by the hepatitis B virus, the hepatitis C virus (responsible for most cases of what formerly was called non-A, non-B hepatitis), the AIDS virus (HIV-1) (Ch. 22), and, in immunocompromised hosts, the cytomegalovirus, are the major offenders.

The fraction of adults having infectious hepatitis or AIDS viruses in the bloodstream is high among populations living under conditions of poor sanitation and among drug addicts who make a practice of sharing the needles with which they indulge their habits. For these reasons, the probability that a unit of blood will be infected with hepatitis virus is heavily dependent on the population from which it was obtained. In general, blood banks that use blood products from volunteer donors tend to have a lower infection transmission rate than do blood banks that pay their donors. A reason for this difference is the fact that blood is one commodity that drug addicts can sell to finance their habits.

With the great advances that have come in understanding the structure and pathogenicity of the hepatitis B and C and AIDS viruses in recent years, it has become increasingly possible to use immunological methods to detect evidence of prior infection of the donor as evidenced by the presence of antibodies against hepatitis B and C, cytomegalovirus, or HIV-1. In patients who are carriers of hepatitis B, virus particles or parts thereof are present in sufficiently high concentrations in blood that sensitive immunochemical tests can efficiently detect them, and tests for antibodies to hepatitis C detect most patients who would transmit this disease by transfusion. The risk of hepatitis transmission can be lowered even further by screening donated blood for elevations in enzyme activities such as alanine aminotransferase that are characteristically increased in the blood of patients with liver inflammation.

In the case of AIDS, the virus exists at such low levels in blood that it makes little sense to try to detect it. The current approach to HIV testing, therefore, uses the serological assays for anti-HIV antibodies described in Chapter 22. Although these tests are very reliable, there persists a small "window of vulnerability" of possibly several months in which a person recently exposed to HIV has yet to generate antiviral antibodies. This window can be closed further by maintaining as small as possible a pool of frequent donors who have repeatedly been tested for antibodies against HIV or hepatitis viruses.

Fractionation of blood into components can serve to some extent to reduce the risk of infection. The hepatitis virus is remarkably hardy and survives the normal vicissitudes of blood storage including freezing and thawing. However, the prolonged storage attendant in the processing of blood for plasma, plasma albumin, and immunoglobulins causes the virus to become nonviable with time or to be removed during the fractionation process. Cytomegalovirus and HIV-1 reside in white blood cells, so that removal of intact white blood cells that occurs during freezing of red blood cells lowers the risk of infusing these viruses. Researchers are presently evaluating the effectiveness of filtration and centrifugation procedures to remove leukocytes from whole blood and red cell preparations for standard transfusion practice. Preliminary evidence suggests that these techniques do reduce viral contamination of transfused blood.

Unfortunately, most coagulation protein fractions are so enriched for the hepatitis virus that these fractions are associated with a high risk of infection. A safe and effective hepatitis B vaccine is now available, however, and whenever possible, patients requiring blood protein concentrates should be vaccinated before their first factor infusions. Other methods available to reduce the risk of infection from blood protein fractions include application of organic solvents, steam pasteurization, and additional purification by means of monoclonal antibodies. The techniques vary in expense and are currently undergoing evaluation. Blood proteins manufactured by recombinant genetic technology are likely to be safe. The major problem now is to make their preparation less expensive. In the United States today, even with precautions in effect, the risk of infection increases cumulatively with each unit of whole blood infused. The absolute risk in a given situation varies with the locale and the sources of blood. It can be appreciated that after therapy of massive hemorrhage or open heart surgery, the risk of infection is relatively high. A hopeful prospect for such patients is the use of autotransfusion. The patient anticipating modest blood loss during elective surgery can donate blood on several occasions before surgery and take iron tablets to stimulate new red cell production. For massive hemorrhage, surgeons are now using devices to remove debris from blood leaking into body cavities during trauma and surgery and reinfusing this blood into the patient's circulation.

SUGGESTED READINGS

Adams PT, Davenport RT, Reardon DA, Roth MS (1992) Detection of circulating donor white blood cells in patients receiving multiple transfusions. Blood 80:551

Beutler E (1993) Platelet transfusion: the 20,000/ml trigger. Blood 81:1411

Cumming PD, Wallace EL, Schorr JB, Dodd RY (1989) Exposure of patients to human immunodeficiency virus through the transfusion of blood components that test antibody-negative. N Engl J Med 321:941

Donahue JG, Munoz A, Ness PM et al (1992) The declining risk of post-transfusion hepatitis C virus infection. N Engl J Med 327:369

Garratty G (1986) Red Cell Antigens and Antiboies. American Association of Blood Banks, Arlington, VA

Kim CLV, Chérif-Zahar B, Raynal V et al (1992) Multiple Rh messenger RNA isoforms are produced by alternative splicing. Blood 80:1074

Lane TA (1992) Leukocyte-reduced blood components. Ann Intern Med 117:2608

Mollison PL, Engelfriet CP, Contreras M (1993) Blood Transfusion in Clinical Medicine. 9th Ed. Blackwell, Oxford, UK

Rossi EC, Simon TL, Moss GS (1991) Principles of Transfusion Medicine. Williams & Wilkins, Baltimore

Seeff LB et al (1992) Long-term mortality after transfusion-association non-A, non-B hepatitis. N Engl J Med 327:1906

Strauss RG (1993) Therapeutic granulocyte transfusion in 1993. Blood 81:1675

Surgenor DM, Wallace EL, Hao SHS, Chapman RH (1990) Collection and transfusion of blood in the United States, 1982–1988. N Engl J Med 322:1646

32

Bone Marrow Transplantation

The replacement of failed, abnormally functioning, or malignant bone marrow with normal marrow is a relatively recent achievement. Its accomplishment and increasing utility grew out of the following developments. First, except for *autologous marrow transplantation* (i.e., the procedure of saving a patient's own marrow stem cells and infusing them back to the donor at a later time), it was necessary to overcome the problems of graft rejection and graft-versus-host disease (GVHD) to permit transplantation of marrow from another individual (*allogeneic transplantation*). Second, it was necessary to gain sufficient experience with the procedure to learn what factors affect the outcome. This information, together with careful documentation of the natural history of diseases in which marrow grafting was contemplated, have begun to inform us as to when and for whom marrow transplantation is indicated. More than anything else, however, the development of bone marrow transplantation represents the heroic efforts of a dedicated clinical investigator, Dr. E. Donnall Thomas, who persevered through years of failure until the procedure came to be standard practice around the world. For this work Thomas received the Nobel Prize in Physiology and Medicine in 1989. Although growing in successes and scope, bone marrow transplantation requires a considerable investment in hospital personnel, space, support resources, and laboratory exper-

tise. It is therefore currently a high-technology activity of hematology.

First used for aplastic anemia and severe combined immune deficiencies, more recent uses of total marrow reconstitution with allogeneic bone marrow have been as therapy for genetic diseases, myelodysplastic and myeloproliferative disorders, and leukemia. Genetic bone marrow disorders treated by means of this approach have included the Wiskott-Aldrich syndrome (Ch. 20), severe congenital anemia or neutropenia (Ch. 22), and severe neutrophil functional disorders (Ch. 18). Bone marrow transplantation was initially attempted in patients with acute leukemia after several relapses, but more recently it has been employed as earlier therapy for acute myelogenous leukemia (Ch. 23), for young adult patients with acute lymphatic leukemia in remission (Ch. 25), for multiple myeloma (Ch. 29), and for selected patients with paroxysmal nocturnal hemoglobinuria, myelofibrosis, and chronic granulocytic leukemia (Ch. 22). In these settings, an obvious additional requirement is the need to destroy completely the malignant or genetically abnormal stem cells from the recipient's bone marrow. Transplantation with autologous bone marrow after intensive cytoreductive therapy is being evaluated presently for the treatment of solid tumors.

IMMUNOLOGY OF BONE MARROW TRANSPLANTATION

Histocompatibility

The factors determining the probability of engraftment of bone marrow from another person are more or less the same as those that influence the acceptance of kidney or other solid organ allografts. The principal factors are the ability to avoid or suppress the expression of a cell-mediated immune response against the graft, or by the graft against the host. In these immune responses, the structures recognized as nonself by the immune system, primarily T lymphocytes, are histocompatibility antigens on the surfaces of the cells of engrafted organs. As described in Chapter 19, these antigens, first identified on the surfaces of lymphocytes, are designated human lymphocyte antigens, or HLA. The reactivity of anti-HLA antibodies with lymphocytes is documented by their capacity to bind to target lymphocytes and fix

the entire complement cascade to the lymphocyte membrane, thereby causing it to leak. This leakage can be detected by measuring the release of intracellular constituents labeled with radioactive chromium or by observing for the seepage of certain dyes into the cell from the extracellular medium. The result of years of cooperative effort involving many laboratories that accumulated antisera and reacted them with lymphocytes of several generations of multiple families has generated a descriptive panel of HLA antibodies that define corresponding antigens. This information has been supplemented with data on the genetic distribution of various cellular enzymes and plasma proteins known to be coded by particular genes. On the basis of this collection of data, it is evident that HLA are encoded by DNA on the short arm of the sixth chromosome. The positions of different HLA variants on this chromosome have been mapped (Fig. 32-1).

The HLA system has been divided serologically into four major groups: HLA-A, HLA-B,

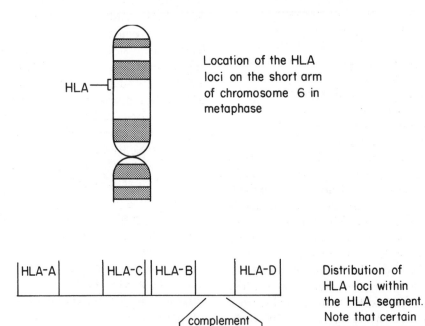

Location of the HLA loci on the short arm of chromosome 6 in metaphase

Distribution of HLA loci within the HLA segment. Note that certain complement protein loci are also within this region.

Fig. 32-1. Chromosome 6 map showing loci relevant for histocompatibility.

HLA-C, and HLA-D. Groups A through C, the class I major histocompatibility complex (MHC) antigens, are defined by complement-fixing reactions. A particular HLA phenotype expressed on cell surfaces is the result of codominant mendelian inheritance. For example, if the maternal HLA type is ab and the paternal type is cd, the offspring can end up ac, ad, bc, or bd. The inheritance of HLA is complicated by genetic crossovers that, as expected, occur in proportion to the distance between the alleles on the sixth chromosome. The D allele of the HLA system, which represents class II MHC proteins, is further subdivided serologically into groups DR, DQ, and DW. It is historically different from the others because its definition was based on a more complex biological phenomenon, the *mixed lymphocyte response* (MLR). In other words, the cell surface configuration expressed by this allele is too subtle to be recognized by specific complement-fixing antibodies. Rather, its detection has required the active participation of lymphocytes. If B lymphocytes of one person are genetically different at the D determinant from those of another person and are mixed with the nonidentical person's T lymphocytes, several days' cultivation of the mixture of lymphocytes will cause the T lymphocytes to undergo a blastogenic response. This response is detected by means of a stimulation of incorporation of radioactive thymidine into the lymphocyte DNA.

The MLR is especially important for bone marrow transplantation, because HLA compatibility is required both for the complement fixation-determined antigens and the MLR-related antigens in order for an acceptable probability of engraftment to occur. In the developed countries, in which the average family size is small, the chances are about two in three that an individual will not have suitably histocompatible (HLA- and MLR-matched) siblings. To address this problem, a national registry has been established to permit transplant centers to identify unrelated but HLA-matched donors for recipients lacking sufficiently histocompatible siblings or other relatives. This registry must be extremely large (> 100,000 donors) for a recipient to have a finite chance of identifying a match.

Moreover, even "perfect" matching of nonidentical twins with respect to the HLA and MLR antigens does not invariably ensure engraftment or prevent GVHD. Clearly, as yet undefined antigens must evoke immunological recognition, therefore, except for identical twins, some degree of immunosuppression is necessary to ensure successful transplantation. Nevertheless, improvements in immunosuppressive therapy have permitted the transplantation of marrow from increasingly less well-matched donors. In the future, more precise matching may result from the use of molecular genetics, testing compatibility by comparing restriction fragment length polymorphisms using probes for particular loci in the MHC complex. It is noteworthy that bone marrow allotransplantation differs from solid organ transplantation in the requirement for more stringent histocompatibility; grafts from unrelated donors of kidneys, livers, and hearts require initial immunosuppression, but are quite successful and after a time can persist in the recipient following withdrawal of immunosuppressive therapy.

Technology of Marrow Grafting

Insofar as most candidates for marrow transplantation suffer from immunodeficiency or decreased numbers or function of phagocytes, they are susceptible to infection. Therefore, an initial supportive effort is often required to eradicate existing infection and to place the patient in a protected environment in which further infection can be avoided. If thrombocytopenia and bleeding are occurring as part of the underlying disease, appropriate transfusions are given, although only if absolutely necessary in order to minimize immunization against antigens that could compromise the graft.

Hematopoietic stem cells can "home" from the blood to the bone marrow. For reconstitution of lymphoid stem cells, as few as a half million to 1 million nucleated bone marrow cells will suffice. To establish an entire hematopoietic stem, 10 times more cells are needed. These numbers of cells can be obtained from 50 to 500 ml of bone marrow. This quantity of marrow cells is easily derived from multiple aspirates of the pelvic bone marrow. The procedure must be performed with the subject under general or regional anesthesia. The donor must therefore be able to tolerate regional or general anesthesia during which marrow is obtained. For this reason, the donor must understand that some risk, albeit small, accompanies the procedure and that the benefits of donation are strictly emotional and social. When infants and small children are potential donors, physicians have used the legal court system to evaluate the risks and benefits of donation. In these proceedings, a court-appointed lawyer acts as guardian for the child. In most cases the judges have ruled that the knowledge apparent later in life that a child tried to save the life of a sibling was sufficiently positive psychologically for the child to warrant the small risks involved. Donors must, of course, be screened for diseases transmitted by blood, such as acquired immunodeficiency syndrome (AIDS), hepatitis, and cytomegalovirus infection.

The anticoagulated bone marrow samples procured are strained through steel mesh to remove bone spicules and fat aggregates; they are then infused into the histocompatible recipient. The preparation required of the recipient for this infusion depends on the disease being treated and on the degree of immunological compatibility between donor and recipient.

Immunosuppressive treatment precedes the transplant, and except for therapy of aplastic anemia, in which the recipient bone marrow is empty, it is necessary to eradicate the preexisting marrow (in, say, congenital blood diseases) or leukemic or other malignant cells. These immunosuppressive and cytoreductive treatments are referred to as *conditioning regimens*. The immunosuppressive therapy employed usually involves administration of an aklylating agent together with total body irradiation and is highly effective. To destroy the recipient's

marrow or neoplastic cells, combination chemotherapy and total body irradiation therapy, according to principles discussed in Chapter 21, are applied. Since the therapy is followed by bone marrow reconstitution, limiting the toxicity of cytotoxic treatment can be avoided, permitting very aggressive treatment regimens that have a good chance of killing the target cells. Clearly the earlier in a neoplastic disease the patient is transplanted, the smaller the tumor burden and the lower the incidence of drug resistance.

In all patients receiving bone marrow transplants but especially when establishing immunological competency in the patient with severe combined immune deficiency, a major problem in the immunodeficient recipient is *GVHD. Acute GVHD* can affect many organ systems, and usually manifests by fever, diarrhea and a maculopapular skin rash, frequently on the palms and soles; eczematous changes in the skin are also observed. Evidence of liver dysfunction is common. Bone marrow from donors in whom T-cell precursors secrete the cytokine interleukin-2 (IL-2) is especially prone to cause acute GVHD in recipients, suggesting that such donors either should be avoided or more aggressive immunosuppressive treatment applied. Some of the manifestations of GVHD may arise from elaboration of cytokines, such as tumor necrosis factor (TNF) and IL-1.

Chronic GVHD leads to hepatic dysfunction, mucosal ulcerations, lichenification of the skin, and death in a third of cases. Therefore, the strategy is to administer immunosuppressive drugs, generally methotrexate and/or cyclosporin (Chs. 20 and 21), after the beginning of engraftment, giving enough treatment to try to prevent GVHD without compromising the growth and differentiation of the lymphoid graft.

In the case of replacement of narrow hematopoietic stem cells to a failed bone marrow, vigorous immunosuppression is necessary to inhibit graft rejection and GVHD. Immunosuppressive drugs such as corticosteroids, cyclosporin, methotrexate, and alkylating agents are commonly used, and new agents such as thalidomide are being evaluated (Ch. 21). A technique used to gain initial immunosuppression without compromising the viability of the graft is to give a transfusion of "buffy coat" cells from the donor before the marrow infusion, followed by an immunosuppressive drug. The buffy coat is the leukocyte- and platelet-rich interface between the red cells and plasma of a unit of whole blood after centrifugation. The goal is to expose the recipient's immune system to any antigens in donor blood cells that might be foreign. The lymphoid cells responding to the antigens begin to undergo "blast" transformation, a state in which they have an increased susceptibility to toxic therapy. This flushing out of potentially reactive lymphocytes permits them to be exposed to a vigorous dose of immunosuppressive therapy at a time when this treatment does not compromise the graft. Even after infusion of the marrow, at some point immunosuppressive treatment in more moderate amounts is given to suppress rejection and GVHD, which occurs in about 40 percent of transplant patients. Another strategy is to deplete cytotoxic T-cells from a donor's bone marrow aspirated for reconstitution of a recipient.

After conditioning and infusion of the donor's marrow, a period of waiting and supportive care follows. In the case of severe combined immune deficiency, donor T lymphocytes appear in the blood within 2 weeks of transplantation. By 1 to 2 months, the recipient demonstrates the capacity to mount specific immune responses, and immunoglobulins are synthesized. These patients often end up with *mixed chimerism*, that is, the recipient's B cells coexist with donor T cells. In most other transplant settings, recovery of full immune function takes much longer, from 1 to 2 years. Natural killer and B cells reach normal blood concentrations within a month, but B-cell function lags behind the numbers. T-cell reconstitution is slower and, again, functional recovery is also delayed.

In the setting of transplantation for marrow failure, genetic disease, or leukemia, the appearance of reticulocytes and nucleated erythrocytes at about the sixth to tenth day heralds the beginning of expression of a successful graft. A special consideration is the situation of transplantation, when donor and recipient ABO blood types are incompatible (Ch. 31). In this case, the isohemagglutinin titers of the recipient are tested, and, if low, small amounts of donor red cells given following marrow infusion to absorb the isohemagglutinins present and protect the developing erythroid cells. Subsequent transfusions must be of the donor's ABO type. Patients with high isohemagglutinin titers (>1/32) require plasmapheresis to remove the antibodies. This is easily accomplished since the isohemagglutinins are of the IgM class (Ch. 31).

Phagocyte precursors appear at about 7 to 10 days, and mature cells are evident between 14 and 28 days. Platelets appear last, by about 4 weeks. Hematopoietic hormones (Ch. 1) can accelerate the emergence of mature blood cells from an engrafted marrow and are being studied with regard to clinical results. Investigators, however, are concerned about using them in patients being treated for myeloproliferative disorders. The failure of a graft to "take" usually but not always means that immunological rejection has occurred. In this circumstance, a second attempt at transplantation with more vigorous immunosuppression may then be tried.

The increase in peripheral blood counts that occurs after a transplantation attempt may not necessarily indicate engraftment. Rarely, the bone marrow recovers in idiopathic aplastic anemia after immunosuppressive therapy, possibly because the cause of such cases is an autoimmune reaction against the patient's own hematopoietic stem cells. In acute leukemia and for genetic disorders there is the possibility that the recovery of peripheral blood cells is actually a result of insufficient sterilization of the host marrow and reflects a return of the recipient's own blood cells. To document engraftment, it is possible to use a number of genetic markers of peripheral blood cells. If the transplant is from male to female or vice versa, the appearance or disappearance of the Y chromosome is useful, although it has been found that sex-matched transplants fare nearly two times better than mismatched ones. Other tests for engraftment involve detecting changes in cell surface antigens such as blood groups by immunological procedures or the presence of donor restriction fragment length polymorphisms of donor origin in the recipient cells.

Complications of Bone Marrow Transplantation

In the initial phase of the transplant, the major problems are those associated with pancytopenia, namely, infection and bleeding. During this time multiple transfusions and antibiotics are given and surveillance procedures performed for detection of infection. Subsequently, acute and then chronic GVHD become principal complications. These can sometimes be difficult to differentiate from gastrointestinal infections occurring in the setting of the immunodeficiency associated with transplantation. If acute GVHD ensues despite the prophylactic treatment described above, therapy is initiated with corticosteroids, cyclosporin, or antithymocyte antibodies (antithymocyte globulin). Chronic GVHD is managed with corticosteroids, cyclosporin, and supportive care.

Other problems are systemic effects of chemotherapy, radiation, and infection such as hemorrhagic cardiomyopathy, interstitial pneumonitis with pulmonary failure, veno-occlusive disease of the liver (especially in patients with preexisting liver disease), and second neoplasms. Cytomegalovirus infection is an especially troublesome complication, being a major contributor to significant pulmonary disease. One approach to this infection is to screen blood products for cytomegalovirus in addition to the usual blood-borne pathogens. In many recipients, however, the infection represents reactivation of latent virus, and to address this problem, prophylactic therapy with the antiviral agents acyclovir or gancyclovir appears to be successful. In rare cases leukemia has developed in the cells of the graft following a successful transplant.

The overriding factor currently determining the success of a transplant is the availability of a histocompatible donor. A second consideration is the recipient's age. The older the recipient, the higher the incidence of GVHD; the ability of the patient to withstand the complications of bone marrow failure declines with age as well. At present about half of patients with aplastic anemia who have received marrow transplants survive for 2 to 3 years, whereas about 20 percent of untransplanted patients with this disease are alive after these intervals. These figures are mainly applicable to relatively young persons, because engraftment is rare (and therefore rarely attempted) in patients over 40 years of age. The survival data are best for patients under 20 years of age treated in large referral centers that perform many transplants.

An infrequent consequence of marrow transplantation, also encountered in other immunodeficiency settings, is an uncontrolled proliferation of B cells, possibly induced by Epstein-Barr virus. This proliferation can result in an infectious mononucleosis syndrome that remits or can induce a chronic condition and even malignant lymphoma. In the severe cases following bone marrow transplantation, some therapeutic success has resulted from infusion of anti-B-cell antibodies.

Despite the risks, complications, and intensive resource requirements, bone marrow transplantation can be considered an acceptable alternative to the progression of fatal or severely debilitating hematologic diseases, and the majority of appropriately selected patients enjoy good quality of life following a successful transplant procedure.

Future Possibilities of Marrow Allotransplantation

Although the concept has been proved that it is possible to restore normal hematopoiesis in patients with hemoglobinopathies by bone marrow transplantation, some conservative authorities believe that only patients with life-threatening or severely debilitating diseases should be treated with bone marrow transplantation. If progress continues in surmounting immunological and other problems besetting bone marrow allografting, however, the objections will recede, and the uses of the treatment will expand. Marrow transplantation may be useful in restoring metabolic pathways to patients with certain inborn errors of metabolism and with storage diseases. As the knowledge of the immune system increases, more sophisticated immunological engineering may permit engraftment of marrow across histocompatibility barriers without immunosuppression. This achievement would dramatically increase the number of patients able to benfit from the procedure.

AUTOLOGOUS MARROW THERAPY

Destruction of hematopoietic stem cells with resulting bone marrow failure is often a consequence of intensive therapy of hematological and nonhematological malignancy. This complication can limit the amount of antitumor treatment. In theory, if bone marrow stem cells could be removed before administration of chemotherapy or irradiation and returned to the patient afterward for engraftment, this limitation could be circumvented. The fact that it is now possible to preserve bone marrow stem cells indefinitely in a frozen state and the lack of immunological barriers to autotransplantation are attractive features of this therapeutic approach. However, two problems limit the success of this technology. First, the toxicity of anticancer therapy in high doses is such that organs other than the blood can be irreversibly damaged. Therefore, even if very high doses of treatment are given and the patient is hematologically reconstituted with autologous marrow, the treatment causes unacceptable damage to other organs. Second, there is the possibility that the patient's bone marrow contains tumor stem cells as well as normal hematopoietic stem cells. The malignant cells, however, may be less viable than normal cells during cryopreservation and also

are amenable to attack by ex vivo chemotherapy or monoclonal antibody techniques. These issues notwithstanding, autologous bone marrow transplantation has been studied and shown to be effective in patients in first remission for acute myelogenous and acute lymphatic leukemias and in Hodgkin's disease and is being evaluated for other hematologic neoplasms and for solid tumors.

BONE MARROW TRANSPLANTATION AND GENE THERAPY

An exciting and imminent direction for autologous bone marrow treatment is the insertion of genes into bone marrow stem cells. This genetic engineering should be applicable to patients with congenital hemolytic disorders and other genetic diseases and for new approaches to neoplastic disease. For example, autotransplantation of mouse bone marrow transfected with the human multidrug resistance gene *MDR1* (Ch. 21) yielded animals able to withstand treatment with high levels of the chemotherapeutic drug taxol. The transfected gene in the setting of the chemotherapy served both for selection of the modified cells and for protection from chemotherapy. Problems to be surmounted for this approach to be widely useful include on the one hand designing vectors for inserting genes that do not cause viral disease and do not damage host DNA and on the other hand obtaining sufficient expression levels of the gene product introduced to be clinically useful. As mentioned in Chapter 20, relatively low levels of adenosine deaminase in lymphoid cells are adequate to overcome the immunosuppression resulting from enzyme deficiency, so that this disease is a good candidate for gene therapy.

SUGGESTED READINGS

Antin JH, Ferrara JLM (1992) Cytokine dysregulation and acute graft-versus host disease. Blood 80:2964

Browne PV, Lawler M, Humphries P, McCann SR (1991) Donor-cell leukemia after bone marrow transplantation for severe aplastic anemia. N Engl J Med 325:710

Champlin R (1993) Preparative regimens for autologous bone marrow transplantation. Blood 81:277

Chao NJ, Schmidt GM, Niland JG et al (1993) Cyclosporine, methotrexate, and prednisone compared with cyclosporine and prednisone for prophylaxis of acute graft versus host disease. N Engl J Med 329:1225

Chao NJ, Tierney DK, Bloom JR et al (1992) Dynamic assessment of quality of life after autologous bone marrow transplantation. Blood 80:825

Goodman JL et al (1992) A controlled trial of fluconazole to prevent fungal infections in patients undergoing bone marrow transplantation. N Engl J Med 326:845

Goodrich JM, Mori M, Gleaves CA et al (1991) Early treatment with gancyclovir to prevent cytomegalovirus disease after allogeneic bone marrow transplantation. N Engl J Med 325:1601

Horowitz MM, Przepiorka D, Champlin RE et al (1992) Should HLA-identical sibling bone marrow transplants for leukemia be restricted to large centers? Blood 79:2271

Kernan NA, Bartsch G, Ash RC et al (1993) Analysis of 462 transplantations from unrelated donors facilitated by the national marrow donor program. N Engl J Med 328:593

Lucarelli G et al (1990) Bone marrow transplantation in patients with thalassemia. N Engl J Med 322:417

McDonald GB, Sharma P, Matthews DE et al (1985) The clinical course of 53 patients with venooclusive disease of the liver after marrow transplantation. Transplantation 39:603

Santos GE (1983) The history of bone marrow transplantation. Clin Haematol 12:611

Sorrentino BP, Brandt SJ, Bodine D et al (1992) Selection of drug-resistant bone marrow cells in vivo after retroviral transfer of human MDR1. Science 257:99

Theobald M, Nierle T, Bunjes D et al (1992) Host-specific interleukin-2-secreting donor T-cell precursors as predictors of acute graft-versus-host disease in bone marrow transplantation between HLA-identical siblings. N Engl J Med 327:1613

Turhan AG, Humphries K, Phillips GL et al (1989) Clonal hematopoiesis demonstrated by X-linked DNA polymorphisms after allogeneic bone marrow transplantation. N Engl J Med 320:1655

Welch HG, Larson EB (1989) Cost effectiveness of bone marrow transplantation in acute nonlymphocytic leukemia. N Engl J Med 321:807

Index

Note: Page numbers followed by an *f* indicate figures, and those followed by a *t* indicate tables.

action of, 7, 8f, 8t, 21, 22f, 23
in aplastic anemia, 364
deficiency of
in HIV infection, 331
in kidney dysfunction, 99
in polycythemia vera, 367
production of
autonomous, 180–181
excessive, polycythemia in, 179–181
recombinant, therapy with, 11, 100
E-selectins, in neutrophil function, 283, 283f
Esophageal varices, in hemochromatosis, 56
Esophageal web, in iron deficiency anemia, 53, 54f
Essential thrombocythemia, 369–370
Ethanol ingestion. *See* Alcohol use and abuse.
Ethanol paracoagulation test, in fibrinolysis evaluation, 202
Ethylenediaminetetraacetic acid, as anticoagulant, 3
Etoposide, 351
Euglobin lysis time, in fibrinolysis evaluation, 201–202, 203f
Exons, of globin gene, 139, 139f
Extrinsic pathway, in clotting cascade, 194, 195f
Eye, sickle cell anemia manifestations in, 169

FAB (French-American-British) classification
acute lymphocytic (lymphatic) leukemia, 395, 396, 396t
acute myelogenous leukemia, 379–381, 380t
Fab region, of immunoglobulin, 266, 266f
in blood cell destruction, 432, 433
Fabricius, bursa of, 309
Factor 1, in complement system, 269
Factor B, in complement system, 268, 269f
Factor D, in complement system, 268, 269f
Factor H, in complement system, 269
Factor II. *See* Prothrombin.
Factor V
deficiency of, 208t
receptors for, 221
released from platelets, 218, 218t
Factor V/VIII inactivating complex, 198, 199f
Factor VII
activated (VIIa)
in factor X activation, 191–192, 191f
neutralization of, 198, 199f
activation of, 189–190, 190f
disseminated intravascular coagulation and, 234f
deficiency of, 208t
Factor VIII
deficiency of, 203, 204f, 205–207, 208t
in factor IX activation, 191
half-life of, 206
porcine, 206–207
receptors for, 221
replacement therapy with, 206–207
separation of, from plasma, 447
synthesis of, 196–197

von Willebrand factor-rich, 226
in von Willebrand's disease, 225–227, 225t, 226f
Factor VIII antigen. *See* von Willebrand factor.
Factor VIII coagulant, 196–197, 225
Factor IX
activation of, 191, 191f
deficiency of (hemophilia B), 207, 208t
Factor X
activated, neutralization of, 198, 199f
activation of, 190, 190f, 191–192, 191f
deficiency of, in amyloidosis, 277
Factor XI
activation of, 190, 190f
deficiency of, 208t
Factor XII
activation of, disseminated intravascular coagulation and, 234f
deficiency of, 207
determination of, 195
in factor XI activation, 190, 190f
Factor XIII, deficiency of, 208t
Fanconi's anemia, 361
leukemia predisposition in, 377
Fatigue
in iron deficiency anemia, 52
in radiation therapy, 347
Fava beans, hemolysis from, 129, 133
F cells, fetal hemoglobin in, 137, 138f
Fc region, of immunoglobulins, 266, 266f, 285
in blood cell destruction, 433, 439, 440–441
Febrile agglutinins, 441
Feline sarcoma virus, 338
Ferriheme, in hemoglobin clearance, 122, 123f
Ferritin
iron storage in, 44, 44f, 46, 47f, 48
in iron deficiency, 51–52, 52f
levels of, in hemochromatosis, 58f, 59
Ferrochelatase
deficiency of, in porphyria, 71t
in heme synthesis, 65, 66t
Ferrokinetics, 48–49, 49f
of aplastic anemia, 362–363
of hemolytic anemia, 108, 108f
of ineffective erythropoiesis, 73, 73f
fes oncogene, 338
Fetal hemoglobin. *See* Hemoglobin F.
Fetus
anticoagulant effects on, 251
dead retained, disseminated intravascular coagulation in, 235, 236
hematopoiesis in, 10
hemolysis in, 437–438
immune system development in, 323
isoantibodies in, 431
Fever, in Hodgkin's lymphoma, 408–409
Fibrin
in coagulation, 2
D-D dimers of, 201, 202f, 256
degradation products of, 200–202, 202f